Chinese Medicine: Modern Applications of Traditional Formulas

Chinese Medicine: Modern Applications of Traditional Formulas

Edited by Penelope Williams

SYRAWOOD
PUBLISHING HOUSE
New York

Published by Syrawood Publishing House,
750 Third Avenue, 9th Floor,
New York, NY 10017, USA
www.syrawoodpublishinghouse.com

Chinese Medicine: Modern Applications of Traditional Formulas
Edited by Penelope Williams

International Standard Book Number: 978-1-68286-490-6 (Hardback)

Cataloging-in-Publication Data

Chinese medicine : modern applications of traditional formulas / edited by Penelope Williams.
p. cm.
Includes bibliographical references and index.
ISBN 978-1-68286-490-6
1. Medicine, Chinese. 2. Traditional medicine--China. 3. Alternative medicine. I. Williams, Penelope.
R601 .C45 2017
615.5--dc23

Printed in China.

TABLE OF CONTENTS

Preface IX

Chapter 1 **TCM Database@Taiwan: The World's Largest Traditional Chinese Medicine Database for Drug Screening *In Silico*** 1
Calvin Yu-Chian Chen

Chapter 2 **Registration Quality Assessment of Acupuncture Clinical Trials** 6
Jing Gu, Ye Zhao, Xiaogang Wang, Jianjun Jiang, Jinhui Tian, Kehu Yang

Chapter 3 **Gender Differences in Traditional Chinese Medicine use among Adults in Taiwan** 16
Chun-Chuan Shih, Chien-Chang Liao, Yi-Chang Su, Chin-Chuan Tsai, Jaung-Geng Lin

Chapter 4 **Characterization of Rheumatoid Arthritis Subtypes using Symptom Profiles, Clinical Chemistry and Metabolomics Measurements** 23
Herman A. van Wietmarschen, Weidong Dai, Anita J. van der Kooij, Theo H. Reijmers, Yan Schroën, Mei Wang, Zhiliang Xu, Xinchang Wang, Hongwei Kong, Guowang Xu, Thomas Hankemeier, Jacqueline J. Meulman, Jan van der Greef

Chapter 5 **Efficacy and Safety of Traditional Chinese Medicine for Diabetes** 31
Linong Ji, Xiaolin Tong, Hongyuan Wang, Haoming Tian, Huimin Zhou, Lili Zhang, Qifu Li, Yizhong Wang, Hongmei Li, Min Liu, Hongjie Yang, Yanbin Gao, Yan Li, Quanmin Li, Xiaohui Guo, Gangyi Yang, Zhongai Zhang, Zhiguang Zhou, Guang Ning, Yingli Chen, Sanjoy Paul, for the Evidence-Based Medical Research of Xiaoke Pill Study Group

Chapter 6 **An Epidemiological Study of Concomitant use of Chinese Medicine and Antipsychotics in Schizophrenic Patients: Implication for Herb-Drug Interaction** 41
Zhang-Jin Zhang, Qing-Rong Tan, Yao Tong, Xue-Yi Wang, Huai-Hai Wang, Lai-Ming Ho, Hei Kiu Wong, Yi-Bin Feng, Di Wang, Roger Ng, Grainne M. McAlonan, Chuan-Yue Wang, Vivian Taam Wong

Chapter 7 **Traditional Chinese Medicine in Cancer Care: A Review of Controlled Clinical Studies Published in Chinese** 50
Xun Li, Guoyan Yang, Xinxue Li, Yan Zhang, Jingli Yang, Jiu Chang, Xiaoxuan Sun, Xiaoyun Zhou, Yu Guo, Yue Xu, Jianping Liu, Alan Bensoussan

Chapter 8 **Colorimetric Grading Scale can Promote the Standardization of Experiential and Sensory Evaluation in Quality Control of Traditional Chinese Medicines** 61
Jia-bo Wang, Ling-na Zeng, Qing-ce Zang, Qian-feng Gong, Bao-cai Li, Xue-ru Zhang, Xiaohui Chu, Ping Zhang, Yan-ling Zhao, Xiao-he Xiao

Chapter 9 **Altered Hub Configurations within Default Mode Network following Acupuncture at ST36: A Multimodal Investigation Combining fMRI and MEG** 70
Youbo You, Lijun Bai, Ruwei Dai, Hao Cheng, Zhenyu Liu, Wenjuan Wei, Jie Tian

Chapter 10 ***In Silico* Investigation of Potential Src Kinase Ligands from Traditional Chinese Medicine** 82
Weng Ieong Tou, Calvin Yu-Chian Chen

Chapter 11 **Assessing the Quality of Reports about Randomized Controlled Trials of Acupuncture Treatment on Mild Cognitive Impairment** 97
Xiao Lu, Shang Hongcai, Wang Jiaying, Hu Jing, Xiong Jun

Chapter 12 **Favorable Circulatory System Outcomes as Adjuvant Traditional Chinese Medicine (TCM) Treatment for Cerebrovascular Diseases in Taiwan** 103
Hsienhsueh Elley Chiu, Yu-Chiang Hong, Ku-Chou Chang, Chun-Chuan Shih, Jen Wen Hung, Chia-Wei Liu, Teng-Yeow Tan, Chih-Cheng Huang

Chapter 13 **HPLC–MS/MS Analysis of a Traditional Chinese Medical Formulation of Bu-Yang-Huan-Wu-Tang and its Pharmacokinetics after Oral Administration to Rats** 111
Lee-Hsin Shaw, Lie-Chwen Lin, Tung-Hu Tsai

Chapter 14 **Epidemiology, Quality and Reporting Characteristics of Systematic Reviews of Traditional Chinese Medicine Interventions Published in Chinese Journals** 124
Bin Ma, Jiwu Guo, Guoqing Qi, Haimin Li, Jiye Peng, Yulong Zhang, Yanqin Ding, Kehu Yang

Chapter 15 **Electroacupuncture for Moderate and Severe Benign Prostatic Hyperplasia** 130
Yang Wang, Baoyan Liu, Jinna Yu, Jiani Wu, Jing Wang, Zhishun Liu

Chapter 16 **Sub-Typing of Rheumatic Diseases Based on a Systems Diagnosis Questionnaire** 136
Herman A. van Wietmarschen, Theo H. Reijmers, Anita J. van der Kooij, Jan Schroën, Heng Wei, Thomas Hankemeier, Jacqueline J. Meulman, Jan van der Greef

Chapter 17 **Assessment of the Reporting Quality of Randomized Controlled Trials on Treatment of Coronary Heart Disease with Traditional Chinese Medicine from the Chinese Journal of Integrated Traditional and Western Medicine** 146
Fang-fang Fan, Qin Xu, Qi Sun, Sheng-jun Zhao, Ping Wang, Xue-rui Guo

Chapter 18 **Study on the Main Components Interaction from *Flos Lonicerae* and *Fructus Forsythiae* and their Dissolution In Vitro and Intestinal Absorption in Rats** 155
Wei Zhou, Xiaobin Tan, Jinjun Shan, Shouchuan Wang, Ailing Yin, Baochang Cai, Liuqing Di

Chapter 19 **A Network Pharmacology Study of Chinese Medicine QiShenYiQi to Reveal its Underlying Multi-Compound, Multi-Target, Multi-Pathway Mode of Action** 168
Xiang Li, Leihong Wu, Wei Liu, Yecheng Jin, Qian Chen, Linli Wang, Xiaohui Fan, Zheng Li, Yiyu Cheng

Chapter 20 **A Systems Biology-Based Approach to Uncovering the Molecular Mechanisms Underlying the Effects of Dragon's Blood Tablet in Colitis, Involving the Integration of Chemical Analysis, ADME Prediction, and Network Pharmacology**........179
Haiyu Xu, Yanqiong Zhang, Yun Lei, Xiumei Gao, Huaqiang Zhai, Na Lin, Shihuan Tang, Rixin Liang, Yan Ma, Defeng Li, Yi Zhang, Guangrong Zhu, Hongjun Yang, Luqi Huang

Chapter 21 **Screening Active Components from Yu-Ping-Feng-San for Regulating Initiative Key Factors in Allergic Sensitization**........191
Dandan Shen, Xuejian Xie, Zhijie Zhu, Xi Yu, Hailiang Liu, Huizhu Wang, Hongwei Fan, Dawei Wang, Guorong Jiang, Min Hong

Chapter 22 **Full Toxicity Assessment of Genkwa Flos and the Underlying Mechanism in Nematode *Caenorhabditis elegans***........202
Yan Qiao, Yunli Zhao, Qiuli Wu, Lingmei Sun, Qinli Ruan, Yanyan Chen, Meng Wang, Jinao Duan, Dayong Wang

Chapter 23 **Methodological Reporting of Randomized Trials in Five Leading Chinese Nursing Journals**........212
Chunhu Shi, Jinhui Tian, Dan Ren, Hongli Wei, Lihuan Zhang, Quan Wang, Kehu Yang

Chapter 24 **Practitioner Perspectives on Strategies to Promote Longer-Term Benefits of Acupuncture or Counselling for Depression**........219
Hugh MacPherson, Liz Newbronner, Ruth Chamberlain, Stewart J. Richmond, Harriet Lansdown, Sara Perren, Ann Hopton, Karen Spilsbury

Permissions

List of Contributors

Index

PREFACE

Chinese Medicine is a popular form of alternative medicine. Some of the significant treatments under this field are acupuncture, herbal medicine, etc. It is an ancient form of medicine based on the philosophy of Yin and Yang. This book attempts to understand the multiple branches that fall under the discipline of Chinese medicine and how such concepts have practical applications. While understanding the long-term perspectives of the topics, the book makes an effort in highlighting their impact as a modern tool for the growth of the discipline. Scientists and students actively engaged in this field will find this book full of crucial and unexplored concepts.

After months of intensive research and writing, this book is the end result of all who devoted their time and efforts in the initiation and progress of this book. It will surely be a source of reference in enhancing the required knowledge of the new developments in the area. During the course of developing this book, certain measures such as accuracy, authenticity and research focused analytical studies were given preference in order to produce a comprehensive book in the area of study.

This book would not have been possible without the efforts of the authors and the publisher. I extend my sincere thanks to them. Secondly, I express my gratitude to my family and well-wishers. And most importantly, I thank my students for constantly expressing their willingness and curiosity in enhancing their knowledge in the field, which encourages me to take up further research projects for the advancement of the area.

Editor

1

TCM Database@Taiwan: The World's Largest Traditional Chinese Medicine Database for Drug Screening *In Silico*

Calvin Yu-Chian Chen[1,2,3]*

1 School of Chinese Medicine, China Medical University, Taichung, Taiwan, 2 Department of Bioinformatics, Asia University, Taichung, Taiwan, 3 Department of Computational and Systems Biology, Massachusetts Institute of Technology, Cambridge, Massachusetts, United States of America

Abstract

Rapid advancing computational technologies have greatly speeded up the development of computer-aided drug design (CADD). Recently, pharmaceutical companies have increasingly shifted their attentions toward traditional Chinese medicine (TCM) for novel lead compounds. Despite the growing number of studies on TCM, there is no free 3D small molecular structure database of TCM available for virtual screening or molecular simulation. To address this shortcoming, we have constructed TCM Database@Taiwan (http://tcm.cmu.edu.tw/) based on information collected from Chinese medical texts and scientific publications. TCM Database@Taiwan is currently the world's largest non-commercial TCM database. This web-based database contains more than 20,000 pure compounds isolated from 453 TCM ingredients. Both cdx (2D) and Tripos mol2 (3D) formats of each pure compound in the database are available for download and virtual screening. The TCM database includes both simple and advanced web-based query options that can specify search clauses, such as molecular properties, substructures, TCM ingredients, and TCM classification, based on intended drug actions. The TCM database can be easily accessed by all researchers conducting CADD. Over the last eight years, numerous volunteers have devoted their time to analyze TCM ingredients from Chinese medical texts as well as to construct structure files for each isolated compound. We believe that TCM Database@Taiwan will be a milestone on the path towards modernizing traditional Chinese medicine.

Editor: Andreas Hofmann, Griffith University, Australia

Funding: The research was supported by grants from the National Science Council of Taiwan (NSC 99-2221-E-039-013-), China Medical University (CMU99-S-02) and Asia University (CMU98-ASIA-09). This study is also supported in part by Taiwan Department of Health Clinical Trial and Research Center of Excellence (DOH99-TD-B-111-004) and Taiwan Department of Health Cancer Research Center of Excellence (DOH99-TD-C-111-005). The funders had no role in study design, data collection and analysis, decision to publish, or preparation of the manuscript.

Competing Interests: The author has declared that no competing interests exist.

* E-mail: ycc@mail.cmu.edu.tw; ycc929@MIT.EDU

Introduction

For thousands of years, traditional Chinese medicine (TCM) holds an important role in medical diagnosis and treatments in Eastern Asia. However, due to lack of systematic investigation and poor understanding of TCM regimens, TCM is less recognized in the Western society. Recently, increasing effort has been devoted to study TCM, from which a large number of bioactive compounds have been isolated and studied. Hence, there is a need to establish a database to organize the enormous amounts of TCM data and make the virtual screening of TCM ingredients easily accessible.

Although there are many websites detailing information for TCM sources, traditional usage from ancient material medica texts, and processing and storage procedures, these databases, such as The Chinese medicine sampler (http://www.chinesemedicinesampler.com) and Dictionary of Chinese Herbs (http://alternativehealing.org), contain little information of TCM ingredients at molecular level. The TCMGeneDIT database [1] is an effective search engine for TCM-related literature, but the information on the TCM constituents is not well organized. Other databases, including TCMD [2], Chinese Traditional Medicinal Herbs Database [3], and TCM-ID [4], provide general TCM information and 3D structures of TCM ingredients. However, these databases are either inaccessible or highly restricted for information sharing. To date, the ZINC database [5] is currently the largest free 3D molecule database. However, there is no TCM related database similar to the scale of ZINC yet. In the hope of building a complete TCM ingredient library, we construct the TCM Database@Taiwan (http://tcm.cmu.edu.tw/).

In the past, our laboratory has performed screening for multiple TCM components and has successfully discovered novel lead compounds, such as anti-viral, anti-inflammation, anti-cancer, stroke prevention compounds, and hypnotic medications [6–17]. By constructing TCM Database@Taiwan, we can further facilitate the virtual screening process in the experiment design for the TCM lead drug discovery. We firmly believe that the constituents from TCM are the sources to derive novel pharmaceutical compounds.

Results and Discussion

TCM Database@Taiwan (http://tcm.cmu.edu.tw) is currently the largest non-commercial TCM database available for download. This web database is designed in both English and traditional Chinese languages. All 3D structures are constructed in mol2 format and are readily used for virtual screening.

TCM organization

Right now, the database contains 20,000 ingredients from 453 different herbs, animal products, and minerals TCM regimens. In the near future, the database will further record folk herb ingredients. The

TCM database is organized by proposed actions of Chinese medicines (Table S1). There are a total of twenty-two different drug classes and some are further divided into subclasses based on clinical applications recorded in TCM monographs. It should be noted that our TCM classification is based on traditional Chinese theories including the Yin-yang, the human Meridan/Channel system, the Five Elements theory, and the Zang Fu organ theory. It should also be noted that TCM listed under certain classes, such as parasites elimination, dampness reduction and itchiness relief medicinal, and topical application medicinal, contain toxic ingredients and are no longer prescribed in clinics. These ingredients are present in the TCM database for the completeness of TCM records. These data do not imply endorsement for any clinical or private use of the toxic TCM compounds nor for any animal products present in the database.

Search and Display

An overview of available search options and download options is shown in Figure 1. TCM Database@Taiwan can be browsed by simple and advanced search options. The simple search option enables users to browse the website either by TCM medicine or by TCM ingredients (Figure 2). The search-by-TCM-medicine option allows users to select the intended drug action group and then the desired TCM medicine. The search-by-TCM-chemical-composition option allows users to find possible TCM sources of the given molecule. This search result is directly linked to the TCM compound webpage without the need to specifying TCM action group.

For each search options, the result is organized in a "TCM profile" that provides the identified TCM compound(s) and the associated references. Clicking on a TCM compound in the profile will display the compound's 2D and 3D structures, as well as its molecular properties in a new page. Users can download the structure of the molecule in cdx (2D) or mol2 (3D) format at the bottom of the TCM compound webpage. In addition, users can also click on the links to browse other Chinese medicines that contains the selected TCM compound.

The advanced search option incorporates a molecular drawing interface (ChemAxon) for structure search (Figure 3). Users can also specify structure types, including exact search and substructure search, whichever best describes users' needs. Moreover, users can perform searches by specifying the molecular properties, such as molecular weight and ALogP. Both of the advanced search options can be used alone or in conjunction. The result will return molecule(s) that satisfy the input specification in a tabular format with name and 2D representation. For users who prefer search by Chinese medicine names and other TCM information, a website search engine is available at top of every page.

Download Interface

The TCM ingredients are organized by their drug action classes and their original sources. Users can download a specific drug class or a specific TCM or the whole TCM database on Download page.

Sharing TCM Constituents

As technology advances, new TCM ingredients have been isolated and studied each day. Therefore, we implemented an upload function for scientists who are interested in sharing their findings on Chinese medicines. Users may upload their own molecules to the TCM database server in mol2 format. The uploaded molecules will be reviewed and incorporated into the TCM database.

Overall, TCM Database@Taiwan is constructed in the hope to create the most complete TCM library and to strengthen the TCM research network to date. In addition, this web-based database is implemented with virtual screening and molecular simulation functions. For both biochemists studying TCM and medicinal chemists designing novel lead compounds, this database serves as a useful resource for virtual screening as well as for the references in biochemical assays. In the future, we will incorporate genetic algorithm (GA) and support vector machine (SVM) for further TCM classifications based on molecular properties. We

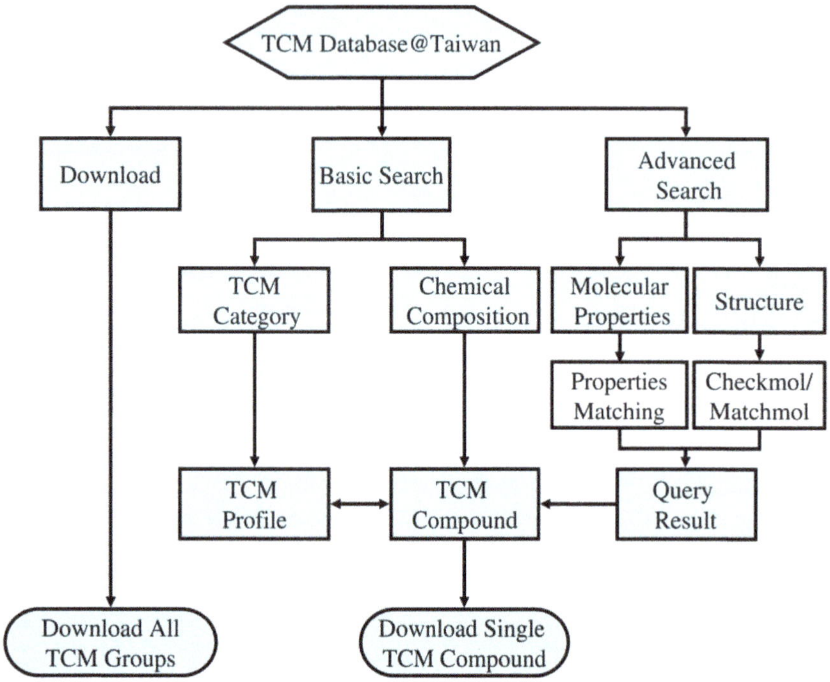

Figure 1. Search flowchart and available download options in TCM database.

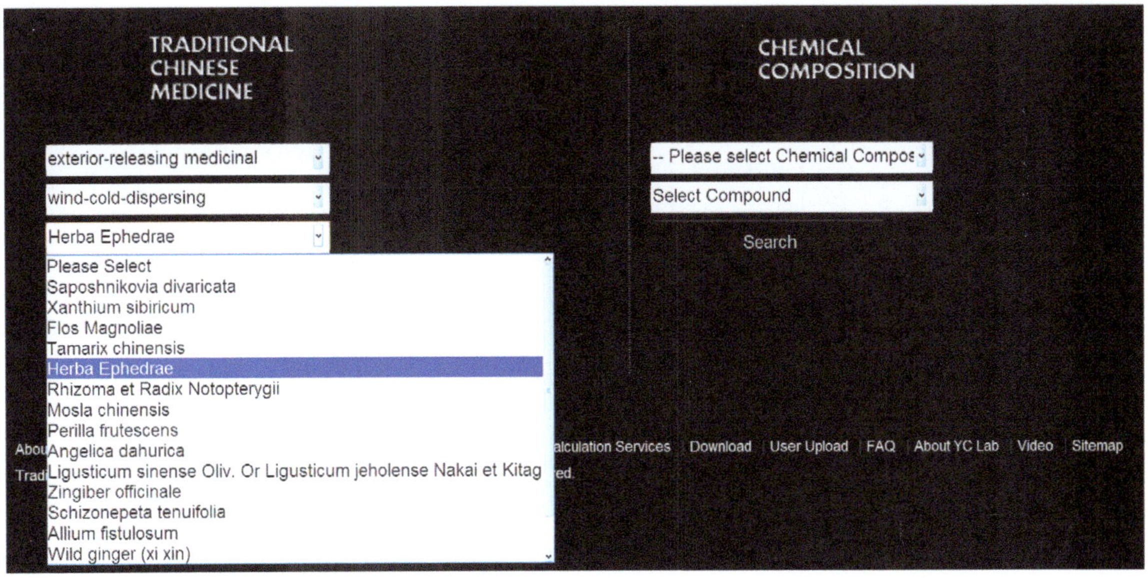

Figure 2. The search tool available in the TCM database. (a) search by TCM category and (b) search by chemical composition.

expect the construction of TCM Database@Taiwan to become a milestone for modern TCM researches.

Methods

The TCM herbs, animal products and minerals listed in the TCM Database @Taiwan were originated from Chinese medical texts and dictionaries [18–22]. In addition, the TCM constituents were collected manually from published results available on Medline [23] and ISI Web of Knowledge (http://apps.isiknowledge.com). The data were organized into twenty-two major classes based on their proposed therapeutic actions recorded in Chinese medical texts [24–26]. The 2D and 3D structures of TCM constituents were built by ChemBioOffice 2008 (CambridgeSoft, Cambridge, MA). The 3D structures were energy minimized in MM2 force field. Physicochemical properties,

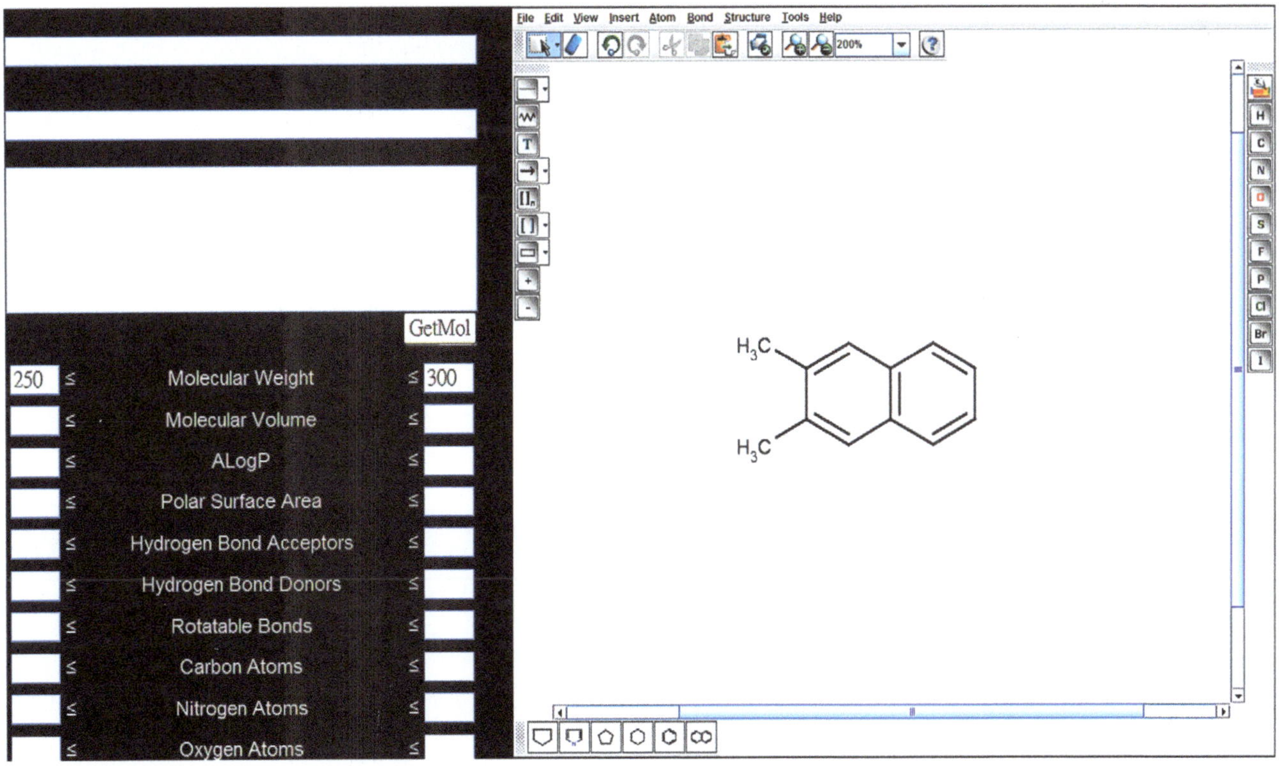

Figure 3. The advance search interface.

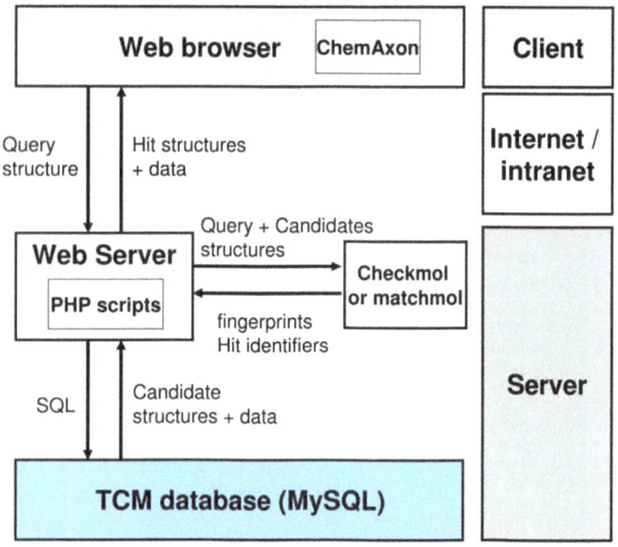

Figure 4. The infrastructure of the TCM database. The design is adapted from Norbert Haider's MolDB5R.

including ALogP and polar surface area, were calculated using ChemBioOffice.

With efficiency and stability as our main concern, we implemented our database on a Linux server, then use MySQL5.0, Apache, and hypertext preprocessor (PHP) for database and web server development. For friendly user interfaces, we used ChemAxon MarvinView applet (https://www.chemaxon.com) for 2D and 3D representation. In addition, we applied MarvinSketch tool from ChemAxon for structure drawing in the advanced search option.

In the advanced search section, the search engine was developed based on the Norbert Haider's MolDB5R package [27]. The infrastructure of the advanced search engine is shown in Figure 4. For search-by-specifying-molecular-properties, a search script written in PHP is used to search and retrieve TCM compounds that satisfied all the input properties. Two programs, checkmol and matchmol, are used to perform the background structure searching and matching process. The queried structure is read by the checkmol program to generate molecular descriptors, which is then used in the preliminary search in the TCM database. The matchmol program is responsible for full structure comparison of the input structures from checkmol. For additional structure search options, such as substructure search, the matchmol program treat one compound as "needle" and other molecule(s) as "haystack" to determine the best-fit substructure of another structure. All the search options in the advanced search section can be used in conjunction. By specifying both molecular properties and query structure scaffold, an additional data screening process is performed to ensure that all the input criteria are met.

Supporting Information

Table S1 Summary of medicines present in each TCM class. The English translation of each class is taken from WHO publication.
(DOC)

Acknowledgments

I am grateful to hundreds of student volunteers who devoted their time checking the TCM compounds from the references and drawing these compounds for more than eight years and National Center of High-performance Computing for computer time and facilities. I also thank the professional suggestion by Drs. Chung Y Hsu, Kun-Lung Chang, Fuu-Jen Tsai of China Medical University, Nobel Laureate Ferid Murad, and professor Marc of Harvard University.

Author Contributions

Conceived and designed the experiments: CYCC. Performed the experiments: CYCC. Analyzed the data: CYCC. Contributed reagents/materials/analysis tools: CYCC. Wrote the paper: CYCC.

References

1. Fang YC, Huang HC, Chen HH, Juan HF (2008) TCMGeneDIT: a database for associated traditional Chinese medicine, gene and disease information using text mining. BMC Complement Altern Med 8: 58.
2. He M, Yan XJ, Zhou JJ, Xie GR (2001) Traditional Chinese medicine database and application on the Web. J Chem Inf Comput Sci 41: 273–277.
3. Qiao XB, Hou TJ, Zhang W, Guo SL, Xu SJ (2002) A 3D structure database of components from Chinese traditional medicinal herbs. J Chem Inf Comput Sci 42: 481–489.
4. Chen X, Zhou H, Liu YB, Wang JF, Li H, et al. (2006) Database of traditional Chinese medicine and its application to studies of mechanism and to prescription validation. Br J Pharmacol 149: 1092–1103.
5. Irwin JJ, Shoichet BK (2005) ZINC - A free database of commercially available compounds for virtual screening. J Chem Inf Model 45: 177–182.
6. Huang HJ, Lee KJ, Yu HW, Chen CY, Hsu CH, et al. (2010) Structure-Based and Ligand-Based Drug Design for HER 2 Receptor. J Biomol Struct Dyn 28: 23–37.
7. Chen CY, Chen CYC (2010) Insights into designing the dual-targeted HER2/HSP90 inhibitors. J Mol Graph Model 29: 21–31.
8. Huang HJ, Chen CY, Chen HY, Tsai FJ, Chen CYC (2010) Computational screening and QSAR analysis for design of AMP-activated protein kinase agonist. J Taiwan Inst Chem Eng 41: 352–359.
9. Chen CYC (2010) Virtual Screening and Drug Design for PDE-5 Receptor from Traditional Chinese Medicine Database. J Biomol Struct Dyn 27: 627–640.
10. Chen CYC (2010) Bioinformatics, chemoinformatics, and pharmainformatics analysis of HER2/HSP90 dual-targeted inhibitors. J Taiwan Inst Chem Eng 41: 143–149.
11. Chen CY, Huang HJ, Tsai FJ, Chen CYC (2010) Drug design for Influenza A virus subtype H1N1. J Taiwan Inst Chem Eng 41: 8–15.
12. Chen CYC (2009) Computational screening and design of traditional Chinese medicine (TCM) to block phosphodiesterase-5. J Mol Graph Model 28: 261–269.
13. Chen CY, Chang YH, Bau DT, Huang HJ, Tsai FJ, et al. (2009) Ligand-Based Dual Target Drug Design for H1N1: Swine Flu- A Preliminary First Study. J Biomol Struct Dyn 27: 171–178.
14. Huang HJ, Yu HW, Chen CY, Hsu CH, Chen HY, et al. (2010) Current developments of computer-aided drug design. J Taiwan Inst Chem Eng 41: 623–635.
15. Chen CYC (2009) Pharmacoinformatics approach for mPGES-1 in anti-inflammation by 3D-QSAR pharmacophore mapping. J Taiwan Inst Chem Eng 40: 155–161.
16. Chen CYC (2009) De novo design of novel selective COX-2 inhibitors: From virtual screening to pharmacophore analysis. J Taiwan Inst Chem Eng 40: 55–69.
17. Chen CYC (2009) Chemoinformatics and pharmacoinformatics approach for exploring the GABA-A agonist from Chinese herb suanzaoren. J Taiwan Inst Chem Eng 40: 36–47.
18. Chen G, Li S (1992) Ben cao gang mu tong shi = General explanation of Compendium of materia medica. Beijing Shi: Xue yuan chu ban she. 2 v. (10, 18, 13, 2323 p., 2342, 2369 p. of plates) p.
19. Zhong N, Zhao G, Dai S, Chen R (2006) Zhong yao da ci dian. Shanghai: Shanghai ke xue ji shu chu ban she. 2 v. (2, 2, 15, 3875 p.) p.
20. Miao X, Zheng J (2002) Shennong ben cao jing shu. Beijing: Zhong yi gu ji chu ban she. 777 p.
21. Lü X (2002) Zhong yao jian bie da quan. Changsha Shi: Hunan ke xue ji shu chu ban she. pp 2, 3, 658.
22. Fang Y, Zhang Z, Miao X (1991) Shang han lun tiao bian. Shanghai: Shanghai gu ji chu ban she: Xin hua shu dian Shanghai fa xing suo fa xing. pp 2, 858.

23. Sayers EW, Barrett T, Benson DA, Bolton E, Bryant SH, et al. (2010) Database resources of the National Center for Biotechnology Information. Nucleic Acids Res 38: D5–D16.
24. Shen L, Li S (1998) Ben cao gang mu cai se tu pu. Beijing Shi: Hua xia chu ban she. pp 4, 21, 471.
25. Yang S (1998) The divine farmer's materia medica: a translation of the Shen Nong Ben Cao Jing. Boulder, CO: Blue Poppy Press. pp xvi, 198.
26. Yao D, Zhang J, Zhonghua RG. Guangzhou Shi: Guangdong ke ji chu ban she: Jing xiao Guangdong sheng xin hua shu dian. pp 3, 519.
27. Haider N (2010) Functionality Pattern Matching as an Efficient Complementary Structure/Reaction Search Tool: an Open-Source Approach. Molecules 15: 5079–5092.

2

Registration Quality Assessment of Acupuncture Clinical Trials

Jing Gu[1,2], Ye Zhao[1], Xiaogang Wang[1], Jianjun Jiang[3], Jinhui Tian[1], Kehu Yang[1]*

1 Evidence-Based Medicine Center, Institute of Integrated Traditional Chinese and Western Medicine, School of Basic Medical Sciences, Lanzhou University, Lanzhou, Gansu, China, **2** Institute of Integrated Traditional Chinese and Western Medicine, Gansu University of Traditional Chinese Medicine, Lanzhou, Gansu, China, **3** Second School of Clinical Medicine of Lanzhou University, Lanzhou, Gansu, China

Abstract

Background: Registration can help with transparency of acupuncture clinical trials (ACTs) by making protocol information and results available to the public. Recently, the number of registered ACTs has increased greatly, but only a few researchers have focused on the quality of ACTs registration. This review provides the first assessment of the registration quality of ACTs and the baseline information for future development.

Methods: All records of ACTs registered in the World Health Organization (WHO) International Clinical Trials Registry Platform (ICTRP) were collected. Data was extracted and input to Excel spreadsheets. The current 20 items of the WHO Trial Registration Data Set (TRDS) and the special prepared items for acupuncture intervention details were used to assess the registration quality of ACTs.

Results: A total of 740 records, found in 11 registries, were examined. The number of registered ACTs increased rapidly and involved a number of different diseases. The completeness of 20 items was not too poor due to 16 of them had a higher reported percentage (>85%). The completeness of the 20 items was different among registries. For example, the average registration percentage of 20 items in Clinicaltrials.gov, ChiCTR, ISRCTN and ANZCTR were 89.6%, 92.2%, 82.4% and 91.6% respectively. Detailed information regarding acupuncture intervention was seriously insufficient. Among the 740 registration records, 89.2% lacked information on the style of acupuncture, 80.8% did not contain details regarding the needles used, 53.5% lacked information on the treatment regimen and 76.2% did not give details of other interventions administered with acupuncture.

Conclusions: The overall registration quality of ACTs is not high enough due to the serious lack of information on the specifics of acupuncture intervention. It is vital that a number of special items be set regarding acupuncture in order to develop a suitable system for the registration of ACTs.

Editor: Lamberto Manzoli, University of Chieti, Italy

Funding: The authors have no support or funding to report.

Competing Interests: The authors have declared that no competing interests exist.

* E-mail: yangkhebm2006@126.com

Introduction

As an alternative medicine methodology, acupuncture has proved effective for the treatment of many diseases and symptoms of disease, such as chronic pain, drug addiction, stroke rehabilitation, asthma and chemotherapy-induced nausea and vomiting [1,2]. Acupuncture has been shown to provide definite curative effects and to cause fewer adverse reactions than some other treatment modalities and has been approved by the WHO and by many other medical and health institutions in some western countries [3–6], and is now practiced widely around the world.

Due to the availability of increased research funding, acupuncture clinical trials (ACTs) have been extensively conducted in many countries in recent decades. As a result, the number of papers related to acupuncture is growing rapidly. Many researchers have not only summarized the clinical efficacy and safety of acupuncture, but have also expressed concern regarding the quality of ACTs. These studies revealed that ACTs had many problems, such as poor methodological quality, unscientific research protocols, and repeated trials of acupuncture [7]. Moreover, the report quality of ACTs was low [8]. Information regarding acupuncturists' qualifications, adverse reactions and follow-up was missing [9]. Problems with publication bias had also extended to ACTs. Vickers reported that all ACTs from mainland China, Hong Kong, Taiwan and Japan were reported to be effective [10]. Additionally, all acupuncture treatments reported in China and Russia (or the former Soviet Union) were reported to be valid. Obviously, the high proportion of positive results reported in these countries was unusual, which could be attributed to publication and selective reporting bias [11]. Based on the above findings, the results of acupuncture trails were found to be unconvincing and unreliable.

The protocol of study is a predefined written document to state the structure of a research project and guide the implementation. A typical protocol has the following elements: background information and scientific rationale, objectives, study design, study population, study procedure, statistical consideration, subject confidentiality, informed consent process, literature references and supplements/appendices. WHO International Clinical Trials Registry Platform (ICTPR) has put key protocol information about each trial in public domain. These information make us learn about general characteristics of trails before it is reported. The registration of clinical trial required that soon after the trial was completed, its salient data be entered onto registries. This would bring negative data to light. Recently, the number of registered ACTs has been greatly increasing. According to a single web portal provided by the WHO International Clinical Trials Registry Platform (ICTPR), the number of registered ACTs has climbed to 740 [12], 520 of which were registered after 2008.

Thus far researchers have focused mainly on the quality of trial registration [13–15], however, to our knowledge, no study has yet examined the registration quality of ACTs. It has also been unclear whether existing general registered items reflect the characteristics of acupuncture intervention and are suitable for ACTs. Therefore, the objective of this study is to summarize and evaluate the quality of ACTs registration with the current 20 items of the WHO trial registration data set (TRDS) [16] and the special prepared items for acupuncture intervention details, which will provide the baseline information for the future development of ACTs registration.

Methods

Source of Data

Using the ICTRP Search Portal (http://apps.who.int/trialsearch/Default.aspx), we researched the registration data sets of WHO registries. Registries included the following: Australian New Zealand Clinical Trials Registry (ANZCTR), Chinese Clinical Trial Register (ChiCTR), ClinicalTrials.gov, Clinical Trials Registry-India (CTRI), Cuban Public Registry of Clinical Trials (RPCEC), EU Clinical Trials Register (EU-CTR), German Clinical Trials Register (DRKS), Iranian Registry of Clinical Trials (IRCT), ISRCTN, Japan Primary Registries Network (JPRN), Pan African Clinical Trial Registry (PACTR), Sri Lanka Clinical Trials Registry (SLCTR), the Netherlands National Trial Register (NTR), Clinical Research Information Service (CRiS) public of Korea (KCT), Brazilian Clinical Trials Registry (ReBec).

Search Strategy

WHO ICTRP prodives us with 'standard search' and 'advanced search'. We selected 'standard search' (to input "acupuncture", "needling", "acupressure", "moxibustion", "auriculotherapy" and "acupoint" into the ICTRP Search Portal (http://apps.who.int/trialsearch/Default.aspx)) without any restriction to focus on the sensitivity of retrieval, expand the scope of search results and improve the recall ration. The search was conducted on data sets from the inception of the registries up to 23 July 2012.

Inclusion Criteria

All records of ACTs that were registered in the WHO ICTRP were included. Acupuncture interventions might have been administered singly or with other interventions. For trials with multiple records, data from the record with the earliest registration date was chosen.

Data Extraction and Analysis

Information of registered ACTs was collected from all of the chosen records which imported into the portal and additional information was viewed through a hyperlink to the record in the source registry (i.e. the registry that provided the data) that was published by ICTRP. A small pilot project designed to test the assessment of framework, and the training and competence of the data extractors, was performed prior to data extraction. Three researchers (Jing GU, Xiaogang WANG and Ye Zhao) extracted the data from 20 random records independently. Results of the pilot were discussed by Kehu Yang and Jing GU and the framework was subsequently adapted.

Two researchers (Jing GU and Ye ZHAO) extracted the data from each record independently. Disagreements were settled through discussion after data extraction. Data was input into a standardized form that was mainly composed of two parts: (1) the minimum 20 items of the WHO TRDS (Text S1) and (2) information related to acupuncture interventions: 1) styles of acupuncture, 2) needling details, 3) treatment regimen, and 4) other interventions administered along with the acupuncture.

Each item was assessed as "yes" (described in records) or "no" (not described in records). Conditions that were studied were classified according to the International Classification of Diseases (ICD-10) by two researchers (Jing GU and Ye Zhao). Discrepancies were resolved by consulting relevant clinical experts.

Descriptive statistics (frequency, percentage) were used to summarize data. Analysis was performed by Microsoft EXCEL software (version Microsoft Excel 2007; http://office.microsoft.com/zh-cn/) and SPSS ware (version 13.0; http://www.spss.com).

Results

A total of 914 registration records were retrieved in the registries. We excluded 174 records and included 740 records of ACTs (Figure 1, Text S2). Information from the registration of 740 trials was collected manually from the registered records.

General Characteristics

1. Year distribution of registration. All of the 740 acupuncture trials were registered during the period of 1999 to 2012. The number of registrations increased from 4 in 1999 to a peak of 149 in 2011. Registration for 2012 was still in process, so the final number was not yet available (Figure 2).

2. The registration quantity of each registry. ACTs were found in the following 11 registries: ClinicalTrials.gov (376), ChiCTR (107), ISRCTN (100), ANZCTR (70), IRCT (46), JPRN (14), KCT (13), EU-CTR (4), DRKS (3), NTR (4) and ReBec (3); No registration records were found in CTRI, RPCEC, PACTR, and SLCTR.

3. Types of diseases. Information was gathered concerning the diseases treated. Of these, 734 (99.2%, 95% CI 98.2–99.6%) records mentioned health condition(s) or problem(s), of which 38 (5.2%, 95% CI 3.8–7.0%) indicated that the participants were otherwise healthy people or did not specify. The most common conditions were "symptoms, signs and abnormal clinical and laboratory findings" (152 (20.7%, 95% CI 17.9–23.8%)). "Diseases of the musculoskeletal system and connective tissue" (100 (13.6%, 95% CI 11.3–16.3%) and "mental and behavioral disorders" (84 (11.4%, 95% CI 9.3–14.0%)) were of special concern (Table 1).

20 Items of WHO TRDS

The completeness of the 20 items of the WHO TRDS was checked. The overall report percentage of these 20 items varied from 38.6% to 100%. Information on the primary register and trial ID, date of registration in primary register and public title, was present in all registration records. Most registration records (>85%) mentioned the following items: source(s) of monetary or material support, primary sponsor, contact for public queries,

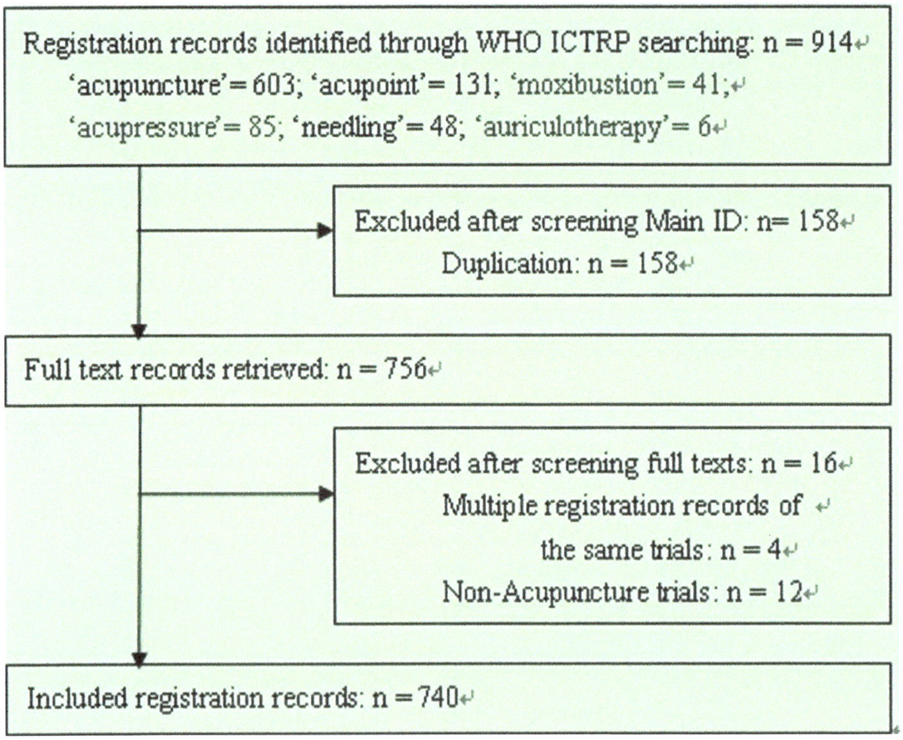

Figure 1. Flow chart of registration records identified, included and excluded.

scientific title, countries of recruitment, health condition(s) or problem(s) studied, intervention(s), key inclusion and exclusion criteria, study type, target sample size, recruitment status, primary outcome(s) and date of first enrollment. More than half of registration records provided items of secondary ID, key secondary outcomes and contact for scientific queries. Less than half of registration records provided information of secondary sponsor(s) (Table 2).

The four centers that had the largest number of registered ACTs were Clinical Trials.gov, ChiCTR, ISRCTN and ANZCTR, and the average registration rate of 20 items were 89.6%, 92.2%, 82.4%, and 91.6% respectively (Table 2).

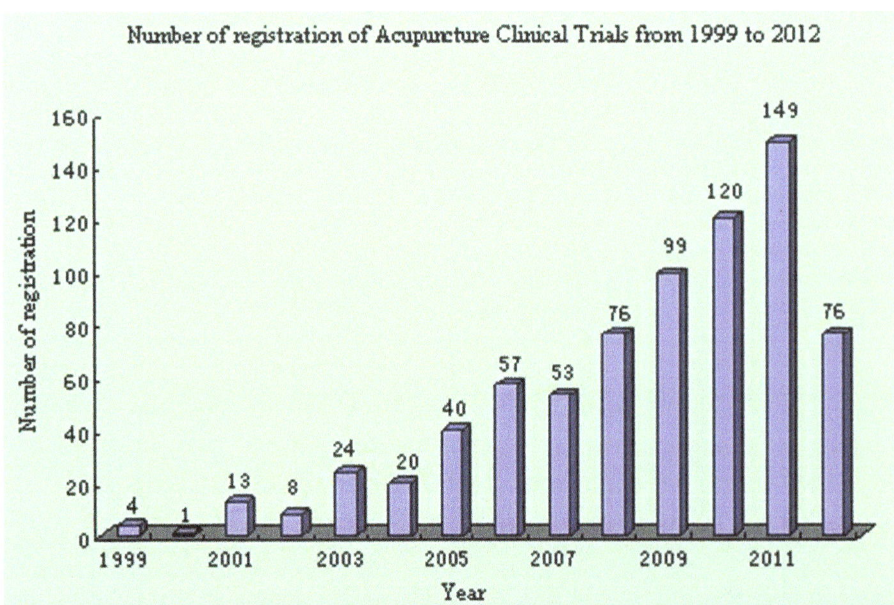

Figure 2. Number of registration of acupuncture clinical trials from 1999 to 2012.

Table 1. Types of diseases.

Types of Diseases (Common ICD-10[a])	Number (%) of n = 734, (95% CI)
Symptoms, signs and abnormal clinical and laboratory findings, not classified elsewhere	152 (20.7, 17.9–23.8)
Diseases of the musculoskeletal system and connective tissue	100 (13.6, 11.3–16.3)
Mental and behavioural disorders	84 (11.4, 9.3–14.0)
Diseases of the genitourinary system	50 (6.8, 5.2–8.9)
Diseases of the digestive system	46 (6.3, 4.7–8.3)
Diseases of the nervous system	45 (6.1, 4.6–8.1)
Pregnancy, childbirth and the puerperium	43 (5.9, 4.4–7.8)
Diseases of the circulatory system	41 (5.6, 4.1–7.5)
Diseases of the respiratory system	32 (4.4, 3.1–6.1)
Neoplasms	31 (4.2, 3.0–5.9)
Endocrine, nutritional and metabolic diseases	22 (3.0, 2.0–4.5)
Infectious and parasitic diseases	15 (2.0, 1.2–3.4)
Injury, poisoning and certain other consequences of external causes	14 (1.9, 1.1–3.2)
Diseases of the eye and adnexa	13 (1.8, 1.0–3.0)
Diseases of the skin and subcutaneous tissue	5 (0.7, 0.3–1.6)
Diseases of the ear and mastoid process	3 (0.4, 0.1–1.3)
Not specified or healthy people	38 (5.2, 3.8–7.0)

[a]Common ICD-10: International Classification of Diseases 10.

Information regarding eligibility criteria for participants was also gathered. A total of 615 (83.1%, 95% CI 80.2–85.6%) records mentioned diagnostic criteria, of which 567 were based solely on "western medicine (diseases)", 17 were based solely on "traditional medicine syndrome" and 31 used both "western disease" and "traditional medicine syndrome" diagnostic criteria. Exclusion criteria were reported in 693 (93.6%, 95% CI 91.6–95.2%) records, and most (>90%) provided information regarding the age and sex of participants (Table 3).

Intervention Specifics of ACTs

Quality of registration of acupuncture intervention specifics was also checked. These intervention specifics are shown in Tables 4 and 5.

Style of acupuncture was reported in 80 (10.8%, 95% CI 8.8–13.3%) trials (Table 4). They covered the following seven types: "traditional Chinese medicine acupuncture", "ear acupuncture", "moxibustion", "western style acupuncture" "Japanese medicine acupuncture", "Korean medical acupuncture" and "tongue acupuncture" (Table 5). The lowest reported percentage of this item was 0% from JPRN, EU-CTR, DRKS, ReBec and NTR while the highest was 38.5% from KCT (Table 4).

Details regarding needling could potentially contain seven items: names or location of points used (uni/bilateral), number of needle insertions per subject per session, depth of insertion, response sought (e.g. de qi or muscle twitch response), needle retention time, needle type (diameter, length, and manufacturer or material) and needle stimulation (e.g. manual, electrical). The average report percentage of these seven items was 19.2% and the lowest reported percentage was 0% (Table 4). Regarding needle stimulation, 35.0% had electrical stimulation, 14.9% had manual stimulation and 8.4% had laser stimulation (Table 5).

Treatment regimen, which refers to information of number, frequency and duration of treatment sessions, was present in 344 (46.5%, 95% CI 42.9–50.1%) trials (Table 4). EU-CTR had the lowest reported percentage (0%) of this item while ReBec, KCT and ANZCTR had the higher reported percentage (>75%) (Table 4).

Details of other interventions administered along with acupuncture were reported in 176 (23.8%, 95% CI 20.9–27.0%) trials (Table 4). They covered the following five types interventions: "western medicine", "traditional Chinese medicine", "exercises rehabilitation, massage, moxibustion, cupping, or similar", "cognitive behavioral therapy, life style advice, or similar", and "other interventions (routine nursing, conventional therapy, etc.)" (Table 5). EU-CTR, ReBec and NTR had the lowest reported percentage (0%) of this item (Table 4).

Discussion

A small number of studies have assessed the registration quality of clinical trials, and only one study was related to ACTs [17]. However, that study only investigated the status quo of the registration for ACTs, but did not report on its quality. In the present study, we retrieved all registered records of ACTs and evaluated the overall quality in order to identify possible deficiencies in ACTs registration and to provide feasible recommendations for development.

We reviewed some of the same variables reported in previous research done by Yang et. al. (2008) [17]. In that study, 206 registration records of ACTs were searched between 1999 and 2008 [17]. In the current study, results retrieved from the WHO ICTRP indicated that the registration number of ACTs has been increasing rapidly in recent years and has reached 740 as of July, 2012. In our research, there are 11 register centers where we can find ACTs while there were only 3 in the Yang study [17]. Similar to previous studies, ClinicalTrials.gov still have the largest number of ACTs while the number of ACTs in ChiCTR has increased from just 5, four years ago [17], to 107, surpassing ISRCTN and ANZCTRN and making it the second biggest registration center. This rapid increase in the number of registration centers that have

Table 2. 20 items of WHO TRDS.

20 Items	Overall	Clinical Trials.gov	ChiCTR	ISRCTN	ANZCTR	IRCT	JPRN	EU-CTR	DRKS	ReBec	KCT	NTR
	N[a] (%) of n = 740, (95% CI)	N[a] (%) of n = 376, (95% CI)	N[a] (%) of n = 107, (95% CI)	N[a] (%) of n = 100, (95% CI)	N[a] (%) of n = 70, (95% CI)	N[a] (%) of n = 46, (95% CI)	N[a] (%) of n = 14, (95% CI)	N[a] (%) of n = 4, (95% CI)	N[a] (%) of n = 3, (95% CI)	N[a] (%) of n = 3, (95% CI)	N[a] (%) of n = 13, (95% CI)	N[a] (%) of n = 4, (95% CI)
Primary Register and Trial ID[b]	740 (100.0, 98.9–100.0)	376 (100.0, 97.9–100.0)	107 (100.0, 93.0–100.0)	100 (100.0, 92.6–100.0)	70 (100.0, 89.7–100.0)	46 (100.0, 85.1–100.0)	14 (100.0, 63.4–100.0)	4 (100.0, 32.6–100.0)	3 (100.0, 26.6–100.0)	3 (100.0, 26.6–100.0)	13 (100.0, 61.6–100.0)	4 (100.0, 32.6–100.0)
Date of Registration in Primary Registry	740 (100.0, 98.9–100.0)	376 (100.0, 97.9–100.0)	107 (100.0, 93.0–100.0)	100 (100.0, 92.6–100.0)	70 (100.0, 89.7–100.0)	46 (100.0, 85.1–100.0)	14 (100.0, 63.4–100.0)	4 (100.0, 32.6–100.0)	3 (100.0, 26.6–100.0)	3 (100.0, 26.6–100.0)	13 (100.0, 61.6–100.0)	4 (100.0, 32.6–100.0)
Secondary ID[b]	445 (60.1, 56.6–63.6)	345 (91.8, 88.5–94.1)	0 (0.0, 0.0–7.0)	77 (77.0, 67.8–84.2)	10 (14.3, 7.9––24.6)	0 (0.0, 0–14.9)	0 (0.0, 0.0–36.6)	4 (100.0, 32.6–100.0)	3 (100.0, 26.6–100.0)	3 (100.0, 26.6–100.0)	0 (0.0, 0.0–38.4)	3 (75.0, 23.8–96.6)
Source(s) of Monetary or Material Support	730 (98.6, 97.5–99.3)	374 (99.5, 97.9–99.9)	106 (99.1, 93.7–99.9)	100 (100.0, 92.6–100.0)	68 (97.1, 89.3–99.3)	46 (100.0, 85.1–100.0)	14 (100.0, 63.4–100.0)	1 (25.0, 3.4–76.2)	3 (100.0, 26.6–100.0)	3 (100.0, 26.6–100.0)	12 (92.3, 60.9–98.9)	3 (75.0, 23.8–96.6)
Primary Sponsor	737 (99.6, 98.8–99.9)	374 (99.5, 97.9–99.9)	107 (100.0, 93.0–100.0)	100 (100.0, 92.6–100.0)	70 (100.0, 89.7–100.0)	46 (100.0, 85.1–100.0)	14 (100.0, 63.4–100.0)	4 (100.0, 32.6–100.0)	3 (100.0, 26.6–100.0)	3 (100.0, 26.6–100.0)	13 (100.0, 61.6–100.0)	3 (75.0, 23.8–96.6)
Secondary Sponsor(s)	286 (38.6, 35.2–42.2)	144 (38.3, 33.5–43.3)	95 (88.8, 81.3–93.5)	0 (0.0, 0.0–7.4)	27 (38.6, 28.0–50.4)	1 (2.2, 0.3–13.9)	0 (0.0, 0.0–36.6)	0 (0.0, 0.0–67.4)	1 (33.3, 4.3–84.6)	3 (100.0, 26.6–100.0)	13 (100.0, 61.6–100.0)	2 (50.0, 12.3–87.7)
Contact for Public Queries	711 (96.1, 94.4–97.3)	351 (93.4, 90.3–95.5)	107 (100.0, 93.0–100.0)	100 (100.0, 92.6–100.0)	70 (100.0, 89.7–100.0)	46 (100.0, 85.1–100.0)	14 (100.0, 63.4–100.0)	0 (0.0, 0.0–67.4)	3 (100.0, 26.6–100.0)	3 (100.0, 26.6–100.0)	13 (100.0, 61.6–100.0)	4 (100.0, 32.6–100.0)
Contact for Scientific Queries	397 (53.6, 50.0–57.2)	137 (36.4, 31.7–41.4)	107 (100.0, 93.0–100.0)	0 (0.0, 0.0–7.4)	70 (100.0, 89.7–100.0)	46 (100.0, 85.1–100.0)	14 (100.0, 63.4–100.0)	0 (0.0, 0.0–67.4)	3 (100.0, 26.6–100.0)	3 (100.0, 26.6–100.0)	13 (100.0, 61.6–100.0)	4 (100.0, 32.6–100.0)
Public Title	740 (100.0, 98.9–100.0)	376 (100.0, 97.9–100.0)	107 (100.0, 93.0–100.0)	100 (100.0, 92.6–100.0)	70 (100.0, 89.7–100.0)	46 (100.0, 85.1–100.0)	14 (100.0, 63.4–100.0)	4 (100.0, 32.6––100.0)	3 (100.0, 26.6–100.0)	3 (100.0, 26.6–100.0)	13 (100.0, 61.6––100.0)	4 (100.0, 32.6–100.0)
Scientific Title	638 (86.2, 83.5–88.5)	353 (93.9, 91.0–95.9)	106 (99.1, 93.7–99.9)	34 (34.0, 25.4–43.8)	70 (100.0, 89.7–100.0)	46 (100.0, 85.1––100.0)	2 (14.3, 3.6–42.7)	4 (100.0, 32.6–100.0)	3 (100.0, 26.6–100.0)	3 (100.0, 26.6–100.0)	13 (100.0, 61.6––100.0)	4 (100.0, 32.6–100.0)
Countries of Recruitment	723 (97.7, 96.3–98.6)	364 (96.8, 94.5–98.2)	103 (96.3, 90.5–98.6)	100 (100.0, 92.6––100.0)	70 (100.0, 89.7–100.0)	46 (100.0, 85.1–100.0)	14 (100.0, 63.4–100.0)	4 (100.0, 32.6–100.0)	2 (66.7, 15.4–95.7)	3 (100.0, 26.6–100.0)	13 (100.0, 61.6–100.0)	4 (100.0, 32.6–100.0)
Health Condition(s) or Problem(s) Studied	734 (99.2, 98.2–99.6)	374 (99.5, 97.9–99.9)	103 (96.3, 90.5–98.6)	99 (99.0, 93.2–99.9)	70 (100.0, 89.7–100.0)	46 (100.0, 85.1–100.0)	14 (100.0, 63.4–100.0)	4 (100.0, 32.6–100.0)	3 (100.0, 26.6–100.0)	3 (100.0, 26.6–100.0)	13 (100.0, 61.6–100.0)	4 (100.0, 32.6–100.0)
Intervention(s)	737 (99.6, 98.8–99.9)	376 (100.0, 97.9–100.0)	104 (97.2, 91.7–99.1)	100 (100.0, 92.6–100.0)	70 (100.0, 89.7–100.0)	46 (100.0, 85.1–100.0)	14 (100.0, 63.4–100.0)	4 (100.0, 32.6–100.0)	3 (100.0, 26.6–100.0)	3 (100.0, 26.6–100.0)	13 (100.0, 61.6–100.0)	4 (100.0, 32.6–100.0)
Key Inclusion and Exclusion Criteria	720 (97.3, 95.8–98.2)	374 (99.5, 97.9–99.9)	107 (100.0, 93.0–100.0)	82 (82.0, 73.2–88.4)	70 (100.0, 89.7–100.0)	46 (100.0, 85.1–100.0)	14 (100.0, 63.4–100.0)	4 (100.0, 32.6–100.0)	3 (100.0, 26.6–100.0)	3 (100.0, 26.6–100.0)	13 (100.0, 61.6–100.0)	4 (100.0, 32.6–100.0)
Study Type	736 (99.5, 98.6–99.8)	376 (100.0, 97.9–100.0)	107 (100.0, 93.0–100.0)	99 (99.0, 93.2–99.9)	70 (100.0, 89.7–100.0)	46 (100.0, 85.1–100.0)	14 (100.0, 63.4–100.0)	4 (100.0, 32.6–100.0)	3 (100.0, 26.6–100.0)	0 (0.0, 0.0–73.4)	13 (100.0, 61.6–100.0)	4 (100.0, 32.6–100.0)
Date of First Enrollment	739 (99.9, 99.0–100.0)	376 (100.0, 97.9–100.0)	107 (100.0, 93.0–100.0)	100 (100.0, 92.6–100.0)	70 (100.0, 89.7–100.0)	46 (100.0, 85.1–100.0)	14 (100.0, 63.4–100.0)	4 (100.0, 32.6–100.0)	2 (66.7, 15.4–95.7)	3 (100.0, 26.6––100.0)	13 (100.0, 61.6–100.0)	4 (100.0, 32.6–100.0)
Target Sample Size	703 (95.0, 93.2–96.4)	352 (93.6, 90.7–95.7)	103 (96.3, 90.5–98.6)	95 (95.0, 88.5–97.9)	70 (100.0, 89.7–100.0)	46 (100.0, 85.1–100.0)	13 (92.9, 63.0–99.9)	1 (25.0, 3.4–76.2)	3 (100.0, 26.6–100.0)	3 (100.0, 26.6–100.0)	13 (100.0, 61.6–100.0)	4 (100.0, 32.6–100.0)
Recruitment Status	738 (99.7, 98.9–99.9)	376 (100.0, 97.9–100.0)	107 (100.0, 93.0–100.0)	100 (100.0, 92.6–100.0)	70 (100.0, 89.7–100.0)	46 (100.0, 85.1–100.0)	14 (100.0, 63.4–100.0)	4 (100.0, 32.6–100.0)	3 (100.0, 26.6–100.0)	3 (100.0, 26.6–100.0)	13 (100.0, 61.6–100.0)	4 (100.0, 32.6–100.0)
Primary Outcome(s)	677 (91.5, 89.2–93.3)	325 (86.4, 82.6–89.5)	106 (99.1, 93.7–99.9)	91 (91.0, 83.6–95.3)	70 (100.0, 89.7–100.0)	46 (100.0, 85.1––100.0)	13 (92.9, 63.0–99.9)	4 (100.0, 32.6–100.0)	3 (100.0, 26.6–100.0)	3 (100.0, 26.6–100.0)	13 (100.0, 61.6–100.0)	3 (75.0, 23.8–96.6)

Table 2. Cont.

20 Items	Overall	Clinical Trials.gov	ChiCTR	ISRCTN	ANZCTR	IRCT	JPRN	EU-CTR	DRKS	ReBec	KCT	NTR
	N[a] (%) of n = 740, (95% CI)	N[a] (%) of n = 376, (95% CI)	N[a] (%) of n = 107, (95% CI)	N[a] (%) of n = 100, (95% CI)	N[a] (%) of n = 70, (95% CI)	N[a] (%) of n = 46, (95% CI)	N[a] (%) of n = 14, (95% CI)	N[a] (%) of n = 4, (95% CI)	N[a] (%) of n = 3, (95% CI)	N[a] (%) of n = 3, (95% CI)	N[a] (%) of n = 13, (95% CI)	N[a] (%) of n = 4, (95% CI)
Key Secondary Outcomes	495 (66.9, 63.4–70.2)	237 (63.0, 58.0–67.8)	78 (72.9, 63.7–80.5)	72 (72.0, 62.4–79.9)	58 (82.9, 72.2–90.0)	25 (54.3, 40.0–68.0)	4 (28.6, 11.1–56.1)	1 (25.0, 3.4–76.2)	1 (33.3, 4.3–84.6)	3 (100.0, 26.6–100.0)	13 (100.0, 61.6–100.0)	3 (75.0, 23.8–96.6)
Total per Registry (%)	(89.0, 86.5–91.0)	(89.6, 86.1–92.3)	(92.2, 85.4–96.0)	(82.4, 73.7–88.7)	(91.6, 82.5–96.2)	(87.8, 74.9–94.6)	(81.4, 53.3–94.4)	(73.8, 23.2–96.3)	(90.0, 17.2–99.7)	(95.0, 9.6–100.0)	(94.6, 61.3–99.5)	(91.2, 24.5–99.7)

[a]N = Number.
[b]ID = Identifying Number.

Table 3. Eligibility criteria for participants.

Category	Number (%) of n = 740, (95% CI)
Diagnostic Criteria	615 (83.1, 80.2–85.6)
Western Medicine (diseases)	567 (76.6, 73.4–79.5)
Traditional Medicine	17 (2.3, 1.4–3.7)
Using both Disease and Syndrome	31 (4.2, 3.0–5.9)
Exclusion Criteria	693 (93.6, 91.6–95.2)
Age	682 (92.2, 90.0–93.9)
Sex	679 (91.8, 89.5–93.5)
Male	14 (2.1[a], 1.2–3.5)
Female	145 (21.4[a], 18.4–24.6)
Both	520 (76.6[a], 73.2–79.6)

[a]n = 679.

ACTs indicates that ACTs registration has become much more common. Although the number of ACTs in ChiCTR is far less than in ClinicalTrials.gov, the rapid growth is obvious, considering it has only been four years since it was established. Therefore it is possible that ChiCTR will become the principle registration center for ACTs in the future. Previous studies reported that the diseases of registered ACTs were limited [17,18]. In contrast, our study found that the types of diseases studied with ACTs are becoming more varied which will be helpful to better develop acupuncture clinical research.

Each registration record was also analyzed and the quality of ACT registration assessed using the following two guidelines: (1) the completeness of 20 items of WHO TRDS and (2) whether the related information of acupuncture intervention was present in the registration records according to specially preparedspecific items.

The contents of clinical trial registrations should contain the basic information about the trial's implementation. The 20 items of the WHO TRDS [16], regarded as the minimum requirement for trial registration, comprehensively covers this basic information. Therefore, ensuring the completeness of the 20 items is the first step in assessing the quality of ACT registration. Complete registration of 20 items minimizes the chance that relevant information will be omitted. This is of importance since missing or uninformative items required by the WHO TRDS may impair the fulfillment of registration promise. In the current study 20 items of the 740 records were reviewed and appraised for completeness. Our results indicated that most items (16 items) had higher percentages (>85%) of completeness. However, information regarding secondary sponsor(s), contact for scientific queries, secondary ID and key secondary outcomes were insufficient. There are two possible reasons for the omission of relevant information. One is that not every participant is willing to provide all 20 items due to academic or commercial interests [19]; the other is that not every registered trial had all of the 20 items [14]. For example, secondary ID or secondary sponsors do not routinely exist in some clinical trials so that the total percentage of these corresponding entries might be lower.

The completeness of 20 items varied among the 11 registries. Clinicaltrials.gov, the center with the largest number of registered ACTs, did not have the highest registration quality while instead we found that ChiCTR had the highest in the registration quality. The completeness of the 20 items in different register centers may be related to the establishment time of centers. Specifically, the 20 items of the WHO TRDS was announced in 2007 so that those

Table 4. Special items for acupuncture intervention details.

Special Items for Acupuncture Intervention Details	Overall	Clinical Trials.gov	ChiCTR	ISRCTN	ANZCTR	IRCT	JPRN	EU-CTR	DRKS	ReBec	KCT	NTR
	N[a] (%) of n=740, (95% CI)	N[a] (%) of n=376, (95% CI)	N[a] (%) of n=107, (95% CI)	N[a] (%) of n=100, (95% CI)	N[a] (%) of n=70, (95% CI)	N[a] (%) of n=46, (95% CI)	N[a] (%) of n=14, (95% CI)	N[a] (%) of n=4, (95% CI)	N[a] (%) of n=3, (95% CI)	N[a] (%) of n=3, (95% CI)	N[a] (%) of n=13, (95% CI)	N[a] (%) of n=4, (95% CI)
Style of Acupuncture[b]	80 (10.8, 8.8–13.3)	42 (11.2, 8.4–14.8)	12 (11.2, 6.5–18.7)	8 (8.0, 4.1–15.2)	11 (15.7, 8.9–26.2)	4 (8.7, 3.3–21.0)	0 (0.0, 0.0–36.6)	0 (0.0, 0.0–67.4)	0 (0.0, 0.0–73.4)	0 (0.0, 0.0–73.4)	5 (38.5, 17.0–65.6)	0 (0.0, 0.0–67.4)
Needling Details[c]	(19.2, 16.5–22.2)											
Names or Location of Points	216 (29.2, 26.0–32.6)	95 (25.3, 21.1–29.9)	28 (26.2, 18.7–35.3)	16 (16.0, 10.0–24.5)	36 (51.4, 39.9–62.9)	29 (63.0, 48.4–75.6)	5 (35.7, 15.7–62.4)	0 (0.0, 0.0–67.4)	0 (0.0, 0.0–73.4)	1 (33.3, 4.3–84.6)	9 (69.2, 40.9–88.8)	0 (0.0, 0.0–67.4)
Number of Needle Insertions per Session	169 (22.8, 20.0–26.0)	82 (21.8, 17.9–26.3)	17 (15.9, 10.1–24.1)	15 (15.0, 9.2–23.4)	27 (38.6, 28.0–50.4)	19 (41.3, 28.1–55.9)	3 (21.4, 7.1–49.4)	0 (0.0, 0.0–67.4)	0 (0.0, 0.0–73.4)	1 (33.3, 4.3–84.6)	5 (38.5, 17.0–65.6)	0 (0.0, 0.0–67.4)
Depth of Insertion	47 (6.4, 4.8–8.4)	25 (6.6, 4.5–9.7)	3 (2.8, 0.9–8.3)	7 (7.0, 3.4–14.0)	5 (7.1, 3.0–16.0)	2 (4.3, 1.1–15.8)	1 (7.1, 1.0–37.0)	0 (0.0, 0.0–67.4)	0 (0.0, 0.0–73.4)	1 (33.3, 4.3–84.6)	3 (23.1, 7.6–52.2)	0 (0.0, 0.0–67.4)
Response Sought	58 (7.8, 6.1–10.0)	27 (7.2, 5.0–10.3)	6 (5.6, 2.5–11.9)	4 (4.0, 1.5–10.2)	15 (21.4, 13.4–32.6)	2 (4.3, 1.1–15.8)	0 (0.0, 0.0–36.6)	0 (0.0, 0.0–67.4)	0 (0.0, 0.0–73.4)	1 (33.3, 4.3–84.6)	3 (23.1, 7.6–52.2)	0 (0.0, 0.0–67.4)
Needle Retention Time	216 (29.2, 26.0–32.6)	95 (25.3, 21.1–29.9)	21 (19.6, 13.2–28.2)	15 (15.0, 9.2–23.4)	43 (61.4, 49.6–72.0)	28 (60.9, 46.2–73.8)	2 (14.3, 3.6–42.7)	0 (0.0, 0.0–67.4)	0 (0.0, 0.0–73.4)	1 (33.3, 4.3–84.6)	11 (84.6, 54.9–96.1)	0 (0.0, 0.0–67.4)
Needle Type[d]	84 (11.4, 9.3–13.8)	50 (13.3, 10.2–17.1)	3 (2.8, 0.9–8.3)	7 (7.0, 3.4–14.0)	15 (21.4, 13.4–32.6)	1 (2.2, 0.3–13.9)	0 (0.0, 0.0–36.6)	0 (0.0, 0.0–67.4)	0 (0.0, 0.0–73.4)	1 (33.3, 4.3–84.6)	7 (53.8, 28.2–77.6)	0 (0.0, 0.0–67.4)
Needle Stimulation	205 (27.7, 24.6–31.0)	101 (26.9, 22.6–31.6)	30 (28.0, 20.4–37.3)	17 (17.0, 10.8–25.7)	33 (47.1, 35.8–58.8)	10 (21.7, 12.1–35.9)	5 (35.7, 15.7–62.4)	1 (25.0, 3.4–76.2)	0 (0.0, 0.0–73.4)	2 (66.7, 15.4–95.7)	4 (30.8, 12.0–59.1)	0 (0.0, 0.0–67.4)
Treatment Regimen[e]	344 (46.5, 42.9–50.1)	184 (48.9, 43.9–54.0)	18 (16.8, 10.9–25.1)	38 (38.0, 29.0–47.9)	54 (77.1, 65.9–85.5)	30 (65.2, 50.5–77.5)	3 (21.4, 7.1–49.4)	0 (0.0, 0.0–67.4)	1 (33.3, 4.3–84.6)	3 (100.0, 26.6–100)	12 (92.3, 60.9–98.9)	1 (25.0, 3.4–76.2)
Other Interventions[f]	176 (23.8, 20.9–27.0)	80 (21.3, 17.4–25.7)	28 (26.2, 18.7–35.3)	25 (25.0, 17.5–34.4)	21 (30.0, 20.4–41.7)	8 (17.4, 8.9–31.1)	1 (7.1, 1.0–37.0)	0 (0.0, 0.0–67.4)	1 (33.3, 4.3–84.6)	0 (0.0, 0.0–73.4)	4 (30.8, 12.0–59.1)	0 (0.0, 0.0–67.4)

[a]N = Number.
[b]Style of acupuncture (e.g. Traditional Chinese Medicine,Japanese,Korean,Western medical,Five Element,ear acupuncture, etc).
[c]Needling details can contain seven items: names or location of points used (uni/bilateral), number of needle insertions per subject per session, depth of insertion, response sought (e.g. de qi or muscle twitch response), needle retention time, needle type (diameter, length, and manufacturer or material) and needle stimulation (e.g. manual, electrical).The total percentage of the seven items was 19.2%.
[d]Needle Type (e.g. diameter, length, and manufacturer or material).
[e]Treatment regimen, refers to number, frequency and duration of treatment sessions.
[f]Other interventions administered to the acupuncture group (e.g. moxibustion, cupping, herbs, exercises, lifestyle advice).

Table 5. Descriptive information of some acupuncture special items.

Category	Number (%) of n, (95% CI)
Style of Acupuncture	**n = 97**
Traditional Chinese Medicine Acupuncture	33 (34.0, 25.3–44.0)
Ear Acupuncture	28 (28.9, 20.7–38.6)
Moxibustion	14 (14.4, 8.7–22.9)
Western Style Acupuncture	13 (13.4, 7.9–21.7)
Japanese Medicine Acupuncture	5 (5.2, 2.2–11.8)
Korean Medical Acupuncture	2 (2.1, 0.5–7.9)
Tongue Acupuncture	2 (2.1, 0.5–7.9)
Needle Stimulation of the Acupuncture	**n = 309**
Electrical	108 (35.0, 29.8–40.4)
Manual	46 (14.9, 11.3–19.3)
Laser	26 (8.4, 5.8–12.1)
Not specified or other stimulation	129 (41.7, 36.4–47.3)
Details of other Interventions Administered to Acupuncture	**n = 176**
Western Medicine	67 (38.1, 31.2–45.5)
Traditional Chinese Medicine	13 (7.4, 4.3–12.3)
Exercises, Rehabilitation, Massage,Moxibustion, Cupping, etc.	37 (21.0, 15.6–27.7)
Cognitive Behavioural Therapy, Life Style Advice, etc.	9 (5.1, 2.7–9.5)
Other Interventions (Routine nursing, Conventional Therapy, etc.)	50 (28.4, 22.2–35.5)

centers established after this announcement would have set the items according to the WHO TRDS. Thus, the items from those centers would have a higher percentage of registration than the centers established prior to 2007. For example, ChiCTR, which was established after 2007, was found to have better completeness and quality of the 20 items.

In the current study we also have determined that for each register center, there were several items that contained woefully inadequate information. This may have been caused by the absence of related items in that specific center. For instance, ISRCIN has no area for information about 'secondary sponsor(s)' [14], and no record contained relevant information. Similarly, the item 'secondary sponsor' was not found in IRCT [14], and only 2.2% records provided relevant information. This speculation is supported by previous research by Liu's [14]. Liu mentioned that, although the data sets of each registry were based on the 20 items, there were still slight differences among registries due to the increase or reduction of some items so that there are different registration rates in different centers.

Unlike general clinical intervention, acupuncture is a special medical technique that treats patients by inserting thin needles into acupoints. Acupuncture clinical practice is mainly concerned with acupuncture theory, acupoints, unique acupuncture manipulation methods, and acupuncture instruments [20]. The "quality" of an intervention in the sense of "how well made is the intervention" is a preclinical not a clinical issue for drugs, biologics, or devices, but for procedures such as acupuncture, intervention quality is a clinical issue. There are many factors which can influence its curative effect and safety. Arguably more information thoroughly describing the acupuncture intervention should be required in the registration of ACTs, just as in the registration of drug, biological and vaccine trials, information on the dose, frequency, route of administration and duration of treatment are needed [16,21]. As an open-source, the information of ACTs registration should be detailed enough to make trials as transparent as possible.

Since acupuncture is a unique medical technique, it is not appropriate to evaluate the quality of its intervention specifics with existing evaluation criterion for general intervention measures. As demonstrated by previous studies, special items that describe the intervention details of acupuncture should be added to the registration of item sets [17]. Further assessment on the quality of ACTs registration could potentially be accomplished using these special items. We developed items and evaluation criterion that contain the following four facets: style of acupuncture, needling details, treatment regimen and other interventions administered with acupuncture. We validated these items for quality evaluation of acupuncture intervention details in reference to the Standards for Reporting Interventions in Controlled Trials of Acupuncture (STRICTA) [22]. As is known to all, the intervention details of acupuncture are totally included by STRICTA. However, unlike the trial report, trial registration is a demonstration of the protocol before implementation while the trial report is the demonstration of the process and details about the trial after completion. Therefore, instead of using all of the items published by STRICTA, we integrated the suggestions of intervention from acupuncturists, clinical expert, methodologists and producers of systematic reviews and chose only those items related with intervention that should be included in a protocol of acupuncture research (the protocol without these information will miss the accuracy of the implementation of trails and the results will be unreliable.). However, we found that information on the details of acupuncture intervention is seriously insufficient. Possible reasons for this may be: (1) these special items were not included in 20 items and the registration centers lacked registration requirements for them. Therefore, these items failed to catch the attention of registrants and registrants neglected the description of acupuncture intervention details or (2) the selection of acupoints and acupuncture manipulation takes great skill and heavy reliance on experience, therefore many clinical acupuncture practitioners keep this information private and are reluctant to share technical details. These limitations cause ACTs to be less transparent.

Acupuncture is a part of Traditional Chinese Medicine (TCM). The necessity of acupuncture intervention and selection of acupoints are based on TCM's syndromes. However, most acupuncture researchers focus on 'western disease' for their diagnostic criteria rather than 'TCMs' syndromes'. In the current study, we found that only 6.5% (2.3% + 4.2%) of ACTs registration records provided information about TCM's syndrome in their diagnostic criteria. To comply with the principles of selection of treatment based on the differential diagnosis of TCM, we strongly propose that diagnostic criteria contain information on both western disease and TCM's syndrome in the registration of ACTs.

After the publication of the announcement of International Committee of Medical Journal Editors (ICMJE) [23], the Ottawa Statement and Declaration of Helsinki [24,25], and with the establishment of the WHO ICTRP, the importance of registration has been gradually accepted so that now, clinical trial registration has become a part of the current research paradigm internationally. With increasing numbers and attention in recent years, ACTs should be encouraged to register in order to improve public confidence in clinical effectiveness. Registration could bring the following benefits to the clinical research of acupuncture. First, registration promotes the inspection of study design and provides technical guidance for the clinical trial [26]. Second, whether the key part of clinical trial was reported or not, a registered protocol can be used as a basis for supervision. Registration will also increase the transparency of the clinical trials, so it can be ensured that the reported information from clinical research is complete, true and valid [24,27] while potential biases are reduced as much as possible. Third, registration of ACTs helps to avoid repeating research and/or wasting resources. Fourth, as a precondition of ACTs being published in journals with high impact factors [18], registration could facilitate the communication of the results from ACTs. Therefore, further quantitative and qualitative improvements are needed in ACTs registration.

Although the quality of ACTs registration was fair in regard to the completeness of the 20 items according to our research, the serious lack of information on acupuncture intervention specifics lowered its overall quality greatly, which made trial registration fail to fulfill its promise of promoting research transparency [28–30].

It is very necessary to establish special registration system for ACTs because of the specificity of acupuncture, just like STRICTA – a special version of CONSORT [31] – is made for acupuncture RCTs. Modifying the existing registration system to include criteria (or items) specific to acupuncture could facilitate developing a registration system for ACTs. The first step would be to establish a registration data set suitable for ACTs. We propose that those items used to assess acupuncture intervention details in the current study be added on the basis of the 20 items. The second step would be to establish a special registry center for ACTs.

There were several limitations in the current study. First, assessment of the registration quality of ACTs in different centers according to the completeness of 20 items may be lacking fairness since the 20 items of the WHO TRDS were not announced until 2007. Therefore, those centers established after 2007 may have a higher registration quality since they could more easily meet the standards set by the WHO TRDS. Second, there are likely many clinical trials that are not registered in the WHO ICTRP, so that it would be impossible for our study to include all of the ACTs that are registered throughout the world.

In conclusion, the overall registration quality of ACTs was not high enough due to the serious lack of information on the specifics of acupuncture intervention. Further improvements are needed in this field. This could be achieved by optimizing the WHO TRDS to include those additional items related to acupuncture. It is extremely vital to establish a number of special items regarding acupuncture intervention to develop a suitable system for the registration of ACTs.

Supporting Information

Text S1 The minimum 20 items of the WHO trial registration data set (WHO TRDs).
(DOC)

Text S2 Main ID of all included registration records.
(DOC)

Author Contributions

Conceived and designed the experiments: JG KY X-GW YZ J-HT. Performed the experiments: JG YZ J-JJ. Analyzed the data: X-GW JG YZ J-HT. Contributed reagents/materials/analysis tools: JG KY X-GW YZ J-HT. Wrote the paper: JG X-GW.

References

1. Richardson PH, Vincent CA (1986) Acupuncture for the treatment of pain: a review of evaluative research. Pain 24: 15–40.
2. National Institutes of Health (1998) NIH Consensus Conference. Acupuncture. JAMA 280: 1518–24.
3. NIH Consensus Development Program (1997) Acupuncture–Consensus Development Conference Statement. Available: http://consensus.nih.gov/1997/1997Acupuncture107html.htm. Accessed 2012 Aug 26.
4. World Health Organization (2003) Acupuncture: Review and Analysis of Reports on Controlled Clinical Trials. Available: http://www.who.int/medicinedocs/en/d/Js4926e/#Js4926e. Accessed 2012 Aug 29.
5. US National Center for Complementary and Alternative Medicine (2006) Acupuncture. Available: http://nccam.nih.gov/health/acupuncture/. Accessed 2012 Nov 7.
6. National Health Service (2012) Acupuncture: Evidence for its effectiveness. Available: http://www.nhs.uk/Conditions/Acupuncture/Pages/Evidence.aspx. Accessed 2012 Aug 14.
7. Sun Yong (2011) Analysis of clinical studies of acupuncture. CJCM 3: 69–70.
8. Xu L, Li J, Zhang M, Ai C, Wang L (2008) Chinese authors do need CONSORT: reporting quality assessment for five leading Chinese medical journals. Contemp Clin Trials 29: 727–731.
9. Geng LL, Lin RS, Sun XY, Wu L, Zhong MM, et al. (2008) Critical appraisal of randomized clinical trials in Chinese Acupuncture and Moxibustion from 2000 to 2006. Zhongguo Zhen Jiu 28: 439–43.
10. Vickers A, Goyal N, Harland R, Rees R (1998) Do certain countries produce only positive results? A systematic review of controlled trials. Controll Clin Trials 19: 159–166.
11. Lao LX (2008) Acupuncture clinical studies and evidence-based medicine–an update. Zhen Ci Yan Jiu 33: 53–61.
12. WHO International Clinical Trials Registry Platform (ICTRP). Available: http://apps.who.int/trialsearch/Default.aspx. Accessed 2012 Jul 23.
13. Viergever RF, Ghersi D (2011) The quality of registration of clinical trials. PLoS One 6: 1–8.
14. Liu X, Li Y, Yu X, Feng J, Zhong X, et al. (2009) Assessment of registration quality of trials sponsored by China. J Evid Based Med 2: 8–18.
15. Sekeres M, Gold JL, Chan AW, Lexchin J, Moher D, et al. (2008) Poor reporting of scientific leadership information in clinical trial registers. PloS One 3: e1610.
16. WHO Trial Registration Data Set (TRDS). Available: http://www.who.int/ictrp/network/trds/en/index.html. Accessed 2012 Jul 28.
17. Yang DQ, Tu Y (2008) Investigation of registration of international acupuncture clinical trials. Available: http://www.cnki.net/kcms/detail/Detail.aspx?dbname = CDMDTOTAL&filename = 2008113899.nh&filetitle. Accessed 2012 Jul 29.
18. Li ZJ, Liu ML, Wang JN, Liang FR (2012) Method and current situations on acupuncture clinical trial registration in the world. Zhen Ci Yan Jiu 37: 86–7.

19. Reveiz L, Krleza-Jerić K, Chan AW, de Aguiar S (2007) Do trialists endorse clinical trial registration? Survey of a Pubmed sample. Trials 8: 30.
20. Wu B, Liu Y, He J (2002) (Evidence based medicine and the present situation and enlightenment of acupuncture clinical research. Journal of Clinical Acupuncture and Moxibustion 18: 1–2.
21. De Angelis CD, Drazen JM, Frizelle FA, Haug C, Hoey J, et al. (2005) Is this clinical trial fully registered? A statement from the international committee of medical journal editors. Croat Med J 46: 499–501.
22. MacPherson H, Altman DG, Hammerschlag R, Youping L, Taixiang W, et al. (2010) Revised Standards for Reporting Interventions in Clinical Trials of Acupuncture (STRICTA): extending the CONSORT statement. PLoS Med 7(6): e1000261.
23. International Committee of Medical Journal (2004) Clinical Trial Registration: A statement from the International Committee of Medical Journal Editors. Available: http://www.icmje.org/clin_trial.pdf. Accessed 2012 Jun 28.
24. Krleza-Jeric K, Chan AW, Dickersin K, Sim I, Grimshaw J, et al. (2005) Principles for international registration of protocol information and results from human trials of health related interventions: Ottawa statement (part 1). BMJ 330(7497): 956–958.
25. World Medical Association (2008) Declaration of Helsinki. Available: http://www.wma.net/en/30publications/10policies/b3/index.html. Accessed 2012 Jun 28.
26. Wang L, Jiang J, Li X (2007) Promote the whole level of Chinese medical journals through the mechanism of registry and publicity of clinical experiment. Xian Dai Qing Bao 27: 221–22.
27. Ghersi D, Pang T (2009) From Mexico to Mail: four years in the history of clinical trial registration. J Evid Based Med 2(1): 1–7.
28. Dwan K, Altman DG, Arnaiz JA, Bloom J, Chan AW, et al. (2008) Systematic review of the empirical evidence of study publication bias and outcome reporting bias. PLoS One 3(8): e3081.
29. Scherer RW, Langenberg P, von Elm E (2007) Full publication of results initially presented in abstracts. Cochrane Database Syst Rev 18(2): MR000005.
30. Chalmers I, Glasziou P (2009) Avoidable waste in the production and reporting of research evidence. Lancet 374(9683): 86–9.
31. Begg C, Cho M, Eastwood S, Horton R, Moher D, et al. (1996) Improving the quality of reporting of randomized controlled trials. The CONSORT statement. JAMA 276(8): 637–9.

3

Gender Differences in Traditional Chinese Medicine Use among Adults in Taiwan

Chun-Chuan Shih[1,2,3]☯, Chien-Chang Liao[4,5,6,7]☯, Yi-Chang Su[2], Chin-Chuan Tsai[1], Jaung-Geng Lin[2]*

1 The School of Chinese Medicine for Post-Baccalaureate, I-Shou University, Kaohsiung County, Taiwan, **2** Graduate Institute of Chinese Medicine, College of Chinese Medicine, China Medical University, Taichung, Taiwan, **3** Taipei Chinese Medical Association, Taipei, Taiwan, **4** Department of Anesthesiology, Taipei Medical University Hospital, Taipei, Taiwan, **5** School of Medicine, Taipei Medical University, Taipei, Taiwan, **6** Center for Health Research, Taipei Medical University Hospital, Taipei, Taiwan, **7** Management Office for Health Data, China Medical University Hospital, Taichung, Taiwan

Abstract

Objectives: The increasing use of complementary, alternative medicine (CAM) and traditional Chinese medicine (TCM) has attracted attention. We report on the gender difference in TCM use among the general population in Taiwan in a population-based, cross-sectional study.

Methods: We collected data on socio-demographic factors, lifestyle and health behavior from the 2001 Taiwan National Health Interview Survey. The medical records of interviewees aged 20–69 years were obtained from National Health Insurance claims data with informed consent. The prevalence of TCM use and the average frequency of TCM use were compared between women and men.

Results: Among 14,064 eligible participants, the one-year prevalence of TCM use for women and men was 31.8% and 22.4%, respectively. Compared with men, women had a higher average TCM use frequency (1.55 visits vs. 1.04 visits, $p<0.001$). This significant difference remained evident after excluding gender-specific diseases (1.43 visits vs. 1.03 visits, $p<0.001$). The average TCM use frequency was significantly higher in women than in men across all age groups. TCM use correlates differed for women and men. Marital status (odds ratio [OR] = 1.55, 95% confidence interval [CI] = 1.30–1.85), family income and unhealthy lifestyle (OR = 1.50, 95% CI = 1.30–1.74) were factors associated with TCM use in men but not in women.

Conclusions: In Taiwan, women used more TCM services than men and the gender differences in the TCM use profile persisted across age groups.

Editor: David W. Dowdy, Johns Hopkins Bloomberg School of Public Health, United States of America

Funding: This study was supported in part by a grant from Committee on Chinese Medicine and Pharmacy, Department of Health, Taiwan (grant number CCMP98-RD-038), China Medical University Hospital (grant number 1MS1), Taiwan Department of Health Clinical Trial and Research Center for Excellence (grant number DOH100-TD-B-111-004) and Taiwan Department of Health Cancer Research Center of Excellence (grant number DOH100-TD-C-111-005). The funders had no role in study design, data collection and analysis, decision to publish, or preparation of the manuscript.

Competing Interests: The authors have declared that no competing interests exist.

* E-mail: jglin@mail.cmu.edu.tw

☯ These authors contributed equally to this work.

Introduction

The increasing use of complementary and alternative medicine (CAM) in recent decades has been documented in many studies in both Asian and Western countries [1–5]. In the United Kingdom an estimated 46% for lifetime use of one or more CAM therapies has been reported in a population-based survey [3]. In Israel, the percentage of the Jewish population aged 45–75 years who consulted CAM providers during the previous year increased from 6% in 1993 to 10% in 2000 [4]. A high prevalence of CAM use has also been observed in Scandinavian countries [5]. This interesting phenomenon has attracted physicians' attention. Many physicians recognize that their patients are interested in CAM therapies and some physicians are interested in learning more about CAM [6,7].

The utilization of traditional Chinese medicine (TCM) is common in Taiwan, Asian countries and immigrant Asians in western countries [8–19]. It was estimated that the one-month, one-year, and six-year utilizations of TCM services in Taiwan were 10.4%, 28.4%, and 62.5%, respectively [12,20]. This pattern of medical pluralism has been investigated in Taiwan [11]. The growing use of TCM in western countries has also been reported [21–23]. Previous reports have focused on the prevalence of TCM use and associated factors. Women were found to have higher TCM use than men [12,20,24–27]. However, few studies investigated the nature of this gender difference in TCM utilization.

Using the National Health Interview Survey (NHIS) and data from the National Health Insurance (NHI) system, this study reports on factors associated with TCM use among adults aged 18 years and older in Taiwan and focuses particularly on the gender difference in TCM usage. The objective of this study is to clarify the gender difference in TCM utilization in Taiwan. This study also provides women's healthcare information on CAM for health professionals.

Materials and Methods

Ethics Statement

This study is based in part on data from the 2001 NHIS approved by the Bureau of Health Promotion, Department of Health and National Health Research Institutes. The Bureau of Health Promotion, Department of Health obtained written informed consent from eligible NHIS participants. The data were analyzed anonymously and all clinical investigations were conducted according to the principles expressed in the Declaration of Helsinki.

Study Design

The 2001 NHIS was a cross-sectional household survey with a representative sample of the non-institutionalized population. Interviewees were all residents of Taiwan, and interviewers completed the interviews in participants' homes. All interviewees were selected from the household census in Taiwan. In addition to personal and socio-demographic information, a face-to-face interview survey also collected information regarding individuals' personal health factors (e.g., disease history and lifestyle), environmental health factors (e.g., exposure to second-hand smoke and home safety), and medical service use (e.g., patterns of medical service use and insurance). Interviews for the population-based survey were completed for 22,121 individuals in 5,798 households at the end of 2001 [28]. About 87% (n = 19,143) of the interviewees gave informed consent for us to link their information with the NHI claims data to retrieve information on medical service use in 2001, including TCM visits. Among the 19,143 participants who agreed to the linking, 14,064 (73.5%) adults between 20 and 69 years old were included in our analysis. Adults in this age group were selected for two reasons: we assumed people in this age group usually made independent decisions about their health care-seeking behaviors and we observed that gender differences were not significant for people aged 70 or older.

Both NHIS data and NHI claims data from 2001 were used in this study. With the written informed consent of eligible NHIS participants that allowed the linking of their NHI data, the 2001 NHIS data were linked to the 2001 NHI claims data. Information about prevalence and frequency of TCM use was drawn from the 2001 NHI claims data. The data were limited to visits to ambulatory TCM medical facilities contracted with the Bureau of National Health Insurance in Taiwan, including 2 public TCM hospitals, 42 private TCM hospitals and 2,544 private TCM clinics in 2001 [29]. Socio-demographic data (including age, gender, education, occupation, family income, ethnicity, religion, and marital status), use of folk therapy (FT), regular health checkups and unhealthy lifestyle (including smoking, alcohol use, and betel nut chewing) were derived from the NHIS data. The FT utilization question in the questionnaire is as follows: In the past one month, have you undergone any therapy such as Gua Sha (skin scraping), Tuina (massage and kneading), Baguan (vacuum bottle therapy), bone setting, spine alignment, Qigong, divination, written charms, sharman, talisman, incense ash or other FT to ease physical discomfort in some non-medical places? (Legal traditional Chinese medicine and western medicine excluded).

Table 1. Characteristics of study participants among men and women.

		Use of TCM			
		Female, n (%)		Male, n (%)	
Age, years	20–29	1798	(33.4)	1751	(21.9)
	30–39	1742	(32.8)	1736	(23.8)
	40–49	1720	(32.2)	1650	(23.2)
	50–59	1093	(32.0)	1012	(20.8)
	60–69	820	(25.4)	742	(20.4)
Education, years	0	711	(24.5)	192	(14.6)
	1–9	2554	(31.8)	2409	(21.9)
	10–12	2166	(32.2)	2210	(22.5)
	≥13	1736	(34.4)	2076	(23.5)
Occupation	Unemployed	872	(30.2)	1703	(20.7)
	Homemaker	2355	(29.3)	12	(25.0)
	Skilled, Unskilled	3207	(33.8)	3790	(22.3)
	Profession	712	(34.0)	1353	(24.5)
Family income, NTDs	<30,000	1304	(29.2)	1162	(18.7)
	30,000–49,999	1584	(31.8)	1578	(23.6)
	50,000–99,999	2943	(33.0)	2831	(24.1)
	≥100,000	1266	(31.9)	1263	(20.7)
Religion	No religion	1904	(29.3)	1857	(21.3)
	Traditional religions	3346	(32.7)	3393	(22.4)
	Buddhist	1493	(35.2)	1259	(24.5)
	Others[a]	417	(24.5)	366	(19.7)
Marital status	Married	4933	(31.1)	4570	(23.9)
	Other status	2240	(33.5)	2321	(19.3)
Indigenous		208	(19.2)	189	(18.5)
Use of folk therapy		518	(44.4)	307	(36.5)
Have regular health checkup		1089	(34.6)	1114	(24.8)
Number of unhealthy lifestyles	None	6084	(32.0)	1905	(25.8)
	One	829	(32.6)	1831	(23.0)
	Two or three	256	(25.4)	3153	(19.9)
Urbanization	Low	2442	(28.4)	2469	(19.2)
	Moderate	3232	(32.1)	3036	(22.8)
	High	1499	(37.0)	1386	(27.1)
Density of TCM physicians	Low	2222	(31.8)	2274	(20.3)
	Moderate	1468	(32.6)	1365	(24.4)
	High	3483	(31.6)	3252	(22.9)

TCM, traditional Chinese medicine; NTDs, New Taiwan Dollars.
[a]Others: Including Protestantism, Catholicism or Islam.

Definitions and Measures

TCM. TCM includes herbal medicines, acupuncture, moxibustion, bone reduction, traditional trauma treatment, traditional dislocation treatment, traditional fracture treatment, Tuina, Baguan, and other therapies. TCM practitioners are registered TCM physicians and practice in a hospital or clinic. TCM in Taiwan is legal, and TCM physicians can advertise the medical benefits of TCM according to medical laws in Taiwan [12].

Folk therapy (FT). FT use is defined as utilization of FT within the past month. The types of FT studied include Gua Sha (skin scraping), Tuina (massage and kneading), Baguan (vacuum bottle therapy), bone setting, spine alignment, Qigong, divination,

Table 2. The average frequency of TCM visits per year for women and men by age groups.

	Average frequency of TCM visits per year					
	All diseases			Diseases excluding gender-specific diseases		
Age group	Women	Men		Women	Men	
All ages	1.55	1.04	p<0.001	1.43	1.03	p<0.001
20–29	1.46	0.84	p<0.001	1.27	0.83	p<0.001
30–39	1.63	0.99	p<0.001	1.44	0.98	p<0.001
40–49	1.60	1.05	p<0.001	1.50	1.05	p<0.001
50–59	1.71	1.31	p<0.001	1.66	1.30	p<0.001
60–69	1.31	1.23	p<0.05	1.30	1.20	p<0.05

TCM, traditional Chinese medicine. All p-values were estimated using Wilcoxon rank sum tests.

written charms, shaman consultation, talismans, incense ash, and other related therapies. The difference between TCM and FT lies in their legality. Legislation from the Department of Health in Taiwan has declared that FT practitioners cannot claim any medical benefits from FT. FT practitioners do not have certifications or legal licenses and they do not work in clinical settings in Taiwan [12].

Urbanization. There are 359 townships and city districts in Taiwan. We calculated the population density (persons/km^2) by dividing the population (persons) by the area (km^2) for each of these administrative units according to the statistics from Minister of Interior, Taiwan. The first, second, and third tertiles were considered areas of low, moderate and high urbanization, respectively [12,30].

Density of TCM physicians. We calculated the density of TCM physicians (TCM physicians/10,000 persons) by using the number of TCM physicians per 10,000 persons for each of the administrative units. The first, second, and third tertiles were considered areas of low, moderate, and high TCM physician density, respectively [12].

Unhealthy lifestyle. A high prevalence of cigarette smoking, alcohol drinking, and betel quid chewing has been found in Taiwan [31]. People with the habit of smoking tobacco (included some times of smoking in lifetime; or less than 5 package in lifetime; or more than 5 package in lifetime), drinking alcohol (current drinkers included any types of alcohol drinks) and/or chewing areca were considered to have unhealthy lifestyles that are associated with cancer and other diseases [11,12].

Statistical Analysis

The proportion of TCM use was compared between women and men using Chi-square tests. We used Wilcoxon rank sum tests to analyze the difference in average use frequency between men and women. A multivariate logistic regression analysis was performed to analyze the factors associated with TCM services use for women and men. These covariates included age, education, family income, occupation, urbanization, religion, ethnicity, marital status, use of folk therapy, regular checkups, unhealthy lifestyle and density of TCM physicians. To precisely clarify the gender difference in TCM visits, gender-specific diseases (Table S1 and Table S2) were excluded from the comparisons of the number of visits and treatments sought between men and women. All analyses were performed using Statistical Analysis Software (SAS), version 9.1 (by SAS Institute Inc., Cary, North Carolina, U.S.A.). A two-sided probability value of <0.05 was considered significant.

Results

Table 1 shows the characteristics of study participants by gender. The prevalence of TCM use among women and men was 31.8% and 22.4%, respectively (p<0.05). Compared with men, women had a higher average frequency of TCM use (1.55 visits per years vs. 1.04 visits per year, p<0.001). This significant difference was present across all age groups and remained evident after excluding the gender-specific diseases (1.43 visits per year vs. 1.03 visits per year, p<0.001) (Table 2). The frequency of TCM use among women and men increased with age in most of the age groups and decreased sharply in the 60–69-year-old group. This ascending trend was even more noticeable after excluding gender-specific diseases. The peak number of TCM visits was in the 50–59-year-old group for both genders, and the lowest number of TCM visits was observed in the 20–29-year-old group, followed by the 60–69-year-old group after excluding gender-specific diseases.

In the multivariate analysis, the following groups were more likely to have visited licensed TCM clinics and practitioners: women aged 30–39 or 50–59 years old who were non-indigenous, were Buddhists, had used FT in the month prior to the interview, lived in areas where the density of TCM practitioners was moderate or high, or lived in areas with low or moderate levels of urbanization. Years of education, occupation, family income, regular health checkups and unhealthy lifestyle were not significantly associated with TCM use. In men, age, family income, marital status, FT use, regular health checkups, and unhealthy lifestyle were associated with TCM use. Men with the following characteristics were more likely to see TCM practitioners: 20–29 years old, average family income less than 100,000 NTDs per month, married, FT users, use of regular health checkups and one or no indicators of unhealthy lifestyle. In addition, a higher density of TCM practitioners and a moderate level of urbanization were also associated with the likelihood of TCM use for men (Table 3).

In the Table 4, females (OR = 1.50, 95% CI = 1.34–1.67), younger people (OR = 1.22, 95% CI = 1.01–1.48), use of FT (OR = 1.78, 95% CI = 1.53–2.08) and having no unhealthy lifestyle (OR = 1.37, 95% CI = 1.21–1.56) were factors associated with TCM use among adults in Taiwan. People living in areas with high density TCM physicians (OR = 1.66, 95% CI = 1.46–1.88) or low-urbanized area (OR = 1.30, 95% CI = 1.16–1.46) were more like to use TCM than the comparison group.

Table 3. Factors associated with TCM use among women and men in multiple logistic models.

Factors		Use of TCM			
		Women, OR (95% CI)		Men, OR (95% CI)	
Age, years	20–29	1.28	(0.97–1.67)	1.37	(1.02–1.83)
	30–39	1.30	(1.00–1.68)	1.25	(0.96–1.63)
	40–49	1.23	(0.96–1.58)	1.07	(0.83–1.39)
	50–59	1.33	(1.04–1.70)	0.91	(0.70–1.19)
	60–69	1.00	(Reference)	1.00	(Reference)
Education, years	0	1.00	(Reference)	1.00	(Reference)
	1–9	1.20	(0.93–1.56)	1.63	(0.94–2.86)
	10–12	1.18	(0.89–1.57)	1.47	(0.83–2.61)
	≥13	1.28	(0.94–1.73)	1.43	(0.80–2.56)
Occupation	Unemployed	1.00	(Reference)	1.00	(Reference)
	Homemaker	0.93	(0.76–1.14)	1.00	(0.21–4.85)
	Skilled, Unskilled	1.09	(0.90–1.31)	0.94	(0.80–1.11)
	Profession	1.01	(0.79–1.28)	1.01	(0.82–1.24)
Family income, NTDs	<30,000	1.00	(0.83–1.21)	1.04	(0.83–1.30)
	30,000–49,999	1.07	(0.90–1.27)	1.29	(1.06–1.56)
	50,000–99,999	1.07	(0.93–1.25)	1.26	(1.06–1.49)
	≥100,000	1.00	(Reference)	1.00	(Reference)
Religion	No religion	1.08	(0.82–1.44)	1.11	(0.78–1.58)
	Traditional religions	1.28	(0.97–1.69)	1.18	(0.84–1.67)
	Buddhist	1.40	(1.05–1.87)	1.33	(0.93–1.90)
	Others	1.00	(Reference)	1.00	(Reference)
Marital Status	Married	0.90	(0.78–1.03)	1.55	(1.30–1.85)
Ethnicity	Non-indigenous	1.65	(1.06–2.57)	0.80	(0.49–1.30)
Use of folk therapy	Yes	1.65	(1.36–2.00)	2.00	(1.56–2.55)
Have regular health checkup	Yes	1.15	(0.99–1.33)	1.18	(1.01–1.39)
Have unhealthy lifestyle	No	1.17	(0.85–1.61)	1.50	(1.30–1.74)
	One	1.20	(0.85–1.69)	1.25	(1.08–1.45)
	Two or three	1.00	(Reference)	1.00	(Reference)
Density of TCM physicians[a]	Low	1.00	(Reference)	1.00	(Reference)
	Moderate	1.27	(1.10–1.48)	1.33	(1.13–1.57)
	High	1.64	(1.38–1.95)	1.69	(1.40–2.04)
Urbanization	Low	1.45	(1.24–1.69)	1.19	(1.01–1.41)
	Moderate	1.20	(1.03–1.41)	1.31	(1.10–1.55)
	High	1.00	(Reference)	1.00	(Reference)

[a]TCM physicians per 10000 residents.
CI, confidence; OR, odds ratio; TCM, traditional Chinese medicine.

Table 5 presents the distribution of disease categories for which TCM was sought for both women and men. The top five diseases associated with TCM use by women were diseases of the respiratory system (19.1%); diseases of the musculoskeletal system and connective tissue (18.1%); injury and poisoning (16.5%); symptoms, signs and ill-defined conditions (15.0%); and diseases of the genitourinary system (11.7%). The men's disease profile differed slightly from the women's, with diseases of the musculoskeletal system and connective tissue (19.4%) being most prevalent, followed by diseases of the respiratory system (18.9%); injury and poisoning (18.9%); symptoms, signs and ill-defined conditions (13.2%); and diseases of the digestive system (12.4%). Compared with women, men were less likely to go to TCM physicians for genitourinary problems (2.7% vs. 11.7%); the disparity was still apparent after excluding gender-specific diseases (1.6% vs. 4.7%).

Discussion

Using data from this population based nationwide survey we found that women had higher TCM use than men. The factors associated with TCM use were different between women and men. In addition, we investigated the gender difference in TCM use even after excluding gender-specific diseases. One of the strengths of this study is its use of combined NHIS and NHI data, which provided reliable information on medical care usage to minimize recall bias. To the best of our knowledge, this study is the first to

Table 4. Factors associated with TCM use in multivariate logistic regressions.[a]

Factors	Use of TCM	
	OR	(95%CI)
Gender, female vs. male	1.50	(1.34–1.67)
Age, years		
20–29 vs. 60–69	1.22	(1.01–1.48)
30–39 vs. 60–69	1.21	(1.01–1.46)
40–49 vs. 60–69	1.12	(0.94–1.33)
50–59 vs. 60–69	1.10	(0.92–1.32)
Education, years		
1–9 vs. 0	1.26	(1.00–1.58)
10–12 vs. 0	1.19	(0.93–1.51)
≥13 vs. 0	1.24	(0.97–1.60)
Family income, NTDs		
<30,000 vs. ≥100,000	1.00	(0.83–1.21)
30,000–49,999 vs. ≥100,000	1.11	(0.99–1.19)
50,000–99,999 vs. ≥100,000	1.16	(1.02–1.31)
Ethnicity		
Non-indigenous vs. indigenous	1.16	(0.84–1.59)
Religion		
No religion vs. Others	1.08	(0.87–1.34)
Traditional religions vs. Others	1.22	(0.99–1.51)
Buddhist vs. Others	1.36	(1.09–1.69)
Marital Status		
Married vs. others	1.12	(1.01–1.24)
Use of folk therapy		
Yes vs. no	1.78	(1.53–2.08)
Have regular health checkup		
Yes vs. no	1.16	(1.05–1.30)
Have unhealthy lifestyle		
No vs. two or three	1.37	(1.21–1.56)
One vs. two or three	1.27	(1.12–1.45)
Density of TCM physicians[b]		
Moderate vs. low	1.29	(1.16–1.44)
High vs. low	1.66	(1.46–1.88)
Urbanization		
Low vs. high	1.30	(1.16–1.46)
Moderate vs. high	1.25	(1.12–1.40)

CI, confidence; OR, odds ratio; TCM, traditional Chinese medicine.
[a]Additional adjusted for occupation which is not significant in the model.
[b]TCM physicians per 10000 residents.

exclude gender-specific diseases in a comparison of TCM use between women and men.

There is reasonably consistent evidence that women are somewhat more likely than men to use TCM [32]. MacPherson et al. analyzed 9,408 acupuncture patients in the United Kingdom (UK) and found that 74% were female [23]. Among schizophrenic patients in Hong Kong, females were more likely to use TCM compared with males (OR = 1.32, 95% CI = 1.09–1.62) [13]. Among Korean American elderly, a higher proportion of women visited TCM centres than men in the past 6 months (21.0% vs. 9.3%, $p<0.001$) [14]. A higher proportion (80%) of TCM was investigated in Singaporean children but the sex difference in TCM use was not reported [17]. In Hong Kong, TCM is used by more women than men (OR = 1.58, 95% CI = 1.28–1.97) [18]. Using the NHI database, Chen et al. found that women had higher TCM use than men [29]. However, the results of that study were not adequately adjusted for socio-demographic factors. Chang et al. did not exclude gender-specific diseases and reported that the odds of using TCM were higher in females than in males [20]. Another population-based survey failed to investigate the gender difference in TCM use [24]. A study documented that women had higher self-reported TCM use than men, but these results may have been limited due to recall bias in medical usage [12]. Among patients with inflammatory bowel disease, women were more likely to use TCM than men [33]. The findings from our study were similar to previous reports that documented the gender difference in the TCM utilization [12–14,18,20,23,29,34]. Compared with men, women were more likely to use TCM in this study (OR = 1.5). To avoid both recall bias in medical usage and inadequate adjustment for confounding factors, we linked data from the NHIS with the NHI claims database and we found that women had higher TCM use than men even after excluding gender-specific diseases. Unlike previous reports, this study investigated age-specific gender difference in TCM use.

Many studies investigated the higher rate of TCM use in women. [12–14,18,20,23,29,34] However, limited information was available on differences in the average TCM use frequency between men and women. Chen et al. reported the frequency of TCM use in Taiwan. However, their study did not compare the average TCM use frequency between women and men [29]. In a population-based survey, the average TCM use frequency was 2.26±2.29 visits among people who had used TCM in Taiwan [12]. Our study is the first to report that women had higher TCM use frequency than men in Taiwan; the average number of TCM visits for women and men were 1.55 and 1.04, respectively. We also investigated the gender difference in TCM use frequency across every age stratum.

Our results showed disproportionate TCM use among women for the genitourinary system disease category (11.7% for women vs. 2.7% for men). Even after excluding gender-specific diseases in the analysis, TCM use in this disease category was still higher in women than in men. The female predominance in TCM use observed both in various studies and in medical settings has been attributed to women's preference for using TCM therapies for their gynecological problems, including infertility, premenstrual syndrome or postmenstrual discomfort. The considerable reduction in the percentage of TCM use among women attributable to genitourinary system-related illnesses after excluding gender-specific diseases suggests that illnesses specific to women's health accounted for a significant portion of TCM use by women. In terms of health care consumption, women are strong supporters and consumers of TCM services.

In keeping with other reports, [11,12,24,25,29] we found that younger adults were more likely to use TCM than the elderly. Ethnicity and cultural factors, such as religion and FT use, were identified as factors associated with TCM use, thus suggesting a distinct user profile for women in Chinese society compared with women in western societies. Culture related variables are also important in determining TCM use among the older Chinese immigrants in Canada [16]. In fact, with the exception of highly religious measures (e.g., subduing demons, drawing divinatory lots for medicine or taking incense ash), procedures such as skin scraping, vacuum bottle therapy, bone setting, herbal plasters, massage and osteopathic spinal manipulation were all common

Table 5. The distribution of disease categories for which TCM was sought among women and men.

Disease	Proportion (%)			
	All diseases		Excluding gender-specific diseases	
	Women	Men	Women	Men
Diseases of the respiratory system	19.1	18.9	20.6	19.2
Diseases of the musculoskeletal system and connective tissue	18.1	19.4	19.7	19.6
Injury and poisoning	16.5	18.9	17.9	19.1
Specific symptoms, signs and ill-defined conditions	15.0	13.2	16.3	13.3
Diseases of the genitourinary system	11.7	2.7	4.7	1.6
Diseases of the digestive system	10.2	12.4	11.0	12.6
Diseases of the skin and subcutaneous tissue	3.2	3.2	3.4	3.2
Endocrine, nutritional and metabolic diseases and immune disorders	1.5	2.6	1.6	2.6
Diseases of the circulatory system	1.4	3.3	1.5	3.4
Diseases of the nervous system	1.4	2.0	1.5	2.0
Diseases of the sense organs	0.9	1.4	0.9	1.4
Mental disorders	0.4	0.8	0.5	0.8
Infectious and parasitic diseases	0.4	0.8	0.4	0.8
Malignant neoplasia	0.2	0.3	0.1	0.3
Complications of pregnancy, childbirth and the puerperium	0.1	0.0	-	-
Congenital anomalies	0.1	0.0	0.1	0.0
Other neoplasia	0.0	0.2	0.0	0.2

TCM, traditional Chinese medicine.

treatments applied by TCM practitioners in medical settings. There might be some cultural purposes rather than medical incentives behind these healthcare seeking behaviors that are worthy of further investigation. The higher odds of TCM use in areas with a higher density of TCM practitioners for women seem to support the argument that more resources will engender more medical services consumption. Women living in highly urbanized areas had higher TCM use in this study. In general, urbanization is positively correlated with the density of medical services. People living in highly urbanized areas have more opportunities to access various conventional or unconventional therapies [11,12,20].

There are several possible reasons why women had higher TCM use than men. First, women have better knowledge, attitudes and practices for self-care than men. Women are higher users of health care services in general, including CAM and acupuncture, and they are often the primary agents in family health care utilization decisions [21]. It has also been reported that women have more help-seeking behaviors than men [35]. Compared with men, women are more likely to use any form of health care. This tendency might be amplified when considering TCM use [36]. Second, we suggested that women had more opportunities to use TCM for maintaining regular menstruation, [37] promoting health during pregnancy [38-41], and treating post-menopausal syndrome in climacteric age [42]. Third, women may use acupuncture treatment to reduce body weight, waist circumference and body mass index to improve their body image [34,43]. Furthermore, the opportunity cost of accessing medical care is often lower in women than in men. The proportion of women who are homemakers or without a job is higher than in men. As a result, women have more opportunities to use medical care services.

There are some limitations to this study. First, the cross-sectional study design could not provide information about whether TCM use is increasing or decreasing over time or whether the characteristics of TCM users are changing. Second, recall bias in socio-demographic factors and health behaviors may potentially jeopardize the validity of epidemiologic results. Although some researchers have found differences with regard to characteristics between people who gave consent and those who did not [44], we believe this phenomenon did not bias our results significantly because we found that age and gender distributions were comparable between those who consented and those who refused (not shown in the tables). Another limitation is that NHI system coverage more than 95% TCM services are available all over Taiwan. This means that this study may underestimate the utilization of TCM. In addition, the influence of common practices of CAM in the western countries such as heomeopathy, chiropractic or engery therapy on the TCM utilization in Taiwanese people needed to be further evaluated.

In conclusion, we found that women in Taiwan had higher TCM service use than men and the gender difference in the TCM profile use persisted. This study may provide some clinical implications for CAM that are important to health professionals worldwide. More comprehensive data is needed to clarify the causes of the gender difference in TCM use.

Supporting Information

Table S1 Male-specific diseases according to International Classification of Diseases, Clinical Modification in the Ninth Edition (ICD-9-CM).
(DOC)

Table S2 Female-specific diseases according to International Classification of Diseases, Clinical Modification in the Ninth Edition (ICD-9-CM).
(DOC)

Acknowledgments

This study is based (in part) on data from the National Health Interview Survey Original Database provided by the Bureau of Health Promotion, Department of Health, Executive Yuan and National Health Research Institutes. The interpretation and conclusions contained herein do not represent those of Bureau of Health Promotion, Department of Health, Executive Yuan and National Health Research Institutes.

Author Contributions

Conceived and designed the experiments: CCS CCL YCS CCT JGL. Performed the experiments: CCS CCL YCS CCT JGL. Analyzed the data: CCS CCL. Contributed reagents/materials/analysis tools: CCS CCL YCS CCT JGL. Wrote the paper: CCS CCL YCS CCT JGL. Final approval of the version to be published: CCS CCL YCS CCT JGL.

References

1. Eisenberg DM, Davis RB, Ettner SL, Appel S, Wilkey S, et al. (1998) Trends in alternative medicine use in the United States, 1990–1997: results of a follow-up national survey. JAMA 280: 1569–1575.
2. Tindle H, Davis R, Phillips R, Eisenberg D (2005) Trends in use of complementary and alternative medicine by US adults: 1997–2002. Altern Ther Health Med 11: 42–49.
3. Thomas K, Nicholl J, Coleman P (2001) Use and expenditure on complementary medicine in England: a population based survey. Complement Ther Med 9: 2–11.
4. Shmueli A, Shuval J (2004) Use of complementary and alternative medicine in Israel: 2000 vs. 1993. Isr Med Assoc J 6: 3–8.
5. Hanssen B, Grimsgaard S, Launsø L, Fønnebø V, Falkenberg T, et al. (2005) Use of complementary and alternative medicine in the Scandinavian countries. Scand J Prim Health Care 23: 57–62.
6. Davis MP, Darden PM (2003) Use of complementary and alternative medicine by children in the United States. Arch Pediatr Adolesc Med 157: 393–396.
7. Sikand A, Laken M (1998) Pediatricians' experience with and attitudes toward complementary/alternative medicine. Arch Pediatr Adolesc Med 152: 1059–1064.
8. Barnes PM, Bloom B, Nahin RL (2008) Complementary and Alternative Medicine Use Among Adults and Children: United States, 2007 National Center for Health Statistics.
9. Buettner C, Kroenke CH, Phillips RS, Davis RB, Eisenberg DM, et al. (2006) Correlates of use of different types of complementary and alternative medicine by breast cancer survivors in the nurses' health study. Breast Cancer Res Treat 100: 219–227.
10. Buono MD, Urciuoli O, Marietta P, Padoani W, Leo DD (2001) Alternative medicine in a sample of 655 community-dwelling elderly. J Psychosom Res 50: 147–154.
11. Shih CC, Su YC, Liao CC, Lin JG (2010) Patterns of medical pluralism among adults: results from the 2001 National Health Interview Survey in Taiwan. BMC Health Serv Res 10: 191.
12. Shih CC, Lin JG, Liao CC, Su YC (2009) The utilization of traditional Chinese medicine and associated factors in Taiwan in 2002. Chin Med J 122: 1544–1548.
13. Zhang ZJ, Tan QR, Tong Y, Wang XY, Wang HH, et al. (2011) An epidemiological study of concomitant use of Chinese medicine and antipsychotics in schizophrenic patients: implication for herb-drug interaction. PLoS One 6: e17239.
14. Kim M, Han HR, Kim KB, Duong DN (2002) The use of traditional and Western medicine among Korean American elderly. J Community Health 27: 109–120.
15. Chen JX, Hu LS (2006) Traditional chinese medicine for the treatment of chronic prostatitis in China: a systematic review and meta-analysis. J Altern Complement Med 12: 763–769.
16. Lai D, Chappell N (2007) Use of Traditional Chinese Medicine by older Chinese immigrants in Canada. Fam Pract 24: 56–64.
17. Loh CH (2009) Use of traditional Chinese medicine in Singapore children: perceptions of parents and paediatricians. Singapore Med J 50: 1162–1168.
18. Chung V, Wong E, Woo J, Lo SV, Griffiths S (2007) Use of traditional chinese medicine in the Hong Kong special administrative region of China. J Altern Complement Med 13: 361–367.
19. Wu AP, Burke A, LeBaron S (2007) Use of traditional medicine by immigrant Chinese patients. Fam Med 39: 195–200.
20. Chang LC, Huang N, Chou YJ, Lee CH, Kao FY, et al. (2008) Utilization patterns of Chinese medicine and Western medicine under the National Health Insurance Program in Taiwan, a population-based study from 1997 to 2003. BMC Health Serv Res 8: 170.
21. Upchurch DM, Burke A, Dye C, Chyu L, Kusunoki Y, et al. (2008) A sociobehavioral model of acupuncture use, patterns, and satisfaction among women in the United States, 2002. Women Health Issues 18: 62–71.
22. Burke A, Upchurch DM, Dye C, Chyu L (2006) Acupuncture use in the United States: findings from the National Health Interview Survey. J Altern Complement Med 12: 639–648.
23. MacPherson H, Sinclair-Lian N, Thomas K (2006) Patients seeking care from acupuncture practitioners in the UK: a national survey. Complement Ther Med 14: 20–30.
24. Shih SF, Lew-Ting CY, Chang HY, Kuo KN (2008) Insurance covered and non-covered complementary and alternative medicine utilisation among adults in Taiwan. Soc Sci Med 67: 1183–1189.
25. Daly M, Tai CJ, Deng CY, Chien LY (2009) Factors associated with utilization of traditional Chinese medicine by white collar foreign workers living in Taiwan. BMC Health Serv Res 9: 10.
26. Chung VCH, Lau CH, Yeoh EK, Griffiths SM (2009) Age, chronic non-communicable disease and choice of traditional Chinese and western medicine outpatient services in a Chinese population. BMC Health Serv Res 9: 207.
27. Pu CY, Lan VM, Lan CF, Lang HC (2008) The determinants of traditional Chinese medicine and acupuncture utilization for cancer patients with simultaneous conventional treatment. Eur J Cancer Care 17: 340–349.
28. Shih YT, Hung YT, Chang HY, Liu JP, Lin HS, et al. (2003) The design, contents, operation and the characteristics of the respondents of the 2001 National Health Interview Survey in Taiwan. Taiwan J Public Health 22: 419–430.
29. Chen FP, Chen TJ, Kung YY, Chen YC, Chou LF, et al. (2007) Use frequency of traditional Chinese medicine in Taiwan. BMC Health Serv Res 7: 11.
30. Liao CC, Li TC, Lin RS, Sung FC (2006) Urban and rural difference in prevalence and incidence of stroke in 2000 in Taiwan. Taiwan J Public Health 25: 223–230.
31. Liao CC, Wang HY, Lin RS, Hsieh CY, Sung FC (2005) Colorectal and prostate cancer screening practices among men in Taiwan. Taiwan J Public Health 24: 209–216.
32. Chi CH, Lee JL, Lai JS, Chen CY, Chang SK, et al. (1996) The practice of Chinese medicine in Taiwan. Soc Sci Med 43: 1329–1348.
33. Chen YC, Chen FP, Chen TJ, Chou LF, Hwang SJ (2008) Patterns of traditional Chinese medicine use in patients with inflammatory bowel disease: a population study in Taiwan. Hepatogastroenterology 55: 467–470.
34. Hsu CH, Wang CJ, Hwang KC, Lee TY, Chou P, et al. (2009) The effect of Auricular acupuncture in obese women: a randomized controlled trial. J Womens Health 18: 813–818.
35. Oliver MI, Pearson N, Coe N, Gunnell D (2005) Help-seeking behaviour in man and women with common mental health problem: cross-sectional study. Br J Psychiatr 186: 297–301.
36. Bishop FL, Lewith GT (2008) Who uses CAM? A narrative review of demographic characteristics and health: factors associated with CAM use. Evid Based Complement Alternat Med 7: 11–18.
37. Yeh LLL, Liu JY, Lin KS, Liu YS, Chiou JM, et al. (2007) A randomised placebo-controlled trial of a traditional Chinese herbal formula in the treatment of primary dysmenorrhoea. PLoS ONE 2007; 2: e719.
38. Chang PJ, Tseng YC, Chuang CH, Chen YC, Hsieh WS, et al. (2010) Use of Sheng-Hua-Tang and health-related quality of life in postpartum women: a population-based cohort study in Taiwan. Int J Nurs Stud 47: 13–19.
39. Chuang CH, Chang PJ, Hsieh WS, Tsai YJ, Lin SJ, et al. (2009) Chinese herbal medicine use in Taiwan during pregnancy and the postpartum period: a population-based cohort study. Int J Nurs Stud 46: 787–795.
40. Chuang CH, Hsieh WS, Guo YL, Tsai YJ, Chang PJ, et al. (2007) Chinese herbal medicines used in pregnancy: a population-based survey in Taiwan. Pharmacoepidemiol Drug Saf 16: 464–468.
41. Chuang CH, Doyle P, Wang JD, Chang PJ, Lai JN, et al. (2006) Herbal medicines used during the first trimester and major congenital malformations: an analysis of data from a pregnancy cohort study. Drug Saf 29: 537–548.
42. Yang YH, Chen PC, Wang JD, Lee CH, Lai JN (2009) Prescription pattern of traditional Chinese medicine for climacteric women in Taiwan. Climacteric 12: 541–547.
43. Hsu CH, Hwang KC, Chao CL, Chang HH, Chou P (2005) Electroacupuncture in obese women: a randomized, controlled pilot study. J Womens Health 14: 434–440.
44. Huang N, Shih SF, Chang HY, Chou YJ (2007) Record linkage research and informed consent: who consents? BMC Health Serv Res 7: 18.

4

Characterization of Rheumatoid Arthritis Subtypes Using Symptom Profiles, Clinical Chemistry and Metabolomics Measurements

Herman A. van Wietmarschen[1,2*], Weidong Dai[3], Anita J. van der Kooij[4], Theo H. Reijmers[1,5], Yan Schroën[2,6], Mei Wang[2,7], Zhiliang Xu[8], Xinchang Wang[9], Hongwei Kong[3], Guowang Xu[3*], Thomas Hankemeier[1,5], Jacqueline J. Meulman[4], Jan van der Greef[1,2,7,10]

1 Division of Analytical Biosciences, LACDR, Leiden University, Leiden, The Netherlands, **2** Sino-Dutch centre for Preventive and Personalized Medicine, Zeist, The Netherlands, **3** CAS Key Laboratory of Separation Science for Analytical Chemistry, Dalian Institute of Chemical Physics, Chinese Academy of Sciences, Dalian, China, **4** Mathematical Institute, Leiden University, Leiden, The Netherlands, **5** Netherlands Metabolomics Centre, Leiden University, Leiden, The Netherlands, **6** Oxrider, Education and Research, Nieuwegein, The Netherlands, **7** SU BioMedicine, Utrechtseweg, Zeist, The Netherlands, **8** College of Life Science Company Limited, Hangzhou, China, **9** Zhejiang Xinhua hospital Rheumatology and Immunology Department, HangZhou, China, **10** TNO Netherlands Organization for Applied Scientific Research, TNO Pharma, Zeist, The Netherlands

Abstract

Objective: The aim is to characterize subgroups or phenotypes of rheumatoid arthritis (RA) patients using a systems biology approach. The discovery of subtypes of rheumatoid arthritis patients is an essential research area for the improvement of response to therapy and the development of personalized medicine strategies.

Methods: In this study, 39 RA patients are phenotyped using clinical chemistry measurements, urine and plasma metabolomics analysis and symptom profiles. In addition, a Chinese medicine expert classified each RA patient as a Cold or Heat type according to Chinese medicine theory. Multivariate data analysis techniques are employed to detect and validate biochemical and symptom relationships with the classification.

Results: The questionnaire items 'Red joints', 'Swollen joints', 'Warm joints' suggest differences in the level of inflammation between the groups although c-reactive protein (CRP) and rheumatoid factor (RHF) levels were equal. Multivariate analysis of the urine metabolomics data revealed that the levels of 11 acylcarnitines were lower in the Cold RA than in the Heat RA patients, suggesting differences in muscle breakdown. Additionally, higher dehydroepiandrosterone sulfate (DHEAS) levels in Heat patients compared to Cold patients were found suggesting that the Cold RA group has a more suppressed hypothalamic-pituitary-adrenal (HPA) axis function.

Conclusion: Significant and relevant biochemical differences are found between Cold and Heat RA patients. Differences in immune function, HPA axis involvement and muscle breakdown point towards opportunities to tailor disease management strategies to each of the subgroups RA patient.

Editor: Amr H. Sawalha, University of Michigan, United States of America

Funding: This study has been supported by the International cooperation project (No. 2009DFA41250) from the State Ministry of Science & Technology of China and the key foundation (No. 20835006), the creative research group project (No. 21021004) from National Natural Science Foundation of China and the Osteo- and Rheumatoid Arthritis Foundation. The funders had no role in study design, data collection and analysis, decision to publish, or preparation of the manuscript.

Competing Interests: Dr. Mei Wang is employed by SUBiomedicine, Dr. Zhiliang Xu is employed by the College of Life Science Company Ltd. and Prof. Jan van der Greef is employed by TNO. This does not alter the authors' adherence to all the PLoS ONE policies on sharing data and materials.

* E-mail: h.vanwietmarschen@lacdr.leidenuniv.nl (HvW); xugw@dicp.ac.cn (GX)

These authors contributed equally to this work.

Introduction

Discovering subtypes of rheumatoid arthritis (RA) patients is considered a key research area for the improvement of response to therapy [1,2]. RA is a heterogeneous disease which is illustrated by the very good response of some patients to a biological therapy, but a complete lack of response in a large number of other patients [3]. Another striking observation is that in a large group of RA patients low disease activity or remission can be achieved using a single conventional disease-modifying anti-rheumatic drug (DMARD), which contrasts with the current viewpoint to offer aggressive therapy in an early stage of the disease to all patients [4]. Personalized medicine aims to provide the information that allows targeting the right treatment option to the right patient [5]. The first step in this approach is to find relevant subtypes of patients for which a different treatment strategy would clearly be beneficial.

Several subtypes of RA patients have been identified based on particular clinical and molecular features [6,7]. Markers such as disease duration and age have been identified that predict response to treatment [8,9]. Although some molecular markers have been found to predict functional and structural outcomes, these markers rarely find their way into clinical practice. One reason is the difficulty to translate markers found in trial populations to routinely measurable and cost-effective predictors for individuals [10]. This indicates that there is a need to develop new robust and reliable clinically applicable tools to identify subtypes of patients.

Discovery of novel relevant subtypes of RA patients could be improved by using prior knowledge. In this study a Chinese perspective on subtypes of RA patients is used to focus the analysis of the data. According to this perspective RA patients can be divided in two groups (Cold RA and Heat RA) which are treated very differently in Chinese medical practice [11,12].

Cold and Heat are general concepts used in Chinese medicine to distinguish between two types of reactions of the body to some disturbance [13]. A Cold reaction is characterized by pallor, intolerance of cold, absence of thirst, loose stools, clear profuse urine, a pale tongue and a slow pulse. A Heat reaction is characterized by flushed face, fever, thirst, irritability, restlessness, constipation, deep-colored urine, reddened tongue and a rapid pulse [14]. These two types of reactions are expressed in any type of disease to a certain extend. However, Cold and Heat are especially important for rheumatoid arthritis because this disease is perceived in classical Chinese medicine as the result of an invasion of three out of the four existing external pathogens: Wind, Cold, Heat and Damp [13].

Some work has been done to elucidate biological mechanisms related to Cold and Heat types of RA patients. In 2009 we measured 64 differently expressed genes in CD4 positive T-cells of RA patients. This set of genes was enriched for the immune system functions and especially for apoptosis regulation. In Heat RA patients apoptosis related genes were upregulated while in Cold patients apoptosis resitance genes were upregulated [11]. Additionally, a number of plasma metabolite concentrations was significantly different between Cold and Heat RA. Later, genes related to calcium signaling, cell adhesion, PPAR signaling and fatty acid metabolism were found in CD4 positive T-cells of Heat RA patients [15]. Toll-like receptor signaling related genes were found in the T-cells of Cold RA patients. In a similar study, Cold RA was related to Alanine, aspartate and tyosine metabolism and Heat RA to the MAPK pathway, Wnt signaling and insulin signaling, also found by measuring gene expression in CD4 positive T-cells [16]. A GC-MS analysis of Cold and Heat RA plasma revealed elevated plasma levels of glycochenodeoxycholate, proline, saturated and mono-unsaturated phosphatidylcholine (PC) but decreased levels of urea, free fatty acid (FFA) and polyunsaturated PC in Heat RA compared to Cold RA [17].

Recently it was shown that Cold RA patients respond much better to a combination therapy with diclofenac, methotrexate and sulfasalazine than Heat RA patients [18]. However, in clinical studies and clinical practice the features of Cold and Heat might be valued differently by each Chinese medicine practitioner. To improve acceptance of this classification in Western clinical practice it is important to standardize the classification. Further characterization of the physiological, constitutional and biological differences between the Cold and Heat subtypes of RA patients is valuable for increasing our understanding of the disease mechanism.

In this study a systems biology strategy is employed to study the differences between Cold and Heat types of RA patients, classified by a Chinese medicine expert. Data were collected on symptoms, clinical blood parameters and urine metabolites. Multivariate statistics were employed to discover the most discriminating features for the two groups. In particular, a categorical principal component analysis [19,20] was used for the questionnaire and clinical chemistry data and partial least squares discriminant analysis is used for the metabolomics data [21]. The questionnaire was used to determine symptom patterns related to Cold and Heat RA that could be used in clinical practice to determine these subtypes in an objective manner. The metabolomics and clinical results were related to biological processes and related to current understanding of the heterogeneity of rheumatoid arthritis.

Subjects and Methods

Subjects

Female subjects were recruited in the Zhejiang Xinhua Hospital in 2010. The institutional review board of the hospital gave written approval and judged that the study was conducted according to the ethical guidelines. A doctor explained the details of the study to the subjects and ensured written informed consent of each subject. All eligible subjects were diagnosed by a rheumatologist as rheumatoid arthritis patients according to the ACR criteria [22]. Inclusion criteria were a female gender due to the much higher prevalence of RA in women and age >18 years. Each patient was classified by the same Chinese medicine expert as either a Heat subtype or a Cold subtype. When the subtype was unclear the patient was not included in the study. General information such as age, disease duration, medication, etc. was collected using a standard form. Student's t-Test (two-tailed) was used to evaluate the differences between the two groups. Furthermore, a symptom questionnaire was completed by all the patients. Blood and urine samples were taken from each patient after fasting overnight for routine clinical measurements and metabolomics analysis.

Symptom Questionnaire

A short version of a recently developed systems diagnosis questionnaire was used in this study [23]. The 106 item questionnaire was shortened to 57 items by two Chinese medicine experts to target it more directly to Cold and Heat related symptoms. The final version of the questionnaire contained items related to five categories of symptoms: breathing, digestion, climate, quality of the symptoms and pain. The questionnaire was translated into Chinese. An English language version of the questionnaire is added as supplementary information (Text S1). The consistency of the data was checked and the data were recoded [23].

Clinical Measurements

Routine clinical chemistry measurements were conducted on fasting blood samples by the Zhejiang Xinhua Hospital. These measurements consisted of the complete blood count and the following serum measurements: uric acid (URIC), creatinine (CREA), blood urea nitrogen (BUN), triglycerides (TG), cholesterol (CHOL), total protein (TP), albumin (ALB), globulines (BIB), aspartate aminotransferase (AST), alanine aminotransferase (ALT), creatine kinase (CK), creatine kinase-MB (CKMB), lactate dehydrogenase (LDH), immunoglobulin A (IGA), Immunoglobulin G (IGG), immunoglobulin M (IGM), complement 3 (C3), complement 4 (C4), antistreptolysin O (ASO), rheumatoid factor (RHF), c-reactive protein (CRP), anti-cyclic citrullinated protein antibodies (CCP). The results of each clinical parameter were uniformly binned into 19 categories to increase the robustness [19].

Metabolomics Measurements

Urine samples were prepared for Ultra Fast LC/MS-IT-TOF (Shimadzu, Japan) analysis [24]. The technical variation of the analysis over time was monitored by a pooled quality control (QC) sample strategy [25]. The analysis was performed on a Ultra Fast LC/MS-IT-TOF with gradient elution using 0.1% formic acid in water as mobile phase A and 0.1% formic acid in acetonitrile as mobile phase B. For the LC a T3 column (ACQUITY UPLC HSS T3 1.8um, 2.1×100 mm, Waters) was used. Ion mode was switched between positive and negative mode between each scan [24].

Sample preparation for the plasma metabolomics analysis was conducted as follows: 200 µL plasma was mixed with 800 µL acetonitrile, then the mixture was centrifuged at 14000 rpm (Biofuge Stratos, Thermo Scientific, USA) for 10 min at 4°C. The supernatant was freeze-dried and redissolved with 200 µL of 20% acetonitrile.

Chromatographic separation was performed on a BEH C8 column (10 cm×2.1 mm, 1.7 µm, Waters, USA) using a Thermo Fisher Accela LC system. The gradient duration was 31 min at a flow rate of 300 µL/min with mobile phase (A) 0.1% formic acid solution and (B) acetonitrile. The injection volume was 6 µL. The samples were analyzed randomly and the same QC strategy was used as in the urine analysis.

An LC-MS method was used to measure the plasma metabolites. The LTQ-Orbitrap XL (Thermo-Fisher Scientific) settings were as follows: capillary temperature 325°C, source voltage 4.5 kV, capillary voltage 49 V for ESI+analysis; capillary temperature 325°C, source voltage −3.5 kV, capillary voltage −40 V for ESI- analysis. The mass range was set at 100–1000 m/z. The resolution of the Orbitrap was set at 30000.

The urine metabolomics measurements resulted in a list of features after preprocessing the data using Profiling Solution (Shimadzu, Japan) [24]. The plasma metabolomics data were processed by SIEVE software (V1.2, Thermo-Fisher Scientific) for peak picking and peak alignment. The parameter of MZ width was set at 0.01 Da and RT width was set at 0.6 min. Gradient peaks were removed. Features not present in at least 80% of the samples in one class were removed. Zeros were replaced by the smallest measured value divided by 2, the urine data were mean centered and the plasma data was autoscaled. Principal component analysis was then used to screen the data for outliers (objects with scores deviating from the scores of the bulk of the samples) [26], to determine the stability of the analysisover time (by comparing the scores of the QC samples) and monitor possible batch effects (by checking possible time trends in the scores of the objects).

Statistical Analysis

Questionnaire and clinical chemistry data. The focus of the data analysis is to identify questionnaire items and clinical parameters that distinguish between the subgroups of RA patients classified by the CM expert. A forced classification approach [27] using Nonlinear Principal Component Analysis (NLPCA) was chosen. NLPCA is a Principal Component Analysis method that is suitable for variables with mixed measurement level and variables that may have nonlinear relationships to each other [19]. The possibility to capture nonlinear relationships is important because the human body is a nonlinear system expressing complex behavior [28]. Such complex behavior has been observed in the immune system that plays a key role in rheumatoid arthritis. For instance cytokine dose response curves show an initial threshold and stable attractors have been found in cytokine systems [29]. More important is the ability of NLPCA to deal with the questionnaire data that are measured on an ordinal scale or as binary data. The questionnaire data analysis approach using NLPCA is described in detail in a previous paper [23].

NLPCA uses an 'optimal scaling' approach to find quantifications for categorical variables and optimal transformations for interval variables, which means that the percentage of variance of the transformed variables accounted for by the principal components is maximal [30]. The questionnaire items and clinical parameters were all included in a single NLPCA analysis allowing the interpretation of relationships between questionnaire items and clinical parameters.

The use of a the classification variable with a very large weight, here 1000 will cause the objects to cluster together into subclouds in the object space. The weight was chosen such that the objects of both classes were separated completely. As the classification variable is a binary variable, one principal component is sufficient to describe the class differences. In this study we used CATPCA in SPSS version 17.0 [31].

An important consideration in NLPCA is the analysis level chosen for the variables [20]. For the questionnaire variables the analysis level was kept the same as the measurement level (39 ordinal and 3 nominal). Subsequently the presence of nonlinear relationships between the clinical chemistry variables and the classification variable was examined by comparing numerical, spline ordinal and spline nominal transformations of the clinical chemistry variables (i.e., from most restricted to least restricted transformations). A substantial increase in the total variance accounted for (total VAF) due to an analysis level with more degrees of freedom then verifies that a less restrictive model is more appropriate.

After choosing the appropriate analysis level, variables with a proportion variance accounted for (VAF) >0.20 were selected for further analysis to increase the stability of the model and to focus on the most important variables. Leave two out cross validation was used to estimate the classification error of the model. In this approach two objects are reserved as a validation set while a NLPCA model is built using the other 37 objects. The class of the two left out objects is then predicted using the NLPCA model. This procedure is repeated until each of the objects is left out once and the class of each object is predicted. An overall classification error is subsequently calculated and a final model is built using all the available objects. Permutation testing was used to check whether this final model is different from a model based on a random classification.

Metabolomics data. A partial least squares discriminant analysis (PLS-DA) model was built for both the urine and plasma data set to find the most discriminating features between the Cold RA and Heat RA groups, a standard, well accepted technique used in the metabolomics field to discover characteristic differences between groups [32]. A separate model for the urine and plasma data was built to examine the performance of a metabolite profile measured in one compartment in a single analysis. Such a profile would be much easier to develop into a diagnostic tool that can be applied in a clinical setting than a combination of two metabolomics profiles.

A tenfold double cross-validation scheme was followed by permutation testing (250 times) [33]. The inner loop of the cross-validation scheme is used to estimate the optimal number of principal components. In this inner loop two objects are left out to validate the number of principal components. The outer loop is used to estimate the error rate of the model. Again, in the outer loop two objects are left out to independently estimate the error rate. Variables were selected using a jack-knifing procedure in which variables with a standard error in the regression vector above a threshold were removed from the dataset. This threshold is decreased stepwise until the error rate of the model starts to increase. The model with the lowest error rate is then chosen as the optimal model and a final model is then built for the corresponding set of variables and including all the objects. Subsequently, the significance of the resulting model is determined by permutation testing. The same double cross-validation procedure is used to build a model of the same data set but with a permuted classification. After 250 times permuting the classification, the classification error of the 250 models resulting models is compared with the classification error of the model based on the correct classification. The error rate of the correct classification model should be lower than 95% of the distribution of error rates resulting from the permuted classifications.

Identification of the most discriminating features indicated by the PLS-DA model was then attempted for both the urine and plasma model [34]. Evidence for the identity of features was accumulated by integrating information on the following: accurate mass of the ions and some fragments, retention time, HMDB database and in house human urine compound lists. The identification of some compounds was then verified by authentic standards. Finally, a biological interpretation was sought for the most discriminating features.

Results

Subjects

In total 50 patients were enrolled in the study. Eleven of these patients did not fulfill the inclusion criteria and were removed from the analysis. Seven of those eleven patients were male and therefore excluded, of two persons there was no RA diagnosis available, one patient was in the hospital for other reasons and therefore excluded and finally one person was excluded from this analysis because the symptom questionnaire was not completed. Finally, 20 RA patients of the Cold subtype and 19 of the Heat subtype were retained in the study.

Table 1 shows the patient characteristics per group expressed as the means of the age, disease duration, height and weight. None of these characteristics were significantly different (p-value <0.05) between the Cold RA and Heat RA patient groups. 34 patients received western medication such as methotrexate, sulfasalazine, other DMARD's and NSAID's. 36 patients received Chinese herbal medicine.

Clinical and Symptom Differences between RA Subtypes

After merging scoring categories containing less than 7 observations, 15 variables were left with only a single category. There is no variation between the objects for these variables which were therefore removed from the analysis: 'Sudden shortness of breath', 'Amount of phlegm', 'Sticky phlegm', 'Colored phlegm', 'Tender lower abdomen', 'Aggravated with pressure', 'Smelly diarrhea', 'Chills S', 'Chills F', 'Fever with Chills', 'Pain aggravates at night', 'Stabbing pain', 'Sharp pain', 'Deep pain', 'Heavy pain'. After recoding, the data set used for further analysis contained 42 variables.

In the forced classification model the use of a 2nd degree (quadratic) nonmonotonic spline (nominal analysis level) with 2 interior knots for the clinical measurements shows substantially larger variance accounted for (11.8%) than a monotonic spline (ordinal analysis level) (8.2%), indicating a nonmonotonic relationship between the measurements. Also, a two interior knot spline shows a larger variance (11.8%) than a one interior knot spline (9.8%) (more knots allow for more freedom in the transformation). Therefore a 2nd degree spline nominal analysis level with two interior knots was chosen for the clinical chemistry variables. A new model was then built using this analysis level and used to select variables with a proportion of VAF >0.20. A model was subsequently built including the 18 selected variables. The model using splines with 2 interior knots for the clinical chemistry variables was then compared once more with a model using one interior knot. The results showed that the increase in total VAF in the model with 2 interior knots was mostly due to the variable MCHC. Therefore the final analysis level of the clinical variables was adjusted to a 2nd degree spline with 1 interior knot, except for MCHC which was set to 2 interior knots. The final model had a total VAF of approximately 21% (see Table 2 for the loadings of the 18 variables). The transformation plots of the clinical chemistry variables of this model are included as supplementary information (Figure S1). Leave two out cross validation resulted in a classification error of 15%, which is substantially lower than the expected error rate based on random classification (which is 50%).

RA patients that are classified as Heat by the Chinese medicine expert are characterized with higher optimal quantifications on average on the symptoms 'red joints', 'swollen joints', 'warm feeling', 'warm joints', 'dull pain' and 'pain that worsens with

Table 1. Patient characteristics.

	Cold (n = 20)	Heat (n = 19)	p
Age (years)	51±13 (24–74)	54±11 (34–77)	0.44
Disease duration (months)	90±90 (4–240)	100±100 (24–348)	0.44
Height (cm)	159±4 (150–167)	160±4 (155–170)	0.50
Weight (kg)	58±18 (40–120)	58±9 (37–75)	0.97

*Range is given in parenthesis.

Table 2. Discriminating symptoms and clinical measurements.

Variable name	Loading
b17 MCHC	0.580
v40 Red joints	0.544
v39 Swollen joints	0.540
b37 IGG	0.504
v25 Warm feeling	0.495
b8 LY#	0.490
v41 Warm joints	0.490
v56 Dull pain	0.438
v50 Pain worsens by warmth and movement	0.399
b27 CHOL	0.370
b38 IGM	0.359
b19 PLT	0.285
b25 BUN	−0.374
b32 ALT	−0.419
v19 Cold feeling	−0.457
v29 Aversion to cold	−0.472
b18 RDW	−0.475
b44 CCP	−0.495

warmth and movement', and with higher levels of the optimally scaled clinical parameters mean corpuscular hemoglobin concentration (MCHC), IgG, lymphocyte number (LY#), IgM, platelet count (PLT) and cholesterol. Cold RA patients are best characterized with higher optimal quantifications on average on the symptoms 'cold feeling' and 'aversion to cold', and higher levels of the optimally scaled clinical variables blood urea nitrogen (BUN), alanine aminotransferase (ALT), red blood cell distribution width (RDW) and anti-cyclic citrullinated protein antibodies (CCP).

Both groups of patients have a similar average score on the symptoms 'pain' and 'stiff joints' as well as on the clinical parameters rheumatoid factor and c-reactive protein.

Urine and Plasma Metabolite Differences between RA Subtypes

Urine samples of 14 of the 19 Heat RA and 14 of the 20 Cold RA patients included in the analysis described above were collected successfully for the LC-MS analysis. In total 11 urine samples were either not collected at the hospital or the samples were not send to the laboratory for metabolomics analysis. PLS-DA analysis resulted in a final model containing 793 features. A classification error of 14% was obtained by a double cross-validation procedure. Permutation testing indicated that the error rate of this model is significantly ($p<0.05$) different from the distribution of models based on permuted classifications.

The tentative identification of the top 50 most discriminating metabolites resulted in three metabolites that were verified by comparing authentic standards with the samples: acetylcarnitine, riboflavin and pantothenic acid. Thirteen of the top features measured in positive ion mode as well as the acetylcarnitine standard showed the same neutral loss of mass 59.0747 by fragmentation, which is highly indicative of acylcarnitine compounds [35,36]. The retention times of the features showing this loss was increasing with the mass, indicating higher mass features were less polar. This agrees with the fact that larger mass acylcarnitines have longer fatty acid chains and are therefore less polar. Furthermore, several glucuronides and soy isoflavones are suspected, but the identity was not further determined (Table 3).

Table 3. Top discriminating urine metabolites.

Importance	Compound	2Log Cold/ Heat[c]
1	C8:1 acylcarnitine[b]	−0.73
3	C10:3 acylcarnitine[b]	−0.70
11	C8+OH acylcarnitine[b]	−0.89
13	acetylcarnitine[a]	−0.75
15	riboflavin[a]	−2.40
16	C11:1 acylcarnitine[b]	−0.98
21	pantothenic acid[a]	−0.92
27	C6:DC acylcarnitine[b]	−0.55
31	C5 acylcarnitine[b]	−1.21
32	C10:2 acylcarnitine[b]	−0.53
38	C8:2 acylcarnitine[b]	−1.19
41	C10:1 acylcarnitine[b]	−0.23
45	C9:3 acylcarnitine[b]	−2.26
49	C10:3 acylcarnitine isotope[b]	−0.66
50	C6:2:DC acylcarnitine[b]	0.42

[a]verified with authentic standard.
[b]verified with characteristic 59 neutral loss, retention time order, accurate mass.
[c]Calculated 2Log of the ratio between average levels in Cold and Heat patients.

An LC-MS analysis of the plasma samples of 11 Cold RA and 14 Heat RA patients from the same set of patients that are used in the urine metabolomics and questionnaire analysis was performed. Three plasma samples were not available for analysis. Positive ion mode features were not included in the multivariate analysis because the QC samples were not stable. The PLS-DA analysis resulted in a model containing 214 features (classification error of 28%). Permutation testing indicated that the error rate of this model is significantly ($p<0.05$) different from the distribution of models based on permuted classifications. Some of the top 50 features resulting from the PLS-DA model could be identified with authentic standards (Table 4).

Discussion

The subtypes of RA patients are characterized by four sets of features: clinical symptoms (questionnaire items), clinical chemistry measurements in blood, metabolite measurements in urine and in plasma. One hypothesis is that the Cold RA and Heat RA groups have a different inflammatory status. Of the most discriminating symptoms in the analysis, 'warm joints', 'swollen joints' and 'red joints' indicate a difference in inflammatory status. However, c-reactive protein (CRP), an important inflammation marker, was not retained in the final model because of a low proportion of total variance accounted for, based on the two groups. Rheumafactor (RF), an important marker for RA disease activity [37], was not retained in the model either. On the other hand, the lymphocyte numbers are higher in Heat RA patients, although this level is not considered elevated and indicative of inflammation in standard evaluation [38]. A comparable average disease duration of 90 and 100 months for the two groups suggests that not one of the groups can be considered an early arthritis or early aggressive arthritis group. These observations indicate that the severity of inflammation might be different between the groups when the joint symptoms are considered despite similar levels of rheumatoid factor and c-reactive protein.

Swollen joint counts are routinely used to establish disease activity in rheumatoid arthritis [39]. In Table 5 the percentages of Cold and Heat patients with a positive score on zero to three of the symptoms 'warm joints', 'swollen joints' or 'red joints' are given. Even though high scores on the three symptoms are indicative for the Heat group of RA patients, 40% of the Cold patients also have a positive score on at least one of the three symptoms (frequencies of the scored categories per class are included as supplementary information Figure S2 and the raw symptom score data for 'swollen joints', 'warm joints' and 'red joints' is included as supplementary Table S1). The data indicate that the same number of patients in both groups are in pain and score a similar severity of pain (data not shown). These symptom observations indicate that the Heat RA group has much more joint problems than the Cold RA group. It would be interesting to further study the role these joint symptoms could play in sub-typing RA.

Our study shows that the important symptoms for the sub-typing are 'warm feeling', 'pain worsens by warmth and movement', 'cold feeling' and 'aversion to cold'. This is in agreement with a previous study in which a systems diagnosis of 49 patients with rheumatic diseases revealed 'aversion to cold', 'aversion to heat' and 'cold feeling' as highly relevant for the Cold and Heat ranking of the subjects [23]. The symptom 'aversion to cold' and coldness in general was found by others as well [12,40]. Our study and other studies of the biology of Cold and Heat types

Table 4. Top discriminating plasma metabolites.

Importance	Compound[a]	2Log Cold/Heat[b]
2	Dehydroepiandrosterone sulfate (DHEA sulfate)	−0.96
4	4-Methyl-2-oxovaleric acid	−0.25
6	Indoxyl sulfate	−0.44
10	Uric acid	−0.25
11	Cholesterol sulfate	−0.65
13	3-Methyl-2-oxovaleric acid	−0.26
47	Tryptophan	−0.23
50	Alpha-ketoisovaleric acid	−0.13

[a]all compounds are verified with an authentic standard.
[b]Calculated Log of the ratio between average levels in Cold and Heat patients.

of RA patients lead to the hypothesis that the currently unclear effectiveness of cold and heat therapy might be improved by targeting it to the right sub-type [41–43].

Anti-citrullinated protein antibody (CCP) is extensively studied as a predictor of disease progression in RA [44]. In our multivariate model, CCP levels were higher in RA Heat patients suggesting that there might be a difference in disease progression between the two subtypes. The clinical parameters with the highest positive loadings were MCHC and IgG, while RDW showed the highest negative loading next to CCP. Some relationships between the Cold and Heat subtype and clinical measurements are nonlinear (see supplementary Figure S1 for the transformations of the variables). High as well as low serum levels off MCHC result in a positively transformed value, which is related to the Heat class. The highest levels of IgG are related to the Cold RA type, while lower levels are not so clearly Cold or Heat related. Blood urea nitrogen (BUN) levels increase in plasma with serious kidney damage [45]. Higher or lower levels of BUN are related to the Heat RA group, average levels are related to the Cold RA group. Alanine aminotranferase (ALT) is an important parameter to distinguish Cold and Heat patients, which has been found to be related to insuline resistance and atherosclerosis risk in RA patients [46].

The metabolomics analysis in this study revealed higher urine levels of 11 acylcarnitines in the Heat group of RA patients. The enzyme carnitine palmitoyltransferase I (CTP I), located in the outer mitochondrial membrane, transfers acyl groups from coenzyme A to carnitines allowing the transport of fatty acids into the mitochondria for β-oxidation. Plasma carnitine levels are maintained by a combination of dietary intake, endogenous synthesis by the liver and kidneys and active renal reabsorption.

Table 5. Warm, swollen & red joint scores.

# Symptoms	Cold*	Heat*
0	60	26
≥1	40	74
≥2	10	74
3	5	63

*Percentages of subjects showing a positive score on a minimum of 0, 1, 2 or 3 of the symptoms.

Acylcarnitines can leave the mitochondria, enter the blood stream and can be excreted in urine [47].

Significantly lower total carnitine and acylcarnitine excretion in urine of RA patients compared to healthy controls has been reported, while free carnitine levels in urine and plasma are equal in both groups [48,49]. Because dietary intake of carnitines was equal in both groups, an impaired carnitine synthesis was suggested which is controlled by skeletal muscle breakdown. Decreased muscle mass and increased muscle turnover are observed in RA patients, which might be explained by a reduced CTP I activity. This was confirmed by a decreased creatinine and 3-methylhistidine excretion [49]. In this study we find that the levels of a range of acylcarnitines are lower in the Cold RA group than in the Heat RA group. These findings suggest that Cold RA patients have less muscle mass and/or a more pronounced muscle breakdown than RA Heat patients. A limitation of this study is that the plasma acylcarnitine levels are not known. Further studies should therefore be performed to validate the hypothesis that Cold and Heat subtypes of RA patients are related to muscle mass or muscle breakdown.

Decreased urine pantothenic acid and acylcarnitine levels have been shown to indicate an increase in beta-oxidation in patients using PPARα agonist drugs [50]. Peroxisome proliferator-activated receptors (PPAR) activate fatty acid and cholesterol catabolism in the liver, activate gluconeogenesis and regulate amino acid metabolism. In addition, PPAR activates CTP I and CTP II activity. We report lower levels of pantothenic acid and acylcarnitine levels in Cold RA patients which might therefore indicate a difference in the activation of PPAR between the groups.

Interestingly, CTP I activity is inhibited by omega-6 fatty acids while an increased ratio of omega-3 versus omega-6 fatty acids consumption stimulates fatty acid oxidation regulated by CTP I activity [51]. A decrease in CTP I activity also seems to play a role in Chronic Fatigue Syndrome patients. In these patients supplementation with carnitine and acylcarnitine was found to decrease fatigue symptoms [52]. These findings suggest that fatigue in rheumatoid arthritis might be related to a decreased CTP I activity and a changed carnitine homeostasis. Fatigue is one of the most important factors in the disease experience of RA patients [53]. Our findings indicate that urine acylcarnitine levels are an important discriminator between two subtypes of RA patients, which might explain differences in the experience of fatigue. These findings also suggest that carnitine and acylcarnitine supplementation might be beneficial for Cold RA patients and less so for Heat RA patients. Further confirmatory studies should be conducted to prove this hypothesis and develop this targeted treatment option.

Significantly lower DHEAS levels have been reported in premenopausal RA patients and are correlated to low morning cortisol levels and high IL-6 levels indicating a suppression of HPA-axis function [54]. Decreased HPA-axis function is associated with a decreased stress response which results in an inadequate response to stress factors. It is hypothesized that this inadequate response can lead to autoimmune and inflammatory disorders [54]. This study shows a higher DHEAS levels in Heat RA patients compared to Cold RA patients suggesting that the Cold RA group has a more suppressed HPA-axis function. A text mining study [55] has shown that diseases related to Cold according to Chinese medicine theory are more related to hormone function disturbances and Heat related diseases to immune function disturbances, which is in agreement with our findings.

This study provides metabolite, symptom and clinical chemistry profiles for two subtypes of rheumatoid arthritis. The profiles indicate a number of biological processes that seem to be regulated differently in the two groups. RA therapy could be optimized for the two groups in various ways. This study suggests differences in the effects of carnitine and acylcarnitine supplementation for the two groups as well as differences in the effects of hormone treatments such as prednison. We think that the better characterization and biological understanding of Cold and Heat RA offered in this study can be used to tailor therapy to each subgroup. Additionally, this study offers a new subtype to include in studies aiming for an improvement of response to treatment. Finally, the mechanism and effect of specific Cold RA and Heat RA treatment options used in Chinese medicine should be studied and might be integrated in standard disease management strategies by using a standardized Cold RA and Heat RA diagnostic profile.

Supporting Information

Figure S1 Transformation plots of the clinical chemistry variables. On the x-axis the categories of the original discretized variables are represented while on the y-axis the optimally scaled quantifications are shown. A negative quantification corresponds to the Cold classification and a positive quantification to the Heat classification.
(JPG)

Figure S2 Frequencies of scored categories per class.
(JPG)

Table S1 Raw data of 'swollen joints', 'warm joints' and 'red joints' scores acquired by the symptom questionnaire. Patients were asked to give a score between 1 and 7. For the construction of Table 5 the positive scores, scores higher than 1, were counted for the Cold RA and Heat RA group. In Table S1 mean ranks for the Cold RA and Heat RA groups are given for each symptom and the differences between the groups are evaluated with the Mann-Whitney U test. The scoring of the three symptoms is significantly different between the Cold RA and Heat RA group.
(DOC)

Text S1 Symptoms questionnaire.
(DOC)

Acknowledgments

The authors would like to thank Carina de Jong-Rubingh, Sabina Bijlsma and Frans van der Kloet for contributing to the data analysis. We thank Suzan Wopereis for her contribution to the interpretation of the results. Also we thank Koko Wei for her efforts to facilitate the collaboration with the Chinese partners.

Author Contributions

Conceived and designed the experiments: HAW JG THR JJM. Performed the experiments: XW WD. Analyzed the data: HAW THR YS JJM AJK. Contributed reagents/materials/analysis tools: ZX HK TH XW GX MW. Wrote the paper: HAW WD. Conducted patient recruitment: XW ZX GX HK MW.

References

1. Glocker MO, Guthke R, Kekow J, Thiesen H-J (2006) Rheumatoid arthritis, a complex multifactorial disease: on the way toward individualized medicine. Med Res Rev 26: 63–87.
2. Isaacs JD, Ferraccioli G (2011) The need for personalised medicine for rheumatoid arthritis. Ann Rheum Dis 70: 4–7.
3. Smolen JS, Aletaha D (2005) Challenges of predicting treatment response in patients with rheumatoid arthritis. Nat Clin Pract Rheumatol 1: 62–63.
4. Maillefert J-F, Puéchal X, Falgarone G, Lizard G, Ornetti P, et al. (2010) Prediction of response to disease modifying antirheumatic drugs in rheumatoid arthritis. Joint Bone Spine 77: 558–63.
5. van der Greef J, McBurney RN (2005) Innovation: Rescuing drug discovery: in vivo systems pathology and systems pharmacology. Nat Rev Drug Discov 4: 961–7.
6. van Baarsen LG, Wijbrandts CA, Rustenburg F, Cantaert T, van der Pouw Kraan TC, et al. (2010) Regulation of IFN response gene activity during infliximab treatment in rheumatoid arthritis is associated with clinical response to treatment. Arthritis Res Ther 12(1): R11.
7. van der Pouw Kraan TCTM, Wijbrandts CA, van Baarsen LGM, Voskuyl AE, Rustenburg F, et al. (2007) Rheumatoid arthritis subtypes identified by genomic profiling of peripheral blood cells: assignment of a type I interferon signature in a subpopulation of patients. Ann Rheum Dis 66: 1008–14.
8. Anderson JJ, Wells G, Verhoeven AC, Felson DT (2000) Factors predicting response to treatment in rheumatoid arthritis: the importance of disease duration. Arthritis Rheum 43: 22–29.
9. Wolfe F, Cathey MA (1991) The effect of age on methotrexate efficacy and toxicity. J Rheumatol 18: 973–977.
10. Conaghan PG (2011) Predicting outcomes in rheumatoid arthritis. Clin Rheumatol 30 Suppl 1: S41–47.
11. van Wietmarschen H, Yuan K, Lu C, Gao P, Wang J, et al. (2009) Systems biology guided by Chinese medicine reveals new markers for sub-typing rheumatoid arthritis patients. J Clin Rheumatol 15: 330–337.
12. He Y, Lu A, Zha Y, Yan X, Song Y, et al. (2007) Correlations between symptoms as assessed in traditional chinese medicine (TCM) and ACR20 efficacy response: a comparison study in 396 patients with rheumatoid arthritis treated with TCM or Western medicine. J Clin Rheumatol 13: 317–21.
13. Ni M (1995) The Yellow Emperor's Classic of Medicine: A New Translation of the Neijing Suwen With Commentary. Boston, MA: Shambhala.
14. Jiang WY (2005) Therapeutic wisdom in traditional Chinese medicine: a perspective from modern science. Trends in pharmacological sciences, 26(11), 558–563.
15. Lu C, Xiao C, Chen G, Jiang M, Zha Q, et al. (2010) Cold and heat pattern of rheumatoid arthritis in traditional Chinese medicine: distinct molecular signatures indentified by microarray expression profiles in CD4-positive T cell. Rheumatology international 32(1): 61–8.
16. Jiang M, Xiao C, Chen G, Lu C, Zha Q, et al. (2011) Correlation between cold and hot pattern in traditional Chinese medicine and gene expression profiles in rheumatoid arthritis. Frontiers of medicine 5(2): 219–28.
17. Gu Y, Lu C, Zha Q, Kong H, Lu X (2012) Plasma metabonomics study of rheumatoid arthritis and its Chinese medicine subtypes by using liquid chromatography and gas chromatography coupled with mass spectrometry. Mol BioSyst 8: 1535–1543.
18. Lu C, Zha Q, Chang A, He Y, Lu A (2009) Pattern Differentiation in Traditional Chinese Medicine Can Help Define Specific Indications for Biomedical Therapy in the Treatment of Rheumatoid Arthritis. J Altern Complement Med 15: 1021–1025.
19. Meulman JJ, van der Kooij AJ, Heiser WJ (2004) Principal components analysis with nonlinear optimal scaling transformations for ordinal and nominal data. In: Kaplan D. The Sage handbook of quantitative methodology for the social sciences. SAGE. p. 49–70.
20. Linting M, Meulman J, Groenen P, van der Kooij A (2007) Nonlinear principal components analysis: Introduction and application. Psychol Methods 12: 336–358.

21. Barker M, Rayens W (2003) Partial least squares for discrimination. J Chemometr 17: 166–173.
22. Arnett FC, Edworthy SM, Bloch DA, McShane DJ, Fries JF, et al. (1988) The American Rheumatism Association 1987 revised criteria for the classification of rheumatoid arthritis. Arthritis Rheum 31: 315–24.
23. van Wietmarschen HA, Reijmers TH, van der Kooij AJ, Schroën J, Wei H, et al. (2011) Sub-typing of rheumatic diseases based on a systems diagnosis questionnaire. PloS One 6: e24846.
24. Dai WD, Wei C, Kong HW, Jia ZH, Han JK, et al. (2011) Effect of the traditional Chinese medicine tongxinluo on endothelial dysfunction rats studied by using urinary metabonomics based on liquid chromatography-mass spectrometry. J Pharmaceut Biomed 56, 86–92.
25. Gika HG, Theodoridis GA, Wingate JE, Wilson DE (2007) Within-day reproducibility of an HPLC–MS-based method for metabonomic analysis: application to human urine. J Proteome Res 6: 3291–3303.
26. Vandeginste BGM, Massart DL, Buydens LMC, De Jong S, Lewi PJ (1998) Handbook of Chemometrics and Qualimetrics Part B. Amsterdam: Elsevier p.374.
27. Nishisato S (1984) Forced classification: A simple application of a quantification method. Psychometrika 49: 25–36.
28. Higgins J (2002) Nonlinear systems in medicine. The Yale journal of biology and medicine 75: 247–260.
29. Callard R, George AJ, Stark J (1999) Cytokines, chaos, and complexity. Immunity 11(5): 507–513.
30. Linting M, van der Kooij A (2012) Nonlinear Principal Components Analysis With CATPCA: A Tutorial. J Pers Assess 94(1): 12–25.
31. Meulman JJ, Heiser WJ (2009) SPSS Categories 17.0. Chicago, Il.: SPSS Inc.
32. Bijlsma S, Bobeldijk I, Verheij ER, Ramaker R, MacDonald IA, et al. (2006) Large-scale human metabolomics studies: a strategy for data (pre-) processing and validation. Anal Chem 78(2): 567–74.
33. Hendriks MMWB, Smit S, Akkermans WLMW, Reijmers TH, Eilers PHC, et al. (2007) How to distinguish healthy from diseased? Classification strategy for mass spectrometry-based clinical proteomics. Proteomics 7: 3672–3680.
34. Kind T, Fiehn O (2010) Advances in structure elucidation of small molecules using mass spectrometry. Bioanalytical Reviews 2: 23–60.
35. Paglia G, D'Apolito O, Corso G (2008) Precursor ion scan profiles of acylcarnitines by atmospheric pressure thermal desorption chemical ionization tandem mass spectrometry. Rapid Commun Mass Spectrom 22: 3809–3815.
36. McClellan JE, Quarmby ST, Yost RA (2002) Parent and neutral loss monitoring on a quadrupole ion trap mass spectrometer: screening of acylcarnitines in complex mixtures. Anal Chem 74: 5799–5806.
37. van der Heijde DM, van 't Hof MA, van Riel PL, Theumisse LA, Lubberts EW, et al. (1990) Judging disease activity in clinical practice in rheumatoid arthritis: first step in the development of a disease activity score. Ann Rheum Dis 49: 916–920.
38. George-Gay B, Parker K (2003) Understanding the complete blood count with differential. J. Perianesth Nurs 18: 96–114.
39. Ritchie DM, Boyle JA, McInnes JM, Jasani MK, Dalakos TG, et al. (1968) Clinical studies with an articular index for the assessment of joint tenderness in patients with rheumatoid arthritis. Q J Med 37: 393–406.
40. Ryu H, Lee H, Kim H, Kim J (2010) Reliability and Validity of a Cold–Heat Pattern Questionnaire for Traditional Chinese Medicine. J Altern Complem Med 16: 663–667.
41. Robinson V, Brosseau L, Casimiro L, Judd M, Shea B, et al. (2002) Thermotherapy for treating rheumatoid arthritis. Cochrane Database Syst Rev.
42. Verhagen AP, Bierma-Zeinstra SMA, Cardoso JR, de Bie RA, Boers M, et al. (2003) Balneotherapy for rheumatoid arthritis. Cochrane Database Syst Rev 4: CD000518.
43. Kang G-L, Li S, Zhang J-F (2008) Entropy-based model for interpreting life systems in traditional chinese medicine. Evid-Based Compl Alt 5: 273–279.
44. van der Helm-van Mil AHM, Verpoort KN, Breedveld FC, Toes REM, Huizinga TWJ (2005) Antibodies to citrullinated proteins and differences in clinical progression of rheumatoid arthritis. Arthritis Res Ther 7: R949–58.
45. Kazory A (2010) Emergence of blood urea nitrogen as a biomarker of neurohormonal activation in heart failure. Am J Cardiol 106: 694–700.
46. Dessein PH, Woodiwiss AJ, Joffe BI, Norton GR (2007) Aminotransferases are associated with insulin resistance and atherosclerosis in rheumatoid arthritis. BMC Cardiov Dis 7: 31.
47. Sewell AC, Böhles HJ (1995) Acylcarnitines in intermediary metabolism. Eur J Pediatr 154: 871–877.
48. Jones MG, Goodwin CS, Amjad S, Chalmers RA (2005) Plasma and urinary carnitine and acylcarnitines in chronic fatigue syndrome. Clin Chim Acta 360: 173–177.
49. Krähenbühl S, Willer B, Brühlmann P, Hoppeler H, Stucki G (1999) Carnitine homeostasis in patients with rheumatoid arthritis. Clin Chim Acta 279: 35–45.
50. Patterson AD, Krausz KW, Li F, Ho CC, Gonzalez FJ, et al. (2009) Human Urinary Metabolomic Profile of PPARr Induced Fatty Acid -Oxidation research articles. J Proteome Res 4293–4300.
51. Guebre-Egziabher F, Rabasa-Lhoret R, Bonnet F, Bastard J-P, Desage M, et al. (2008) Nutritional intervention to reduce the n-6/n-3 fatty acid ratio increases adiponectin concentration and fatty acid oxidation in healthy subjects. Eur J Clin Nutr 62: 1287–1293.
52. Reuter SE, Evans AM (2011) Long-chain acylcarnitine deficiency in patients with chronic fatigue syndrome. Potential involvement of altered carnitine palmitoyltransferase-I activity. J Intern Med 270: 76–84.
53. Khan NA, Spencer HJ, Abda E, Aggarwal A, Alten R, et al. (2012) Determinants of discordance in patient's and physician's rating of rheumatoid arthritis disease activity. Arthrit Care Res 64: 206–214.
54. Cutolo M, Villaggio B, Foppiani L, Briata M, Sulli A, et al. (2000) The hypothalamic-pituitary-adrenal and gonadal axes in rheumatoid arthritis. Ann Ny Acad Sci 917: 835–43.
55. Li S, Zhang ZQ, Wu LJ, Zhang XG, Li YD, et al. (2007) Understanding ZHENG in traditional Chinese medicine in the context of neuro-endocrine-immune network. IET Syst Biol 1: 51–60.

5

Efficacy and Safety of Traditional Chinese Medicine for Diabetes: A Double-Blind, Randomised, Controlled Trial

Linong Ji[1]*, Xiaolin Tong[2], Hongyuan Wang[3], Haoming Tian[4], Huimin Zhou[5], Lili Zhang[6], Qifu Li[7], Yizhong Wang[8], Hongmei Li[9], Min Liu[10], Hongjie Yang[11], Yanbin Gao[12], Yan Li[13], Quanmin Li[14], Xiaohui Guo[15], Gangyi Yang[16], Zhongai Zhang[17], Zhiguang Zhou[18], Guang Ning[19], Yingli Chen[1], Sanjoy Paul[20]*, for the Evidence-Based Medical Research of Xiaoke Pill Study Group¶

1 Peking University People's Hospital, Beijing, China, **2** China Academy of Chinese Medicial Sciences Guang'anmen Hospital, Beijing, China, **3** Peking University School of Public Health, Beijing China, **4** Sichuan University West China Hospital, Chengdu, China, **5** The First Hospital of Hebei Medical University, Shijiazhuang, China, **6** The Third Affiliated Hospital of Peking University of Traditional Chinese and Western Medicine, Beijing, China, **7** The First Affiliated Hospital of Chongqing Medical University, Chongqing, China, **8** The Central Hospital of China Aerospace Corporation, Beijing, China, **9** China Meitan General Hospital, Beijing, China, **10** The First Affiliated Hospital of Guangzhou University of Traditional Chinese Medicine, Guangzhou, China, **11** Shanghai University of Traditional Chinese Medicine Yueyang Hospital of Integrated Traditional Chinese and Western Medicine, Shanghai, China, **12** Beijing University of Traditional Chinese Medicine Dongfang Hospital, Beijing, China, **13** Zhongshan University Sun Yai-sen Memorial Hospital, Zhongshan, China, **14** General Hospital of PLA Second Artillery, Beijing, China, **15** Peking University First Hospital, Beijing, China, **16** The Second Affiliated Hospital of Chongqing Medical University, Chongqing, China, **17** Nanjing Hospital of Traditional Chinese Medicine, Nanjing, China, **18** The Second Xiangya Hospital of Central South University, Changsha, China, **19** Shanghai Jiaotong University Ruijin Hospital, Shanghai, China, **20** Queensland Clinical Trials and Biostatistics Centre, School of Population Health, University of Queensland, Queensland, Australia

Abstract

Background: Treatment of diabetes mellitus with Traditional Chinese Medicine has a long history. The aim of this study is to establish the safety and efficacy of traditional Chinese medicine combined with glibenclamide to treat type 2 diabetes mellitus.

Methods: In a controlled, double blind, multicentre non-inferiority trial, 800 patients with unsatisfactory glycemic control (fasting glucose 7–13 mmol/L and HbA1c 7–11%) were randomly assigned to receive Xiaoke Pill, a compound of Chinese herbs combined with glibenclamide, or Glibenclamide in two study groups – drug naive group, and patients previously treated with metformin monotherapy (metformin group). Outcome measures at 48 weeks were the incidence and rate of hypoglycemia, mean difference in HbA1c, and proportion of patients with HbA1c<6.5%.

Findings: In drug naïve group, the total hypoglycemia rate and the mild hypoglycemic episode in the Xiaoke Pill arm were 38% ($p = 0.024$) and 41% ($p = 0.002$) less compared to Glibenclamide arm; in Metformin group, the average annual rate of hypoglycemia was 62% lower in Xiaoke Pill arm ($p = 0.003$). Respective mean changes in HbA1c from baseline were −0.70% and −0.66% for Xiaoke Pill and Glibenclamide, with a between-group difference (95% CI) of −0.04% (−0.20, 0.12) in the drug naïve group, and those in metformin group were −0.45% and −0.59%, 0.14% (−0.12, 0.39) respectively. The respective proportions of patients with a HbA1c level <6.5% were 26.6% and 23.4% in the drug naïve group and 20.1% and 18.9% in the metformin group.

Interpretation: In patients with type 2 diabetes and inadequate glycaemic control, treatment with Xiaoke Pill led to significant reduction in risk of hypoglycemia and similar improvements in glycemic control after 48 weeks compared to Glibenclamide.

Trial Registration: Chinese Clinical Trial Register number, ChiCTR-TRC-08000074

Editor: Jianping Ye, Pennington Biomedical Research Center, United States of America

Funding: This work was supported by grants from National Basic Research Program of China (973 program, No. 2011CB504001), National High Technology Research and Development Program (863 program, No. 2006AA02A409), and Guangzhou Zhongyi Pharmaceutical. The funders had no role in study design, data collection and analysis, decision to publish, or preparation of the manuscript.

Competing Interests: The authors have declared that no competing interests exist. Several authors have received speaking honoraria from several pharmaceutical companies as follows: Dr. Ji reports receiving consulting and lecture fees from Eli Lilly, Bristol-Myers Squibb, Novartis, Novo Nordisk, Merck, Bayer, Takeda, Sanofi-Aventis, GlaxoSmithKline, Roche, Johnson & Johnson, boehingeringelheim, and Guangzhou Zhongyi Pharmaceutical, and grants from Guangzhou Zhongyi Pharmaceutical and Bayer. Dr. Q Li reports receiving consulting and lecture fees from Eli Lilly, Novo Nordisk, and Sanofi-Aventis. Dr. Tian reports receiving lecture fees from Bristol-Myers Squibb, Novo Nordisk, Bayer, and Sanofi-Aventis. Dr. Y. Li reports receiving consulting fees from Novartis, Novo Nordisk, and Sanofi-Aventis and lecture fees from Novo Nordisk and Sanofi-Aventis. Dr. Guo reports receiving consulting fees from Novartis, Sanofi-Aventis, and Guangzhou Zhongyi Pharmaceutical and lecture fees from Sanofi-Aventis, Guangzhou Zhongyi Pharmaceutical, and Novo Nordisk. Dr. Y. Gao reports receiving consulting fees from Novartis, Sanofi-Aventis, and Guangzhou Zhongyi Pharmaceutical and lecture fees from Sanofi-Aventis, Guangzhou Zhongyi Pharmaceutical, and Novo Nordisk. Dr. M. Liu reports receiving lecture fees from Eli Lilly, Novo Nordisk, and Bayer. This does not alter the authors' adherence to all the PLOS ONE policies on sharing data and materials.

* E-mail: jiln@bjmu.edu.cn (LJ); s.paul@sph.uq.edu.au (SP)

¶ Investigators in Evidence-Based Medical Research of Xiaoke Pill Study are listed in Appendix S1.

Introduction

Treatment of diabetes mellitus with Traditional Chinese Medicine (TCM) has a long history of more than 2,000 years in China [1]. Diabetes has been described as "Xiaoke (wasting-thirst)" in Traditional Chinese Medicine [2,3]. The classic symptoms and signs of "Xiaoke" include sweet urine, dry mouth, thirst, polydipsia, polyorexia, polyphagia, emaciation, and fatigue [4–7]. Evidence for glucose-lowing effect of TCM is based mainly on animal studies [8]. Large-scale, direct comparison of TCM and well established allopathic glucose lowering drugs in terms of safety (such as hypoglycemia: one of the most common symptoms during treatment of diabetes) and efficacy has been lacking [9–12]. In addition, there is no evidence if TCM has any additional benefits compared with western medicine. One of the major difficulties in studying TCM is the standardizing the dose of TCM in large scale and long-term clinical study.

In China, some diabetes medications are compound preparations of Chinese herbs combined with allopathic medicine such as glibenclamide. One such widely used preparation is Xiaoke Pill [11], which contains 0.25microgram of glibenclamide per pill [12]. The herb components include Radix Puerariae, Radix Rehmanniae, Radix Astragali, Radix Trichosanthis, Stylus Zeae Maydis, Fructus Schisandrae Sphenantherae, and Rhizoma Dioscoreae. These were selected from two ancient TCM formulas for Xiaoke – "Yuquan San" [13] and "Xiaoke Fang" [14]. The selection of those herb components for the treatment of diabetes was based on theory of TCM. Prior studies published in medical journals in China showed significant improvement in diabetes symptoms in favor of Xiaoke Pill. However, the efficacy and safety of Xiaoke Pill has not been evaluated with randomized, double blind, and placebo controlled study.

The Xiaoke Pill is produced with modern pharmaceutical technologies, which ensure the equal quantity of each herb component and glibenclamide in each pill. Therefore, this medicine is suitable for study the efficacy and safety of TCM if controlled properly by glibenclamide.

Evidence-Based Medical Research of Xiaoke Pill is a 52-week, multicentre, double-blind, double-dummy controlled clinical trial to assess the safety and efficacy of Xiaoke Pill compared with glibenclamide alone in patients with inadequate glycemic control and stratified into two groups: newly diagnosed drug naïve patients, and patients treated with metformin for at least three months.

Methods

Ethics Statement

The protocol was approved by the Ethics Review Committee affiliated with each study center, and was implemented in accordance with provisions of the Declaration of Helsinki and Good Clinical Practice guidelines. The full names of each ethics committee were listed as follows:

Ethics Committee of The First Hospital of Hebei Medical University, Ethics Committee of The Third Affiliated Hospital of Peking University of Traditional Chinese and Western Medicine, Ethics Committee of Sichuan University West China Hospital, Ethics Committee of The First Affiliated Hospital of Chongqing Medical University, Ethics Committee of The Central Hospital of China Aerospace Corporation, Ethics Committee of Peking University People's Hospital, Ethics Committee of China Meitan General Hospital, Ethics Committee of The First Affiliated Hospital of Guangzhou University of Traditional Chinese Medicine, Ethics Committee of Shanghai University of Traditional Chinese Medicine, Ethics Committee of China Academy of Chinese Medical Sciences Guang'anmen Hospital, Ethics Committee of Beijing University of Traditional Chinese Medicine Dongfang Hospital, Ethics Committee of Zhongshan University Sun Yai-sen Memorial Hospital, Ethics Committee of General Hospital of PLA Second Artillery, Ethics Committee of Peking University First Hospital, Ethics Committee of The Second Affiliated Hospital of Chongqing Medical University, Ethics Committee of Nanjing Hospital of Traditional Chinese Medicine, Ethics Committee of The Second Xiangya Hospital of Central South University, Ethics Committee of Shanghai Jiaotong University Ruijin Hospital.

All the participants provided their written informed consents to participate in this study.

Study Design

The study consisted of a screening visit, a 4-weeks run-in period, and 48 weeks of follow up (4-weekly) after randomization. Patients deemed eligible at screening entered a 4 weeks run-in period, reinforced by diet and exercise recommendations, to achieve an entry plasma glucose level between 126–234 mg/dl (7–13 mmol/L) and glycated hemoglobin level between 7–11%. At the beginning of the 4-week run-in period, we gave the patients diet and exercise recommendations according to 2007 China Type 2 Diabetes Clinical Practice Guidelines. At the end of the run-in period, according to the protocol, we recorded if the patients control diet and do exercise or not as we recommended. During the run-in period, it will maintain the same normal dose of metformin for patients treated with metformin. Eligible patients were separately randomized to receive double blind and double dummy mono therapy(drug naïve group, n = 400) or add on therapy (metformin group, n = 400) with Xiaoke Pill (Guangzhou Zhongyi Pharmaceutical, Guangzhou, China) or Glibenclamide tablet (Tianjin Pacific Pharmaceutical, Tianjin, China). Of the 18 participant centers in China, 6 were located in TCM hospitals. Statistics Analysis System (SAS) software was used to randomly divide the subjects who have been determined as eligible through screening in the run-in period (Details of Randomization and Blinding were in Supplementary material).

The study management committee consisted of 6 academic members who designed the trial, and one sponsor representative. Data were held by School of Public Health, Peking University, and were independently analyzed by the Queensland Clinical Trials & Biostatistics Centre, University of Queensland.

Study Population

Through a protocol defined screening process, 1076 patients were initially screed and those were deemed suitable for inclusion in the study. Patients with type 2 diabetes, aged 21–70 years, who met the following inclusion criteria were recruited for the study:1) Drug naïve patients with body mass index (BMI) within 18 kg/m^2~28 kg/m^2; 2) Patients who received treatment with metformin at a stable dose ≥750 mg/day for at least 3 months before screening, with BMI within 18 kg/m^2~35 kg/m^2; 3) Stable body weight within at least 3 months before screening; 4) Poor glycemic control with fasting plasma glucose (FPG) between 126–234 mg/dl (7.0–13 mmol/L) and glycated hemoglobin (HbA1c)>7.0% at screening. Exclusion criteria included FPG≥13 mmol/L or HbA1c≥11%, more than 3 episodes of severe hypoglycemia within 6 months before screening, allergic to sulfonylureas or their ingredients, treatment with glucose-lowing agents other than metformin or insulin within 3 months before screening or with exogenous insulin for more than 1 week within 3 months before screening, a history of heart disease within 1 year before screening, a history of abnormal kidney function or serum creatinine levels reaching the upper limit of normal, alanine aminotransferase (ALT) or aspartate aminotransferase (AST)>2.5 times the upper limit of normal, suffering from acute or chronic hepatitis, hemoglobin disease or chronic anemia, or underlying conditions that could lead to poor compliance.

Treatment

Metformin doses for patients in the metformin group were maintained by single brand metformin tablet (250 mg/tablet, Beijing Union Pharmaceutical Factory) provided by the study group at enrollment dose levels throughout the study period. The starting dose for Glibenclamide was 1.25 mg/day (half glibenclamide tablet), and for Xiaoke Pill the dose was 5 pills per day. Following the label of Xiaoke Pill, the maximal daily doses were 7.5 mg/day, and 30pills/day, respectively. Study medicines were adjusted every 4 weeks according to FPG levels: 4.4–7.0 mmol/L - no adjustment; >7.0 mmol/L - addition of 5 pills of Xiaoke Pill and/or half tablet of Glibenclamide; <4.4 mmol/L - reduction of 5 pills of Xiaoke Pill and/or half tablet of Glibenclamide. Dosage titration was at the discretion of the investigator, if poorly tolerated.

Clinical and Biochemical Measurements

Vital signs and any diabetic complication were recorded at every study visit. Anthropometric measurements were taken at baseline and at each of the 13 follow up visits. HbA1c for preliminary screening was measured at participating centers with National Glycohemoglobin Standardization Program (NGSP) certified methods. FPG levels were measured by glucose oxidase method every 4 weeks at participating centers. HbA1c, urinary albumin-creatinine ratio, immunoreactive insulin, C-peptide, high-sensitivity C-reactive Protein (hsCRP), adiponectin and lipids were measured centrally at randomization and 3 monthly intervals. HbA1c was measured by high-performance liquid chromatography (Ultra2 HbA1c Detector, PRIMUS Corporation, USA, normal range: 4 to 6%). An immunonephelometry method was used to measure urinary albumin-creatinine ratio, C-reactive protein, levels of low-density lipoprotein cholesterol (LDL-C), high-density lipoprotein cholesterol (HDL-C), and triglyceride (COBAS Integra 400 Plus System, Roche Diagnostics Ltd. Basel, Switzerland). Immunoreactive insulin and C-peptide were measured by electrochemiluminescence immuno assay (Elecsys 2010 system, Roche Diagnostics Ltd, Basel, Switzerland)). Adiponectin was measured by Enzyme-linked immunosorbent assays (ELISA) [15]. Liver function tests, complete blood count, urine routine assay, kidney function test, twelve-lead ECG, and physical examination were measured or performed at participating centers at recruitment, 24, and 48 weeks after randomization. All study drugs were withheld on the morning of testing.

Scoring of TCM Symptoms of Diabetes

TCM symptoms of diabetes were evaluated blindly at each visit in 320 study subjects (80 in each treatment arm) who were located at the TCM hospitals only. The symptoms included dry throat and mouth, lack of strength, polyphagia, polydipsia, shortness of breath, vexing heat in the chest, palms and soles, palpitations, insomnia, yellowish urine, and constipation. The questionnaire-based scoring of *TCM symptoms of diabetes* (Table S1) was based on the modification of "Table for quantitative grading of diabetes symptoms" [16]. Each symptom was graded into four categories and assigned a score from 0 to 3 (3 = most severe category).

Safety and Efficacy Outcomes

The objectives of the trial were to assess the safety and efficacy of Xiaoke Pill compared with glibenclamide alone in patients with inadequate glycemic control and stratified into two groups: newly diagnosed drug naïve patients, and patients treated with metformin for at least three months.

The safety and efficacy outcomes were incidence of hypoglycemia and the change in HbA1c level at 48 weeks respectively. Secondary endpoints included the changes in fasting glucose level, proportion of patients with HbA1c<6.5%, time to reach HbA1c<6.5%, and, β-cell function, insulin resistance levels, fasting lipid profiles, and the TCM symptoms score.

Safety Assessments

Safety and tolerability were assessed through the analysis of adverse events, laboratory evaluations, and vital signs. Patients were counseled regarding the symptoms of hypoglycemia and requested to immediately perform a finger-stick glucose measurement if any symptoms occurred. Hypoglycemic events were classified as 'mild' if the patient had symptoms or a self-measured capillary glucose level (CG)<63 mg/dL (3.5 mmol/L); 'severe' if the patient had symptoms with CG<50 mg/dL (2.8 mmol/L), and third party assistance was required; "nocturnal hypoglycemia" if hypoglycemia occurred between falling asleep in the evening and breakfast.

Statistical Analysis

Xiaoke Pill was regarded as non-inferior to treatment with Glibenclamide only if, after 48 weeks of treatment, the upper limit of the two-sided 95% CI for the difference in mean HbA1c change was less than 0.4%. A sample size of 400 patients was estimated to provide more than 90% power to test the hypothesis that Xiaoke Pill treatment was non-inferior to treatment with Glibenclamide in each of the study groups, assuming a 20% early discontinuation rate, and an expected inter-patient SD of 1.2%.

The primary analysis was conducted in the intention-to-treat (ITT) population, with supportive per-protocol (PP) analysis [17]. Twenty five imputations for missing clinical and biochemical measurements were performed using multiple-imputation technique based on Bayesian MCMC method [18]. The highest proportion of missing data on longitudinal measurements was only 4%. To account for center-level clustering, the study centers were included as random effect in all regression models. For normal continuous variables, mixed linear regression models were used [19]. Mixed-effect logistic regression models were used to analyze categorical outcomes, with adjustment for baseline data. The 'unstructured' covariance structure was used for all mixed-effect models. The primary efficacy end point was change from baseline HbA1c at week 48; end point analysis at week 24 was exploratory. Difference in the estimated marginal means between the treatment arms along with bootstrapped 95% CI was estimated to draw inference on non-inferiority. The proportion of patients with hypoglycemia was analyzed using a generalized binomial model without adjustment for covariates. For the comparison of hypoglycemia rates, generalized regression models with zero-inflated negative binomial distribution were used.

The insulin sensitivity and insulin resistance measures, and the study doses were analyzed with the use of generalized mixed-effect models with gamma distribution. The symptom score data were analyzed using non-parametric quintile regression, with treatment comparisons at median levels of the symptom scores. All regression fits were bootstrapped for 1000 times to obtain the bootstrapped standard errors. Time to reach HbA1c<6.5% was summarized

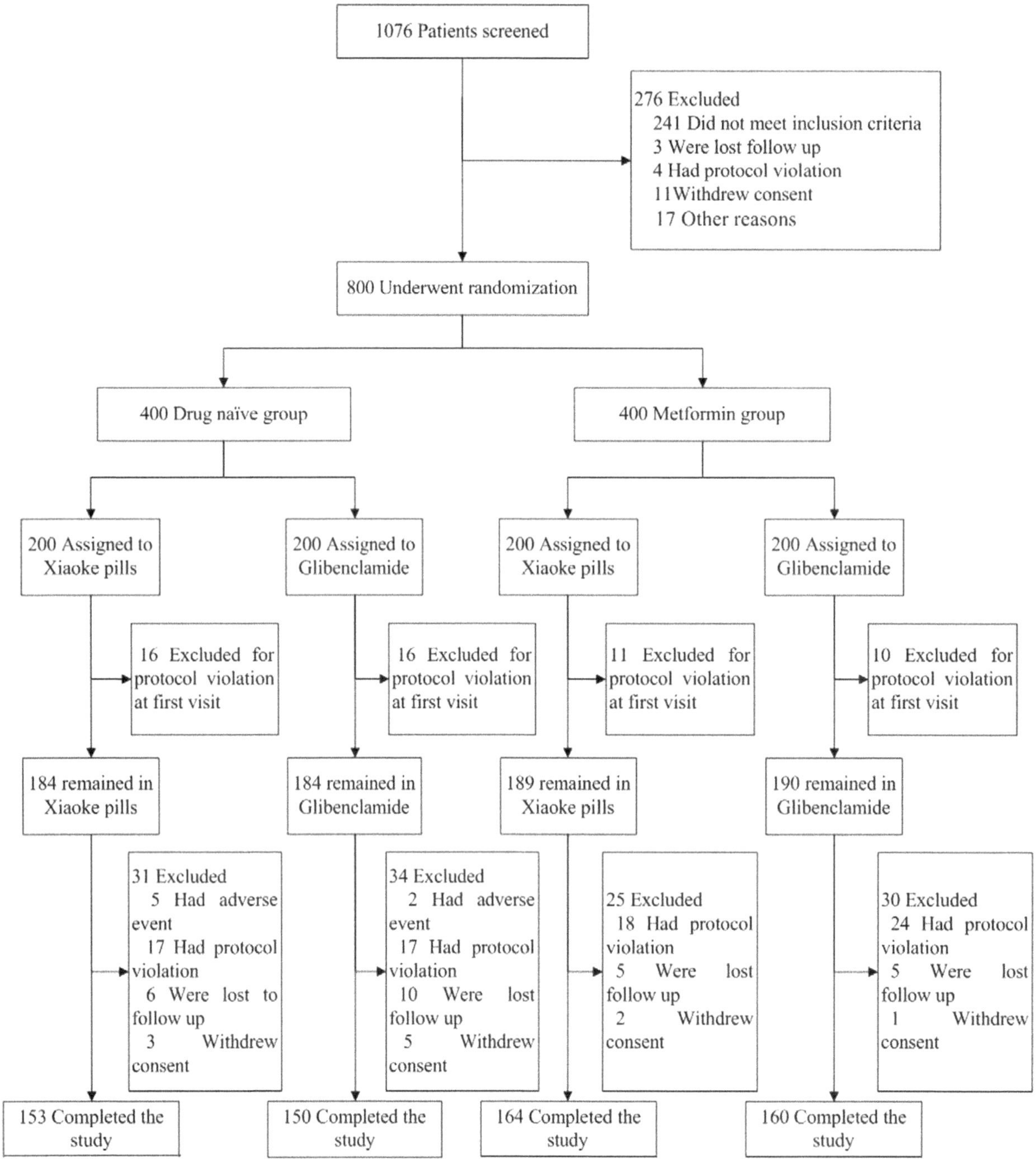

Figure 1. Enrollment and Outcomes.

using Kaplan–Meier estimates. SAS 9.2 (SAS Inc.) and STATA 11 software were used for all statistical analyses.

The protocol for this trial and CONSORT checklist are available as supporting information (Protocol S1 and Checklist S1). Trial Registration: Chinese Clinical Trial Register number, ChiCTR-TRC-08000074.

Results

Study Characteristics

The patients were enrolled between Dec 20th, 2007 and Oct 17th, 2008. 1076 patients who met the inclusion criteria were recruited for the study. After the end of run-in, 800 patients who still meet the inclusion criteria were randomly divided into the drug naïve and metformin study groups (Fig. 1). The respective mean ±SD ages were 53.7±8.6 and 54.7±8.8 years. The median (IQR) duration of diabetes in metformin group was 3 (1.0, 6.3) years; based on Mann-Whitney U tests, no significant differences were observed in the baseline variables between the two treatments in two study groups (Table 1). The total numbers of patients who did not complete the study did not differ significantly – 16.8% and 18.5% in Xiaoke Pill and Glibenclamide arms, respectively, within drug naïve group (n = 65); and 13.6% and 16.3%, respectively, within metformin group (n = 55). Demo-

Table 1. Characteristic of the Patients at Baseline.

Variable	Drug Naïve Group			Metformin Group		
	Xiaoke Pill (n = 184)	Glibenclamide (n = 184)	p	Xiaoke Pill (n = 189)	Glibenclamide (n = 190)	p
Demographics Characteristics						
Age — yr	54±9	54±8	0.91	54±8	55±9	0.94
Male — no. (%)	104(56.5)	106(57.6)	0.83	100(52.9)	92(48.4)	0.38
Patient in CTH— no. (%)	76(41.3)	74(40.2)	0.87	74(39.2)	76(40.0)	0.85
Excercise— no. (%)	135(73.4)	147(79.9)	0.14	146(77.2)	156(82.1)	0.24
Diet— no. (%)	138(75.0)	155(84.2)	0.028	157(83.1)	166(87.4)	0.24
Anthropometric Characteristics						
Weight (kg)	67.1±9.5	66.8±10.5	0.51	68.7±10.4	67.1±11.0	0.48
Body-mass index (kg/m^2)	24.5±2.2	24.4±2.5	0.69	25.4±2.9	25.0±3.1	0.63
Waist-Hip Ratio	0.9±0.1	0.9±0.1	0.89	0.9±0.1	0.9±0.1	0.90
Blood Pressure — mm Hg						
Systolic	126±12	125±14	0.36	125±12	126±13	0.49
Diastolic	78±8	78±9	0.59	78±8	77±8	0.54
Anti-Hypertensive— no. (%)	33(17.9)	28(15.2)	0.48	38(20.1)	31(16.3)	0.34
Metabolic Characteristics						
FPG—mmol/L	9.16±1.74	8.98±1.59	0.31	8.91±1.56	9.09±1.84	0.29
Glycated hemoglobin—%	7.92±1.47	7.85±1.54	0.57	7.68±1.39	7.90±1.51	0.18
Fasting insulin—mIU/L[a]	8.10 (4.98–11.84)	7.96 (5.31–11.69)	0.87	8.40 (5.31–12.13)	7.60 (5.30–11.92)	0.46
HOMA- IS	38.40±31.11	39.76±33.85	0.53	37.96±26.82	38.01±32.36	0.41
HOMA-IR	4.13±4.19	4.19±3.73	0.11	3.75±2.58	3.92±3.50	0.17
Lipids						
Total cholesterol —mmol/L	4.99±0.98	4.97±1.17	0.87	5.14±2.08	4.96±0.94	0.26
High-density lipoprotein— mmol/L	1.1±0.3	1.1±0.3	0.49	1.1±0.3	1.2±0.3	0.53
Low-density lipoprotein— mmol/L	3.20±0.85	3.06±0.92	0.12	2.96±0.87	3.03±0.87	0.23
Triglycerides— mmol/L[a]	1.65 (1.38–2.31)	1.79 (1.25–2.63)	0.50	1.87 (1.41–2.92)	1.87 (1.47–2.54)	0.46
Ratio of albumin to creatinine[a]	3.53 (0.96–10.40)	3.16 (0.86–11.19)	0.11	3.88 (0.93–11.70)	3.94 (0.86–15.94)	0.28
ALT—U/L[a]	20.4 (15, 30)	22 (15.1, 33)	0.44	23 (16, 34)	23 (16, 31)	0.23
AST—U/L[a]	21 (17, 27.5)	21 (17, 27.6)	0.78	21 (17, 28)	21 (17, 27.7)	0.79
Score of TCM symptoms of diabetes	8 (6,9)	8.5 (6,10)	0.27	8.5 (7,12)	8 (6,11)	0.22

[a]Median (Inter Quartile Range).

graphic, anthropometric, and metabolic characteristics of these lost-to-follow-up patients did not differ from those who completed the study.

The glibenclamide doses per day were similar in the two treatment arms during 48 weeks of follow-up (Fig. 2 I&J). The mean ± SD dose of metformin was 1140±340 mg and 1130±360 mg, in Xiaoke Pill and Glibenclamide arms, respectively. The baseline distributions of HbA1c and FPG were similar in both study groups (Fig. 2 A& B, 2 E & F).

Outcome in Drug Naïve Group

All safety analyses were done on the ITT population. Patients in the Xiaoke Pill arm were 38% less likely to have any hypoglycemia compared to those in the Glibenclamide arm [OR (95% CI): 0.62 (0.42, 0.94), p = 0.024]. The average annual rate of hypoglycemia was 24% lower in patients treated with Xiaoke Pill [Rate Ratio (95% CI): 0.76 (0.49, 1.18)]. Patients in Xiaoke Pill arm were also 41% less likely to have a mild hypoglycemic episode compared to those in the Glibenclamide arm [OR (95% CI): 0.59 (0.42, 0.82), p = 0.002, Table 2].

The maximal reduction in the mean HbA1c level occurred by 24 weeks and then increased marginally for both treatments (Fig. 2 C). The mean change from baseline in HbA1c at week 48 was −0.70% in the Xiaoke Pill group and −0.66% in the Glibenclamide group (Table 2), with a between-group difference (95% CI) of −0.04% (−0.20, 0.12). The upper-limit of the 95% CI for the between-group mean difference met the pre-specified criterion for declaring non-inferiority of Xiaoke Pill to Glibenclamide. In PP subjects, the between-group difference (95% CI) was −0.16 (−0.48, 0.16).

At 48 week, patients were 31% more likely to reduce HbA1c below 6.5% in the Xiaoke Pill group [OR (95% CI): 1.31(0.81, 2.13)]. The proportion of patients with HbA1c<7% was the same in the two treatment arms [89 (48.4%)].The mean (95% CI) weeks to reach HbA1c<6.5% was 29.1 (26.4, 31.8) and 28.0 (25.3, 30.8) weeks, in Xiaoke Pill and Glibenclamide arms respectively. At 48

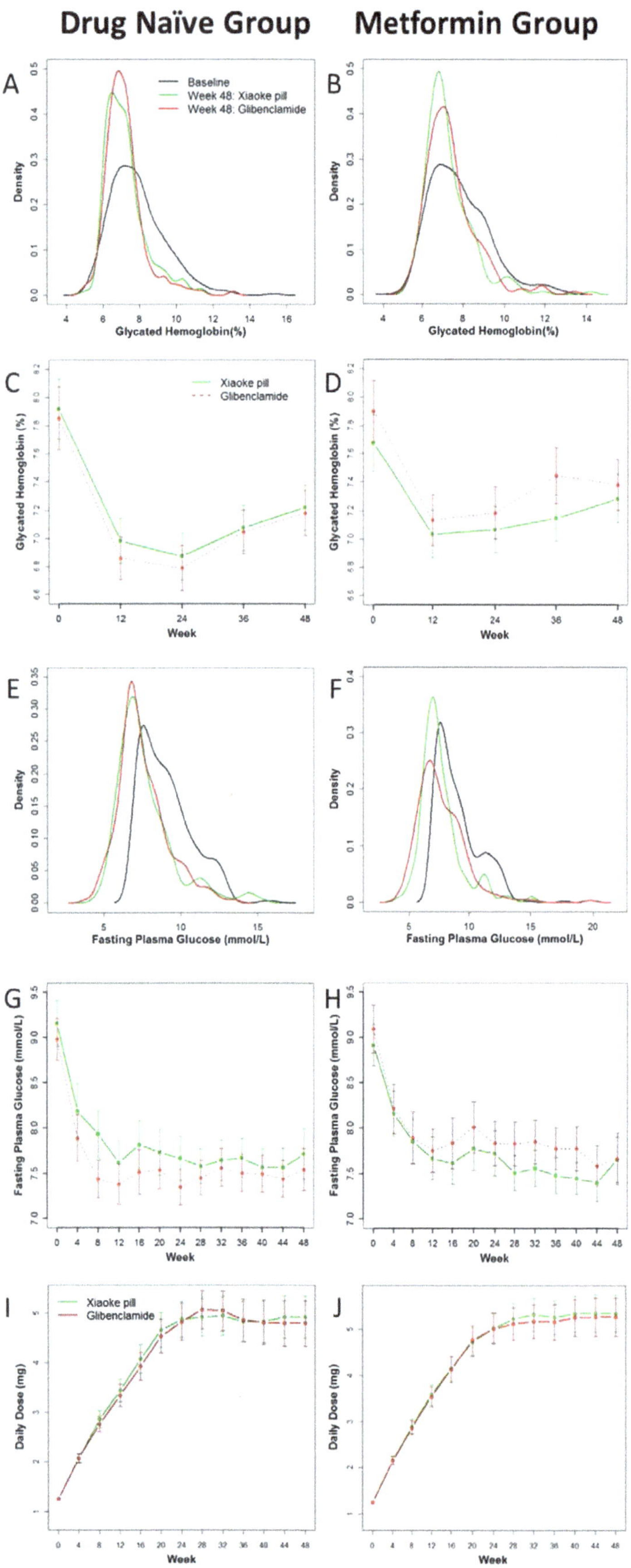

Figure 2. Primary and secondary outcomes over 48 weeks.

Table 2. Outcomes and changes from baseline.

	Treatment Naïve Group			Metformin Group		
	Xiaoke Pill	**Glibenclamide**	**Difference in Mean Change (95% CI)**	**Xiaoke Pill**	**Glibenclamide**	**Difference in Mean Change (95% CI)**
HbA1c— %						
Mean at 24 week (95% CI)	6.84 (6.68, 7.01)	6.77 (6.51, 7.03)		7.05 (6.86, 7.25)	7.17 (6.93, 7.41)	
Absolute change from baseline at 24 week	−1.07 (−1.39, −0.76)	−1.08 (−1.41, −0.74)	0.01 (−0.12, 0.13)	−0.65 (−0.86, −0.45)	−0.78 (−1.12, −0.43)	0.12 (−0.13, 0.38)
Mean at 48 week (95% CI)-ITT	7.20 (7.01, 7.39)	7.18 (6.91, 7.45)		7.27 (7.04, 7.50)	7.36 (7.15, 7.57)	
Absolute change from baseline-ITT	−0.70 (−1.06, −0.34)	−0.66 (−1.05, −0.28)	−0.04 (−0.20, 0.12)	−0.45 (−0.68, −0.22)	−0.59 (−0.94, −0.23)	0.14 (−0.12, 0.39)
Mean at 48 week (95% CI)-PP	6.79 (6.62, 6.96)	6.85 (6.65, 7.04)		6.94 (6.73, 7.15)	6.97 (6.69, 7.24)	
Absolute change from baseline-PP	−0.87 (−1.37, −0.37)	−0.71 (−1.09, −0.33)	−0.16 (−0.48, 0.16)	−0.41 (−0.58, −0.25)	−0.57 (−0.93, −0.21)	0.16 (−0.18, 0.49)
Total hypoglycemia— no. (%)	28(15.2)	39(21.2)		23(12.2)	29(15.3)	
Odd Ratio	0.62(0.42,0.94)		p = 0.024	0.76(0.43,1.35)		p = 0.35
Average Rate/Patient/Year	2.61(1.73)	3.00(1.97)		1.91(1.24)	3.76(2.95)	
Rate Ratio	0.76 (0.48, 1.18)		p = 0.22	0.38 (0.20, 0.71)		p = 0.003
Mild hypoglycemia— no. (%)	26(14.1)	38(20.7)		23(12.2)	28(14.7)	
Odd Ratio	0.59(0.42, 0.82)		p = 0.002	0.80(0.44, 1.44)		p = 0.45
Average Rate/Patient/Year	2.58 (1.50)	2.95 (1.90)		1.87 (1.25)	3.54 (4.01)	
Rate Ratio	0.76 (0.49, 1.18)		p = 0.22	0.40 (0.20, 0.78)		p = 0.007
Nocternal hypoglycemia— no. (%)	3(1.6)	4(2.2)		1(0.5)	8(4.2)	
Odd Ratio	0.75(0.16, 3.33)		p = 0.93	0.12(0.01, 0.98)		p = 0.037
Average Rate/Patient/Year	2 (1)	1.25 (0.5)		1	1.25 (0.71)	
Rate Ratio	-	-		-	-	
N(%)of patients reaching A1c <6.5% at 48 week	49 (26.6)	43 (23.4)		38 (20.1)	36 (18.9)	
Odds Ratio (95% CI)	1.31 (0.81, 2.13)		p = 0.37	1.20 (0.75, 1.92)		p = 0.44
FPG—mmol/L						
Mean at 48 week (95% CI)	7.72 (7.32, 8.11)	7.54 (7.22, 7.86)		7.71 (7.41, 8.01)	7.73 (7.41, 8.04)	
Absolute change from baseline	−1.42 (−1.79, −1.06)	−1.43 (−1.79, −1.06)	0.01 (−0.39, 0.40)	−1.31 (−1.71, −0.90)	−1.48 (−1.87, −1.08)	0.17 (−0.18, 0.51)
N(%)of patients reaching FPG<7 mmol/L	78 (42.4)	82 (44.6)		69 (36.5)	79 (41.6)	
Odds Ratio (95% CI)	1.05 (0.70, 1.58)		p = 0.81	0.72 (0.48,1.08)		p = 0.11
Weight(kg)						
Mean at 48 week (95% CI)	68.09 (65.76, 70.41)	67.75 (65.41, 70.10)		68.99 (66.68, 71.29)	67.91 (64.55, 71.28)	
Absolute change from baseline	0.99 (0.19, 1.79)	1.14 (0.90, 1.38)	−0.15 (−0.89, 0.59)	0.51 (0.08, 0.93)	0.83 (0.48, 1.18)	−0.32 (−0.71, 0.06)
Systolic blood pressure — mm Hg						
Mean at 48 week (95% CI)	126 (124, 128)	126 (124, 129)		125 (123, 127)	128 (124, 131)	
Absolute change from baseline	0.33 (−1.64, 2.29)	1.63 (−0.41, 3.69)	−1.31 (−2.97,0.35)	−0.11 (−2.54, 2.32)	0.82 (−2.07, 3.71)	−0.93 (−3.64, 1.78)
Diastolic blood pressure — mm Hg						
Mean at 48 week (95% CI)	77(75, 78)	77 (76, 79)		78 (76, 79)	78 (76, 79)	
Absolute change from baseline	−0.88 (−2.17, 0.40)	−0.54 (−1.98, 0.91)	−0.35 (−2.33, 1.63)	−0.98 (−2.40, 0.44)	−0.04 (−1.64, 1.56)	−0.94 (−2.98, 1.10)
Total cholesterol —mmol/L						
Mean at 48 week (95% CI)	4.95 (4.80, 5.11)	4.67 (4.51, 4.83)		5.21 (5.02, 5.39)	4.84 (4.64, 5.03)	
Absolute change from baseline	−0.02 (−0.15, 0.11)	−0.30 (−0.54, −0.07)	0.28 (0.02, 0.54)	0.07 (−0.21, 0.34)	−0.13 (−0.28, 0.02)	0.20 (−0.10, 0.49)
Low-density lipoprotein— mmol/L						
Mean at 48 week (95% CI)	2.96 (2.78, 3.15)	2.69 (2.54, 2.84)		2.88 (2.69, 3.08)	2.79 (2.62, 2.97)	

Table 2. Cont.

	Treatment Naïve Group			Metformin Group		
	Xiaoke Pill	Glibenclamide	Difference in Mean Change (95% CI)	Xiaoke Pill	Glibenclamide	Difference in Mean Change (95% CI)
Absolute change from baseline	−0.22 (−0.38, −0.07)	−0.38 (−0.51, −0.23)	0.15 (−0.03, 0.32)	−0.08 (−0.22, 0.06)	−0.31 (−0.46, −0.16)	0.23 (0.06, 0.40)
High-density lipoprotein— mmol/L						
Mean at 48 week (95% CI)	1.06 (1.00, 1.12)	1.05 (1.00, 1.10)		1.07 (1.01, 1.13)	1.12 (1.07, 1.16)	
Absolute change from baseline	−0.08 (−0.11, −0.04)	−0.07 (−0.11, −0.02)	−0.01 (−0.06, 0.03)	−0.02 (−0.07, 0.03)	−0.05 (−0.10, 0.001)	0.03 (−0.03, 0.09)
Triglycerides— mmol/L						
Mean at 48 week (95% CI)	1.97 (1.79, 2.14)	2.03 (1.83, 2.23)		2.43 (2.09, 2.77)	1.87 (1.70, 2.05)	
Absolute change from baseline	−0.12 (−0.30, 0.06)	−0.32 (−0.58, −0.06)	0.20 (−0.09, 0.49)	−0.15 (−0.51, 0.22)	−0.39 (−0.57, −0.20)	0.24 (−0.24, 0.72)
C-peptide— ug/L						
Mean at 48 week (95% CI)	2.22 (1.90, 2.55)	2.34 (2.06, 2.61)		2.29 (2.03, 2.56)	2.08 (1.85, 2.30)	
Absolute change from baseline	−0.12 (−0.37, 0.13)	0.02 (−0.17, 0.21)	−0.14 (−0.41, 0.12)	−0.02 (−0.20, 0.16)	−0.10 (−0.24, 0.05)	0.08 (−0.08, 0.23)
Fasting insulin—mIU/L						
Mean at 48 week (95% CI)	9.50 (8.13, 10.88)	10.68 (9.53, 11.83)		10.07 (9.26, 10.89)	9.74 (8.79, 10.69)	
Absolute change from baseline	−0.53 (−1.53, 0.48)	0.33 (−1.43, 2.10)	−0.86 (−2.79, 1.07)	0.47 (−0.81, 1.75)	−0.10 (−0.81, 0.62)	0.56 (−0.79, 1.92)
HOMA-IR						
Mean at 48 week (95% CI)	3.26 (2.72, 3.80)	3.62 (3.17, 4.06)		3.51 (3.10, 3.91)	3.27 (2.96, 3.58)	
Absolute change from baseline	−0.84 (−1.34, −0.33)	−0.56 (−1.26, 0.14)	0.28 (−0.55, 1.11)	−0.30 (−0.95, 0.34)	−0.72 (−1.09, −0.35)	0.41 (−0.28, 1.10)
HOMA- B						
Mean at 48 week (95% CI)	48.87 (32.94, 64.80)	64.95 (54.69, 75.21)		55.08 (50.66, 59.51)	60.15 (49.18, 71.13)	
Absolute change from baseline	20.50 (12.21, 28.80)	24.77 (14.40, 35.14)	−4.27 (−18.28, 9.74)	16.75 (12.51, 20.99)	21.43 (12.01, 30.85)	−4.68 (−14.75, 5.39)
Score of TCM symptoms of diabetes						
Median (IQR) at 48 week	2 (1,4)	4 (3,5)		3 (2,4)	3.5 (2,5)	
Absolute change from baseline	−5.64 (−6.4, −4.9)	−4.68 (−5.46, −3.89)	−0.96 (−2.08, 0.15)	−6.38 (−7.10, −5.65)	−4.73 (−5.4, −4.03)	−1.65 (−2.66, −0.64)

week, the significant reduction in the FPG level was similar in both treatment arms (Fig. 2E and Table 2).

A significant reduction of total cholesterol by 0.28 mmol/L was observed in the Glibenclamide group (CI of between-group difference: 0.02–0.54 mmol/L). The symptom, as evaluated by the score of *TCM symptoms of diabetes*, was lower in the Xiaoke Pill arm with between-group difference of −0.96 (95% CI: −2.08, 0.15).

Outcome in Metformin Group

Patients in Xiaoke Pill arm were 24% less likely to have any hypoglycemia compared to those in the Glibenclamide arm [OR (95% CI): 0.76 (0.43, 1.35)]. The average annual rate of hypoglycemia was 62% lower in patients treated with Xiaoke Pill [Rate Ratio (95% CI): 0.38 (0.20, 0.71), $p = 0.003$]. There was no significant difference in the incidence of mild hypoglycaemia between the treatment arms. Eight patients reported nocturnal hypoglycemia in the Glibenclamide arm, compared to only one in the Xiaoke Pill arm.

Maximal reduction in the average HbA1c level occurred by 12 week (Fig. 2 C). The mean reduction from baseline in HbA1c at week 48 was 0.45% in the Xiaoke Pill arm and 0.59% in the Glibenclamide arm, with a between group difference (95% CI) of 0.14 (−0.12, 0.39)% (Table 2). The upper-limit of the 95% CI for the between-group mean difference in change from baseline in HbA1c marginally met the pre-specified criterion for declaring non-inferiority of Xiaoke Pill.

At 48 week, 20.1% and 18.9% patients had HbA1c below 6.5% in the Xiaoke Pill and Glibenclamide arm, respectively. The proportion of patients with HbA1c<7% at 48 weeks was higher in the Xiaoke Pill arm [89(47.1%)] compared to those in the Glibenclamide arm [77 (40.5%)], and mean (95% CI) weeks to reach HbA1c<6.5% was 31.1 (28.3, 33.9) and 30.6 (27.8, 33.4) weeks, respectively. The significant reduction in the FPG level was similar in both treatment arms (Fig. 2F and Table 2).

Significant reduction in LDL-C and triglyceride levels, by 0.31 and 0.39 mmol/L, respectively, were observed in the Glibenclamide arm. However, the CI of between-group difference in triglyceride was −0.24, 0.72 mmol/L. The TCM diabetes symptom score was significantly lower in the Xiaoke Pill arm with between-group difference of −1.65 (95% CI: −2.66, −0.64).

Adverse Events

No serious adverse event was reported during the study. The proportions of adverse events, which were reported in only four categories, did not differ significantly (Table S2). For those with dyslipidemia, the average levels of cholesterol and triglyceride did not differ significantly between the treatments.

Discussion

Our study showed that Xiaoke Pill is associated with reduced risk of hypoglycemia and has similar glucose-lowing efficacy as compared with glibenclamide. At the same level of glibenclamide dose and glycemic control, the Xiaoke Pill had clearly demonstrated a reduced incidence and rate of hypoglycemia as compared with glibenclamide, suggesting that the TCM in the Xiaoke Pill had protective effects against hypoglycemia induced by glibenclamide. The herb components in Xiaoke pill include Radix Puerariae, Radix Rehmanniae, Radix Astragali, Radix Trichosanthis, Stylus Zeae Maydis, Fructus Schisandrae Sphenantherae, an d Rhizoma Dioscoreae. A recent study showed Radix astragali, which is one of the TCM components of Xiaoke Pill, could amplify the glucose counter-regulatory response to insulin-induced hypoglycemia in rats [20]. Radix astragali might exert its action directly, or indirectly, in two brain regions, the paraventricular hypothalamus (PVN) and nucleus tractus solitaries (NTS), known to be involved in glucose-sensing during hypoglycemia [20]. One Chinese study found Radix Puerariae could protect neuron from hypoglycemic and hypoxia damage in vitro cell experiment [21]. However, most of the studies focus on the anti-oxidative effect of the traditional Chinese herbs. More studies are needed to interpret the mechanism of TCM's anti-hypoglycemia effect.

Between 4 and 24 weeks of the study, 97 (52.7%) and 95 (51.6%) patients in the treatment naïve group reduced HbA1c below 6.5% in the Xiaoke Pill and Glibenclamide arms, respectively. During same period, 129 (70.1%) and 125 (67.9%) patients reduced FPG below 7 mmol/L. At 48 week, the absolute changes in FPG levels were also similar in the two treatment arms in both study groups (Fig. S1). Our study design allowed comparing the TCM in the Xiaoke Pill to its placebo on top of equal amount of glibenclamide. Given the label limitation on maximum dosage of Xiaoke Pill, the low dose usage of glibenclamide in this trial gave more opportunity of detecting the glucose-lowing effect of TCM.

Five prior studies published in medical journals in China [22–26] showed significant improvement in diabetes symptoms in favor of Xiaoke Pill. These 4–8 weeks open-level studies were mostly single centre studies, and only one study assessed the hypoglycemic events. However, the validity of the design of these studies is questionable, and makes it hard to draw any robust conclusion with regard to safety and efficacy of Xiaoke Pill [27].

Xiaoke Pill was associated with greater improvement in symptoms of diabetes in a pre-specified subgroup analysis. However, caution should be taken in interpreting this result, as improvement in symptoms might also be associated with the reduction of hypoglycemia risk observed in Xiaoke Pill treatment arm. Symptoms associated with hypoglycemia such as fatigue, hunger, and palpitation were included in the score system. Further study is needed to validate this finding with the consideration that this finding might be specific to clinical studies involving glucose lowing agents that could cause hypoglycemia.

No differences were observed in changes in insulin resistance, β-cell function, HDL, triglyceride, blood pressure, hsCRP and adiponectin (data not presented) between Xiaoke Pill and Glibenclamide treatment arms. Such results suggest that TCM in Xiaoke pill had no additional impact on the pathophysiological changes associated with type 2 diabetes.

TCM is used widely in treating type 2 diabetes not only in China, but also in the other parts of the world. But the role of TCM and other herbal medicines in the management of type 2 diabetes is still not established [28]. The absence of scientific understanding has caused skepticism and criticism about TCM, often because of the low methodological quality of trials [8,9,11,29,30]. Furthermore, most of these trials were published in Chinese and were not included in systematic reviews. Selective publication of positive trials is another problem. Over 80% [28] of people in developing countries depend on herbal medicine for basic health care. Thus the evidence for safety and efficacy of TCM use for treatment of diabetes, provided by this study, is a contribution towards reducing entrenched inequity in access to effective care for poor people.

Supporting Information

Table S1 Score of TCM symptoms of diabetes.
(DOC)

Table S2 Adverse Events.
(DOC)

Figure S1 Mean (95% CI) percentage change at 48 weeks from baseline in Glycated Hemoglobin, Fasting Plasma Glucose and Symptom Score.
(DOC)

Checklist S1 CONSORT checklist.
(DOC)

Protocol S1 Trial protocol.
(DOC)

Appendix S1 List of Investigators.
(DOC)

Acknowledgments

We thank all the patients for agreeing to participate in this study. We are grateful to the nurses as well as technicians in the laboratory for their practical work during the study.

Author Contributions

Critically revised the menuscript for important intellectual content: LJ HW HT HZ LZ Qifu Li YW HL ML HY YG YL Quanmin Li XG GY Z. Zhang Z. Zhou GN YC SP Performed the experiments: The Evidence-Based Medical Research of Xiaoke Pill Study Group. Conceived and designed the experiments: LJ XT HT XG ML Qifu Li YL. Performed the experiments: The Evidence-Based Medical Research of Xiaoke Pill Study Investigators. Analyzed the data: LJ YL SP. Contributed reagents/materials/analysis tools: HW SP. Wrote the paper: LJ SP. Critically revised the manuscript for important intellectual content: LJ HW HT HZ LZ Qifu Li YW HL ML HY YG YL Quanmin Li XG GY Z. Zhang Z. Zhou GN YC SP.

References

1. Cheng JT (2000) Review: drug therapy in Chinese traditional medicine. The Journal of Clinical Pharmacology 40: 445–450.
2. Zhang H, Tan C, Wang H, Xue S, Wang M (2010) Study on the history of Traditional Chinese Medicine to treat diabetes. Eur J of Integr Med 2: 41–46.
3. Ni MS (1995) The Yellow Emperor's Classic of Medicine: A New Translation of the NeijingSuwen with Commentary. Boston, MA: Shambhala Publications. 316 p.
4. Cang Chung-Ching HH (1983) Chin Kuei You Lueh. Long Beach: Oriental Healing Arts Institute: 240 p.
5. Hsu HY (1978) Chinese herb therapy for diabetes mellitus. Bull of the Oriental Healing Arts Inst 3: 12–17.
6. Sena M, Chuang G, Tam W, Tam G, Tam C (2009) Survey of biological active molecules in the Chinese traditional herbal formula LiuWeiDiHuangWan for the treatment of Type II Diabetes. FASEB J 23: 900–905.
7. Zhang Y, Ma Y, Zhou W, Chen J, Wei C (2004) Effect of LiuweiDihuang decoction on the function of hypothalamus-pituitary-ovary axis in senescence-accelerated mouse. Int Congress Ser 1260: 421–426.
8. Li WL, Zheng HC, Bukuru J, Kimpe ND (2004) Natural medicines used in the traditional Chinese medical system fortherapy of diabetes mellitus. J Ethnopharmacol 92: 1–21.
9. Liu JP, Zhang M, Wang WY, Grimsgaard S (2004) Chinese herbal medicines for type 2 diabetes mellitus. Cochrane Database Syst Rev 3: CD003642.
10. Xie WD, Zhao Y, Zhang Y (2011) Traditional Chinese Medicines in Treatment of Patients with Type 2 Diabetes Mellitus. Evidence-Based Complementary and Alternative Medicine: 726723.
11. Yeh GY, Eisenberg DM, Kaptchuk TJ, Phillips RS (2003) Systematic review of herbs and dietary supplements for glycemic control in diabetes. Diabetes Care 26: 1277–1294.
12. Ye TS (2006) Record of medical practice. Beijing: People's Medical Publishing House. 553 p.
13. Zhu DX, Yang SZ (1993) The Heart and Essence of Dan-xi's Methods of Treatment. Boulder, CO: Blue Poppy Press. 450 p.
14. Pharmacopoeia Commission (2010) Pharmacopoeia of the People's Republic of China. Beijing: China Medical Science and Technology Press. 1248 p.
15. Li M, Fisette A, Zhao XY, Deng JY, Mi J, et al (2009) Serum resistin correlates with central obesity but weakly with insulin resistance in Chinese children and adolescents. Int J Obes 33: 424–439.
16. Zheng X (2010) Principal Guideline For the Development of New Traditional Chinese Medicine. Beijing: China Medical Science Press. 727 p.
17. Home PD, Jones NP, Pocock SJ, Beck-Nielsen H, Gomis R, et al. (2007) Rosiglitazone RECORD study: glucose control outcomes at 18 months. Diabet Med 24: 626–634.
18. Kenward MG, Carpenter J (2007) Multiple imputation: current perspectives. Stat Methods Med Res 16: 199–218.
19. Demidenko E (2004) Mixed models: theory and applications. Hoboken, NJ: Wiley. 736 p.
20. Sang Z, Zhou L, Fan X, McCrimmon RJ (2010) Radix astragali (huangqi) as a treatment for defective hypoglycemia counterregulation in diabetes. Am J Chin Med 38: 1027–1038.
21. Xu XH, Zheng XX (2008) Effects of Puerarin on the Levels of Calcium and Nitric Oxide in Cultured H ippocampal Neurons during Oxygen-G lucose Deprivation. Chin Pharm J 43: 1308–1312
22. Zhou R, Guo JJ, Yin CM, Li TK (2003) Clinical observations of Xiaoke Wan in treatment of type 2 diabetic patients(Qi and Yin deficiency zheng). Zhong guoYao Wu Yu Lin Chuang 3: 131–132
23. Zhang HZ (1999) Clinical observation into Xiaoke Wan in the treatment of 86 cases of type 2 diabetic patients. Zhong Yi Yao Yan Jiu 15: 19–21
24. Zhao YC, Hou M (1998) Xiaoke Wan in treatment of 200 cases of type 2 diabetic patients. Changchun Zhong Yi Xue Yuan Xue Bao 14: 15
25. Chen G, Ni YD, Lai XM, Liang HQ (2003) Clinical study on Xiaoke Wan in treating type 2 diabetes mellitus with Qiand Yin Defiency. Zhong Yao Xin Yao Yu Lin Chuang Yao Li 14: 84–86
26. Wu JL (2005) Observations into the effects of Xiaoke Wan in treatment of diabetes. Shi Yong Zhong Xi Yi Jie He Lin Chuang 5: 18–19
27. Wang G, Mao B, Xiong ZY, Fan T, Chen XD, et al. (2007) The Quality of Reporting of Randomized Controlled Trials of Traditional Chinese Medicine: A Survey of 13 Randomly Selected Journals from Mainland China. Clin ther 29: 1456–1467
28. European Medicines Agency (2005) Public statement on the risk associated with the use of herbal products containing Aristolochia species. Available: http://www.emea.europa.eu/pdfs/human/hmpc/13838105en.pdf. Accessed 2008 Jul 10.
29. Tang JL, Zhan SY, Ernst E (1999) Review of randomised controlled trials of traditional Chinese medicine. BMJ 319: 160–161.
30. Wang E, Wylie-Rosett J (2008) Review of selected Chinese herbal medicines in the treatment of type 2 diabetes. Diabetes Educ 34: 645–654.

6

An Epidemiological Study of Concomitant Use of Chinese Medicine and Antipsychotics in Schizophrenic Patients: Implication for Herb-Drug Interaction

Zhang-Jin Zhang[1,2*], Qing-Rong Tan[2*], Yao Tong[1], Xue-Yi Wang[3], Huai-Hai Wang[2], Lai-Ming Ho[4], Hei Kiu Wong[1], Yi-Bin Feng[1], Di Wang[1], Roger Ng[5], Grainne M. McAlonan[6], Chuan-Yue Wang[7], Vivian Taam Wong[8]

1 School of Chinese Medicine, Faculty of Medicine, the University of Hong Kong, Hong Kong, China, **2** Department of Psychiatry, Fourth Military Medical University, Xijing Hospital, Xi'an, Shaanxi, China, **3** Mental Health Center, Hebei Medical University, Shijiazhuang, Hebei, China, **4** School of Public Health, the University of Hong Kong, Hong Kong, China, **5** Department of Psychiatry, Kowloon Hospital, Hong Kong, China, **6** Department of Psychiatry, the University of Hong Kong, Hong Kong, China, **7** Capital Medical University, Beijing Anding Hospital, Beijing, China, **8** Chinese Medicine Section, Hospital Authority, Hong Kong, China

Abstract

Background: Herb-drug interactions are an important issue in drug safety and clinical practice. The aim of this epidemiological study was to characterize associations of clinical outcomes with concomitant herbal and antipsychotic use in patients with schizophrenia.

Methods and Findings: In this retrospective, cross-sectional study, 1795 patients with schizophrenia who were randomly selected from 17 psychiatric hospitals in China were interviewed face-to-face using a structured questionnaire. Association analyses were conducted to examine correlates between Chinese medicine (CM) use and demographic, clinical variables, antipsychotic medication mode, and clinical outcomes. The prevalence of concomitant CM and antipsychotic treatment was 36.4% [95% confidence interval (95% CI) 34.2%–38.6%]. Patients using concomitant CM had a significantly greater chance of improved outcomes than non-CM use (61.1% vs. 34.3%, OR = 3.44, 95% CI 2.80–4.24). However, a small but significant number of patients treated concomitantly with CM had a greater risk of developing worse outcomes (7.2% vs. 4.4%, OR = 2.06, 95% CI 2.06–4.83). Significant predictors for concomitant CM treatment-associated outcomes were residence in urban areas, paranoid psychosis, and exceeding 3 months of CM use. Herbal medicine regimens containing Radix Bupleuri, Fructus Gardenia, Fructus Schisandrae, Radix Rehmanniae, Akebia Caulis, and Semen Plantaginis in concomitant use with quetiapine, clozapine, and olanzepine were associated with nearly 60% of the risk of adverse outcomes.

Conclusions: Concomitant herbal and antipsychotic treatment could produce either beneficial or adverse clinical effects in schizophrenic population. Potential herb-drug pharmacokinetic interactions need to be further evaluated.

Editor: Ehsan Syed, Pennsylvania State University, United States of America

Funding: This study was supported by the intramural research fund of the University of Hong Kong and Hospital Authority of Hong Kong. The funders had no role in study design, data collection and analysis, decision to publish, or preparation of the manuscript.

Competing Interests: The authors have declared that no competing interests exist.

* E-mail: zhangzj@hku.hk (ZJZ); tanqingr@fmmu.edu.cn (QRT)

Introduction

With the widespread use of various herbal products which are often concomitantly used with pharmaceutical drugs, herb-drug interactions have become an important issue in drug safety and clinical practice [1,2]. This was initially because of several case studies reporting nephrotoxic and hepatotoxic effects associated with herbal medicine use [3–5]. It is well documented that concomitant use of herbal medicine with conventional drug treatment can alter pharmacokinetic profiles of many classes of pharmaceutical drugs, including psychotropic agents, anticoagulants, oral contraceptives, immunosuppressants, cardiovascular drugs, anti-HIV, anticancer agents and antiepileptics [1,2,6]. However, whether such concomitant treatment with herbal and conventional medicine is associated with clinical outcomes in a defined population of patients remains to be determined.

Most patients with schizophrenia may develop a chronic course and are required for long-term maintenance treatment [7]. Although antipsychotic therapy is a mainstay in the maintenance treatment of schizophrenia, patients still often experience relapse and various adverse events caused by antipsychotic treatment [7]. In order to improve the therapeutic efficacy and reduce adverse side effects related to antipsychotic therapy, herbal medicine and other alternative therapies have been increasingly introduced into the treatment of schizophrenia [8]. This is particularly apparent in Chinese patients who have distinctive perceptions of Chinese medicine (CM), of which herbal materials account for about 85% preparations and products.

Numerous studies have shown therapeutic benefits of herbal medicine for persistent negative symptoms, cognitive impairment, and adverse side effects in schizophrenic patients [8]. Our recent study revealed that herbal medicine could alleviate hyperprolactinemia in schizophrenic patients [9]. Nevertheless, there are also case studies reporting acute and persistent psychosis caused by herbal supplementary use [10,11]. These data suggest that herbal medicine in combination with antipsychotic drugs may produce either positive or negative clinical effects, making it important to examine potential relationships between clinical outcomes and concomitant treatment with herbal and antipsychotic agents in schizophrenia.

The primary objective of this epidemiological survey was to determine the prevalence of CM concomitant use and its associations with demographic, clinical characteristics and treatment outcomes in a random sample of patients with schizophrenia through face-to-face interview using a structured questionnaire.

Methods

Study design and setting

This retrospective, cross-sectional epidemiological study was conducted in 17 psychiatric hospitals and mental health centers in China. The selection of the study sites was based on geographic and sociodemographic variations as previously described [12], with particular consideration of regions, local economic development levels, and overall educational levels, as these variables are heavily related to perceptions and beliefs for CM. The study was approved by Institutional Review Board (IRB) of the University of Hong Kong/Hospital Authority Hong Kong West Cluster and registered at www.HKClinicalTrials.com (HKCTR-874). All participants or their guardians were required to give written informed consent for participating in the survey. The survey was conducted between April 2009 and September 2009.

Population and sample

The study population was confined to patients with schizophrenia who visited psychiatric clinics or were hospitalized during the survey period. Patients who met the following criteria were eligible for the study: (1) aged 15 years or above; (2) had a primary diagnosis of schizophrenia or schizoaffective disorder based on *International Classification of Diseases (ICD), 10th Edition* [13]; (3) had been taking conventional antipsychotic treatment for at least 6 weeks; and (4) patients, their caregivers and/or doctors could provide necessary information about CM use if CM was used.

One key question that the present study attempted to answer was whether concomitant use of CM could affect the clinical outcomes of patients with schizophrenia, particularly adverse outcomes related to concomitant CM and antipsychotic use. Estimation of sample size was therefore based on the prevalence of CM use and the proportion of CM users with worse outcomes (see below). These two indices had been obtained from a pilot survey of 297 patients with schizophrenia [8], showing that nearly 36% of patients concomitantly used CM and 5.7% of CM users experienced worse outcomes, while only 2.8% of non-CM users had worse outcomes. In order to detect a 2.9% difference in the rate of worse outcomes between CM users and non-CM users, with a power (1-β) of 80% and a two-tailed level of $\alpha = 0.05$, 1750 participants were required to detect statistical difference in terms of worse outcomes associated with concomitant CM use. The number of surveyed subjects allocated to each study site was determined based on the volume of visits and annual admission numbers. The selection of eligible patients at each survey site was determined using random number tables.

Study instruments

A specifically designed structured questionnaire was administered in the survey. The questionnaire covered: (1) sociodemographic and clinical characteristics; (2) purpose, advice source, attitude, and awareness of CM use; (3) the concomitant use pattern including individual CMs, conventional medication modes, and duration of the concomitant use; and (4) clinical outcomes. Chinese medicine (CM) is defined as preparations and products in powder, tablet, capsule, soft-gel, or liquid form prepared from single or mixed herbal, mineral, and animal materials or extracts [8]. CM users were defined as those who had been using CM consecutively for at least one month or cumulatively for at least 3 months with no more than 45 days of absence in total and no more than 7 consecutive days of absence when the survey was conducted. Those who never or only occasionally used CM were defined as non-CM users. This definition of the length of CM use was based on CM clinical practice, demonstrating that CM therapy of most chronic mental-emotional conditions requires a considerable period before observable improvements are achieved [14].

Clinical outcomes were classified as improved, worse, and unchanged condition. Improved outcomes were defined as clinically meaningful improvements occurring in the preceding one month on one or more conditions as follows: (1) psychosis; (2) comorbid psychiatric symptoms, mainly anxiety, depression, cognitive impairment, and sleep disorders; (3) adverse side effects associated with antipsychotic therapy, frequently body weight gain, constipation, enuresis, hyperprolactinemia, hypersalivation, leukopenia, and tardive dyskinesia; and (4) comorbid non-psychiatric conditions, such as hypertension and diabetes. Worse outcomes were defined as hospitalization, emergency room visits, or changes in medication modes due to the worsening of psychosis, comorbid symptoms, intolerable side effects, or the occurrence of new comorbid symptoms in the preceding one month. Patients who did not experience either clinically meaningful improvement or worsening in the preceding one month were defined as subjects with unchanged conditions. The assessment of clinical outcomes was conducted by psychiatrists based on changes in the severity and frequency of episodes of related symptoms, physical examination, and laboratory tests as well as reports from patients and their guardians.

Survey procedures

The survey was performed by trained psychiatrists on site with face-to-face interview. To ensure consistency of the survey across sites and over time, two sessions of training workshop were conducted for interviewers who were practicing psychiatry. Upon completion of the training workshops, inter-rater reliability was assessed by calculating interrater agreement coefficients (κ value) for the designed questionnaire. All interviewers had achieved a κ value of at least 0.8 after training sessions. In addition, post-survey interviews were further conducted to verify missing and illogical data.

Data analysis

The prevalence of CM use was calculated using maximum likelihood estimation of logistic regression. Chi-square (χ^2) test was used to determine bivariate associations between CM use and demographic and clinical variables. Binary logistic regression model was further used for multivariate analyses to identify independent factors associated with CM use from the same variable tested in the bivariate analysis. The association between clinical outcomes and CM use was also examined using Chi-square (χ^2) test and binary logistic regression analysis, with adjustment for demographic and clinical variables that were found to be significantly associated with CM use.

Subgroup analyses were conducted in CM-using subjects to further determine associations between clinical outcomes and CM and antipsychotic concomitant use modes. Chi-square test and multinomial logistic regression model were respectively utilized to examine bivariate and multivariate associations of clinical outcomes with demographic and clinical variables. Multinomial logistic regression model was also applied to evaluate associations of clinical outcomes with individual CMs and antipsychotic regimens that were used in at least 5% of CM-using respondents with either improved or worsened conditions, with adjustment for demographic and clinical variables that were shown to be significantly associated with clinical outcomes.

Odds ratio (OR) and 95% confidence interval (95% CI) were obtained from binary and multinomial logistic regression analysis. In association analyses of clinical outcomes, the unchanged outcome served as reference for improved and worse outcome in the calculation of OR values. All analyses were performed with SPSS version 16 software (Chicago, IL, USA). Statistical significance was defined as $p<0.05$ and all tests were two-sided.

Results

The characteristics of the sample

In a total of 1795 eligible subjects surveyed, seven were excluded from the analyses due to missing basic demographic and clinical data (gender, age, and the illness duration). In the remaining 1788 subjects who were included in the final analyses, 51% were males and the mean (±SD) age was 32±12 years. Fifty-three percent were diagnosed with paranoid schizophrenia. These demographic and clinical characteristics were similar to those reported in previous epidemiological surveys of schizophrenic population in China [15].

The characteristics of antipsychotic medication modes

Thirty-five psychotropic drugs were identified. Medication regimens of 99.3% subjects included antipsychotics and 43% had two or more antipsychotics. The remaining 0.7% subjects were medicated with mood stabilizers occasionally combined with antipsychotics. The most commonly used antipsychotics in all subjects were risperidone (50.8%), quetiapine (21.0%), clozapine (17.2%), olanzapine (8.2%), and phenothiazines (7.0%). This medication mode was similar to that previously reported in China [16]. No significant differences were observed in frequency distribution of these antipsychotic regimens between CM- and non-CM-using subjects (see below), except for risperidone monotherapy. For the latter the proportion of CM-using respondents treated was significantly higher than non-CM-using respondents (30.8% vs. 23.4%, $p<0.001$, Chi-square test).

The prevalence and characteristics of CM use

Direct observation showed a prevalence of 37.5% (671/1788) of the concomitant use. Re-calculation using maximum likelihood estimation yielded a similar prevalence of 36.4% (95% CI: 34.2%–38.6%). One hundred and twenty different CM materials used were identified: 92 herbal materials, 12 mineral materials, and 16 animal materials. But 33.7% of CM-using subjects were unable to provide full information about their CM formulae or prescriptions for identifying individual CMs. Only a small portion (6.4%, 43/671) of CM-using patients used single-herbal preparations.

There were 86% of CM-users who used CM therapy initially in order to enhance antipsychotic efficacy, reduce antipsychotic-induced adverse side effects and comorbid psychiatric symptoms (mainly anxiety, depression, cognitive and sleep problems). Sixty-six percent of CM users reported that CM use was recommended by their psychiatrists. Most CMs were prescribed by CM practitioners. Nearly 47% of CM-users were entirely unaware of potential risks of concomitant use of herbal and antipsychotic agents; only 16.4% realized such potential risks. In non-CM-using patients, 35.1% did not know much about CM and 58.1% did not think CM was helpful for their conditions, while only 5.1% were aware of the potential risks of the concomitant treatment.

Demographic and clinical correlates of CM use

Bivariate analysis displayed significant associations of CM use with gender ($p=0.002$), household income ($p=0.001$), the illness duration ($p<0.001$), number of episode ($p<0.001$), and number of hospitalization ($p<0.001$) (Table 1). Multivariate analysis further revealed that CM use was significantly associated with male (OR = 1.32, 95% CI 1.09-1.62, $p=0.006$), residence in rural areas (OR = 1.48, 95% CI 1.18–1.85, $p=0.001$), average (OR = 1.56, 95% CI 1.19–2.06, $p=0.001$) and high (OR = 2.36, 95% CI 1.58–3.53, $p<0.001$) household income, and greater than one year of illness duration (OR = 1.95, 95% CI 1.45–2.63, $p<0.001$).

CM use correlates of clinical outcomes

While 61.1% (410/671) of CM-using patients and 34.3% (383/1117) of non-CM-using patients displayed improved outcomes, 7.2% (48/671) CM users and 4.4% (49/1117) of non-CM users experienced worse outcomes in the preceding one month (Table 2). Chi-square tests showed that clinical outcomes were significantly associated with whether CM was concomitantly used with antipsychotic drugs ($p<0.001$). In a binary logistic regression model, CM users had significantly greater odds of improved (OR = 3.44, 95% CI 2.80–4.24, $p<0.001$) and worse outcomes (OR = 3.15, 95% CI 2.06–4.83, $p<0.001$) compared to non-CM users.

Demographic and clinical correlates of clinical outcomes in CM users

Chi-square tests showed that clinical outcomes were significantly associated with resident areas ($p<0.001$), diagnostic types ($p<0.001$), and duration of CM use ($p=0.007$). Multinomial logistic regression analysis further revealed significant associations of improved outcomes with residence in urban areas (OR = 4.81, 95% CI 3.14–7.36, $p<0.001$), paranoid schizophrenia (OR = 2.65, 95% CI 1.83–3.84, $p<0.001$) and more than 3 months of CM use (OR = 1.35, 95% CI 0.91–1.98, $p=0.036$). In CM users who experienced worse conditions, similar significant multivariate associations were also observed with residence in urban areas (OR = 6.91, 95% CI 3.09–15.43, $p<0.001$), paranoid schizophrenia (OR = 1.89, 95% CI 0.96–3.71, $p=0.012$), and more than 3 months of CM use (OR = 3.28, 95% CI 1.44–7.46, $p=0.005$) (Table 3).

Antipsychotic medication correlates of clinical outcomes in CM users

Five different antipsychotic agents and five antipsychotic treatment regimens that were used in at least 5% of CM-using patients with either improved or worse outcomes were identified (Table 4). Multinomial logistical regression analyses, with adjustment for resident areas, diagnostic types, and duration of CM use, variables that were significantly associated with clinical outcomes, revealed no significant associations with any antipsychotic treatment regimens favoring improve outcomes, but significantly lower odds of improved outcomes were observed in patients whose antipsychotic regimens included olanzapine (OR = 0.48, 95% CI 0.27–0.85, $p=0.035$). There were significantly higher odds of worse outcomes in subjects whose

Table 1. Bivariate and multivariate associations of CM use with demographic and clinical variables in patients with schizophrenia under antipsychotic medication.[a]

Variable	bivariate			Multivariate	
	n	CM use (%)	p	OR (95% CI)	p
Gender			0.002		
Female	879	33.9		1	
Male	909	41.0		1.32 (1.09–1.62)	0.006
Age, yrs			0.108		
<18	92	31.5		1	
18–45	1478	37.1		1.04 (0.58–1.37)	0.899
>45	218	43.1		1.17 (0.71–1.94)	0.540
Marital status			0.109		
Single/divorce/widow	1004	35.9		1	
Married	784	39.7		1.06 (0.86–1.32)	0.589
Education, yrs			0.391		
≤10	1064	36.8		1	
11–13	458	40.2		1.27 (0.99–1.63)	0.062
≥14	266	36.1		1.01 (0.72–1.42)	0.941
Occupation			0.645		
Unemployed	368	38.9		1	
Non-professional	927	37.9		0.92 (0.68–1.24)	0.568
Professional and students	493	35.9		0.81 (0.62–1.08)	0.153
Resident areas			0.135		
Urban	1120	36.2		1	
Rural	668	39.8		1.48 (1.18–1.85)	0.001
Household income [b]			0.001		
Low	330	30.6		1	
Average	1242	37.9		1.56 (1.19–2.06)	0.001
High	216	45.8		2.36 (1.58–3.53)	
<0.001					
Diagnostic subtype			0.143		
Paranoid	942	39.2		1	
Non-paranoid [c]	846	35.7		0.89 (0.73–1.09)	0.245
Duration of the illness, yrs			<0.001		
≤1	396	25.0		1	
>1	1392	41.1		1.95 (1.45–2.63)	
<0.001					
Number of episodes			<0.001		
≤2	895	32.2		1	
>2	893	42.9		1.14 (0.84–1.53)	0.402
Number of hospitalization			<0.001		
≤2	1142	33.9		1	
>2	646	44.0		1.18 (0.88–1.58)	0.270

a. CM, Chinese medicine. Data analyses were based on CM users (n = 671) with non-CM users (n = 1117) as reference. Chi-square test was used for bivariate analysis and binary logistic regression mode for multivariate analysis.
b. Household income was compared to local average levels.
c. Non-paranoid psychosis includes disorganized, undifferentiated, residual, and tonic types of schizophrenia and schizoaffective disorder.

Table 2. Bivariate and multivariate associations between clinical outcomes and CM use in patients with schizophrenia.[a]

Outcomes	Bivariate			Multivariate	
	n	CM users (%)	p	OR (95% CI) [b]	p
			<0.001		
Unchanged	898	23.7		1	
Improved	793	51.7		3.44 (2.80–4.24)	<0.001
Worse	97	49.5		3.15 (2.06–4.83)	<0.001

a. CM, Chinese medicine. Data analyses were based on CM users (n = 671) with non-CM users (n = 1117) as reference. Chi-square test was used for bivariate analysis and binary logistic regression for multivariate analysis.
b. Binary logistic regression analysis was adjusted for sex, resident areas, household income, duration of illness, number of episode, and number of hospitalization, variables significantly associated with CM use as shown in Table 1.

antipsychotic regimens included quetiapine (OR = 1.90, 95% CI 0.88–4.08, p = 0.013), quetiapine alone (OR = 2.16, 95% CI 0.95–4.95, p = 0.031) or clozapine alone (OR = 3.02, 95% CI 0.94–9.70, p = 0.025) (Table 4).

Individual CM correlates of clinical outcomes

Of 120 different CM materials identified, 21 (20 herbal materials and one animal material) were used in at least 5% of CM-using subjects with either improved or worse outcomes (Table 5). Multinomial logistic regression model analysis showed no significant associations of improved outcomes with any individual CMs identified, but the inclusion of Acorus gramineus in CM treatment regimens significantly reduced odds of worse outcomes compared to improved outcomes (OR = 0.11, 95% CI 0.01–0.88, p = 0.037). Significantly higher odds of worse outcomes were observed in subjects whose CM treatment regimens included Radix Bupleuri (OR = 2.49, 95% CI 1.10–5.62, p = 0.028), Fructus Gardenia (OR = 9.16, 95% CI 4.19–20.02, p<0.001), Fructus Schisandrae (OR = 3.90, 95% CI 1.42–10.73, P = 0.008), Radix Rehmanniae (OR = 3.48, 95% CI 1.03–11.70, p = 0.044), Akebia Caulis (OR = 14.6, 95% CI 2.50–31.87, p<0.001), and Semen Plantaginis (OR = 21.10, 95% CI 4.32–103.05, p<0.001). Frequency distributions revealed that concomitant treatment regimens containing these six herbal materials and worse outcome-associated antipsychotics accounted for 59.8% (49/82) of total identified concomitant treatment regimens in patients with worse outcomes (Table 6).

Discussion

In our survey of a representative sample of patients with schizophrenia, nearly 36% of them had concomitant CM and antipsychotic treatment. This prevalence rate of CM use is somewhat lower than that observed in other commonly occurring chronic conditions in Chinese communities [17–19]. In non-CM-using patients, nearly 58% did not believe CM could help their condition, suggesting that the lower prevalence of CM use in schizophrenic population is mainly related to their negative attitude towards this traditional remedy. Unlike patients in Western society where a minority of them informed their doctors of their use of alternative medicine [20,21], CM use in most patients in this study was recommended by their psychiatrists. However, only about one-third of patients were aware of the

Table 3. Bivariate and multivariate associations of clinical outcomes with demographic and clinical variables in schizophrenic patients in Chinese medicine and antipsychotic concomitant treatment.[a]

	Bivariate				Multivariate-IM		Multivariate-WS	
	n	IM (%)	WS (%)	p	OR (95% CI)	p	OR (95% CI)	p
Gender				0.344				
Male	373	62.2	8.0		1		1	
Female	298	59.7	6.0		0.77 (0.53–1.12)	0.173	0.55 (0.28–1.10)	0.091
Age, yrs				0.625				
<18	29	72.4	6.9		1		1	
18–45	548	61.1	7.3		0.76 (0.24–2.43)	0.304	0.73 (0.09–5.81)	0.325
>45	74	57.5	6.4		0.40 (0.14–1.16)	0.231	0.66 (0.10–4.19)	0.438
Marital status				0.349				
Single/divorce/widow	360	58.9	6.9		1		1	
Married	311	63.7	7.4		1.23 (0.83–1.82)	0.816	1.30 (0.63–2.65)	0.478
Education, yrs				0.270				
≤10	391	62.7	8.4		1		1	
11–13	184	58.7	4.9		0.72 (0.46–1.12)	0.183	0.52 (0.21–1.24)	0.299
≥14	96	59.4	6.3		0.92 (0.50–1.69)	0.476	0.90 (0.30–2.73)	0.335
Occupation				0.345				
Unemployed	143	55.2	8.4		1		1	
Non-professional	351	63.3	7.7		1.69 (1.03–2.78)	0.183	1.39 (0.58–3.32)	0.186
Professional/students	177	61.6	5.1		1.17 (0.68–2.02)	0.835	0.70 (0.25–1.93)	0.460
Resident areas				<0.001				
Rural	266	48.9	8.2		1		1	
Urban	405	69.1	5.6		4.81 (3.14–7.36)	<0.001	6.91 (3.09–15.43)	<0.001
Household income [b]				0.302				
Low	101	56.4	11.9		1		1	
Average	471	62.6	6.4		1.57 (0.74–3.29)	0.213	0.66 (0.18–2.41)	0.191
High	99	58.6	6.1		1.41 (0.82–2.42)	0.136	0.44 (0.18–1.06)	0.291
Diagnostic subtype				<0.001				
Non-paranoid [b]	302	50.7	7.2		1		1	
Paranoid	369	69.7	7.0		2.65 (1.83–3.84)	<0.001	1.89 (0.96–3.71)	0.012
Duration of illness, yrs				0.991				
≤1	99	60.6	7.1		1		1	
>1	572	61.2	7.2		1.02 (0.56–1.84)	0.958	1.17 (0.40–3.42)	0.769
Number of episodes				0.747				
≤2	288	60.1	8.0		1		1	
>2	383	61.9	6.5		1.13 (0.65–1.97)	0.663	0.75 (0.27–2.13)	0.594
Number of hospitalization				0.780				
≤2	387	61.8	7.5		1		1	
>2	284	60.2	6.7		0.88 (0.51–1.52)	0.655	0.86 (0.31–2.40)	0.775
Duration of CM use, months				0.007				
1-3	233	58.4	3.9		1		1	
>3	438	62.6	8.9		1.35 (0.91–1.98)	0.036	3.28 (1.44–7.46)	0.005

a. CM, Chinese medicine; IM, improved; WS, worse. Data analyses were based on CM users (N = 671) who had clinical outcomes with improved (n = 410), worse (n = 48), and unchanged (n = 213) conditions. The unchanged condition served as reference. Chi-square test was used for bivariate analysis and multinomial logistic regression for multivariate analysis.
b. The definitions of household income and non-paranoid schizophrenia are the same as Table 1.

potential risks of concomitant treatment with CM. These findings may reflect an underestimation of both potential benefits and risks of CM use among patients and their psychiatrists.

We found that concomitant CM use was significantly associated with male, residence in rural areas, relatively higher household income, longer duration of illness, and more episodes and

Table 4. Multivariate associations between clinical outcomes and antipsychotic medication modes in patients with schizophrenia who were treated concomitantly with CM.[a]

	Improved (n = 410)			Worse (n = 48)		
	%	OR (95% CI)	p	%	OR (95% CI)	p
The most frequently used antipsychotics						
Risperidone	56.1	1.22 (0.86–1.75)	0.900	41.7	0.81 (0.42–1.56)	0.696
Quetiapine	19.5	0.75 (0.49–1.16)	0.463	27.1 [b]	1.90 (0.88–4.08)	0.013
Clozapine	20.7	1.40 (0.90–2.19)	0.542	22.9	1.29 (0.63–2.66)	0.068
Olanzapine	7.1	0.48 (0.27–0.85)	0.035	12.5	0.97 (0.37–2.54)	0.463
Phenothiazines	6.5	0.92 (0.47–1.81)	0.819	2.1	0.25 (0.03–1.95)	0.837
The most frequently used antipsychotic regimens						
Risperidone alone	33.9	1.34 (0.90–1.99)	0.276	33.3	1.14 (0.56–2.31)	0.424
Quetiapine alone [b]	11.7	0.69 (0.41–1.17)	0.063	27.1 [b]	2.16 (0.95–4.95)	0.031
Clozapine + risperidone	6.3	1.43 (0.65–3.17)	0.527	8.3	2.63 (0.74–9.38)	0.064
Clozapine alone	4.6	1.37 (0.60–3.12)	0.438	12.5	3.02 (0.94–9.70)	0.025
Olanzapine alone	4.1	0.57 (0.27–1.22)	0.213	12.5	1.88 (0.66–5.34)	0.399

a. CM, Chinese medicine. Unchanged outcomes (n = 213) served as reference. Multinomial logistical regression analysis was adjusted for resident areas, diagnostic subtype, and duration of CM use, variables significantly associated with clinical outcomes as shown in Table 3.
b. It is noted that all quetiapine-including treatment regimens are quetiapine monotherapy.

hospitalizations. These associations suggest that the men living in rural areas may have greater positive beliefs about CM for their illnesses. Previous studies also showed that people who had persistent and recurrent mental-emotional problems more often sought alternative therapies than populations with other chronic diseases [21,22].

While it was similar in most antipsychotic treatment regimens in CM- and non-CM-using patients, there exist significant bivariate and multivariate associations between CM use and clinical outcomes. Patients in CM concomitant treatment had a significantly greater chance of improved clinical outcomes compared to non-CM use (61.1% vs. 34.3%, OR = 3.44, 95% CI 2.80–4.24). However, a small but significant number of patients treated concomitantly with CM had a greater risk of developing worse outcomes (7.2% vs. 4.4%, OR = 2.06, 95% CI 2.06–4.83). These data clearly indicate that CM concomitant treatment could produce either beneficial or adverse effects on clinical outcome, probably depending on different combinations of CM and antipsychotics.

Furthermore, bivariate and multivariate analyses of CM-using subgroup revealed that both improved and worse outcomes were significantly associated with residence in urban areas, suggesting that patients living in urban areas may have greater impacts with CM therapy than those in rural areas. This is likely due in part to the fact that urban patients generally have more unconventional and conventional treatment options compared to rural patients [16]. This perhaps results in an increase in unpredictable positive and negative clinical effects, as the therapeutic properties of most CM preparations are not yet well identified. Meanwhile, the addition of CM significantly increased the chances of improved outcomes in paranoid patients compared to non-paranoid subtype. Several studies have demonstrated differences in neuropsychological character and clinical response to antipsychotic treatment between paranoid and non-paranoid subtypes [23,24] as well as subtype specificity of genetic profile [25,26]. Thus, the greater chance of alteration in treatment outcomes observed in paranoid patients may reflect a similar subtype difference in clinical effects of CM treatment.

Our results demonstrated that exceeding 3 months of CM use is a significant predictor for both improved and worse clinical outcomes. This finding confirms empirical evidence, suggesting that CM therapy of most chronic conditions requires a considerable duration in order to achieve observable improvement [14]. However, the finding is also consistent with those of case studies, revealing that most nephrotoxic and hepatotoxic effects associated with herbal medicine use are observed after 1–5 months of intake [4,5,27]. Considering difficulties in monitoring herbal toxicity and potential herb-drug interactions due to complex mixtures of unknown and unidentified ingredients in CM, the determination of an optimal length of the treatment might be a feasible strategy in minimizing adverse and toxic effects while maximizing beneficial effects. For this purpose, correlations between different length of CM use and changes in pharmacokinetic profile of conventional drugs may deserve to be further determined.

We found that CM-using patients whose antipsychotic regimens included olanzapine had significantly lower chance of improved outcomes. Meanwhile, quetiapine and clozapine monotherapy significantly heightened the risk of developing worse outcomes, suggesting associations of these three atypical antipsychotics with adverse clinical outcomes when used concomitantly with CM. On the other hand, among seven individual CM materials identified to be significantly associated with clinical outcomes, six were found to be significantly associated with adverse outcomes. They were Radix Bupleuri, Fructus Gardenia, Fructus Schisandrae, Radix Rehmanniae, Akebia Caulis, and Semen Plantaginis. Moreover, the concomitant treatment regimens including these herbal materials and antipsychotics associated with adverse outcomes accounted for nearly 60% of total identified treatment regimens in patients with worse outcomes. These data suggest that the heightened risk of adverse outcomes observed is closely associated with these herbal agents in combination with antipsychotic regimens.

As the identified herbal medicines have been well demonstrated to have high safety profiles [28], the adverse outcomes observed seem to be attributable to herb-drug pharmacokinetic interactions in which the pattern of drug metabolism is altered. Despite lack of information about the interactions between herbal and antipsychotic agents, early case studies reported that ginseng combined with phenelzine and betel nut with fluphenazine caused broad adverse effects in schizophrenic patients [29–31]. Our recent study of bipolar patients also found that combination treatment with the mood stabilizer carbamazepine and an herbal preparation for 26 weeks resulted in a significantly lower level of serum carbamazepine compared to carbamazepine alone, suggesting that the

Table 5. Multivariate associations of clinical outcomes with individual CMs in concomitant use with antipsychotics in schizophrenic patients.[a]

Individual Chinese medicine	Improved (n = 410)			Worse (n = 48)		
	%	OR (95% CI)	p	%	OR (95% CI)	p
Radix Glycyrrhizae (Gan-Cao)	26.8	1.59 (1.06–2.38)	0.232	12.5	0.53 (0.21–1.35)	0.181
Acorus gramineus (Shi-Chang-Pu)	17.3	1.11 (0.66–1.87)	0.699	2.1	0.11 (0.01–0.88)	0.037
Ziziphus jujuba (Suan-Zao-Ren)	14.1	0.63 (0.39–1.01)	0.056	18.8	0.83 (0.36–1.90)	0.660
Curcuma root (Yu-Jin)	13.9	1.76 (0.98–3.17)	0.058	14.6	1.84 (0.70–4.79)	0.214
Radix Angelica Sinensis (Dang-Gui)	13.9	1.03 (0.63–1.70)	0.901	8.3	0.63 (0.21–1.92)	0.422
Poria cocos (Fu-Ling)	13.2	1.30 (0.76–2.24)	0.335	12.5	1.28 (0.48–3.40)	0.620
Radix Bupleuri (Chai-Hu)	12.2	1.14 (0.68–1.93)	0.616	22.9	2.49 (1.10–5.62)	0.028
Radix Polygalae (Yuan-Zhi)	10.0	0.86 (0.50–1.49)	0.599	20.8	1.82 (0.77–4.31)	0.173
Salvia Miltrorrhiza (Dan-Shen)	9.8	0.87 (0.49–1.53)	0.625	10.4	0.92 (0.33–2.61)	0.881
Lumbricus (Di-Long)	9.8	0.95 (0.54–1.68)	0.863	4.2	0.17 (0.02–1.30)	0.088
Rhizoma Atractylodes (Bai-Zhu)	9.8	1.31 (0.69–2.47)	0.408	4.2	0.51 (0.11–2.34)	0.388
Dried tangerine peel (Chen-Pi)	9.5	1.16 (0.63–2.12)	0.635	8.3	0.94 (0.30–2.97)	0.921
Fructus Gardenia (Zhi-Zi)	8.3	1.02 (0.55–1.90)	0.947	45.8	9.16 (4.19–20.02)	<0.001
Flos Carthami (Hong-Hua)	8.3	0.99 (0.57–1.75)	0.984	4.2	0.47 (0.11–2.08)	0.318
Rhizoma Chuan Xiong (Chuan-Xiong)	7.6	0.73 (0.40–1.33)	0.306	4.2	0.38 (0.09–1.69)	0.204
Semen Persicae (Tao-Ren)	7.3	0.92 (0.49–1.75)	0.808	4.2	0.53 (0.12–2.41)	0.413
Magnolia officinalis (Hou-Po)	4.3	0.59 (0.26–1.30)	0.190	8.3	1.05 (0.31–3.52)	0.938
Fructus Schisandrae (Wu-Wei-Zi)	4.1	0.89 (0.38–2.07)	0.782	22.9	3.90 (1.42–10.73)	0.008
Radix Rehmanniae (Di-Huang)	3.4	1.22 (0.49–3.06)	0.669	12.5	3.48 (1.03–11.70)	0.044
Akebia Caulis (Mu-Tong) [b]	1.0	0.49 (0.12–2.04)	0.326	25.0	8.92 (2.50–31.87)	<0.001
Semen Plantaginis (Che-Qian-Zi)	0.7	1.64 (0.17–16.20)	0.671	33.3	21.10 (4.32–103.05)	<0.001

a. CM, Chinese medicine. The unchanged outcomes (n = 213) served as reference. Models were adjusted for resident areas, diagnostic subtype, and duration of CM use, variables significantly associated with clinical outcomes as shown in Table 3.
b. Akebia Caulis includes the two species: Akebia quinata (Thunb.) Decne. and Akebia trifoliate (Thunb.) Koidz.

addition of herbal medicine accelerates carbamazepine metabolism and lowers its blood concentration [32]. Like carbamazepine, most antipsychotic drugs, including clozapine, olanzapine, and quetiapine, are metabolized as substrates for cytochrome P450s (CYPs) [33,34]. Therefore, pharmacokinetic interactions may play an important role in influencing clinical outcomes in patients with

Table 6. Frequency distribution of herbal and antipsychotic concomitant treatment regimens associated with adverse outcome in schizophrenic patients.

	Risperidone alone	Quetiapine alone [a,b]	Clozapine alone [a]	Olanzepine-including [a]	Risperidone +clozapine	Others
Radix Bupleuri	4	1	3	2	1	0
Fructus Gardenia	7	7	2	3	3	0
Fructus Schisandrae	4	4	2	1	0	0
Radix Rehmanniae	2	2	2	0	0	0
Akebia Caulis	4	5	1	1	1	0
Semen Plantaginis	3	7	3	3	0	0
Others [c]	2	0	0	1 [c]	0	1
Subtotal	**26**	**26**	**13**	**11**	**5**	**1**
		49				
Total	**82**					

a. These antipsychotic regimens are significantly associated with adverse outcome as shown in Table 4.
b. It is noted that all quetiapine-including treatment regimens are quetiapine monotherapy.
c. Other herbal material-including regimens were not counted in subtotal regimens associated with adverse outcomes.

schizophrenia under concomitant treatment of herbal and antipsychotic agents observed in the present study.

There are several limitations in the present study. First, as patients who sought CM treatment may have distinctive perceptions about herbal medicine, psychological or "placebo" factors could not be excluded. The use of structured assessment instruments, including symptom scales and laboratory tests, should be helpful in further clarifying treatment effects of CM therapy. Second, since a considerable portion of CM-users were unable to provide full information about their CM formulae, it may lead to an underestimation of individual CMs associated with clinical outcomes. On the other hand, due to difficulties in collecting information about dosages of herbal and antipsychotic agents as well as the quality of herbal preparations, these factors were not considered in the present study. However, it should be noted that there have been extensive reports about severe adverse events caused by overdosing, heavy metal contaminations, and adulterants with conventional drugs of herbal supplements [5,35,36], all of which might account for the presumed adverse effects of herbal and antipsychotic combinations. Fourth, as the majority of CM treatments were recommended by psychiatrists to their patients, obtaining information about psychiatrists' attitudes and knowledge of CM would be helpful in devising safe and effective strategies of concomitant CM and antipsychotics in the treatment of schizophrenia. Finally, although there are many statistically significant results found in the study, "chance significances" may not be excluded. Additional cautions should be paid when the results are considered with reference in future studies.

In conclusion, a relatively small proportion of patients with schizophrenia have concomitant CM and antipsychotic treatment. Such concomitant treatment may heighten the risk of developing worse clinical outcomes in a small number, but increase the chance of improving treatment outcomes in a much greater number of patients. Better identification of the concomitant herbal and antipsychotic treatment regimens that are associated with clinical outcomes provides useful hints for further clarifying herb-drug pharmacokinetic interactions.

Acknowledgments

We thank the following research members for conducting on-site survey and data collection: Yun-Chun Chen, Rui-Guo Zhang, Hua-Ning Wang, Ya-Hong Zhang, and Li Guo at Department of Psychiatry of the Fourth Military Medical University, Zeng-Rong Gong at Xinfeng Psychiatric Hospital of Lintong City, La-Ke Li at Baoji Psychiatric Hospital, Xiang Wang at Yulin Psychiatric Hospital, Zhen Peng at Xianyan Psychiatric Hospital, Ling Dong at Xi'an Dongfang Psychiatric Hospital, Hui Wang at Mianxian Psychiatric Hospital, Bo Zhang at Ankang Psychiatric Hospital, Cui-Xia An, Gui-Xing Jin and Shao-Min Yao at Mental Health Center of Hebei Medical University, Xiao-Dong Zhou at PLA 256 Hospital, Guo-Zheng Li at Xingtai Qiaodong Psychiatric Hospital, Bing-Li Wang at Nangong Minghua Township Hospital, Jun-Jie Feng at Handan Integrative Hospital, Jian-Jie Qiao at Jize Licaozhuang Mental Health Clinic, Xiao-Ying Wang at Langfang Psychiatric Hospital, Shuang-Qian Xie at Hengshui Psychiatric Hospital, Yong-Jun Cui at Cangzhou Anding Hospital, and Zheng Li at Huanghua Anding Psychiatric Hospital. Ms. Lilly Lee helped with data input.

Author Contributions

Conceived and designed the experiments: ZJZ QRT YT XYW. Performed the experiments: QRT XYW HHW CYW. Analyzed the data: LMH HKW DW. Wrote the manuscript: ZJZ QRT YT YBF RN GMM CYW VTW.

References

1. Fugh-Berman A (2002) Herb-drug interactions. Lancet 355: 134–138.
2. Izzo AA, Ernst E (2009) Interactions between herbal medicines and prescribed drugs: an updated systematic review. Drugs 69: 1777–1798.
3. Isnard Bagnis C, Deray G, Baumelou A, Le Quintrec M, Vanherweghem JL (2004) Herbs and the kidney. Am J Kidney Dis 44: 1–11.
4. Vanherweghem JL, Depierreux M, Tielemans C, Abramowicz D, Dratwa M, et al. (1993) Rapidly progressive interstitial renal fibrosis in young women: association with slimming regimen including Chinese herbs. Lancet 341: 387–391.
5. Yuen MF, Tam S, Fung J, Wong DK, Wong BC, et al. (2006) Traditional Chinese medicine causing hepatotoxicity in patients with chronic hepatitis B infection: a 1-year prospective study. Aliment Pharmacol Ther 24: 1179–1186.
6. Yang XX, Hu ZP, Duan W, Zhu YZ, Zhou SF (2006) Drug-herb interactions: eliminating toxicity with hard drug design. Curr Pharm Des 12: 4649–4664.
7. Csernansky JG, Schuchart EK (2002) Relapse and rehospitalisation rates in patients with schizophrenia: effects of second generation antipsychotics. CNS Drugs 16: 473–484.
8. Zhang ZJ, Tan QR, Zhen XC, Tong Y (2010) The potential benefits of herbal medicines for schizophrenia: from empirical observations to clinical trials (chapter 16) In: Hertzman M, Adler L, eds. Clinical Trials in Psychopharmacology. UK: Wiley-Blackwell. pp 311–335.
9. Yuan HN, Wang CY, Sze CW, Tong Y, Tan QR, et al. (2008) A randomized crossover comparison of herbal medicine and bromocriptine against risperidone-induced hyperprolactinemia in patients with schizophrenia. J Clin Psychopharmacol 28: 264–370.
10. Peterson E, Stoebner A, Weatherill J, Kutscher E (2008) Case of acute psychosis from herbal supplements. S D Med 61: 173–177.
11. Przekop P, Lee T (2009) Persistent psychosis associated with salvia divinorum use. Am J Psychiatry 166: 832.
12. Zhang ZX, Zahner GE, Román GC, Liu XH, Wu CB, et al. (2006) Socio-demographic variation of dementia subtypes in China: Methodology and results of a prevalence study in Beijing, Chengdu, Shanghai, and Xian. Neuroepidemiology 27: 177–187.
13. World Health Organization (1992) The ICD-10 classification of mental and behavioural disorders: clinical descriptions and diagnostic guidelines .
14. Maciocia G (1994) The practice of Chinese medicine: the treatment of diseases with acupuncture and Chinese herbs. Edinburgh, UK: Churchill Livingstone. pp 342–385.
15. Xiang YT, Ma X, Cai ZJ, Li SR, Xiang YQ, et al. (2008) Prevalence and socio-demographic correlates of schizophrenia in Beijing, China. Schizophr Res 102: 270–277.
16. Xiang YT, Weng YZ, Leung CM, Tang WK, Ungvari GS (2007) Clinical and social determinants of antipsychotic polypharmacy for Chinese patients with schizophrenia. Pharmacopsychiatry 40: 47–52.
17. Chen Z, Gu K, Zheng Y, Zheng W, Lu W, et al. (2008) The use of complementary and alternative medicine among Chinese women with breast cancer. J Altern Complement Med 14: 1049–1055.
18. Wu B, Liu M, Liu H, Li W, Tan S, et al. (2007) Meta-analysis of traditional Chinese patent medicine for ischemic stroke. Stroke 38: 1973–1979.
19. Ma K, Lee SS, Chu EK, Tam DK, Kwong VS, et al. (2008) Popular use of traditional Chinese medicine in HIV patients in the HAART era. AIDS Behav 12: 637–642.
20. Druss BG, Rosenheck RA (1999) Association between use of unconventional therapies and conventional medical services. JAMA 282: 651–656.
21. Eisenberg DM, Davis RB, Ettner SL, Appel S, Wilkey S, et al. (1998) Trends in alternative medicine use in the United States, 1990-1997: results of a follow-up national survey. JAMA 280: 1569–1575.
22. Eisenberg DM, Kessler RC, Foster C, Norlock FE, Calkins DR, et al. (1993) Unconventional medicine in the United States. Prevalence, costs, and patterns of use. N Engl J Med 328: 246–252.
23. Bersani G, Valeri M, Bersani I, Piazza A, Adorno D, et al. (1989) HLA antigens and neuroleptic response in clinical subtypes of schizophrenia. J Psychiatr Res 23: 213–220.
24. Zalewski C, Johnson-Selfridge MT, Ohriner S, Zarrella K, Seltzer JC (1998) A review of neuropsychological differences between paranoid and nonparanoid schizophrenia patients. Schizophr Bull 24: 127–145.
25. Fanous AH, Kendler KS (2008) Genetics of clinical features and subtypes of schizophrenia: a review of the recent literature. Curr Psychiatry Rep 10: 164–170.
26. Jablensky A (2006) Subtyping schizophrenia: implications for genetic research. Mol Psychiatry 11: 815–836.
27. Tanaka A, Nishida R, Yoshida T, Koshikawa M, Goto M, et al. (2001) Outbreak of Chinese herb nephropathy in Japan: are there any differences from Belgium? Intern Med 40: 296–300.
28. Feng YB, (ed.) (2009) Basic and clinical toxicology of Chinese medicine (Chinese version). Hong Kong: Public House of Commercial Affairs.
29. Deahl M (1989) Betel nut-induced extrapyramidal syndrome: an unusual drug interaction. Mov Disord 4: 330–332.
30. Jones BD, Runikis AM (1987) Interaction of ginseng with phenelzine. J Clin Psychopharmacol 7: 201–202.

31. Shader RI, Greenblatt DJ (1985) Phenelzine and the dream machine—ramblings and reflections. J Clin Psychopharmacol 5: 65.
32. Zhang ZJ, Kang WH, Li Q, Tan QR (2007) The beneficial effects of the herbal medicine Free and Easy Wanderer Plus (FEWP) for mood disorders: double-blind, placebo-controlled studies. J Psychiatr Res 41: 828–836.
33. Sheehan JJ, Sliwa JK, Amatniek JC, Grinspan A, Canuso CM (2010) Atypical Antipsychotic Metabolism and Excretion. Curr Drug Metab 11: 516–25.
34. Wang B, Zhou SF (2009) Synthetic and natural compounds that interact with human cytochrome P450 1A2 and implications in drug development. Curr Med Chem 16: 4066–4218.
35. Ernst E (2002) Toxic heavy metals and undeclared drugs in Asian herbal medicines. Trends Pharmacol Sci 23: 136–139.
36. Ernst E (2004) Risks of herbal medicinal products. Pharmacoepidemiol Drug Saf 13: 767–771.

Traditional Chinese Medicine in Cancer Care: A Review of Controlled Clinical Studies Published in Chinese

Xun Li[1,2], Guoyan Yang[1], Xinxue Li[1], Yan Zhang[3], Jingli Yang[4]☙, Jiu Chang[3]☙, Xiaoxuan Sun[3]☙, Xiaoyun Zhou[5], Yu Guo[5], Yue Xu[6], Jianping Liu[1]*, Alan Bensoussan[2]*

1 Centre for Evidence-based Chinese Medicine, Beijing University of Chinese Medicine, Beijing, China, **2** Centre for Complementary Medicine Research (CompleMED), University of Western Sydney, Sydney, New South Wales, Australia, **3** School of Preclinical Medicine, Beijing University of Chinese Medicine, Beijing, China, **4** School of Management, Beijing University of Chinese Medicine, Beijing, China, **5** School of Acupuncture and Moxibustion, Beijing University of Chinese Medicine, Beijing, China, **6** School of Humanities, Beijing University of Chinese Medicine, Beijing, China

Abstract

Background: Traditional Chinese medicine (TCM) has been widely applied for cancer care in China. There have been a large number of controlled clinical studies published in Chinese literature, yet no systematic searching and analysis has been done. This study summarizes the current evidence of controlled clinical studies of TCM for cancer.

Methods: We searched all the controlled clinical studies of TCM therapies for all kinds of cancers published in Chinese in four main Chinese electronic databases from their inception to November 2011. We bibliometrically analyzed the included studies and assessed the reporting quality.

Results: A total of 2964 reports (involving 253,434 cancer patients) including 2385 randomized controlled trials and 579 non-randomized controlled studies were included. The top seven cancer types treated were lung cancer, liver cancer, stomach cancer, breast cancer, esophagus cancer, colorectal cancer and nasopharyngeal cancer by both study numbers and case numbers. The majority of studies (72%) applied TCM therapy combined with conventional treatment, whilst fewer (28%) applied only TCM therapy in the experimental groups. Herbal medicine was the most frequently applied TCM therapy (2677 studies, 90.32%). The most frequently reported outcome was clinical symptom improvement (1667 studies, 56.24%) followed by biomarker indices (1270 studies, 42.85%), quality of life (1129 studies, 38.09%), chemo/radiotherapy induced side effects (1094 studies, 36.91%), tumor size (869 studies, 29.32%) and safety (547 studies, 18.45%). Completeness and adequacy of reporting appeared to improve with time.

Conclusions: Data from controlled clinical studies of TCM therapies in cancer treatment is substantial, and different therapies are applied either as monotherapy or in combination with conventional medicine. Reporting of controlled clinical studies should be improved based on the CONSORT and TREND Statements in future. Further studies should address the most frequently used TCM therapy for common cancers and outcome measures should address survival, relapse/metastasis and quality of life.

Editor: Wael El-Rifai, Vanderbilt University Medical Center, United States of America

Funding: This work was supported by Program for Innovative Research Team of Beijing University of Chinese Medicine (No.2011-CXTD-09), and grant number 2011ZX09302-006 from the Ministry of Science and Technology of China and 101207007 from the State Administration of Traditional Chinese Medicine. The funders had no role in study design, data collection and analysis, decision to publish, or preparation of the manuscript.

Competing Interests: The authors have declared that no competing interests exist.

* E-mail: jianping_l@hotmail.com (JL); a.bensoussan@uws.edu.au (AB)

☙ These authors contributed equally to this work.

Introduction

With an ageing worldwide population coupled with unhealthy lifestyles and increased medical intervention, the burden of disease and overall mortality has shifted gradually to primarily non-communicable diseases such as cardiovascular disease and cancer [1]. It is estimated that about 12.7 million cancer cases and 7.6 million cancer deaths occurred in 2008 [2], and the World Health Organization (WHO) estimates that 84 million people would die of cancer between 2005 and 2015 [3].

The earliest records of tumors can be traced back to inscriptions on bones and tortoiseshells in the 16th–11th century B.C., and the "malignant sores" with "swelling but without ulceration" recorded by traditional Chinese medicine (TCM) doctors in Qin Dynasty (221-207 B.C.) already presented various theories and approaches to treat cancer. [4].

TCM has increasingly become popular in the West including in cancer patients [5]. Chinese medicine plays an important role in minimizing disability, protecting cancer patients against suffering from complications, and helping patients to live well [6]. Chinese medicine may also assist in supportive and palliative care by reducing side-effects of conventional treatment or improving quality of life [7]. It is estimated the United States National Cancer

Institute (NCI) spends around $120 million each year on CAM related research projects [8].

A recent review of surveys of complementary and alternative medicine use for cancer [9] identified 74 studies over the last 15 years, with 70% of publications occurring after 2005.

Previous reviews of TCM for cancer care in Chinese publications have identified 716 case reports involving 1,198 patients [10], and 1,217 case series reports involving 92,945 patients [11], which showed a large prevalence of a diversity of TCM clinical application for cancer patients. However, controlled clinical studies were not included in these two reviews. In order to catch a more comprehensive picture on TCM clinical usage for cancer care in China, we systematically reviewed Chinese literature to summarize the clinical evidence of controlled clinical studies in this area.

Materials and Methods

Literature Search

We searched four major Chinese electronic databases including China National Knowledge Infrastructure (CNKI) (1911-November 2011), Chinese Scientific Journal Database (VIP) (1989-November 2011), Chinese BioMedical Literature Database (CBM) (1978-November 2011), and Wanfang Database (1994-November 2011).

The Chinese searching terms were zhong yi (Chinese medicine), zhong yao (Chinese medicine/Chinese herbal medicine), zhong yi yao (Chinese medicine), zhong cheng yao (Chinese proprietary medicine), zhen (needling/acupuncture), jiu (moxibustion), tui na (tui na/massage), gua sha (scraping), ba guan (cupping), xue wei (acupoint), qi gong, min zu yao (ethnomedicine), min jian (folk); terms related to cancer disease including ai (cancer), liu (tumor), e (malignant), bai xue (leukemia), gu sui (bone marrow) and lin ba (lymph). Based on pilot searches, we noted improved outcomes by searching for any match with study citation, abstract, keyword or subject word.

Study Selection

Randomized controlled trials (RCT) or non-randomized (clinical) clinical studies (CCS) with at least one group involving TCM treatment for all types of cancer-related patients including malignant tumor, malignant hematologic disease and patients with precancerous condition were included. Controlled studies reporting "random allocation" were regarded as RCT, while controlled studies without mentioning randomization were regarded as CCS, including non-randomized controlled clinical trial (CCT) and prospective/retrospective observational study.

Two authors (XL and GYY) screened the titles and abstracts of the hits from literature searching, and full papers were retrieved by downloading electronic versions (JC, JLY, XYZ, and YG) and hand searching when electronic versions were unavailable (GYY).

Data Extraction

A structured data extraction form was designed (XL and XXL), and 10 authors (YZ, GYY, JLY, YG, XXS, XYZ, JC, XXL, YX and XL) participated in data extraction. The data extraction involved study information as followed:

We extracted bibliometric information, including citation information, publication types and funding information if available.

Clinical related indices consisted: 1) Disease and diagnosis: we recorded the cancer types according to International Statistical Classification of Diseases and Related Health Problems 10th Revision [12]. We extracted clinical-related conditions which the study addressed as the primary diagnosis of the included patients in the studies. Studies about prevention were specially categorized. Studies reported primary diagnosis related to TCM syndrome differentiation were specially recorded. We recorded the reporting completeness of diagnostic criteria, syndrome differentiation (bianzheng) and application of diagnostic gold standard (pathological diagnosis or cytological diagnosis). 2) Treatment and control: We distinguished conventional treatments and TCM, administration routes of TCM information both in treatment group and control group, further classification of herbal medicine and acupoint stimulation, and the reporting of treatment method, dosage and treatment duration for both TCM and conventional medicine. 3) Outcome measures: We extracted and classified clinical-related outcomes. If quality of life was reported, the tool for measuring was extracted if available. If the authors defined the graded effectiveness by combining a number of outcomes, for example, obvious improvement of quality of life and obvious reduction of tumor size meant "very effective" while obvious improvement of quality of life or obvious reduction of tumor size meant "effective", rather than reporting each original outcome, we recorded this as "combined outcome". Whether the author recommended the clinical application as the study report conclusion was also extracted.

We assessed the completeness of reporting according to CONSORT Statement [13] for RCTs and TREND Statement [14] for CCSs. We assessed the reporting of diagnosis criteria, inclusion/exclusion criteria, allocation methods, blinding, details of interventions and level of controls, and use of outcomes measures for quality of life. We identified whether the study was randomized and whether the method of randomization as reported by authors. We identified blinding as either to patients, physicians, evaluators and/or statisticians. If placebo was reported and "double blind" was mentioned, we classified the blinding as "blinding to physicians and patients", while if placebo was reported without mentioning the details of blinding, we classified the blinding as "blinding to the patients".

We summarised well designed (reporting both randomization methods and blinding details) studies reporting positive survival outcomes to identify any significant evidence for the TCM treatments.

All the extraction was verified by one author (XL), and any discrepancies were discussed with the other authors for consensus.

Data Analysis

Data were presented by counts, percentage and frequency. Epidata (Version 13.02) was applied for data extraction, and Microsoft Excel and SPSS for Windows (version 17.0, Chicago, Illinois, USA) were applied for data analysis (XL, XXL, GYY).

Results

Bibliometric Information

A total of 137,510 citations were identified and screened based on searching in the four electronic databases, and 3737 full papers were retrieved. A final 2,964 articles involving 253,434 (10-1700, 85.50±70.59) participants were included after exclusion due to duplication, non-controlled clinical studies, non-cancer related studies or insufficient information (Figure 1).

A total of 2385 RCTs and 579 CCSs were identified. The earliest controlled clinical study was a retrospective clinical report about integrative medicine treating esophageal cancer published in 1984 [15]. The earliest RCTs we identified were one study of herbal injection for cancer pain in 513 advanced-staged cancer patients [16] and another study of herbal decoction for bone

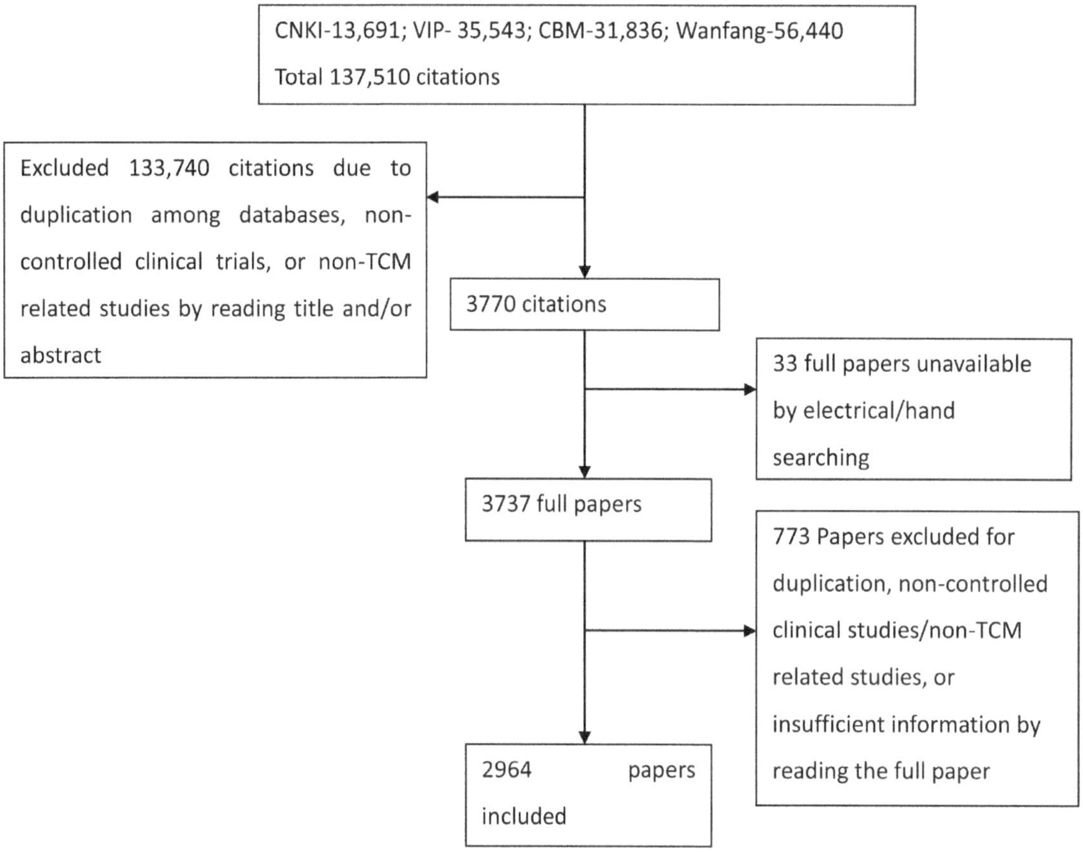

Figure 1. Flow chart of Literature searching and study selection. Presentation of the procedure of literature searching and study selection with numbers of articles at each stage.

marrow and immune function-related side effects induced by chemotherapy involving 40 patients [17], both of which were published in 1985. The quantity of publications increased especially after the year 2000. The publication types were further divided into journal articles, dissertations and conference proceedings. Studies reporting the funding information were specifically summarised in order to present the quantity change tendency, too. (Figure 2).

Participants and Diseases

Among the 2964 controlled clinical studies, 1490 studies focused on the treatment of cancer, and the other studies focused on precancerous condition, cancer-related clinical conditions, post-surgery conditions and radio/chemotherapy induced side effects (Table S2). Leucopenia was the most frequently reported primary diagnosis in radio/chemotherapy-induced side effects (119 studies out of 991), and cancer pain showed the highest frequency in cancer-related conditions (123 studies out of 283).

Out of the total 2964 studies, 292 (9.85%) involving 26,585 (10.49%) patients focused on cancer or cancer-related conditions prevention. Prevention of relapse and/or metastasis took up 16 studies out of 17 for relapse and/or metastasis, occupying the largest percentage (94.12%) of prevention. There were also more studies related to the prevention of radiation injury (61.19%), and prevention of other drug induced side effects (60.00%) than the studies about treatment of the same clinical conditions. (Table S1).

Cancer types were summarised into 17 categories according to ICD-10 (Table S2, Figure 3). Calculating by case numbers and study numbers, the highest prevalence cancer types treated, included in descending order of priority, were respectively lung cancer, liver cancer, stomach cancer, breast cancer, esophagus cancer, colorectal cancer, and nasopharyngeal cancer (Figure 4).

Interventions in Different Groups

Among the total 2964 studies, the majority of 2770 (93.45%) studies reported studies with 2 arms, 175 (5.90%) studies reported 3 arm studies, while 19 (0.64%) reported 4 or more arms in one study.

Interventions in treatment groups involved purely TCM intervention in 836 (28.21%) studies, while TCM combined with conventional treatment in 2128 (71.79%) studies. The interventions in control groups involved purely conventional treatment in 2570 (86.71%) studies, TCM combined with conventional treatment in 204 (6.88%) studies, and purely TCM intervention in 182 (6.14%) studies.

TCM intervention. TCM interventions reported in the total 2964 studies were classified into herbal medicine, acupoint stimulation, dietary therapy, massage, TCM psychological intervention, TCM five element music therapy and qigong. Herbal medicine, including oral decoction, injection, external usage, perfusion, aerosol inhalation, mouth rinsing and nasal feeding, was the most frequently applied intervention in both treatment group (2667 studies, 89.98%) and control group (327 studies, 11.03%). Among all the types of herbal medicine, herbal medicine decoction was the majority. More than half (1145 out of 1720, 66.57%) decoctions were individualized, and most of the studies

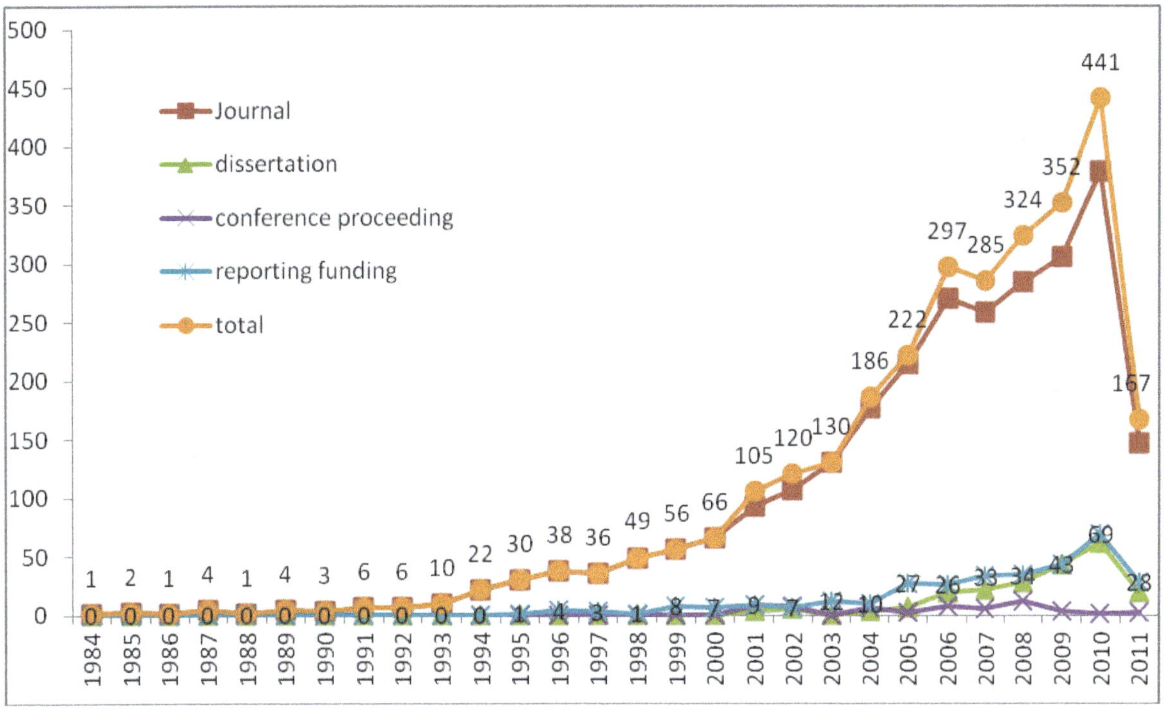

Figure 2. Publication number of controlled clinical studies of TCM for cancer published in Chinese. Presentation of the number of Chinese publication of controlled clinical studies of TCM for cancer in each year. The publication numbers of all the studies, journal articles, conference proceedings, dissertations, and the publications reporting funding information are shown respectively.

reported the detailed ingredients of the decoctions (Table 1). No study reported quality assessment of herbs or final herbal products.

Out of 379 (12.79%) and 56 (1.89%) studies reporting acupoint stimulation as the TCM treatment in treatment groups and control groups respectively, needling acupuncture and acupoint injection were dominating. Most of the studies related to acupoint stimulation reported acupoint composition (treatment group 372 studies, 86.28%, control group 50 studies, 89.29%) (Table 1).

Conventional treatment. Conventional treatment reported in the 2964 studies included chemotherapy, Western medicine as routine treatment, radiotherapy, interventional therapy and surgery. Chemotherapy was the dominating conventional treatment in both treatment group (1170 studies, 54.98% in the 2128 studies reporting TCM+conventional medicine) and control group (1328 studies, 47.87% in the 2774 studies reporting TCM+con-

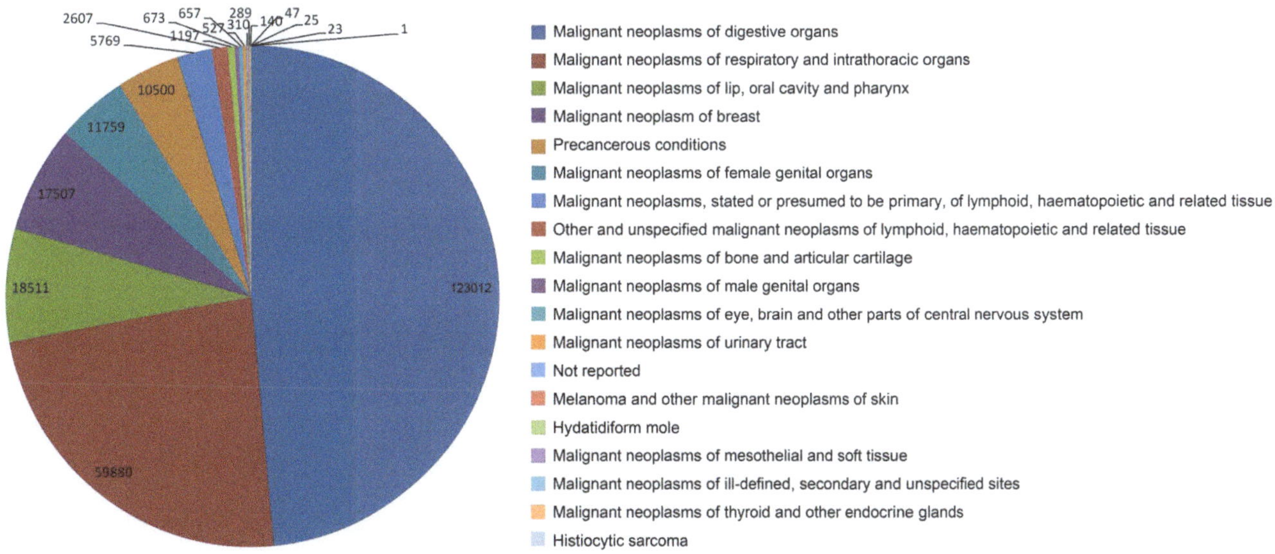

Figure 3. Cancer categories in controlled clinical studies of TCM for cancer published in China. Presentation of the categories of cancers reported in the include studies according to ICD-10.

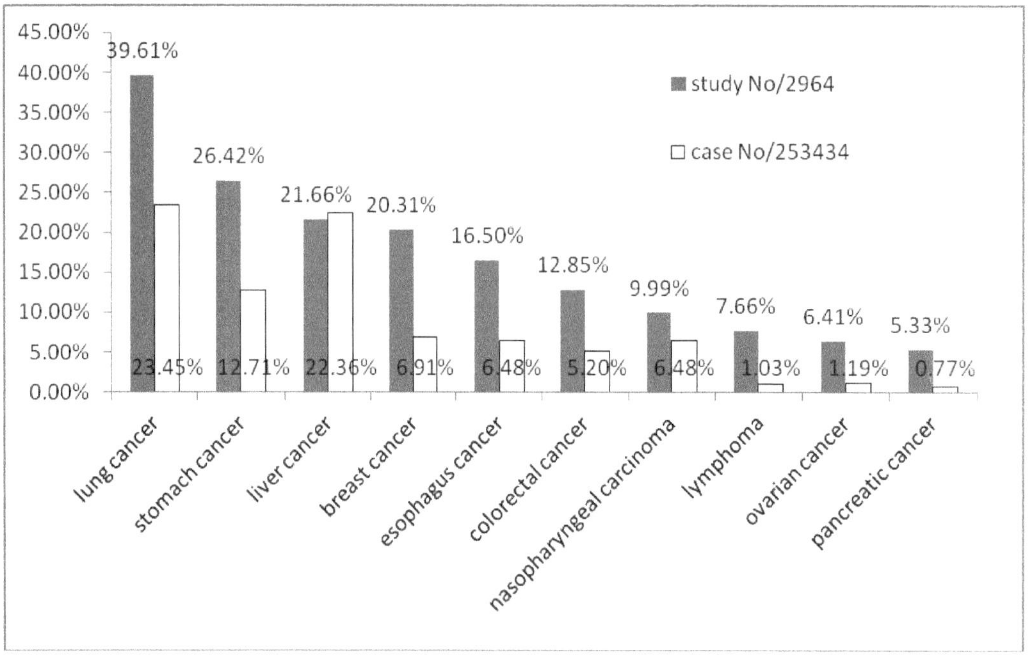

Figure 4. Top 10 cancer types with study numbers. Presentation of the top 10 most frequently reported cancer types calculate by study numbers. The numbers of participants ware also presented.

ventional medicine or conventional medicine only), followed by western medicine or other routine treatments (Table 1).

Control types. There were 25 studies applied placebo and 2 applied sham acupuncture as the control, and another 6 studies did not give any treatment to the patients in the control groups.

Detailed information of the intervention. Most studies reported the details of treatment such as method description, dosage and treatment duration. There were 410 (13.83%) studies failed to present any treatment information for treatment group and 376 (12.69%) for control group (Table 1).

Outcome Measurement

The most-frequently reported outcome measurement was clinical symptom (1667 studies, 56.24%), followed by laboratory indices (1270 studies, 42.85%), quality of life (1129 studies, 38.09%), chemo/radiotherapy induced side effects (1094, 36.91%), tumor size (869 studies, 29.32%) and safety (547 studies, 18.45%). Survival was reported in 433 (14.61%) studies while metastasis and relapse were reported in 109 (3.68%) and 101 (3.41%). Among the total 1129 studies reporting quality of life as the outcome measurement, Karnofsky Score was applied in most of the studies (942 studies, 83.44%). There were 41 studies reported quality of life measured by "QOL Score" without giving any other detailed information, and we could not identify the exact tool by any of the information provided by the publication and references. (Table 2).

There were totally 516 studies (17.41%) reported clinical effectiveness levels graded by several outcomes together without giving adequate information for each of the original outcome. (Table 2).

Overall Recommendation of Treatments

Among the total 2964 studies, 756 (25.51%) studies recommended generalizing the treatment to the broader community based on treatment effectiveness. Commonly seen recommendations included: "this treatment method is very effective with good safety, and is very suitable for generalization in the clinical applications".

Completeness of Reporting

Out of 2964 studies, 2136 (72.06%) reported diagnosis criteria of the included patients, 2315 (78.10%) reported golden standard for cancer diagnosis, such as pathological diagnosis or cytologic diagnosis, 1020 (34.41%) reported inclusion and/or exclusion criteria for the participants, while 1339 (45.18%) reported the stages of cancer.

The reporting rates across different publication types were different in diagnosis criteria, golden standard of cancer, inclusion/exclusion criteria, cancer staging and randomization method. Dissertations more frequently reported all of the detailed information mentioned above. (Table 3, Table 4).

Studies with funding information more frequently reported inclusion/exclusion criteria, cancer staging and blinding details than those without funding information. (Table 3, Table 4).

Reporting of inclusion/exclusion criteria, randomization method and details of blinding increased over time. (Figure 5).

There were 679 (22.91%) studies reported TCM diagnosis based on syndrome differentiation as diagnosis standards as selection criteria, reference for treatment or for outcome measuring.

Randomization. Among the 2385 RCTs, 394 (16.52%) reported adequate randomization methods, such as random table, computer software randomization, drawing lots and throwing coin. There were 33 studies reported "envelope method" or "random envelop "as the randomization method, and we counted them as adequate randomization method, too. Conference proceedings and dissertations had higher rate of reporting randomization methods out of studies mentioning "randomization" (Table 4).

Table 1. Intervention and control for cancer patients in controlled clinical studies of TCM for cancer published in Chinese.

Therapy	Treatment group	% (/2964)	Control group	% (/2964)
Herbal medicine	**2667**	**89.98%**	**327**	**11.03%**
oral medication	2098	70.78%	273	9.21%
decoction (reporting ingredients)	1720 (1631)	58.03%	149 (131)	5.03%
individualized prescription (reporting ingredients)	1145 (1089)	38.63%	103 (90)	3.48%
proprietary herbal products (reporting ingredients)	758 (564)	25.57%	185 (111)	6.24%
hospital prepared herbal medicine (reporting ingredients)	303 (278)	10.22%	22 (19)	0.74%
injection	450	15.18%	51	1.72%
external	200	6.75%	15	0.51%
perfusion	15	0.51%	1	0.03%
aerosol inhalation	5	0.17%	0	0.00%
mouth rinsing	5	0.17%	1	0.03%
nasal feeding	1	0.03%	0	0.00%
Acupoint stimulation (acupoint composition)	**379 (372)**	**12.79%**	**56 (50)**	**1.89%**
needling	131	4.42%	22	0.74%
acupoint injection	122	4.12%	20	0.67%
moxibustion	71	2.40%	5	0.17%
electronic acupuncture	44	1.48%	3	0.10%
acupoint application	28	0.94%	3	0.10%
ear acupuncture	18	0.61%	1	0.03%
acupressure	16	0.54%	0	0.00%
laser or microwave stimulation	4	0.13%	2	0.07%
cupping	2	0.07%	0	0.00%
acupoint nerve stimulation	2	0.07%	0	0.00%
bee-sting therapy	2	0.07%	0	0.00%
point embedding therapy	1	0.03%	0	0.00%
sham acupuncture (control group)			2	0.07%
Other types of TCM intervention	**31**	**1.05%**	**6**	**0.20%**
dietary therapy	15	0.51%	2	0.07%
massage	10	0.34%	3	0.10%
TCM psychological intervention	3	0.10%	0	0.00%
TCM five element music therapy	2	0.07%	0	0.00%
qigong	1	0.03%	1	0.03%
Conventional medicine				
chemotherapy	1170	39.47%	1328	44.80%
radiotherapy	354	11.94%	367	12.38%
western medicine or other routine treatment	622	20.99%	1228	41.43%
interventional therapy	162	5.47%	155	5.23%
surgery	73	2.46%	68	2.29%
Reporting completeness of interventions				
no information about medication duration	410	13.83%	376	12.69%
no information about dosage	133	4.49%	190	6.41%
no information about medication	38	1.28%	114	3.85%

Blinding. A total of 63 studies reported blinding to the participants, and 40 studies out of them (63.49%) reported the people who were blinded, such as participants, physicians, outcome measurers and statisticians. The other 23 studies just mentioned "blinding", "single blinding" or "double blinding" without providing any further information. Again, conference proceeding and dissertations reported the people who were blinded more frequently if "blinding" was mentioned (Table 4).

Significant Evidence of TCM Treatments

There were five studies [18–22] reporting relatively well designed RCTs with positive survival findings using Chinese herbal medicine. One study used herbal extract granules, another

Table 2. Outcome measurements reported in controlled clinical studies of TCM for cancer published in Chinese.

Outcome measurement	No.	Frequency (/2964)
clinical symptom	1667	56.24%
biomarker indices	1270	42.85%
quality of life	1129	38.09%
Karnofsky Score	942	31.78%
EORTC-QLQ	58	1.96%
QOL score without specific information	41	1.38%
FACT	27	0.91%
ECOG Score	5	0.17%
WHOQOL	5	0.17%
SF-36	4	0.13%
self-description	3	0.10%
FLIC Scale	2	0.07%
GQLI (Gastrointestinal Quality of Life Index)	2	0.07%
TCM quality of life scale	2	0.07%
other	15	0.51%
not reported	27	0.91%
chemo/radiotherapy induced side effects	1094	36.91%
tumor size	869	29.32%
safety	547	18.45%
survival	433	14.61%
post-surgery side effects	156	5.26%
body weight	126	4.25%
metastasis	109	3.68%
relapse	101	3.41%
pain	71	2.40%
imaging indexes	47	1.59%
fever	29	0.98%
depression indexes	10	0.34%
appetite	8	0.27%
economic indexes	6	0.20%

used a herbal capsule, and 3 used conventional Chinese herbal decoctions. Two of the studies reported TCM alone as the treatment intervention and the other 3 involved integrative TCM and conventional medicine. (Table S3).

Discussion

This study systematically identified and analyzed controlled clinical studies of TCM for cancer, and included 2964 studies from 1984 to 2011. This is the continuous part of previous reviews on case reports and case series [10,11] with the same topic. Unlike case reports and case series, Chinese publications of controlled clinical studies of TCM for cancer did not commence until 1984. This was consistent with the starting time of clinical trials in China, as a previous searching found that the earliest clinical trial in China started in the end of 1970s, and the first clinical trial in TCM area was a study of Chinese herbal injection for angina published in 1983 [23]. The number of publications increased with time, especially after 2000, which paralleled significant

Table 3. Completeness of Reporting across different types of publications.

	Total No. of the studies	Reporting funding	*Impact of reporting with or without funding reporting (p value) Δ*	Journal articles	Dissertation	*Compared with journal article (chi-square, p value)*	C onference proceeding	*Compared with journal article (chi-square, p value)*
Total	2964	322		2698	209		57	
Diagnosis criteria	2136	242	*0.191*	1895	201	*64.863, <0.001**	40	*<0.001, 0.992*
Golden standard	2315	251	*0.944*	2082	186	*15.821, <0.001**	47	*0.889, 0.425*
Inclusion/exclusion Criteria	1020	158	*<0.001* (OR = 1.99)*	789	204	*403.083, <0.001**	27	*8.796, 0.003**
Staging	1339	169	*0.005* (OR = 1.31)*	1152	154	*75.271, <0.001**	33	*5.295, 0.021*

*: statistically significant difference.
Δ: based on logistic regression.

Table 4. Overall picture of methodology quality of RCT and CCS of TCM for cancer.

	Total No. of the studies	Reporting funding	*Impact of reporting with or without funding reporting (p value) Δ*	Journal articles	Dissertation	*Compared with journal article (chi-square, p value)*	Conference proceeding	*Compared with journal article (chi-square value, p value)*
Total	2964	322		2698	209		57	
RCT	2385	289		2191	157		37	
Randomization method	394	95	*<0.001* (OR = 2.94)*	326	58	*52.134, <0.001**	10	*4.193, 0.041*
Blinding	63	17		53	9		1	
Who is blinded	40	14	*0.069*	34	5	*0.894,0.819***	1	*0.894,0.819***

*statistically significant difference.
**p value of chi-square across journal articles, dissertation and conference proceeding.
Δ: based on logistic regression.

development of controlled clinical studies in China, and also possibly of the establishment of Chinese medical databases. Publication numbers fall in 2011 which may be partially due to the time lag in recording of trials by the databases.

The most frequently reported cancer types were consistent with the most common types of cancer (lung, stomach, liver, colon and breast cancer) causing deaths each year according to WHO [24] and basically consistent with the estimation of the new cancer diagnosis for developing countries (lung & bronchus cancer, stomach cancer, liver cancer, breast cancer and colon & rectum cancer) [2] Leukemia was ranked 10th as calculated by patient cases numbers, and was not ranked within the top 10 cancer types if calculated by study numbers, which was quite different from case series (5th rank) and case reports (2nd rank). One possibility is that the treatment of leukemia is quite individualized, and there tends to be more publications of case series and case reports where more flexible and variable treatments are allowed than strict standardized interventions expected in RCTs. Both clinical observations and controlled clinical trials should be implemented to confirm the effectiveness and safety in the future.

The clinical application of TCM is of high clinical interest not only in the treatment of cancer and cancer related conditions, but also in its prevention. We identified 292 studies involving 26,585 patients using TCM treatment for prevention of relapse/metastasis of cancer or other cancer related conditions. Compared to treatment interventions, TCM seems to have higher impact in the prevention of relapse and/or metastasis, hemorrhage, radiotherapy induced inflammation, radiation injury, chemo/radiotherapy induced nausea and/or vomiting or other gastrointestinal disorder, other chemotherapy included side effects, and other drug-induced side effects. This is consistent with previously identified role of TCM as complementary medicine adjuvant or postal to conventional treatment [6–7,9].

In our literature search, whilst we did not apply any terms directly related to precancerous lesions; we nevertheless identified 98 studies involving 11,759 patients with precancerous conditions. A more comprehensive search with more precise search terms including specific names of each precancerous condition should be implemented for a complete view of studies of TCM in cancer prevention.

Reporting completeness, including recording of inclusion/exclusion criteria, randomization method for RCTs, and recording of blinding improved with time. However, around half of the studies still did not provide adequate information around patient diagnosis and recruitment. This could be directly due to the poor reporting of studies, or indeed that some of these studies were actually retrospective clinical records summary instead of prospective clinical trials although the published article claimed itself as "clinical trial" or "clinical study". It is necessary and essential for a prospective clinical study to recruit participants based on pre-defined standardized diagnosis criteria and clear selection criteria.

As far as the methodology is concerned, according to CONSORT Statement [13], a randomized controlled trial must report the details of randomization methods and blinding if blinding was implemented, and for non-randomized clinical study, TREND (Improving the Reporting Quality of Nonrandomized Evaluations of Behavioral and Public Health Interventions) Statement [14] requires that the authors report whether or not participants, those administering the interventions, and those assessing the outcomes were blinded to study condition assignment. We recommend that future publications give detailed information of randomization methods including sequence generation and randomization concealment and blinding information

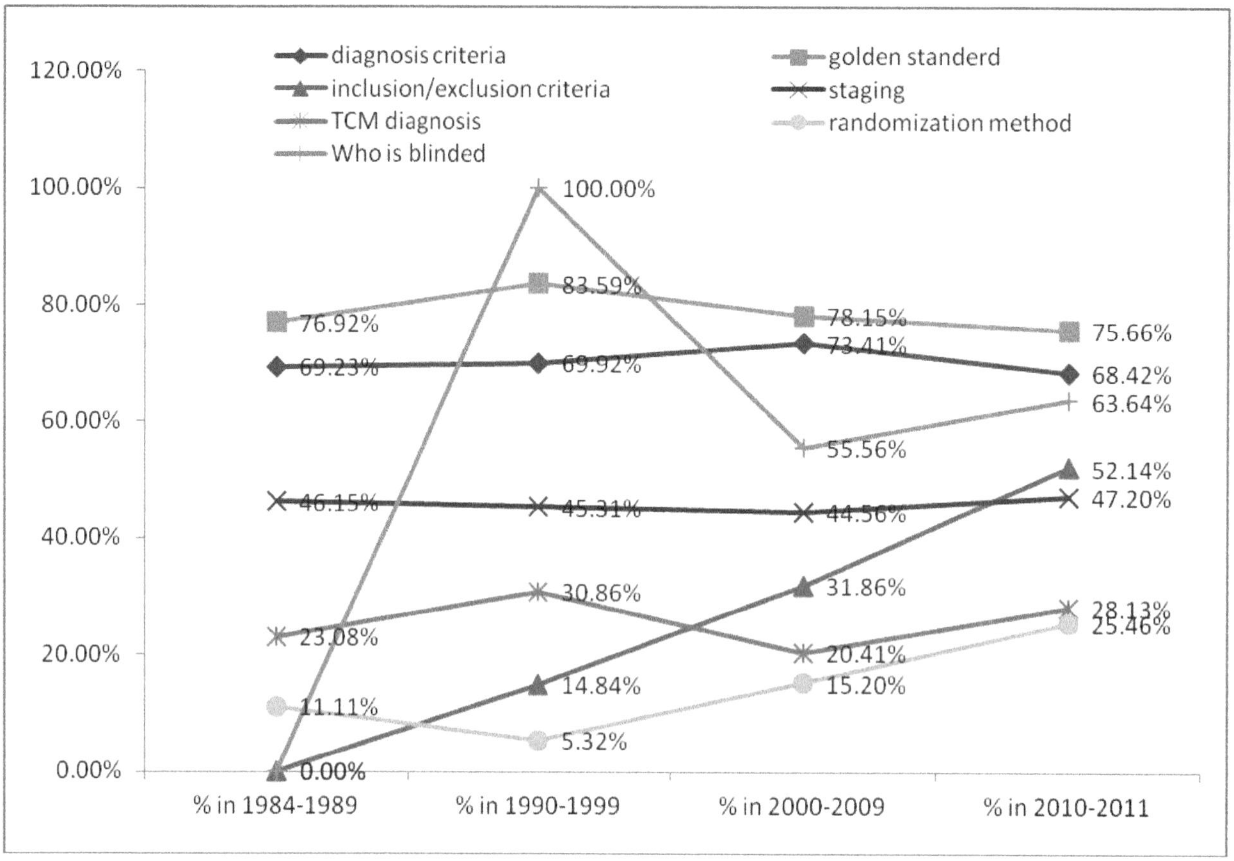

Figure 5. Reporting completeness, randomization methods and blinding across years. Percentage of reporting diagnosis criteria, inclusion/exclusion criteria, TCM diagnosis, golden standard of cancer, cancer staging, randomization method and blinding in the time order. Years are presented by the clusters of 1984–1989, 1990–1999, 2000–2009 and 2010–2011.

including whether blinding is used and who are blinded if available. If the report is based on existing previous data, the article should clearly articulate that it is a retrospective report so as todistinguish itself from prospective clinical studies.

If TCM syndrome differentiation is applied, the standard for judgment should be clearly stated.

Quality of life as one of the most important clinical outcomes and closely related to the patient wellbeing and increasingly included in studies. However the tools for measuring quality of life should have been more thoroughly reported with standard references in order to ensure clearer contribution to clinical decision making and design of further studies.

Funded studies, conference proceedings and dissertations seemed to generate higher report quality, which indicates that peer reviews is important for reporting of clinical studies, and the researchers in China are aware and able to do better research, however many of the Chinese journals haven't paid enough attention to the standard and strict requirement when accepting submissions. It is urgently suggested that journals in China endorse international standards such as CONSORT for randomized controlled trials and TREND for non-randomized controlled trials in their author guidelines to improve the quality of clinical studies and reporting.

More than 20% of the studies failed to provide adequate gold standard diagnosis for cancers, which could creates risks in interpretation of data. As an essential element of cancer studies, we suggest every clinical studyreport clear methods of cancer diagnosis in the future. We searched the Chinese publications based on general searching terms for example zhong yi (Chinese medicine) and zhong yao (Chinese herbal medicine), publications only labeled by the exact treatment such like the name of the herbal formula would have been missed out. More standard labelling is responsible for a more complete searching. We recommend that the future publication have at least one label related to Chinese medicine or herbal medicine for keyword or subject word if the study is TCM-related.

It was difficult to judge whether papers were reports of a prospective clinical studies without adequate information such as randomization methods and inclusion/exclusion criteria. Thus we combined together all clinical studies which involved comparison between different groups of patients receiving different interventions. Whilst most of studies mentioned "randomization", we could not assess more than 2,000 studies for study type (retrospective or prospective), and could not apply strict methodological evaluation as described in Cochrane Handbook [25]. Future studies should focus on specific types of TCM treatment for certain cancer with more detailed evaluation and analysis to ensure conclusions around effectiveness and safety and contribute to evidence-based clinical recommendations.

With regards to reviews of case series and case reports of TCM for cancer, individualized Chinese herbal medicine was the most frequently reported intervention. We suggest that the future studies focus on tailoring of treatment in cancer care.

Among the studies published in Chinese, herbal medicine is the main TCM intervention for cancer, comprising almost 90% in the total 2964 studies, which is also 7 times the number of acupuncture studies. This difference is much larger compared to a review based on English publications (acupuncture in 71 studies while Chinese herbal medicine in 11 studies) [9], which might reflect policy and levels of use of herbal medicine in different countries as well as publication bias. Although most of the included studies involved herbal medicine, there is no study reporting quality assessment of herbs or herbal products. Since the quality of herbal medicine is closely related to the clinical effectiveness and safety, and also essential for the quality of clinical study [26], this issue should be addressed in the future.

There have been a large number of controlled clinical studies of TCM for cancer, especially certain types with higher frequency such as lung cancer, liver cancer, stomach cancer, colorectal cancer, breast cancer, esophagus cancer, nasopharyngeal cancer, cervical cancer, ovarian cancer and pancreatic cancer. Systematic reviews could be implemented in order to access the effectiveness and safety of the TCM treatments for thesis types of cancers so that higher quality of evidence could be brought about based on the existing clinical information, the money and time have been spent, for the contribution to the clinical practice. One literature review of systematic reviews of TCM published in PubMed and Cochrane Library during the year 1999 to 2009 [26] identified 4 systematic reviews of TCM for cancer care including nasopharyngeal cancer, esophageal cancer, unrespectable hepatocellular cancer, and cancer pain respectively. We also identified Cochrane systematic reviews or protocols about Chinese herbal medicine for certain types of cancer including gastric precancerous lesions [27], Chinese herbal medicine for advanced pancreatic cancer [28], Chinese herbal medicine for chemotherapy side effects in colorectal cancer [29], Chinese herbal medicine for side effects of breast cancer [30], and herbal medicine for advanced colorectal cancer [31].

Conclusions

In future standard and adequate reporting of TCM cancer studies is essential. More attention should be paid to reporting clinical outcomes of importance to patient care and clinical decision making including survival times, extent of relapse/ metastasis and quality of life.

Supporting Information

Table S1 Cancer-related clinical condition of the cancer patients treated by TCM in the controlled clinical studies. The study numbers and case numbers of cancer-related clinical conditions of the cancer patients treated by TCM. The clinical diagnosis is further classified as treated by TCM and prevented by TCM.
(DOC)

Table S2 Types of cancer treated by TCM in controlled clinical studies published in Chinese journals. Types of cancer treated by TCM in controlled clinical studies according to the category of. ICD-10 codes of all the cancers are presented in the table.
(DOC)

Table S3 Characteristics of studies with significant evidence of TCM treatments for cancer published in Chinese. The characteristics of 5 RCTs of TCM for cancer reporting randomization methods and blinding information with outcomes of survival, relapse and/or metastasis and quality of life.
(DOC)

Acknowledgments

We thank Associate Prof. Zhaolan Liu and PhD student Qing Li from Centre for Evidence-based Chinese Medicine, Beijing University of Chinese Medicine for their suggestions in statistic analysis, and Prof. Kelvin Chan from Herbal Medicine Group, Faculty of Pharmacy, University of Sydney, and Centre for Complementary Medicine Research, University of Western Sydney for his suggestions in drafting the manuscript.

Author Contributions

Substantial contribution to the study design and manuscript revision: JL AB. Conceived and designed the experiments: JL Xun Li. Performed the experiments: Xun Li GY Xinxue Li YZ JY JC XS XZ YG YX. Analyzed the data: Xun Li GY Xinxue Li. Wrote the paper: Xun Li.

References

1. World Health Organization (2009) Global health risks: mortality and burden of disease attributable to selected major risk.
2. Jemal A, Bray F, Center MM, Ferlay J, Ward E, et al. (2011) Glabal cancer statistics. CA Cancer j Clin 61: 69–90.
3. Danhier F, Feron O, Préat V (2010) To exploit the tumor microenvironment: Passive and active tumor targeting of nanocarriers for anti-cancer drug delivery. J Control Release 148: 135–146.
4. Li PW (2003) Management of cancer with Chinese medicine. Donica Publishing.
5. Boon HS, Olatunde F, Zick SM (2007) Trends in complementary/alternative medicine use by breast cancer survivors: comparing survey data from 1998 and 2005. BMC Womens Health 30: 4.
6. Yoder LH (2005) Let's talk 'cancer prevention'. MedSurg Nursing 14: 195–198.
7. Ernst E (2009) Complementary and alternative medicine (CAM) and cancer: the kind face of complementary medicine. Int J Surg 7: 499–500.
8. Jia L (2012) Cancer complementary and alternative medicine research at the US National Cancer Institute. Chin J Integr Med 18: 325–332.
9. Carmady B, Smith CA (2011) Use of Chinese medicine by cancer patients: a review of surveys. Chin Med 9: 22.
10. Liu J, Li X, Liu J, Ma L, Li X, et al. (2011) Traditional Chinese medicine in cancer care: a review of case reports published in Chinese literature. Forsch Komplementmed 18: 257–263.
11. Yang GY, Li X, Li XL, Wang L, Li J, et al. (2012) Traditional Chinese medicine in cancer care: a review of case series published in the Chinese literature. Evid Based Complement Alternat Med 2012: 751046. Epub 2012 May 31.
12. ICD-10 Version 2010. Available: http://apps.who.int/classifications/icd10/browse/2010/en. Accessed 2012 Nov 3.
13. Schulz KF, Altman DG, Moher D, for the CONSORT Group (2010) CONSORT 2010 Statement: updated guidelines for reporting parallel group randomised trials. Ann Int Med 2010 152: 726–732.
14. Des Jarlais DC, Lyles C, Crepaz N, TREND Group (2004) Improving the reporting quality of nonrandomized evaluations of behavioral and public health interventions: the TREND statement. Am J Public Health 94: 361–366.
15. Bao YH, Fang SY, Li G (1984) [Clinical analysis of integrative medicine for treating pancreatic cancer]. Zhong Xi Yi Jie He Za Zhi (Journal of Integrative Chinese and Western Medicine) 4: 16–18.
16. Xie BH, Huang KJ, Wang FM (1985) [Clinical observation of Chinese herbal medicine plus chemotherapy for pain in advanced stage cancer patients]. Zhong Xi Yi Jie He Za Zhi (Chinese Journal of Integrated Traditional and Western Medicine) 10: 586.
17. Wang TX, Du XG (1985) [The use of Chinese traditional medicine and herbs in prevention of immune-myelo-suggpressive effects in chemotherapy of malignant lymphoma]. Zhong Liu Lin Chuang (Chinese Journal of Clinical Oncology) 2: 144–146.
18. Huang S, Li DY (2011) [Clinical observation of Fufang Zhebei Keli in improving the survival of acute leukemia patients]. Master thesis. Beijing University of Chinese Medicine.
19. Xu ZY, Jin CJ, Shen DE, Li M, Zhou WD, et al. (2007) [Clincal study on treatment of advanced non-small-cellung cancer with Chinese herbal medicine in different stages combined with chemotherapy]. Zhong Guo Zhong Xi Yi Jie He Za Zhi (Chinese Journal of Integrative Traditional and Western Medicine) 27: 874–878.
20. Wang LF, Xu ZY, Jin CJ, Wang ZQ, Deng HB, et al. (2010) [Clinical study on treatment of advanced lung adenocarcinoma with staged Chinese herbal

medicine and chemotherapy]. Zhanghai Zhong Yi Yao Za Zhi (Shanghai Journal of Traditional Chinese Medicine) 6: 41–43.
21. Liu HT, Li JH (2009) [Evidence-based medicine analysis of Chinese herbal medicine in improving survival of post-surgery breast cancer patients]. Zhong Wai Yi Xue Wen Zhai (World Health Digest Medical Periodical) 8: 26–29.
22. Li LN, Liu WS, Xu K, Wu WY, Liu YL, et al. (2003) [Prognostic factor study of traditional Chinese medicine treatment based on syndrome differentiation for treating III,IV stage non-small cell lung cancer]. Shaanxi Zhong Liu Yi Xue (Shaanxi Journal of Oncology Medicine) 11: 44–47.
23. Wu T, Zhan SY, Li LM (2004) [History of the development of epidemiology experimental study]. Chin J Epidemiol (Zhong Hua Liu Xing Bing Xue Za Zhi) 25: 633–636.
24. World Health Organization (2012) Cancer Fact Sheets. Available: http://www.who.int/mediacentre/factsheets/fs297/en/. Accessed 2012 Nov 3.
25. Higgins JPT, Green S (editors) (2011) Cochrane Handbook for Systematic Reviews of Interventions Version 5.1.0 [updated March 2011]. The Cochrane Collaboration.
26. Jiang M, Yang J, Zhang C, Liu B, Chan K, et al. (2012) Clinical studies with traditional Chinese medicine in the past decade and future research and development. Planta Med 76: 2048–2064.
27. Tang X, Liu G, Wang P, Wu T (2008) Chinese herbal medicine alone or combined with vitamins for gastric precancerous lesions (Protocol). Cochrane Database of Systematic Reviews.
28. Ni YH, Li X, Xu Y, Liu JP (2012) Chinese herbal medicine for advanced pancreatic cancer (Protocol). Cochrane Database of Systematic Reviews.
29. Wu T, Munro AJ, Guanjian L, Liu GJ (2005) Chinese medical herbs for chemotherapy side effects in colorectal cancer patients. Cochrane Database of Systematic Reviews.
30. Zhang M, Liu X, Li J, He L, Tripathy D (2007) Chinese medicinal herbs to treat the side-effects of chemotherapy in breast cancer patients. Cochrane Database of Systematic Reviews.
31. Guo Z, Jia X, Liu JP, Liao J, Yang Y (2012) Herbal medicines for advanced colorectal cancer. Cochrane Database of Systematic Reviews.

8

Colorimetric Grading Scale Can Promote the Standardization of Experiential and Sensory Evaluation in Quality Control of Traditional Chinese Medicines

Jia-bo Wang[1,9], Ling-na Zeng[1,2,9], Qing-ce Zang[1,3,9], Qian-feng Gong[3], Bao-cai Li[2], Xue-ru Zhang[1], Xiao-hui Chu[1], Ping Zhang[1], Yan-ling Zhao[1], Xiao-he Xiao[4]*

1 China Military Institute of Chinese Medicine, 302 Military Hospital, Beijing, China, **2** Faculty of Life Science and Technology, Kunming University of Science and Technology, Kunming, China, **3** Pharmacy College, Jiangxi University of Traditional Chinese Medicine, Nanchang, China, **4** Integrative Medicine Center, 302 Military Hospital, Beijing, China

Abstract

Experiential and sensory evaluation is an ancient method that remains important in the current quality control system of Traditional Chinese Medicines (TCMs). The process is rapid and convenient when evaluating the quality of crude materials in TCM markets. However, sensory evaluation has been met with skepticism because it is mainly based on experience and lacks a scientific basis. In this study, rhubarb was selected to demonstrate how color-based sensory evaluation could differentiate the quality of herbal medicines objectively. The colors of the rhubarb samples, expressed as RGB values, were obtained from different parts and forms of the plant, including the plant's surface, fracture surface color, and a powdered form with or without treatment with a color-developing reagent. We first divided the rhubarb samples into three grades based on the total content of five hydroxyanthraquinone derivatives, the major pharmacological components in rhubarb. Then, a three-layer back-propagation artificial neural network (BP-ANN), calibrated with selected training samples, was used to correlate the quality of the rhubarb with its color. The color of the rhubarb powder after coloration attained the highest accuracy (92.3%) in predicting the quality grade of the test samples with the established artificial neural networks. Finally, a standardized colorimetric grading scale was created based on the spatial distribution of the rhubarb samples in a two-dimensional chromaticity diagram according to the colors of the powdered rhubarb after color enhancement. By comparing the color between the scale and the tested samples, similar to performing a pH test with indicator paper, subjects without sensory evaluation experience could quickly determine the quality grade of rhubarb. This work illustrates the technical feasibility of the color-based grading of rhubarb quality and offers references for quantifying and standardizing the sensory evaluation of TCMs, foods and other products.

Editor: Pratibha V. Nerurkar, College of Tropical Agriculture and Human Resources, University of Hawaii, United States of America

Funding: This research is supported by the Industry Research Program of Traditional Chinese Medicine (Nos. 200807020 and 201207002), the National Key Technology Research and Development Program (No. 2012BAI29B02), and the National Science Foundation of China (Nos. 81274026 and 30973947). The funders had no role in study design, data collection and analysis, decision to publish, or preparation of the manuscript.

Competing Interests: The authors have declared that no competing interests exist.

* E-mail: pharmacy302@126.com

9 These authors contributed equally to this work.

Introduction

Experiential and sensory evaluation is a rapid and effective evaluation method that has been used widely in various fields [1–3]. The technique has been used for more than 30 years in the food industry as a quality control test, characterizing the taste and colors of foods, and is becoming increasingly important in food markets [4–6]. A set of unique methods of sensory evaluation have been developed as Traditional Chinese Medicines (TCMs) evolves. Traditional sensory evaluation is based primarily on the human senses to assess shape, size, texture, color, odor and taste. Sensory evaluation remains one of the most effective methods to assess the raw materials used in TCM. Compared with modern quality control methods that involve spectroscopy, chromatography, mass spectrometry and cutting-edge biotechnology, sensory evaluation is convenient, fast and effective [7]. Nevertheless, these high-tech modern methods have been greatly researched, whereas the conventional sensory evaluation methods interest few modern researchers. In China, quality evaluation based on sensory characteristics is widely used in the TCM markets. There are some commercial specifications of TCMs conventionally accepted by the growers, medicinal vendors, TCM physicians and consumers. Also there are *Dao-di* herbs (good quality herbs produced in the native areas) conventionally accepted by practitioners to differentiate the quality of TCMs. Those commercial specifications and the concept of *Dao-di* herbs are generally defined by a set of specific morphological features. Growers of medicinal herbs typically select a superior species or variety to cultivate based on those specific morphological features. Similarly, medicinal vendors classify and price TCMs based on different specifications, and consumers primarily evaluate the quality of a TCM on the basis of sensory characteristics [8]. The repeatabilities of the experiential and sensory assessment by practitioners for the TCMs, like rhubarb and *Coptis chinensis*, etc., have been demonstrated in our previous studies [9,10]. Although traditional sensory evaluation has been regularly applied in China, there are some disadvantages. One concern is whether the sensory evaluation has a scientific foundation and chemical basis. A second issue is how the practice can be applied by people with little sensory evaluation experience, specifically users in the Western world.

Color is one of the most important characteristics in sensory evaluation for TCMs. Some ancient Chinese herbal medicine literature, such as the *Origins of the Materia Medica* (*Ben Cao Yuan Shi*), emphasize the importance of color as an identifier of high quality herbal materials (Figure 1). For example, an *Aucklandia* root (*muxiang* in Chinese) that is cadet blue in color is considered to be superior, mid-grade if yellowish-white, and inferior in quality when characterized by an oleaginous black color [11]. The correlation between color and chemical composition, however, is not well studied. Furthermore, sensory evaluation relies greatly on personal experiences, which are difficult to quantify and standardize. Thus, its application has been restricted. To our knowledge, no previous quantification and standardization of color evaluation for Chinese herbal medicine has been reported.

Rhubarb, an ancient and one of the best known Chinese herbal medicines, has been recognized for centuries in traditional medicine for its pharmacological properties, including its purgative [12], nephric protecting [13,14], liver protecting [15], antimicrobial and hemostatic properties [16]. The major pharmacological components in rhubarb are five hydroxyanthraquinones (HAQs) – aloe-emodin, rhein, emodin, chrysophanol and physcion – which are also quality control markers in the Chinese pharmacopoeia [17]. The quality of rhubarb correlates directly with the content of the five HAQs. Rhubarbs of different grades usually exhibit different colors, such as dark red, brown yellow or yellow. According to traditional sensory evaluation, rhubarbs of good quality are often bright yellow and those of poor quality were often dark yellow or brown. The objectivity and reproducibility of sensory evaluation for rhubarb have been demonstrated using the Delphi method [9]. In this study, rhubarb has been selected as a model drug for its representative color in sensory evaluation.

The overall flowchart of this study is shown in Figure 2. First, we divided the rhubarb samples into three grades based on the total content of the five HAQs. Second, we used the three-layer back-propagation artificial neural network (BP-ANN) to find relationships between the quality and the color of the samples. Finally, we defined a colorimetric grading scale for the quality of rhubarb. By comparing the color of a sample with this scale, similar to matching the color of litmus paper with a color scale to ascertain pH, customers can quickly determine rhubarb quality. To investigate which kind of sample produced the best colors to use for grading rhubarb, colors from the plant surface, fracture surface color and powder, with or without coloration by a color-developing reagent, were analyzed. Through this work, we illustrated the feasibility of color-based grading for rhubarb and developed a practical tool, a standardized colorimetric grading scale, to classify the rhubarb. Furthermore, we provided some references for the quantification and standardization of sensory evaluation of TCMs.

Materials and Methods

Materials

Thirty-four batches of rhubarb were collected from various sources in China (Table 1). All of the voucher specimens were deposited at the China Military Institute of Chinese Materia Medica. The samples were identified by Professor Xiao-He Xiao as the dried roots and rhizomes of *Rheum palmatum* L., *Rheum tanguticum* Maxim. ex Balf. and *Rheum offcinale* Baill. The chemical reagents were analytical grade and obtained from the Beijing Chemical Factory (Beijing, China).

Ethics

No specific permits were required for the described field studies. The aforementioned locations are neither privately-owned nor protected by the Chinese government. And there is no endangered or protected species involved in the specific locations where we collected the rhubarb samples.

Camera System

Images were acquired using a camera system equipped with a standard lightbox, camera, computer, ZoomBrowser EX software, data lines and digital camera (PowerShot G5 Pro 5.0 Megapixel, Canon Inc., Nagasaki, Japan). The standard lightbox consists of a steel framework, fluorescent lamp (LUMILUX, FH14W/865HE, OSRAM Company, München, Germany), ballast and shading-cloth.

Optimization of Shooting Conditions

Exposure time, aperture size, and light sensitivity were optimized to obtain clear images. The optimal camera performance parameters were determined by varying exposure time (1/4, 1/6, 1/8, 1/10, 1/13, 1/15, 1/20, 1/30, 1/40, 1/60, 1/80, 1/100), aperture size (8.0, 7.1, 6.3, 5.6) and ISO light sensitivity value (50 and 100). The results showed that the clearest image with well-balanced brightness and contrast was acquired using the following conditions: an exposure time of 1/10 second, an aperture size of 8.0 and an ISO light sensitivity value of 50.

Sample Coloration and Obtainment of RGB Values

Powder coloration: The powdered rhubarb samples of 0.3 g were weighed respectively and then dispersed into a 96-well plate which is generally used in cell culture and molecular biology experiments. Then an aqueous solution of 0.5% NaOH (0.6 ml) was added to each well to develop the color of the sample. After coloration, pieces of square filter paper (1.5×1.5 cm) were then inserted into the colored powder to absorb the rhubarb solution in the wells, and the filter papers were transferred to the standard lightbox for immediate imaging.

Fractured surface coloration: NaOH solution (0.5%, 0.2 ml) was sprayed onto the fractured surface of each sample of rhubarb. These samples were photographed immediately in the lightbox.

All samples, with or without coloration, were placed in the standard lightbox, and photographs were taken using the optimized shooting conditions described above. Some representative images are shown in Figure 3. All images were saved in the.jpg format. The RGB values were extracted from the images using Photoshop CS4 (Adobe Systems Inc., USA) image processing software.

BP Neural Network Analysis

A BP neural network with one input layer, one hidden layer, and one output layer was established in this study. According to the experimental results, the RGB values were set as three of the evaluation parameters. In this experiment, there were seven initial nodes in the hidden layer, and the number of nodes was defined to be 2N+1, where N is the number of input layer nodes. In the output layer, three nodes were designated to represent the three grades of rhubarb. The hidden layer and input vectors were

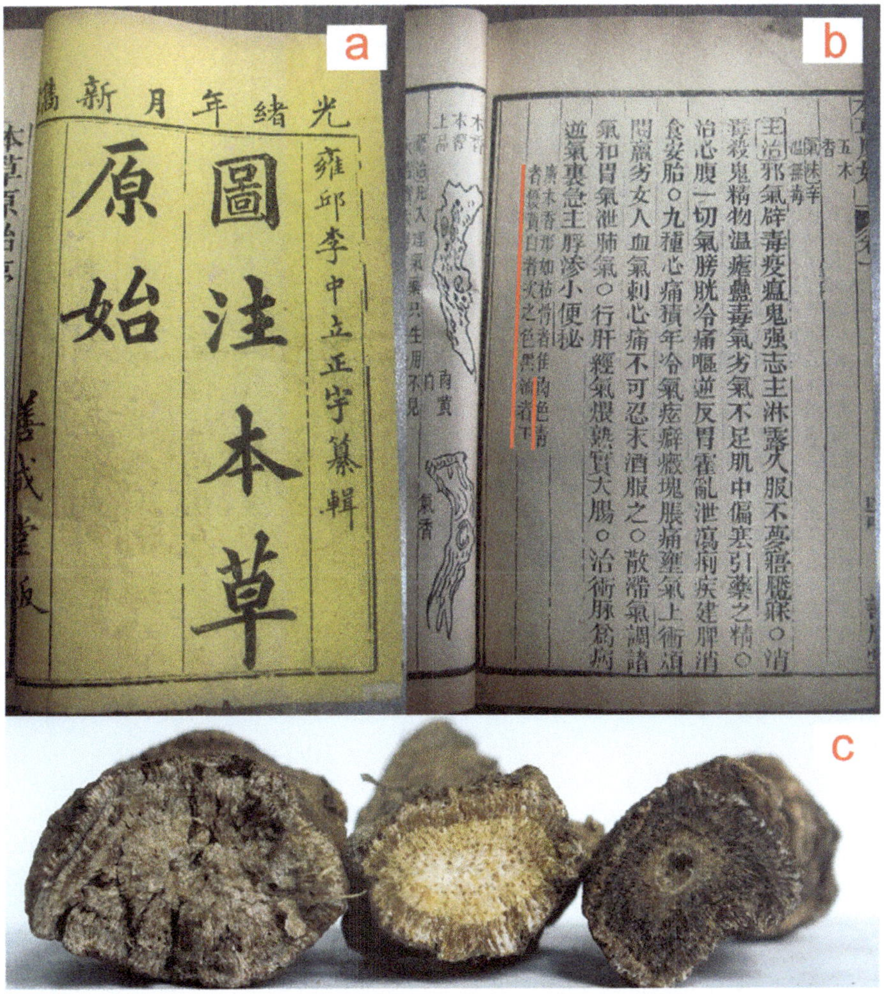

Figure 1. The herbal classic *Origin of the Materia Medica* (*Ben Cao Yuan Shi*) describes the color-based quality evaluation of Chinese herbal materials. a) *Origin of the Materia Medica*, written by Zhong-li Li in 1612 during the Ming Dynasty, has been considered the first of the herbal classics in China, which described the sensory characteristics for identification of commercial herbal materials (the medicinal parts of the plants) in detail rather than the plant morphology. b) The original description in the book for the color-based quality evaluation of *Aucklandia* root (*Aucklandia lappa* Decne, *muxiang* in Chinese). *Aucklandia* root is an herb that has been commonly used to treat gastroenterological diseases in China for over two thousand years. c) Photographs of the *Aucklandia* root samples in different color. The quality of *Aucklandia* root can be placed into three grades based on the color of its fracture surfaces: cadet blue denotes superior quality (left); yellowish-white indicates ordinary quality (middle); and an oleaginous black color suggests inferior quality (right).

connected, and the output layer and input vectors were not. In addition, the training sample set and the desired values were normalized with *Premnmx* from the Matlab toolbox. Finally, the BP network was established using the *Newcf* function and the transfer function of neurons in each layer was *tansig* and *purelin*. The network training function was *trainParam*. After training, the

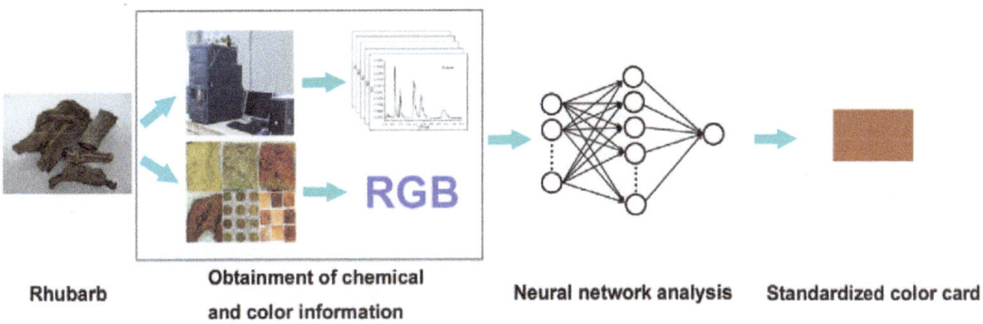

Figure 2. The flowchart for this study.

Table 1. RGB values of the color of the surface, the fracture surface and powder with or without further color development.

No.	Collection place	Grade	Surface color			Fractured surface color						Powder color					
			Without coloration			Without coloration			With coloration			Without coloration			With coloration		
			R	G	B	R	G	B	R	G	B	R	G	B	R	G	B
1	Li, Gansu	2nd	176	141	42	162	142	78	125	38	34	195	148	38	203	85	26
2	Li, Gansu	2nd	159	132	37	152	151	116	127	55	37	154	123	33	167	74	46
3	Li, Gansu	2nd	181	150	47	166	151	100	147	52	31	175	135	27	196	83	35
4	Li, Gansu	2nd	110	82	32	153	154	101	136	54	31	123	88	33	181	79	43
5	Li, Gansu	3rd	90	72	37	202	181	112	198	79	34	144	113	43	216	120	44
6	Li, Gansu	1st	149	125	33	165	150	85	144	80	31	171	131	34	240	163	69
7	Li, Gansu	1st	102	86	47	105	91	42	44	42	44	118	90	31	173	85	46
8	Dali, Yunnan	2nd	146	115	36	155	154	103	119	57	39	166	134	27	233	159	63
9	Dali, Yunnan	3rd	84	70	37	115	107	70	80	42	43	116	87	29	233	172	92
10	Dali, Yunnan	3rd	127	97	34	162	170	130	146	74	28	150	112	12	231	144	46
11	Gansu	2nd	103	86	44	117	107	55	92	47	39	119	92	31	197	114	61
12	Qinghai	1st	128	95	28	126	93	31	94	47	33	132	101	21	143	64	45
13	Xining, Qinghai	2nd	143	112	37	145	142	110	126	57	35	174	125	25	182	95	41
14	Fengjie, Chongqing	3rd	104	84	33	112	109	47	57	53	39	103	81	36	180	101	49
15	Xining,Qinghai	1st	128	97	33	141	140	119	103	53	45	148	101	32	128	58	51
16	Gansu	3rd	129	95	30	158	156	86	115	64	31	145	105	17	188	85	41
17	Shanxi	2nd	142	114	42	124	111	77	132	50	44	170	125	41	181	89	43
18	Gansu	3rd	108	92	53	114	110	42	88	56	36	108	79	27	166	83	46
19	Tibet	1st	106	83	44	127	120	61	101	54	47	126	86	18	156	58	42
20	Shiqu, Sichuan	1st	104	88	47	151	140	92	165	77	26	133	94	19	192	80	32
21	Saichuan, Sichuan	1st	113	95	49	156	115	33	112	44	46	158	112	21	200	91	33
22	Changdu, Tibet	2nd	110	84	33	104	78	50	65	34	38	110	79	24	124	60	55
23	Gansu	2nd	128	109	45	153	151	112	134	67	37	145	95	24	196	99	43
24	Tibet	2nd	111	93	56	146	138	73	115	58	41	133	103	27	198	84	40
25	Beichuan, Sichuan	2nd	82	65	34	139	138	86	105	59	42	111	81	25	166	65	44
26	Liangshan, Sichuan	2nd	99	76	36	164	141	85	157	50	31	143	98	23	202	84	31
27	Guizhou	3rd	109	85	31	117	100	35	67	47	43	109	76	25	185	89	44
28	Yaan, Sichuan	2nd	123	91	26	166	164	135	154	62	33	151	110	22	198	74	36
29	Changdu, Tibet	2nd	93	72	35	140	110	46	107	49	38	125	88	19	182	79	48
30	Gansu	3rd	123	93	28	137	125	49	107	72	38	115	78	19	177	95	82
31	Qinghai	1st	121	82	22	128	111	39	96	53	42	120	87	24	158	70	51
32	Sichuan	2nd	141	102	25	146	122	48	115	45	36	141	100	20	192	81	40
33	Gansu	3rd	115	91	29	129	111	49	100	76	40	125	96	27	188	107	63
34	Qinghai	3rd	102	87	38	108	105	56	64	56	37	123	102	25	213	143	87
	R*		0.192	0.128	−0.020	0.014	−0.101	−0.004	0.056	−0.265	0.131	0.199	0.092	−0.181	−0.388	−0.460	−0.341

*The pearson's correlation coefficient between the color data (R, G or B values) and the total content of HAQs in the samples.

grading standards were saved in the network, and the BP neural network was able to produce a prediction. Although the determined sample grades are discrete numbers (1, 2, or 3) in the training process, the predicted values are continuous real numbers. The grade of an inputted sample could be designated based on the predicted value. For example, if the output value is in the range of (0.51–1.50], the sample should be designated as the grade 1 (Figure 4). Additionally, for the grade 2 and grade 3, the ranges are designated as (1.51–2.50] and (2.51–3.50], respectively. In the results predicted by the BP network, some output values were not in the range of (0.51–3.50]. These numbers were considered incorrect predictions.

The process can be summarized as follows:

(i) Input the quality evaluation parameters of the training samples into the network input nodes.

(ii) Create the BP neural network.

(iii) Select proper training functions and parameters.

(iv) Output the results from the prediction to the output nodes of the network.

(v) Input the three evaluation parameters for the samples.

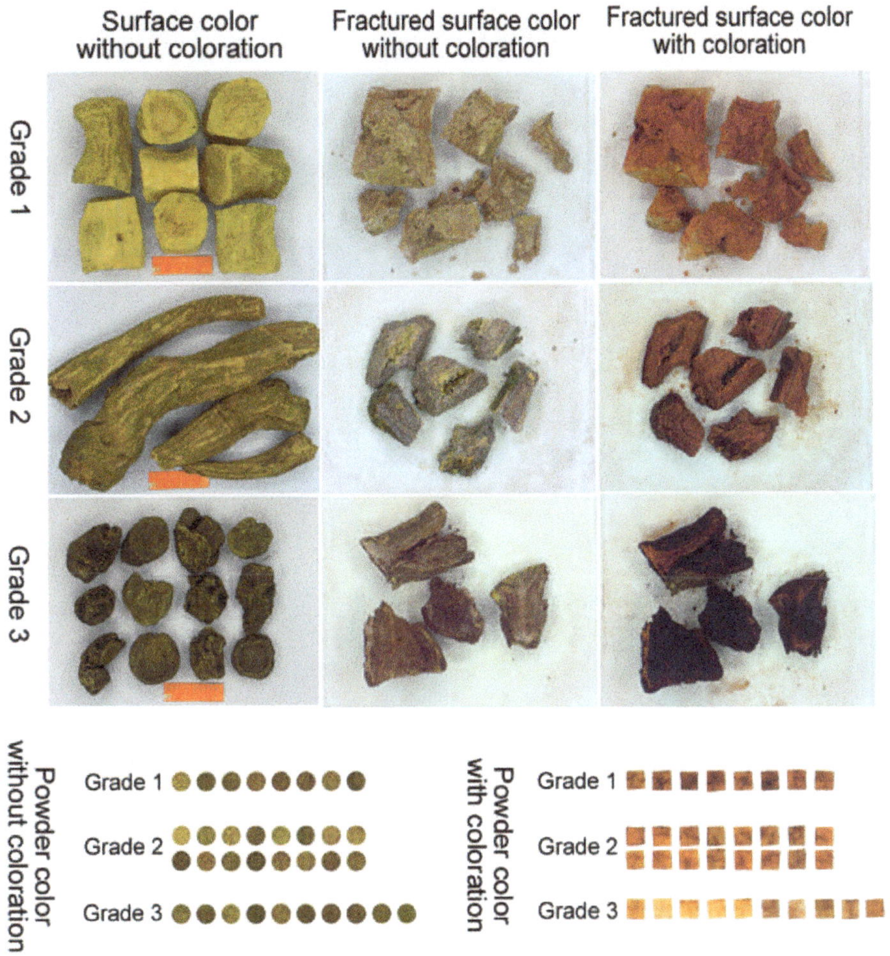

Figure 3. Representative images of rhubarb samples of different grades.

(vi) Proceed through the Matlab simulation.

```
[pn,meanp,stdp,tn,meant,stdt] = prestd(p,t); % normalizing
% establish neural network
net = newcf (minmax(ptr), [21 1], {'tansig' 'purelin'}, 'traingdx', 'learnsom');
% train the neural network
net.trainParam.epochs = 4500;
net.trainParam.goal = 0.000001;
net.trainParam.show = 40;
net.trainParam.lr = 0.05;
[net,tr] = train (net,ptr,ttr,[],[],val,test);
a = poststd(an,meant,stdt); % reverse normalization
% end
```

Color Conversion for Rhubarb Samples

Because the RGB color space consists of three dimensions, it is difficult to use RGB information to summarize the distribution of the rhubarb samples in each quality grade. To distinguish the lower and upper thresholds for grading different rhubarb samples, the RGB values were transformed into the CIE1931 XYZ color space, where the values can be normalized and plotted in a two-dimensional CIE1931xy chromaticity diagram. The formulas used to convert between the CIE XYZ and RGB color spaces are well documented [18,19]. The CIE XYZ color space is deliberately designed so that the Y parameter is a measure of the brightness or luminance of a color. The chromaticity of a color is then specified by the derived parameters x and y, two of the three normalized values which are functions of the three tristimulus values X, Y, and Z.

$$x = \frac{X}{X+Y+Z} \tag{1}$$

$$y = \frac{Y}{X+Y+Z} \tag{2}$$

$$z = \frac{Z}{X+Y+Z} = 1 - x - y \tag{3}$$

The derived color space specified by x and y can represent all of the chromaticities visible to the average person within a two-dimensional chromaticity diagram, which is a widely used tool to specify colors [18].

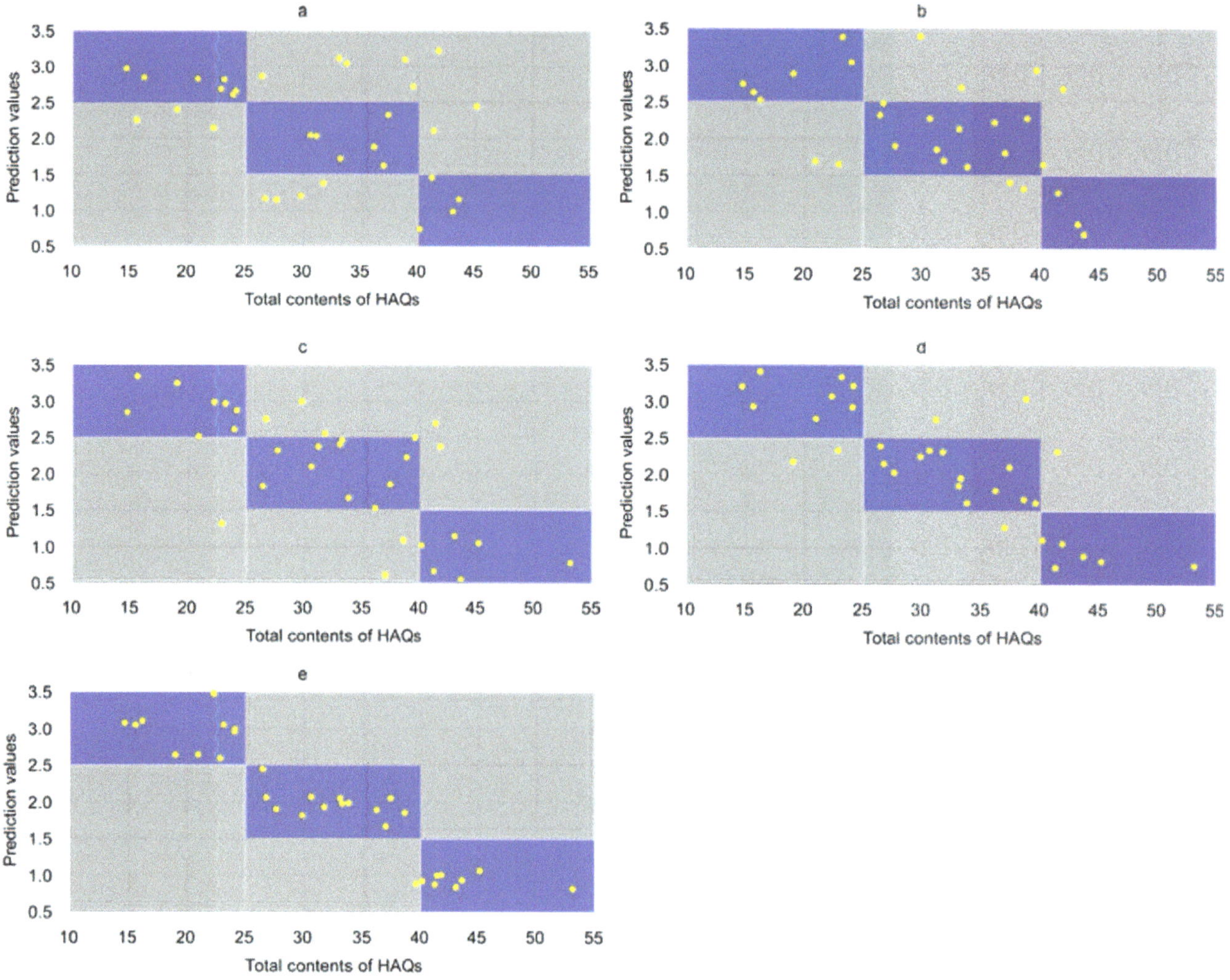

Figure 4. Color-based predictions of the grades of rhubarb samples from the BP network. All the thirty-four samples were counted here, including the training set and the test set. The blue areas indicate correct predictions, and the gray areas indicate incorrect predictions. a, Using the color from the surface of rhubarb without additional coloration as the input parameter, the percentage of correct predictions was 50.0% (17 correct predictions in 34 samples). b, When the colors of the fracture surfaces without development were input, the percent of correct predictions was 64.7% (22 correct predictions in 34 samples). c, When the color-enhanced fracture surfaces were analyzed, the percent of correct predictions was 73.5% (25 correct predictions in 34 samples). d, Using the powder without coloration as the input, the percent of correct predictions was 79.4% (27 correct predictions in 34 samples). e, Analysis of the powder after color development yielded predictions that were 91.2% accurate (31 correct predictions in 34 samples).

Design of the Colorimetric Grading Scale

To establish the color scale for colorimetric grading, we assumed that rhubarb samples of different quality would distribute randomly in a circle centered at the expected color values (points O_1, O_2 and O_3, shown in Figure 5a) for the samples. These values are typically within the radius of the maximum distance from the center in the chromaticity diagram. The centroid (point D) of the triangle that consists of the points O_1, O_2 and O_3 can be assigned as the division point that divides the samples into the different quality grades.

Results

Quality Grade Assignment for the Rhubarb Samples

Before the BP-ANN analysis, the rhubarb samples were divided into three grades according to the total content of the five HAQs (T_{HAQs}) based on the following definitions: grade 1, $T_{HAQs} \geq 40.00$ mg g^{-1}, grade 2, $25.00 < T_{HAQs} < 40.00$ mg g^{-1}, and grade 3, $T_{HAQs} \leq 25.00$ mg·g^{-1} (Table S1).

Color Quantization into RGB Values for the Rhubarb Samples

Images of a sample were captured in the standard lightbox and under natural light at different times (morning, noon, afternoon, evening) during the day using the optimized shooting conditions described above. Table 2 shows the relative standard deviations (RSD) of the R, G and B channels, which were 10.24%, 10.22% and 11.75%, respectively, when shooting under natural light at different time points. In contrast, the RSD for the R, G and B values were 0.94%, 1.13% and 1.81%, respectively, when shooting in the lightbox. The lighting conditions provided by the lightbox enable good reproducibility when acquiring images for color information. In this study, we acquired different colors of the herb, including the outside surface, a fracture surface, and a powder,

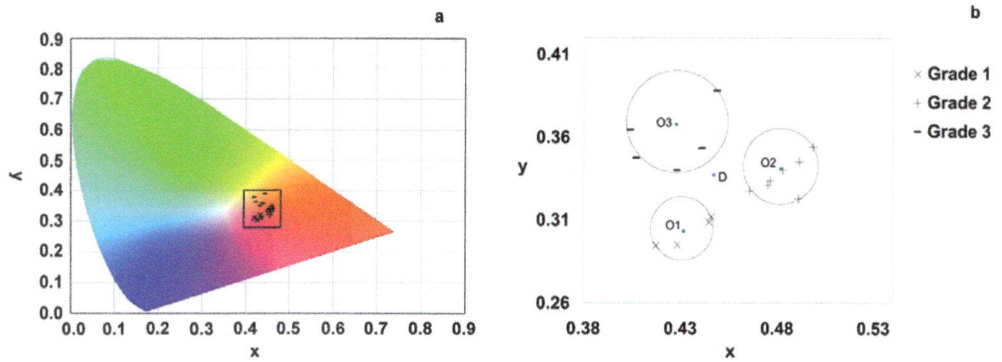

Figure 5. The distribution of the rhubarb samples in each grade in the CIE1931xy chromaticity diagram. a, The overall distribution of the samples in the two-dimensional coordinates overlaying on the CIE1931xy chromaticity diagram. The samples in the grade 1 mainly distribute in the lower left region favoring red-purple; the samples in the grade 2 distribute in the right region toward orange; and the samples in the grade 3 distribute in the upper left region tending toward yellow. b, Schematic diagram describing the geometric calculations for the segmentation points. The diagram represented the magnified region in the panel a.

with or without coloration by a developing reagent (Figure 3). The RGB values from the 34 rhubarb samples are shown in Table 1. The data of surface color with coloration were not listed and excluded from the research because the data varied greatly in different zones of the herb surface.

Neural Network Establishment and Prediction

The neural network was established firstly by processing the training set, and then the other samples were taken as the test set to assess the validity of the predictions and results from the network. We assumed the samples containing intermediate amount of HAQs in a certain quality grade are representative for the whole of the grade. So those samples of T_{HAQS} in the intermediate range (20% less than or greater than the upper or lower limit of each quality grade) were chosen as the training samples: The grade 1 consisted of samples 6, 7, 12, 15, 19, 20 and 21; the grade 2 contained samples 1, 2, 3, 4, 8, 11 and 17; and the grade 3 were samples 5, 9, 10, 14, 16, 27 and 30. After establishment of the BP network, the other thirteen samples out of the training set were input as test samples and predicted. The prediction accuracy by the BP network diversified depending on which form of color of the herb was examined. The prediction accuracy values of each kind of color were: 38.5% (5 correct predictions in 13 test samples) for the surface color, 92.3% (12 correct predictions in 13 test samples) for the powder color after coloration and 69.2% (9 correct predictions in 13 test samples) for the other three kinds of color. In addition, the predictions for the former training samples were also counted and combined with the results of the test samples. The prediction values were plotted with the contents of the five HAQs in Figure 4. It could be found that the color of the rhubarb powder after coloration attained the lowest wrong prediction of the quality grade for all the samples.

Table 2. The reproducibility of the RGB measurements.

Experiment	Under natural light			In standard lightbox		
	R	G	B	R	G	B
1	116	102	57	114	103	56
2	117	103	57	114	103	56
3	117	103	57	114	102	56
4	121	106	51	112	100	54
5	122	106	57	113	102	54
6	120	106	54	111	101	55
7	119	105	54	112	101	53
8	115	98	51	112	100	54
9	123	100	49	112	100	55
10	110	96	49	112	101	55
11	87	77	42	112	101	55
12	105	93	51	114	102	55
13	110	98	53	113	102	54
14	92	89	39	112	101	54
15	96	75	41	111	99	53
RSD (%)	10.24	10.22	11.75	0.94	1.13	1.81

Calculation of the Boundaries that Differentiate Grades of Rhubarb

The sixteen representative samples (sample 12, 15, 19 and 31 in the grade 1; sample 1, 3, 4, 24, 26, 28 and 32 in the grade 2; and sample 9, 10, 14, 33 and 34 in the grade 3) showing the least overlap in their distribution in the chromaticity diagram (i.e., distributed approximately 80% of the possible maximum distance from the center of each quality grade) were selected to determine the boundaries for differentiating the rhubarb grades. The acquired RGB values of the representative samples were converted to values within the CIE 1931xy color space and then plotted in the chromaticity diagram (Figure 5a). The distribution of the three grades of the rhubarb samples separated into distinct regions. According to the calculations described above, the mathematical expectation points (x, y) of each grade are O_1 (0.4315, 0.3031), O_2 (0.4819, 0.3408) and O_3 (0.4277, 0.3677). The division point D (x, y) is defined as the geometric center of the three mathematical expectation points calculated for the three grades and occurs at (0.4470, 0.3372). Figure 5b shows that the rhubarb samples in each grade distribute away from the division point (D) in three directions toward a different color category. The grade 1 tends toward the red-purple region; the grade 2 to the orange region; and the grade 3 to the yellow region. Thus, how the samples distribute can be used to determine the grade of an unknown rhubarb sample, specifically by comparing the color of the

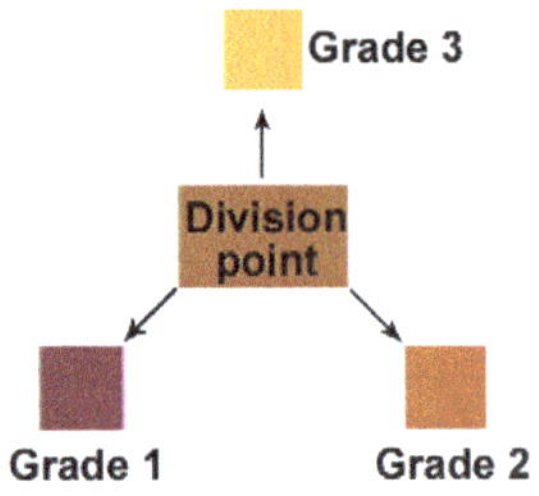

Figure 6. Differences between the color at the division point and the colors of the mathematical expectation points for each grade.

unknown with a colorimetric grading scale created based on the color of the division point (*D*). Corresponding ribbons was drawn using the software from the RGB values of the division point (*D*) and the mathematical expectation points (O_1, O_2, O_3) for each grade (Figure 6).

Discussion

Because of the convenience and speed of sensory evaluation compared with the laboratory analyses of chemical content, the desired color-based grading method would help in assessing the quality of rhubarb in the TCM marketplace. The approach for obtaining the color information is important for sensory evaluation. A colorimeter is a device that is commonly used to measure the color components of solid samples. In our preliminary experiment, we found that measuring the color of rhubarb by colorimeter was difficult because the plant's surface or fracture surface was not smooth and uniformly colored, which decreased the repeatability of the results. Unfortunately, most herbal medicines have various shapes that affect reproducibility. In this study, we used a digital camera to capture images of samples and extracted the color data from these images using Photoshop (Adobe Corporation, USA). Through this approach, the color data of the herbs are consistent with how colors are perceived by human vision. The RGB (red, green, blue) color model is one of the most widely used of the color systems. An additive model in which red, green, and blue light are summed to produce a broad array of colors, the model includes almost all of the colors that can be perceived by the human eye. In this study, the RGB values were used to represent color quantitatively. The RGB values could be converted into visual color, which made it possible to create a color scale that could be used as a reference for grading the quality of rhubarb.

Different concentrations of HAQs display different shades of yellow or red under a neutral or alkaline environment, respectively, which indicates a relationship between the color of the herb and its HAQ content. However, we found that the absolute values of Pearson's correlation coefficients between the contents of the five HAQs and the RGB values ranged from 0.004 to 0.460 (Table 1), showing non-significant linear correlation between the two variables. It could not be found a direct correlation between the color and quality of rhubarb because the RGB values are distributed in a non-linear space. So, we used artificial neural networks (ANNs), generally developed for non-linear mapping, generalization, self-organization and self-learning [20], to find relationships between the quality and the color of the samples. The most popular method used in ANN-based pattern recognition is the back-propagation (BP) trained, first-order neural network [21], which was used in this study. In Figure 4, it could be found that the outside surface color generated the lowest accuracy compared with the fracture surface color and the powder. After additional color development of the samples with a 0.5% NaOH aqueous solution, the rhubarb displayed a red to dark red color based on the Bornträger reaction of the base with the HAQs. Consequently, the coloration of the samples enhanced the accuracy of the network and increased the number of correct predictions for all sample types. The results suggested that measuring surface color of rhubarb is useless to some extent in assessment of its quality, because the color on the outside surface of the rhubarb can be more easily affected over the course of production and storage than the other sources of color data. The ununiformity was another defect of surface color in assessment of its quality. When the rhubarb is ground into powder form, the uniformity of color can be improved. In addition, developing the color of the HAQs has an advantage in reducing interference from other colored substances. Hence, the color-enhanced powder of rhubarb is preferred in color-based assessment of its quality.

The ANN results indicate that there is a positive but non-linear correlation between the quality of rhubarb and its color. However, the neural network is still a machine-based approach. To facilitate the quality assessment of rhubarb, we tried to establish a colorimetric grading scale to visually discriminate rhubarbs of varying quality. The boundaries of each quality grade of rhubarb were calculated according to their distribution in the chromaticity diagram (Figure 5b). The differences between the colors at the division point (*D*) and the colors of the calculated expected values for each grade can be distinguished with the naked eye, which enables the development of a color scale that can be printed on a card and used to grade rhubarb in the field [22]. For widespread use, the colorimetric grading scale could be printed on paper, similar to professional color cards such as Munsell color cards, to minimize the deviation between the theoretical and individually perceived colors.

In summary, the results of this study revealed that color or color parameters (RGB values) provided important information for the classification of quality of TCMs, such as rhubarb. However, the results varied depending on where the color was sampled: at the surface or fracture surface of the rhubarb, and with or without color development. The BP-ANN network achieved the highest percentage of correct predictions when analyzing powdered samples that were chemically processed to express color, which suggests that powders may be the best type of sample for the accurate grading of rhubarb. On the basis of the distribution of several rhubarb samples in the chromaticity diagram, we have designed a colorimetric grading scale to discriminate between rhubarbs of varying quality. By comparing the color of the sample with the colorimetric grading scale on the card, similar to determining pH using litmus paper, customers without experience in sensory evaluation could quickly assess the quality of rhubarb. This work illustrates the technical feasibility of color-based grading of rhubarb quality and provides useful references for the quantification and standardization of sensory evaluation-based quality control for TCMs, foods and other products.

Supporting Information

Table S1 Contents (mg g^{-1}) of the five HAQs in the rhubarb samples.
(DOC)

Text S1 Ultra Peformance liquid chromotography (UPLC) analysis.
(DOC)

Acknowledgments

The authors acknowledge Rui-xian Zhang, Wei Zhang and Su-min Hu for support in searching the ancient herbal books. The authors also acknowledge Ji Zhang for identifying the herb samples.

Author Contributions

Conceived and designed the experiments: XHX JBW. Performed the experiments: JBW LNZ QCZ XRZ. Analyzed the data: XHC LNZ QCZ JBW QFG BCL. Contributed reagents/materials/analysis tools: QFG BCL PZ YLZ. Wrote the paper: JBW QCZ LNZ YLZ.

References

1. Shahidi F, Rubin LJ, D'Souza LA, Teranishi R, Buttery RG (1986) Meat flavor volatiles: A review of the composition, techniques of analysis, and sensory evaluation. Crit Rev Food Sci 24(2): 141–243.
2. Evin F, Siekierski E (2002) Sensory evaluation of heating and air conditioning systems. Energ Buildings 34(6): 647–651.
3. Parpinello GP, Meluzzi A, Sirri F, Tallarico N, Versari A (2006) Sensory evaluation of egg products and eggs laid from hens fed diets with different fatty acid composition and supplemented with antioxidants. Food Res Int 39(1): 47–52.
4. Cunha CR, Dias AI, Viotto WH (2010) Microstructure, texture, colour and sensory evaluation of a spreadable processed cheese analogue made with vegetable fat. Food Res Int 43(3): 723–729.
5. Elortondo FJP, Ojeda M, Albisu M, Salmerón J, Etayo I, et al. (2007) Food quality certification: An approach for the development of accredited sensory evaluation methods. Food Qual Prefer 18(2): 425–439.
6. Parpinello GP, Versari A, Chinnici F, Galassi S (2009) Relationship among sensory descriptors, consumer preference and color parameters of Italian Novello red wines. Food Res Int 42(10): 1389–1395.
7. Zhu SH (2006) Modern commodity studies for traditional Chinese medicine. Beijing: People's Medical Publishing House. p.113.
8. Zhao ZZ, Liang ZT, Guo P (2011) Macroscopic identification of Chinese medicinal materials: Traditional experiences and modern understanding. J Ethnopharmcol 134(3): 556–564.
9. Wang JB, Zhang XR, Chu XH, Huang MJ, Jin C, et al. (2010) Delphi-based study on scientificity of organoleptic evaluation for rhubarb commercial specification. Chin J Chin Mat Med 35(20): 2657–2561.
10. Chu XH, Wang JB, Kong WJ, Zhao XJ, Liu FF, et al. (2011) Study on the reproducibility of organoleptic evaluation of commercial specification of *Rhizoma Coptidis* based on delphi method. World Sci Tech/Modern Tradit Chin Med Mat Med 13(2): 321–327.
11. Li ZL (2007) Origins of the Materia Medica (*Ben Cao Yuan Shi*). Beijing: People's Medical Publishing House.
12. Cuéllar MJ, Giner RM, Recio MC, Máñez S, Ríos JL (2001) Topical anti-inflammatory activity of some Asian medicinal plants used in dermatological disorders. Fitoterapia 72(3): 221–229.
13. Yokozawa T, Suzuki N, Okuda I, Oura H, Nishioka I (1985) Changes in the urinary constituents in rats with chronic renal failure during oral administration of rhubarb extract. Chem Pharm Bull 33, 4508–4514.
14. Wang JB, Zhao YL, Xiao XH, Li HF, Zhao HP, et al. (2009) Assessment of the renal protection and hepatotoxicity of rhubarb extract in rats. J Ethnopharmacol 124, 18–25.
15. Zhao YL, Wang JB, Zhou GD, Shan LM, Xiao XH (2009) Investigations of free anthraquinones from rhubarb against alpha-naphthylisothiocyanate- induced cholestatic liver injury in rats. Basic Clin Pharmacol 104(6), 463–469.
16. WHO Monographs on Selected Medicinal Plants (1999) Geneva: World Health Organization. p.231–240.
17. Pharmacopoeia of the People's Republic of China, First Div. (2010) Beijing: China Medical Science Press. p.22–23.
18. Rossel RAV, Minasny B, Roudier P, McBratney AB (2006) Colour space models for soil science. Geoderma 133(3–4): 320–333.
19. Mendoza F, Dejmek P, Aguilera JM (2006) Calibrated color measurements of agricultural foods using image analysis. Postharvest Biol Tec 41(3): 285–295.
20. Huang Y, Kangas LJ, Rasco BA (2007) Applications of artificial neural networks (ANNs) in food science. Crit Rev Food Sci 47(2): 113–26.
21. Agatonovic-Kustrin S, Beresford R (2000) Basic concepts of artificial neural network (ANN) modeling and its application in pharmaceutical research. J Pharmaceut Biomed 22(5): 717–727.
22. Xiao XH, Wang JB, Zhang XR, Chu XH (2011) The preparation method for the colorimetric grading scale card to discriminate the quality grade of Chinese materia medica. CN102042978A.

Altered Hub Configurations within Default Mode Network following Acupuncture at ST36: A Multimodal Investigation Combining fMRI and MEG

Youbo You[1], Lijun Bai[1]*, Ruwei Dai[1], Hao Cheng[3], Zhenyu Liu[1], Wenjuan Wei[1], Jie Tian[1,2]*

1 Key Laboratory of Molecular Imaging and Functional Imaging, Institute of Automation, Chinese Academy of Sciences, Beijing, China, **2** Life Science Research Center, School of Electronic Engineering, Xidian University, Xi'an, Shaanxi, China, **3** Department of Anesthesiology, Beijing Ditan Hospital affiliated to Capital Medical University, Beijing, China

Abstract

Acupuncture, an externally somatosensory stimulation in the Traditional Chinese Medicine, has been proposed about its modulations on the brain's default mode network (DMN). However, it is still unknown on how the internal brain resting networks are modulated and what inferences can be made about the physiological processes underlying these changes. Combining high spatial resolution of functional magnetic resonance imaging (fMRI) with high temporal resolution of magnetoencephalography (MEG), in the current multimodal study, we sought to explore spatiotemporally whether or not band-specific DMN hub configurations would be induced by verum acupuncture, compared with sham control. Spatial independent component analysis was applied to fMRI data, followed by the discrete regional sources seeded into MEG data. Partial correlation analysis was further adopted to estimate the intrinsic functional connectivity and network hub configurations. One of the most striking findings is that the posterior cingulate cortex is not only validated as a robust DMN hub, but served as a hub only within the delta and gamma bands following the verum acupuncture, compared with its consistently being a DMN hub in sham control group. Our preliminary results may provide a new perspective to lend support for the specificity of neural mechanism underlying acupuncture.

Editor: Xi-Nian Zuo, Institute of Psychology, Chinese Academy of Sciences, China

Funding: This paper is supported by the National Basic Research Program of China (973 Program) under Grant 2011CB707700, the National Natural Science Foundation of China under Grant No. 81227901, 61231004, 30970771, 81000640, 81171314, 30970769, 81071217, the Fundamental Research Funds for the Central Universities (2011JBM226) and NIH (R01HD046526 & R01HD060595), the Beijing Nova program (grant number Z111101054511116), and Beijing Natural Science Foundation (grant number 4122082), the Fellowship for Young International Scientists of the Chinese Academy of Sciences under Grant No. 2010Y2GA03, the Chinese Academy of Sciences Visiting Professorship for Senior International Scientists under Grant No. 2012T1G0036, 2010T2G36, 2012T1G0039. The funders had no role in study design, data collection and analysis, decision to publish, or preparation of the manuscript.

Competing Interests: The authors have declared that no competing interests exist.

* E-mail: tian@ieee.org (JT); bailj4152615@gmail.com (LB)

Introduction

Acupuncture, an ancient healing modality in the Traditional Chinese Medicine, has the therapeutic effects in the treatment of a range of diverse disorders [1–2]. However, it has not gained a proper position so far in the modern biomedical disciplines. This is partly due to the fact that physiological mechanisms underlying acupuncture effects still remain elusive. Among all research interests, one of the most appealing is focused on the unresolved but fundamental issue in which the central representations of peripheral acupuncture stimulation with regard to its functional specificity. In other words, whether exerting acupuncture at certain acupoints can produce functionally specific effects in the brain compared to a sham or placebo control procedure. Although accumulating evidence emerges [3–7], the debate over such acupoint specificity continues [8–10]. In order to promote better acceptance of acupuncture as a viable clinical treatment, it is thus vital and necessary to explore the biological mechanisms of functional specificity underlying acupuncture.

It is remarkable to find that a large proportion of neuroimaging acupuncture researches have been carried out with the utilization of functional magnetic resonance imaging (fMRI). Indeed, its high spatial resolution (on the order of millimeters scale) has prominently paved the way to identify the induced activity of brain regions in the spatial dimension reliably [5]. However, the Blood Oxygen Level Dependent signal detected by fMRI only reflects the neuronal activity indirectly [11–12]. Due to the latency of the hemodynamic response, it is more or less handicapped in the temporal dimension, only examining correlations in the relatively slow neuronal oscillations [13]. Analysis conducted only within this low frequency domain in previous acupuncture researches thereby may be limited to unveil completely the underlying mechanism since most electrophysiological aspects of neural activities took place at a much faster time scale [14]. For instance, working memory is associated with neuron interactions in the theta band, while gamma synchronization is related to perception and consciousness [15–16]. Electrophysiological imaging technology such as magnetoencephalography (MEG), on the contrary, has the ability to bypass the hemodynamic response and measure the magnetic fields induced by synchronized current flows in neuronal assemblies [17]. It can provide a unique window into the neurophysiological processing on the milliseconds time scale [18] so as to capture the detailed temporal profile of neural

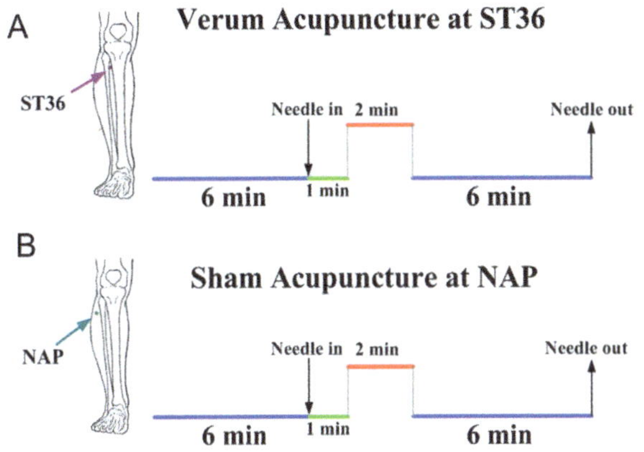

Figure 1. Experimental paradigm. Panel A indicated that acupuncture stimulation was performed at acupoint ST36 on the right leg (Zusanli, arrow pointing to dark pink dot). Panel B indicated that needling was performed at a nearby nonacupoint on the right leg (NAP, arrow pointing to dark cyan dot). The red line refers to needle administration, and the green line represents no acupuncture manipulation with needle inserted, the blue line indicates a 6-minute resting state or post-acupuncture resting state.

responses induced by acupuncture. However, its spatial resolving power does not match that of fMRI [19]. Since fMRI offers excellent spatial resolution with poor temporal resolution, while MEG provides excellent temporal resolution but poor spatial resolution, one feasible idea occurred that more exhaustive understanding of neural processes would be achieved by the combined employment of fMRI for localization and MEG for timing [20–22].

During the last decade, it has been gradually recognized that the brain is a complex network of dynamic systems with abundant functional interactions between local and remote regions [23–26]. One of the fast growing interests is related to the default mode network (DMN), which is identified as the distributed brain regions activated during rest but deactivated when specific goal-directed behavior is needed [27–28]. Accumulating evidence has typically demonstrated that several DMN regions play pivotal roles in connecting other regions and serve as network hubs with significant higher functional connectivity density [23,29]. In particular, recent investigations disclosed that the posterior cingulated cortex (PCC) constitutes one of the strongest DMN hubs in healthy subjects, with the highest degree of connectivity with other regions [29–32]. While substantial information has been gained about the prominent role of the hubs, the issues require more investigations on how these hubs interact with the rest of DMN regions and, more importantly, their alterations induced by acupuncture. The function of DMN has been considered to putatively engaged in self referential mental activity [33], stimulus-independent thoughts [34], and monitoring the environment among others [35] to maintain the body's homeostasis. In practice, the well-identified physical effects of acupuncture needling and its purported clinical efficacy also suggest that acupuncture acts in maintaining a homeostatic balance of the internal state within and across multiple brain networks [36]. Since the whole-brain hubs could be rearranged specifically following verum acupuncture compared with sham stimulation [37], furthermore, it has been increasingly elucidated that acupuncture could modulate spontaneous neural activities in wide resting brain networks, particularly within the DMN and its anticorrelated networks [5,38–40], therefore, further understanding of how such external intervention interacts with internal regulatory processes by regulating the DMN hubs may enlighten us to gain an appreciation of the physiological function and integrated mechanisms involved in acupuncture [5]. In recent electrophysiological studies, it is newly elucidated that functional connectivity between whole-brain regions would be modulated by acupuncture within specific frequency bands [41].

The current study attempted to spatiotemporally explore the specific DMN hub configurations following the verum acupuncture (Stomach Meridian 36, ST36), using sham acupuncture (non-

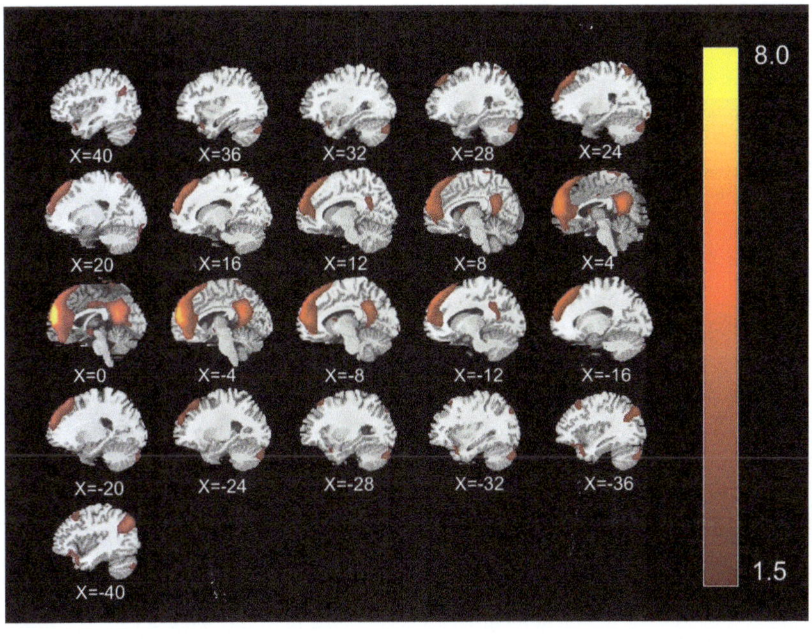

Figure 2. Spatial DMN components of group results extracted from fMRI data. Images are Z statistics overlaid on the average high-resolution scan transformed into standard (MNI 152) space. Red to yellow are Z values, ranging from 1.5 to 8.0.

Table 1. Talairach coordinates of the regional sources used to model the MEG data (P<0.05, FDR corrected).

Regions of Interest	Hem	Talairach x	y	z	Z value	V voxels
MFG	L	−2	57	21	5.54	422
	R	2	57	8	4.94	341
SFG	L	−2	57	23	5.57	495
	R	4	58	25	3.19	742
ACC	L	−2	54	−1	3.71	77
	R	4	47	9	2.75	57
PCC	L	−2	−49	25	3.14	65
	R	2	−50	19	3.36	82
STG	L	−38	17	−19	2.21	56
	R	38	17	−19	2.27	33
AG	L	−49	−63	31	2.43	19
	R	51	−63	31	2.00	16
IPL	L	−46	−50	52	2.40	206
	R	50	−42	56	1.52	15
MTG	L	−49	−63	29	2.41	39
	R	53	−59	25	2.10	22

Abbreviations: Hem, hemisphere; L, left; R, right; MFG, medial frontal gyrus; SFG, superior frontal gyrus; ACC, anterior cingulate cortex; PCC, posterior cingulate cortex/precuneus; STG, superior temporal gyrus; AG, angular gyrus; IPL, inferior parietal lobule; MTG, middle temporal gyrus.

meridian point, NAP) as a control. Moreover, since previous investigations demonstrated the modulation on band-specific functional connectivity among the whole-brain network, it is proposed here that whether such regulations would specifically exist within conventional frequency bands, that is, delta (0.5–4 Hz), theta (4–8 Hz), alpha (8–13 Hz), beta (13–30 Hz) and gamma bands (30–48 Hz). To test this hypothesis, we attempted to employ fMRI for spatially identifying the DMN component and MEG for temporally evaluating the hub configurations so that more comprehensive knowledge would be dug out on the specific physiological mechanism underlying acupuncture.

Table 2. The DMN hub configurations during the resting state (REST), following sham acupuncture (NAP) and verum acupuncture (ST36) within the 5 frequency bands respectively.

Frequency band	Conditions REST	NAP	ST36
Delta	PCC, IPL	PCC, MTG	PCC, SFG
Theta	PCC	PCC, STG	MFG, STG, SFG
Alpha	PCC, ACC,STG, SFG	PCC, ACC,STG, SFG, MFG	STG, SFG
Beta	PCC, ACC, SFG	PCC, ACC, SFG	ACC, SFG
Gamma	PCC	PCC, ACC	PCC, STG

Abbreviations as in Table 1.

Materials and Methods

Subjects

In order to reduce inter-subject difference, 28 right-handed healthy college students (14 males, 14 females, aged 24.5±1.8 years) from a homogeneous group were enrolled. All of them were acupuncture naïve. Participants were screened to exclude individuals with a history of major medical illness, head trauma, neuropsychiatric disorders or used any prescription medications within the last month. All subjects gave written, informed consent after the experimental procedures being fully explained. The Tiantan Hospital Subcommittee on Human Studies approved the methods and procedures, all of which was in accordance with the Declaration of Helsinki.

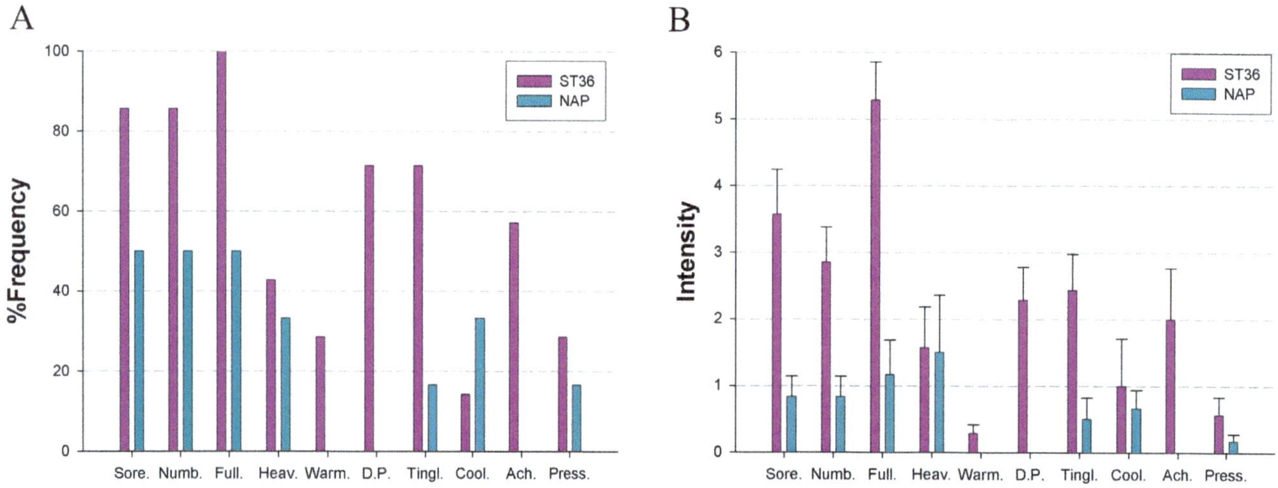

Figure 3. Averaged psychophysical response. A. The percentage of subjects that reported the given sensations. The frequency of aching was found greater following acupuncture at ST36. B. The intensity of sensations measured by average score (with standard error bars) on a scale from 0 denoting no sensation to 10 denoting an unbearable sensation. Sore, soreness; Numb, numbness; Full, fullness; Heav, heaviness; Warm, warmth; DP, dull pain; Tinl, tingling; Cool, coolness; Ach, aching; Press, pressure.

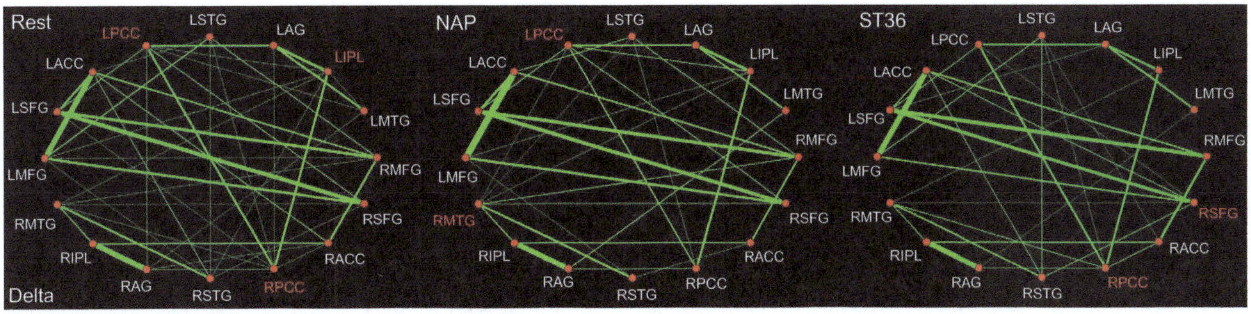

Figure 4. DMN hub configurations preceding acupuncture and following acupuncture at ST36 or NAP within the delta band (P<0.05, FDR corrected). The DMN hubs are indicated in red which are denoted as at least one standard deviation greater than the average degree of the network. The strength of the functional connectivity was expressed by the thickness of the green line. L, left; R, right; MFG, medial frontal gyrus; SFG, superior frontal gyrus; ACC, anterior cingulate cortex; PCC, posterior cingulate cortex/precuneus; STG, superior temporal gyrus; AG, angular gyrus; IPL, inferior parietal lobule; MTG, middle temporal gyrus.

Experimental paradigm

Twenty-eight participants were evenly divided into two groups, one for ST36 and the other for NAP, being matched by age and gender. All participants underwent firstly resting state functional MRI scanning for 6 min, followed by MEG data collection, during which the manual acupuncture was exerted at either ST36 or NAP. The whole MEG data collection lasts for 15 min, with the first 6 min for resting-state scanning and the other 9 min for acupuncture intervention. Both verum and sham manual acupuncture employed the single-block design paradigm, incorporating 2 min needle manipulation, preceded by 1 min rest epoch and followed by 6 min rest (without acupuncture manipulation) scanning. The experimental paradigm of MEG scanning can be found in Fig. 1. All participants were asked to remain relaxed without engaging in any mental tasks. To facilitate blinding, they were also instructed to keep their eyes closed to prevent from actually observing the procedures.

Verum acupuncture was performed at ST36 on the right leg (Zusanli, located four finger breadths below the lower margin of the patella and one finger breadth laterally from the anterior crest of the tibia) [42–43]. Verum acupuncture was delivered using a sterile disposable 38 gauge stainless steel acupuncture needle, 0.2 mm in diameter and 40 mm in length, which was inserted perpendicularly into the skin surface at a depth of 1.5–2.5 cm. Sham acupuncture was initially devised by an experienced and licensed acupuncturist (with 6 years of experience and had been trained to perform in the fMRI settings), with needling at non-meridian point (2–3 cm apart from ST36), with needle depth, stimulation intensity and manipulation procedure all identical to those used in verum acupuncture. A balanced "tonifying and reducing" technique was utilized as twirling the needle clockwise and counter-clockwise equally [44]. Stimulation consisted of rotating the needle clockwise and counterclockwise for 1 min at a rate of 60 times per min. The whole procedure was performed by the same acupuncturist on all participants.

According to Traditional Chinese Medicine, the sensation induced by twirling needles at the acupoints is asserted as "*De-qi*", which is essential to the efficacy of acupuncture [45]. As a concurrent psychophysical analysis, the MGH Acupuncture Sensation Scale (MASS) was utilized in the present study to quantify the subjective *De-qi* sensations [38,46]. The sensation rates ranged from 0 to 10 (0 = no sensation, 1–3 = mild, 4–6 = moderate, 7–8 = strong, 9 = severe and 10 = unbearable sensation). Spreading of any sensation was noted in a binary fashion and coded as follows: 1-spreading reported; 0-spreading not reported.

Table 3. The functional connectivity between the DMN key nodes and their alterations induced by acupuncture within the delta band (0.5–4 Hz).

Functional Connectivity	Delta				
	Rest	**NAP**	***P*-value**	**ST36**	***P*-value**
MFG-SFG	0.3643	0.4011	0.358	0.4299	0.723
SFG-ACC	0.2332	0.3016	0.231	0.1383	0.407
ACC-PCC	0.0546	0	–	0.0779	0.611
PCC-STG	0.0551	0.0710	0.841	0.0709	0.019
STG-AG	0	0	–	0	–
AG-IPL	0.6478	0.6209	0.635	0.6226	0.075
IPL-MTG	0.1289	0.1276	0.839	0.1199	0.699
MTG-MFG	0.0447	0.0817	0.125	0	–
MFG-ACC	0.6874	0.7952	0.575	0.6373	0.193
SFG-PCC	0.1176	0.0954	0.119	0.0953	0.623
ACC-STG	0.0823	0.0818	0.774	0.1167	0.053
PCC-AG	0.2077	0.2081	0.831	0.2145	0.752
STG-IPL	0.0504	0	–	0	–
AG-MTG	0.2146	0.2176	0.856	0.2438	0.648
IPL-MFG	0.0420	0.0632	0.742	0	–
MTG-SFG	0.0670	0.0806	0.248	0.0631	0.617
MFG-PCC	0	0	–	0	–
SFG-STG	0.0477	0	–	0.0975	0.161
ACC-AG	0.0516	0	–	0	–
PCC-IPL	0.2443	0.2363	0.684	0.2482	0.742
STG-MTG	0.2273	0.2622	0.396	0.2133	0.869
AG-MFG	0	0	–	0	–
IPL-SFG	0	0	–	0	–
MTG-ACC	0	0	–	0	–
MFG-STG	0.0755	0.0867	0.636	0.1219	0.195
SFG-AG	0	0	–	0.0475	–
ACC-IPL	0.1461	0.1228	0.395	0.1492	0.953
PCC-MTG	0.0685	0.0504	0.938	0.0843	0.872

The maximum of the 4 pairwise connections obtained between the two ROIs located in both hemispheres was defined as the connectivity between the two nodes (one sample *t*-test, $P<0.05$). Significant alterations induced by acupuncture at ST36 relative to NAP were based on the paired *t*-test ($P<0.05$) or with the emergence/suspension of functional connectivity following acupuncture compared with the resting state.

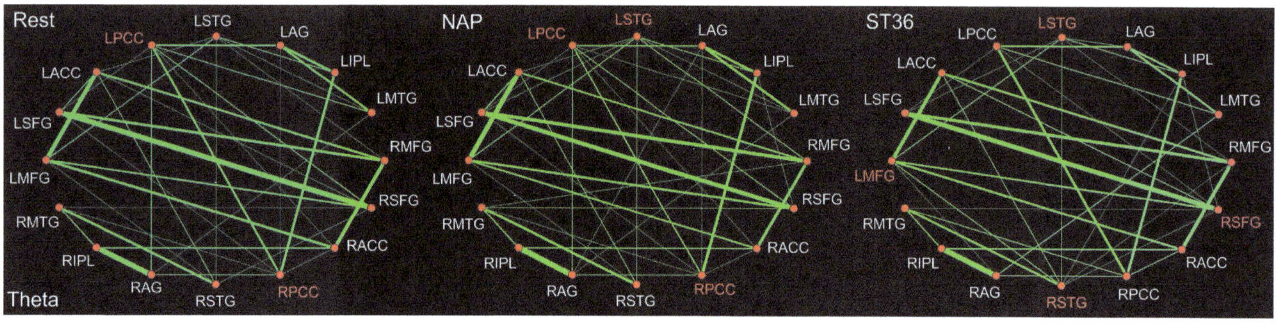

Figure 5. DMN hub configurations preceding acupuncture and following acupuncture at ST36 or NAP within the theta band (P<0.05, FDR corrected). The DMN hubs are indicated in red which are denoted as at least one standard deviation greater than the average degree of the network. The strength of the functional connectivity was expressed by the thickness of the green line. L, left; R, right; MFG, medial frontal gyrus; SFG, superior frontal gyrus; ACC, anterior cingulate cortex; PCC, posterior cingulate cortex/precuneus; STG, superior temporal gyrus; AG, angular gyrus; IPL, inferior parietal lobule; MTG, middle temporal gyrus.

fMRI and MEG data acquisition

All fMRI data were obtained with a 3.0 T MRI system (Allegra; Siemens, Erlangen, Germany). A custom-built head holder and foam padding were used to restricted head movements. The images were parallel to the AC-PC line and covered the whole brain. Thirty-two axial slices were obtained using a T2*-weighted single-shot, gradient-recalled echo planar imaging sequence (FOV = 240 mm×240 mm, matrix = 64×64, thickness = 5 mm, TR = 2000 ms, TE = 30 ms, flip angle = 75°). The total functional scanning was lasted for 6 minutes during the resting state. After the functional run, high-resolution structural information on each subject was also acquired using 3D MRI sequences with a voxel size of 1 mm^3 for anatomical localization (TR = 2700 ms, TE = 2.19 ms, matrix = 384×512, FOV = 256 mm×256 mm, flip angel = 7°, thickness = 1 mm).

The MEG data were recorded when participants comfortably seated inside an electromagnetically shielded room. The cortical responses were recorded with the whole head MEG system (CTF Systems Inc., Port Coquitlam, BC, Canada) consisting of 151 hardware first-order magnetic gradiometers. Two of the original 151 channels were not available due to technical problems during recording for all participants. The whole MEG scanning lasted 15 minutes, incorporating a 6 min resting state recording and followed by above-mentioned 9-min acupuncture procedure (Fig. 1). The head position was monitored during the measurement using head position indicator coils. MEG data were recorded at the sample rate of 600 Hz. The same acquisition settings were used for an empty-room recording without a subject in the MEG room to estimate the background noise [47]. During the recording, participants were instructed to close their eyes to reduce artifact signals due to eye movements, but remain awake as much as possible. The investigator and MEG technician checked the signal on-line and observed the participants using a video monitor. The head position relative to the MEG sensors was measured before and after each recording session by leading small alternating currents through three head position coils attached to the left and right pre-auricular points and the nasion on the subject's head. For all analyzed data sets, head displacements within a recording session were below 5 mm.

fMRI data analysis

The first five volumes of fMRI data were discarded to eliminate non-equilibrium effects of magnetization [48]. All images were subsequently pre-processed using the statistical parametric mapping (SPM5, http://www.fil.ion.ucl.ac.uk/spm/) [49]. Firstly, the image data underwent realignments for head motions using the least-squares minimization. None of subjects had head movements

Table 4. The functional connectivity between the DMN key nodes and their alterations induced by acupuncture within the theta band (4–8 Hz).

Functional Connectivity	Theta				
	Rest	NAP	*P*-value	ST36	*P*-value
MFG-SFG	0.3450	0.3848	0.405	0.3490	0.894
SFG-ACC	0.0922	0.1727	0.105	0.1204	0.142
ACC-PCC	0.0760	0.0691	0.055	0.0841	0.317
PCC-STG	0	0	–	0	–
STG-AG	0	0	–	0.0596	–
AG-IPL	0.6085	0.6289	0.064	0.2721	0.000
IPL-MTG	0.1433	0.1499	0.779	0.1399	0.833
MTG-MFG	0	0.0452	–	0	–
MFG-ACC	0.4756	0.5512	0.772	0.4608	0.132
SFG-PCC	0.0850	0.0883	0.314	0.0694	0.854
ACC-STG	0.0753	0.0841	0.714	0.0929	0.302
PCC-AG	0.2061	0.1669	0.208	0.1778	0.269
STG-IPL	0.0922	0.0818	0.545	0.0895	0.685
AG-MTG	0.2387	0.2929	0.057	0.2614	0.544
IPL-MFG	0	0	–	0	–
MTG-SFG	0.0553	0.0598	0.340	0.0679	0.533
MFG-PCC	0	0	–	0	–
SFG-STG	0.0472	0.0641	0.301	0.0614	0.463
ACC-AG	0.	0	–	0	–
PCC-IPL	0.2790	0.3263	0.091	0.5980	0.000
STG-MTG	0.2744	0.3002	0.628	0.2436	0.921
AG-MFG	0	0	–	0.0455	–
IPL-SFG	0	0.0410	–	0.0498	–
MTG-ACC	0	0	–	0	–
MFG-STG	0.0832	0.0817	0.818	0.0971	0.807
SFG-AG	0	0	–	0	–
ACC-IPL	0.1580	0.1509	0.981	0.1656	0.988
PCC-MTG	0.0773	0.0549	0.716	0.0904	0.998

The maximum of the 4 pairwise connections obtained from the two ROIs located in both hemispheres was defined as the connectivity between the two nodes (one sample *t*-test, $P<0.05$). Significant alterations induced by acupuncture at ST36 relative to NAP were based on the paired *t*-test ($P<0.05$) or with the emergence/suspension of functional connectivity following acupuncture compared with the resting state.

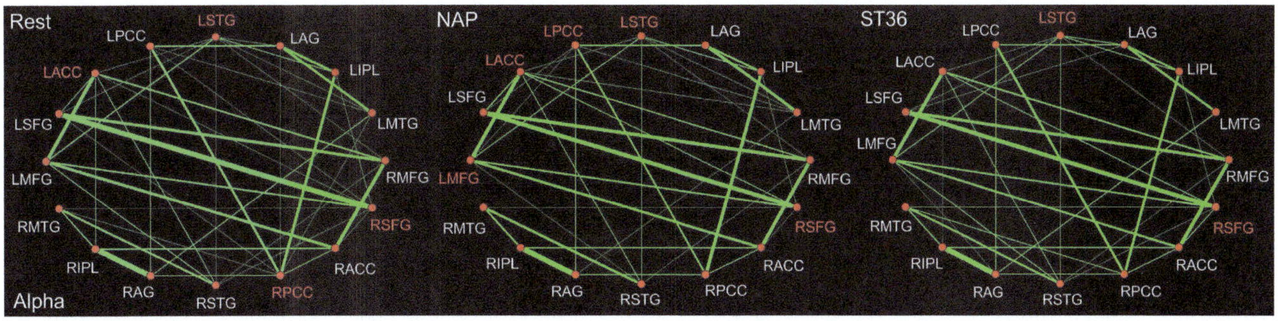

Figure 6. DMN hub configurations preceding acupuncture and following acupuncture at ST36 or NAP within the alpha band (P<0.05, FDR corrected). The DMN hubs are indicated in red which are denoted as at least one standard deviation greater than the average degree of the network. The strength of the functional connectivity was expressed by the thickness of the green line. L, left; R, right; MFG, medial frontal gyrus; SFG, superior frontal gyrus; ACC, anterior cingulate cortex; PCC, posterior cingulate cortex/precuneus; STG, superior temporal gyrus; AG, angular gyrus; IPL, inferior parietal lobule; MTG, middle temporal gyrus.

exceeding 1 mm on any axis or head rotation greater than one degree. A mean image created from the realigned volumes was coregistered with the subject's individual structural T1-weighted volume image. Secondly, the standard Montreal Neurological Institute (MNI) template provided by SPM5 was used in the spatial normalization. Then these data were resampled at 2 mm×2 mm×2 mm and filtered utilizing a finite-impulse response band-pass filter (0.01~0.08 Hz) in order to remove the effect of low-frequency drift and high-frequency noise [50–51]. Subsequently, the functional images were smoothed by a Gaussian kernel with a full width at half maximum of 6 mm (FWHM = 6 mm).

A data-driven method named independent component analysis (ICA), which is able to extract multiple functional connectivity networks [26,52], was performed on the preprocessed data of all subjects using the Group ICA of fMRI Toolbox (GIFT) [53–54]. To reduce the computational load of simply entering all subjects' data into an ICA analysis, two reduction steps were conducted, one on data from each subject and the other on an aggregate data set. In the first round of principal component analysis (PCA), the data for individual subject were dimension-reduced to 52 in the GIFT toolbox. After concatenation across subjects, the dimension was again reduced via the second round of PCA to 33 components estimated by the Minimum Description Length (MDL) criteria, followed by an independent component estimation using Infomax algorithm [54–55]. The mean ICs of all the subjects, the corresponding mean time courses and ICs for each subject were obtained from group ICA separation and back-reconstruction [53]. The maps of these ICs across all subjects were generated for a random effect analysis using a one-sample t-test. Thresholds were set at P<0.05 (correction with the FDR criterion). The intensity values in each spatial map were converted to Z scores to indicate the voxels that contributed most strongly to a particular IC. Voxels with absolute Z-values greater than 1.5 are considered active voxels of the IC [56]. The independent component was selected, which best matched the default mode network as previously reported [26,28]. Every template region was spherical with a radius of 5 mm (varying sphere size had no effect on component identification), and the average value of voxels within the template minus that of voxels outside the template was calculated for each component. Finally, the component with the greatest difference was determined to be the best-fit component and was designated as the DMN. The peak voxels of 8 core regions of interest (ROIs) were subsequently identified within the DMN component. These ROIs mainly include the bilateral medial frontal gyrus (MFG), superior frontal gyrus (SFG), anterior cingulate cortex (ACC), posterior cingulate cortex (PCC), superior temporal gyrus (STG), angular gyrus (AG), inferior parietal lobule (IPL) and middle temporal gyrus (MTG) [50,57–59]. See Fig. 2. Talairach coordinates of peak foci for each ROI are listed in the Table 1.

MEG data analysis

A third-order gradient noise reduction (computed with CTF software) was applied to the MEG signals on line. The raw data were then digitally filtered off-line with a band-pass of 0.5–48 Hz, followed by down-sampled at a rate of 300 Hz. Subsequently, the MEG data were band-passed into bands of interest: delta (0.5–4 Hz), theta (4–8 Hz), alpha (8–13 Hz), beta (13–30 Hz) and gamma band (30–48 Hz) [60–62]. To specifically highlight the temporal dynamics within and across different regions of the default mode network, discrete regional dipole source analysis [63] was applied in each frequency band to create a spatial filter to project into source space using the Brain Electrical Source Analysis (BESA, MEGIS Software GmbH, Germany) software package which implements a least squares algorithm to solve the overdetermined problem and estimate the activity contributed by each source to the scalp-recorded data [64–66]. This methodology overcomes some of the limitations associated with conducting analysis only in the sensor space and allows the spatiotemporal modeling of multiple simultaneous sources over defined intervals [67]. In our study, to represent brain activity within DMN preceding or following acupuncture, relevant fixed regional sources were seeded into a 3-layer spherical head model and source activity was estimated from each subject's continuous scalp data for further analysis [64,68]. Positioning of regional sources drew on the spatial localization of peak voxels in the DMN component obtained in fMRI. Talairach coordinates of these regional sources and proximate cortical structures are listed in Table 1.

Functional connectivity analysis and hub definition

Partial correlation analysis has been proven effective as a measure of the functional connectivity between a given pair of regions by attenuating the contribution of other sources of covariance [69–71]. Besides, partial correlations can be used to build undirected graphs, in which connections (edges) between nodes (vertices) depict their conditional dependence [69,72]. Given a set of N random variables, the partial correlation matrix is a symmetric matrix in which each off-diagonal element is the correlation coefficient between a pair of variables after partialling

Table 5. The functional connectivity between the DMN key nodes and their alterations induced by acupuncture within the alpha band (8–13 Hz).

Functional Connectivity	Alpha				
	Rest	NAP	*P*-value	ST36	*P*-value
MFG-SFG	0.3511	0.3768	0.564	0.3491	0.988
SFG-ACC	0.0997	0.1573	0.066	0.1103	0.078
ACC-PCC	0.0908	0.0778	0.034	0.1063	0.403
PCC-STG	0	0	–	0	–
STG-AG	0.0303	0	–	0.0800	0.148
AG-IPL	0.6003	0.6231	0.262	0.6070	0.768
IPL-MTG	0.1620	0.1753	0.362	0.1583	0.487
MTG-MFG	0	0	–	0	–
MFG-ACC	0.4672	0.3990	0.667	0.4492	0.116
SFG-PCC	0.0489	0.0460	0.912	0	–
ACC-STG	0.0925	0.0929	0.496	0.0908	0.684
PCC-AG	0.2084	0.1649	0.111	0.1593	0.157
STG-IPL	0.1000	0.0991	0.711	0.0984	0.689
AG-MTG	0.2778	0.3513	0.007	0.2971	0.731
IPL-MFG	0	0	–	0	–
MTG-SFG	0.0649	0.0544	0.482	0.0733	0.721
MFG-PCC	0	0.0451	–	0	–
SFG-STG	0.0388	0	–	0.0580	0.299
ACC-AG	0	0	–	0	–
PCC-IPL	0.3218	0.3922	0.197	0.3020	0.606
STG-MTG	0.2581	0.2926	0.501	0.2536	0.616
AG-MFG	0	0	–	0.0524	–
IPL-SFG	0.0604	0.0544	0.697	0.0622	0.696
MTG-ACC	0	0.0556	–	0	–
MFG-STG	0.1160	0.0957	0.155	0.1151	0.889
SFG-AG	0	0	–	0.0543	–
ACC-IPL	0.1708	0.1638	0.479	0.1697	0.749
PCC-MTG	0.0588	0.0508	0.633	0.0955	0.379

The maximum of the 4 pairwise connections obtained from the two ROIs located in both hemispheres was defined as the connectivity between the two nodes (one sample *t*-test, $P<0.05$). Significant alterations induced by acupuncture at ST36 relative to NAP were based on the paired *t*-test ($P<0.05$) or with the emergence/suspension of functional connectivity following acupuncture compared with the resting state.

out the contributions to the pairwise correlation of all other variables included in the dataset [71,73–75]. In our case, it was thus utilized within each frequency band to estimate the correlation coefficient between each pair of regions within DMN, factoring out the contribution to the pairwise correlations of the other 14 brain regions.

To estimate the partial correlation matrix within each frequency band for every participant, covariance matrix S was generated, using the 360s-long MEG data matrix Y on a subject-by-subject basis. Each component of S contains the sample covariance value between two brain regions (j, k) was $s_{j,k} = T^{-1} \sum_{t=1}^{T} (y_j(t)-\bar{y}_j)(y_k(t)-\bar{y}_k)$, where $\bar{y}_j$ denotes the average over time of the observations in a given region, T denotes the number of time points. Afterwards, the off-diagonal elements of the inverted matrix S^{-1} was rescaled to obtain the partial correlation matrix R: $r_{j,k} = -s^{-1}_{j,k} \Big/ \sqrt{s^{-1}_{j,j} s^{-1}_{k,k}}$ [71]. A Fisher's r-to-Z transformation was then applied on the partial correlation matrices in order to improve the normality of the partial correlation coefficients [76]. To test the null hypothesis that the partial correlation was zero between any pair of regions within DMN, we conducted multiple one-sample *t*-tests for the individually estimated partial correlations for each condition. False discovery rate (FDR) procedure was applied to restrict the expected proportion of type I errors to $q<0.05$ [77]. Subsequently, the partial correlation matrices obtained individually were averaged to obtain group mean inter-regional functional connectivity. Due to the lack of consensus as to the best method for defining network hubs, a pragmatic method was applied in which nodes were identified as network hubs if their degree values were at least one standard deviation greater than the average degree of the network [37,78]. Finally, significant alterations of functional connectivity induced by acupuncture for either ST36 or NAP group was evaluated for each band by means of a paired *t*-test with thresholded at $P<0.05$ in SPSS 17.0 software package for Windows.

Results

Psychophysical responses

The prevalence of subjective "*De-qi*" sensations was expressed as the percentage of individuals in the group who reported the given sensations (Fig. 3A). The intensity was expressed as the average score ± standard error (Fig. 3B). The occurrence frequency of all sensations except coolness was found to be greater for acupuncture at ST36 than NAP. The overall stimulus intensities (mean ± SE) were greater for ST36, exhibiting a stronger *De-qi* sensation in verum acupuncture ($P<0.05$, two sample *t*-test).

Band-specific DMN hub configurations

In the present study, the pairwise functional connectivity analysis between the 8 core brain regions within the default mode network were evaluated for each of the 5 conventional frequency bands (delta, theta, alpha, beta and gamma) preceding and following acupuncture, with the aim of exploring the band-specific alterations of DMN hub configurations induced by verum acupuncture at ST36, using a nearby non-acupoint (NAP, sham acupuncture) as a control. The summary of the DMN hub configurations within each frequency band was listed in the Table 2.

For the delta band (0.5–4 Hz), the PCC and IPL were identified as DMN hubs during the resting state (Fig. 4). Following acupuncture, either at ST36 or at NAP, it is of interest to find that little was modulated on the key role played by PCC in the DMN hub configurations. By contrast, the IPL no longer acted as a network hub within the DMN in either group during the post-stimuli acupuncture resting state. In addition, specific acupuncture-induced alterations on hub configuration were also exhibited. To be specific, the right MTG was identified as a hub following sham acupuncture, while the right SFG was spotted following verum acupuncture at ST36. Taken into account the acupuncture-induced alterations of functional connectivity, it can be found that the functional interactions were suspended between STG and IPL, ACC and AG following either sham or verum acupuncture. In the NAP group, the connectivity between ACC and PCC as well as SFG and STG was found to be interrupted. On the contrary, the

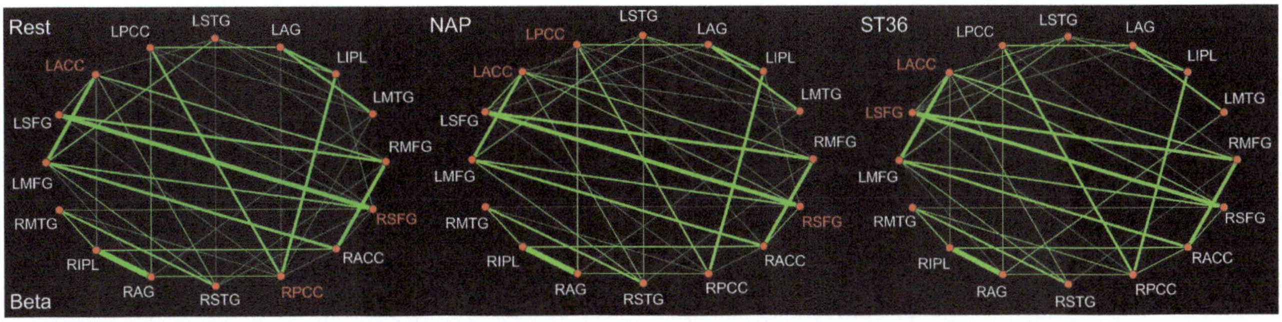

Figure 7. DMN hub configurations preceding acupuncture and following acupuncture at ST36 or NAP within the beta band ($P<0.05$, FDR corrected). The DMN hubs are indicated in red which are denoted as at least one standard deviation greater than the average degree of the network. The strength of the functional connectivity was expressed by the thickness of the green line. L, left; R, right; MFG, medial frontal gyrus; SFG, superior frontal gyrus; ACC, anterior cingulate cortex; PCC, posterior cingulate cortex/precuneus; STG, superior temporal gyrus; AG, angular gyrus; IPL, inferior parietal lobule; MTG, middle temporal gyrus.

Table 6. The functional connectivity between the DMN key nodes and their alterations induced by acupuncture within the beta band (13–30 Hz).

Functional Connectivity	Beta				
	Rest	NAP	*P*-value	ST36	*P*-value
MFG-SFG	0.3274	0.3446	0.725	0.3271	0.957
SFG-ACC	0.0915	0.1372	0.198	0.1281	0.221
ACC-PCC	0.0815	0.0717	0.023	0.0789	0.843
PCC-STG	0	0	–	0	–
STG-AG	0	0	–	0.0575	–
AG-IPL	0.6204	0.6424	0.256	0.6178	0.857
IPL-MTG	0.1534	0.1577	0.392	0.1481	0.631
MTG-MFG	0	0	–	0	–
MFG-ACC	0.4636	0.4153	0.107	0.4319	0.091
SFG-PCC	0.0642	0.0573	0.382	0.0529	0.443
ACC-STG	0.0914	0.0904	0.364	0.0897	0.598
PCC-AG	0.1979	0.1630	0.169	0.1771	0.392
STG-IPL	0.0969	0.0850	0.425	0.0878	0.441
AG-MTG	0.2357	0.3116	0.004	0.2517	0.750
IPL-MFG	0	0	–	0	–
MTG-SFG	0.0539	0.0491	0.793	0.0696	0.159
MFG-PCC	0	0	–	0	–
SFG-STG	0.0360	0	–	0.0458	0.694
ACC-AG	0	0	–	0	–
PCC-IPL	0.3118	0.3708	0.127	0.3059	0.610
STG-MTG	0.2575	0.2738	0.970	0.2535	0.667
AG-MFG	0.0429	0	–	0.0468	0.481
IPL-SFG	0.0446	0.0507	0.537	0	–
MTG-ACC	0	0.0514	–	0	–
MFG-STG	0.1121	0.0987	0.727	0.1020	0.642
SFG-AG	0	0.0458	–	0.0406	–
ACC-IPL	0.1566	0.1609	0.474	0.1405	0.595
PCC-MTG	0.0624	0.0533	0.776	0.0934	0.458

The maximum of the 4 pairwise connections obtained from the two ROIs located in both hemispheres was defined as the connectivity between the two nodes (one sample *t*-test, $P<0.05$). Significant alterations induced by acupuncture at ST36 relative to NAP were based on the paired *t*-test ($P<0.05$) or with the emergence/suspension of functional connectivity following acupuncture compared with the resting state.

relation between MTG and MFG together with IPL and MFG was disconnected following acupuncture at ST36. Meanwhile, there emerged the functional connectivity between the SFG and AG as well as increased interaction between PCC and STG in the ST36 group (Table 3).

Compared with the DMN hub configuration during the resting state in the delta band, it was recognized furthermore that the PCC constituted the only hub within the theta band (4–8 Hz). What's more, the most interesting difference lies in the fact that, following sham acupuncture at NAP, the bilateral PCC were still remained among the core hub regions, however, neither of them served as a hub following the verum intervention at ST36 (Fig. 5). Meanwhile, the STG was emerged to act as a network hub following either ST36 or NAP stimulation. In addition, it was remarkable that the SFG was specifically discerned as a DMN hub for the ST36 group. Following acupuncture at NAP, the connectivity between MTG and MFG was detected to be enhanced, while in the ST36 group, the relations between STG and AG, PCC and IPL, AG and MFG were found to be emerged, while the connectivity between AG and IPL was significantly decreased. Interestingly, the connection between IPL and SFG was detected to be strengthened following either acupuncture (Table 4).

Among the 5 frequency bands, it seems that there are the most hubs within the alpha band (8–13 Hz) during the resting state (Fig. 6), involving the ACC, STG, PCC as well as SFG. In line with the theta band, it is notable that the left STG served robustly as network hubs following either sham or verum acupuncture. Besides, it was also illustrated that the PCC acted as a hub specifically following the sham acupuncture. Moreover, what's different between the theta and alpha band is that the SFG not only emerged as a hub for the ST36 group, but also formed a network hub for the NAP group in the alpha band. In addition, it was noted that the ACC together with MFG formed the DMN hubs following acupuncture at NAP, none of which, on the contrary, was designated for the ST36 group. Moreover, the relations between ACC and PCC, STG and AG as well as SFG and STG were weakened, while the connections between AG and MTG, MFG and PCC, MTG and ACC were found to be strengthened following the sham stimulation. In the ST36 group, the connectivity between SFG and PCC was decreased while the relations between AG and MFG, SFG and AG were increased (Table 5).

To some extent similarity was found for the DMN hub configurations during the resting state between the beta band (13–30 Hz) and the alpha band (Fig. 7). First of all, the PCC was

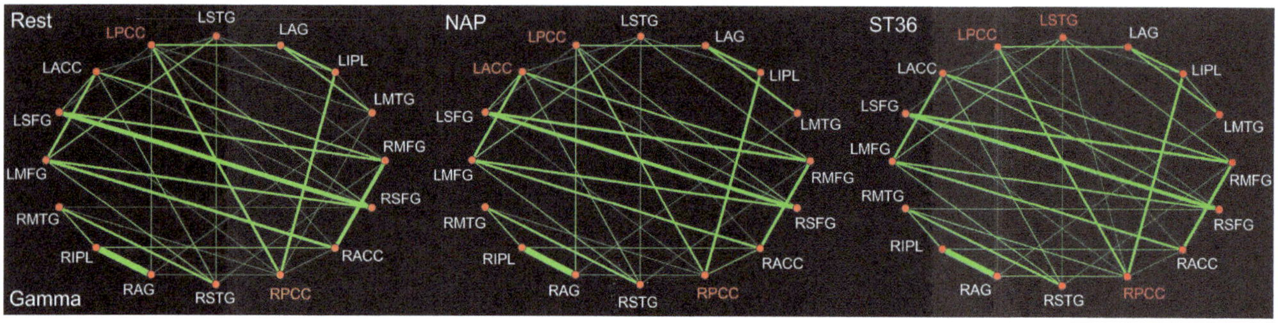

Figure 8. DMN hub configurations preceding acupuncture and following acupuncture at ST36 or NAP within the gamma band ($P<0.05$, FDR corrected). The DMN hubs are indicated in red which are denoted as at least one standard deviation greater than the average degree of the network. The strength of the functional connectivity was expressed by the thickness of the green line. L, left; R, right; MFG, medial frontal gyrus; SFG, superior frontal gyrus; ACC, anterior cingulate cortex; PCC, posterior cingulate cortex/precuneus; STG, superior temporal gyrus; AG, angular gyrus; IPL, inferior parietal lobule; MTG, middle temporal gyrus.

consistently identified as a hub. In addition, the ACC together with SFG was also designated for the beta band. Following either verum or sham acupuncture, it is noticeable that little was influenced on the role played by ACC and SFG for the DMN hub configurations. However, compared with the NAP group, the PCC did not serve as a network hub any more following acupuncture at ST36. There are also some shared alterations of the functional connectivity induced by acupuncture between the beta and alpha band. Following acupuncture at NAP, the connection between ACC and PCC, SFG and STG as well as AG and MFG were detected to be reduced, while the relations between AG and MTG, MTG and ACC, SFG and AG were enhanced. After stimulation at ST36, the connection between IPL and SFG was decreased, while the relations between STG and AG, SFG and AG were illustrated to be increased (Table 6).

In line with other frequency bands, the PCC was as well shown dominantly as the default mode network hub during the resting state within the gamma band (30–48 Hz). Following acupuncture, for either verum or sham stimulation, it is of interest to find that there was little acupuncture-induced modulation over the role played by PCC in the DMN hub configurations (Fig. 8). The PCC as well as the ACC was illustrated to be the network hubs following sham acupuncture. On the contrary, apart from the PCC, the STG was denoted specifically to work as a hub following acupuncture at ST36. Following acupuncture at either NAP or ST36, only a few significant alterations of functional connectivity were demonstrated within the gamma band. For the NAP group, the connection between MTG and SFG was decreased, while the connectivity between MTG and AG was significantly increased. For the ST36 group, significant increased connectivity was detected only between PCC and STG (Table 7).

Discussion

To the best of our knowledge, it is the first study to explore spatiotemporally the acupuncture effects on the DMN hub configurations within conventional frequency bands (delta, theta, alpha, beta and gamma) following stimulation at ST36, using a nearby non-acupoint (NAP) as a control, by combining fMRI and MEG analysis.Results exhibits differential alterations within the hub configurations of the DMN during the post-stimuli acupuncture resting state.

DMN hub configurations during the resting state

Among all DMN core regions, the PCC has been extensively denoted as the pivotal role in connecting other DMN brain regions for transmitting information under the mentioned cognitive processes, or optimizing the connectivity pattern to reduce cost of wiring and resources [23,29–30]. In the present study, by combining fMRI and MEG techniques, we not only confirmed the crucial function of the PCC in the DMN, but further extend previous knowledge about its hub configuration in the frequency domains. It is worthy to mention that the PCC constitutes the most attention-grabbing region as it is the only one which acted as a DMN hub consistently across the 5 conventional frequency bands (delta, theta, alpha, beta and gamma rhythm). Meanwhile, in line with previous fMRI studies, the IPL [79–80] and ACC, SFG [28] were validated as DMN hubs during the resting state. Moreover, with the advantage of MEG in providing amount of details in temporal dimension, it was further revealed that their crucial functions were exerted not across the 5 bands but within specific rhythms, especially with delta band for IPL and alpha, beta bands for both ACC and SFG.

Differential hub configurations following verum and sham acupuncture

Recently a number of noninvasive sham controls have been developed and tested [38,81–82]. While these hold promise in some respects, they also have limitations in what they can be used for, thus they should be used only when it is clear that their use matches the question for which sham treatment model is being selected [83]. Sham acupuncture is proved to a reasonable placebo control in many acupuncture fMRI setting, and can effectively reduce the subjects' bias toward the stimulation. In the current study, we also employed sham acupuncture as a control model. The comparison of the verum acupuncture, compared with the sham control, was expected to reveal the acupoint-specific response in the human brain and the observed differences between these two conditions may constitute a specific physiological effect.

As illustrated in aforementioned results (Fig. 4–8), the PCC constitute one of the most noteworthy DMN hubs with saliently differential alterations following either verum or sham acupuncture. Following sham acupuncture at NAP, the PCC remained to serve consistently as DMN hub across all 5 frequency bands. However, it is interesting to find out that the PCC was to a large extent regulated in specific bands by the verum acupuncture at ST36. Actually, it is only within delta and gamma bands that the PCC still acted as a DMN hub. As implicated typically in previous

Table 7. The functional connectivity between the DMN key nodes and their alterations induced by acupuncture within the gamma band (30–48 Hz).

Functional Connectivity	Gamma				
	Rest	NAP	*P*-value	ST36	*P*-value
MFG-SFG	0.2814	0.2980	0.669	0.2909	0.860
SFG-ACC	0.0775	0.1195	0.584	0.1283	0.092
ACC-PCC	0.0751	0.0760	0.191	0.0698	0.789
PCC-STG	0	0	–	0.0466	–
STG-AG	0	0	–	0	–
AG-IPL	0.6653	0.6769	0.303	0.6568	0.497
IPL-MTG	0.1366	0.1321	0.551	0.1397	0.796
MTG-MFG	0	0	–	0	–
MFG-ACC	0.3825	0.3614	0.495	0.3610	0.239
SFG-PCC	0.0842	0.0868	0.672	0.0718	0.583
ACC-STG	0.1050	0.1060	0.346	0.1039	0.592
PCC-AG	0.1843	0.1504	0.120	0.1756	0.578
STG-IPL	0.0594	0.0424	0.227	0.0517	0.066
AG-MTG	0.1843	0.2440	0.009	0.1883	0.828
IPL-MFG	0	0	–	0	–
MTG-SFG	0.0448	0	–	0.0561	0.125
MFG-PCC	0	0	–	0	–
SFG-STG	0	0	–	0	–
ACC-AG	0	0	–	0	–
PCC-IPL	0.2886	0.3226	0.127	0.2845	0.942
STG-MTG	0.2578	0.2568	0.166	0.2395	0.928
AG-MFG	0	0	–	0	–
IPL-SFG	0	0	–	0	–
MTG-ACC	0	0	–	0	–
MFG-STG	0.1073	0.0953	0.226	0.0930	0.611
SFG-AG	0	0	–	0	–
ACC-IPL	0.1130	0.1176	0.772	0.0976	0.491
PCC-MTG	0.0489	0.0533	0.772	0.0841	0.265

The maximum of the 4 pairwise connections obtained from the two ROIs located in both hemispheres was defined as the connectivity between the two nodes (one sample *t*-test, $P<0.05$). Significant alterations induced by acupuncture at ST36 relative to NAP were based on the paired *t*-test ($P<0.05$) or with the emergence/suspension of functional connectivity following acupuncture compared with the resting state.

neuroimaging studies, the PCC served as not only a DMN hub [28], but a core region for the whole brain network when engaging more brain regions within the whole brain network [23]. Recently, it is speculated that the brain regions are organized into interleaved networks to accomplish various functions or healing effects when a neural intervention is triggered [7]. Since DMN involves a mode of preparedness and alertness of possible changes in the internal milieu as well as external environment, the integrity of connectivity between the DMN and other brain networks may be central to the balance of brain functions [84]. Previous studies have shown alterations in the generalized activity and functional connectivity of the DMN in patients with various kinds of disorders [85–87]. Following stimulation at pain-control acupoints, it is demonstrated as well that there is increased DMN connectivity with pain related regions [40]. This suggests that specific brain networks may facilitate a correspondence between acupuncture stimulation and the central nervous system. Moreover, it has been proven, following acupuncture at vision-related acupoint, that the PCC performed intensive connections with other discrete core regions in vision networks [7]. Taken into account the ST36 is a commonly used acupoint for pain control in clinical practice, it is postulated that PCC would engage extensive interactions with the neural networks for both pain transmission and perception [88–89]. The connectivity was therefore believed to be enhanced between the PCC and those core regions within the pain matrix [90]. As a result, the role as a DMN hub played consistently by the PCC across the 5 frequency bands may be to some extent inhibited, supposed to be reallocated in order to balance the energy for the whole brain network to better exert the analgesia effect. In addition, it is for the first time revealed that the physiological regulations induced by acupuncture were dependent on the specific rhythms of neural activity. Compared with sham acupuncture, the acupuncture-induced modulation for PCC was mainly confined within the theta, alpha and beta bands.

Another striking finding is that, regarding to other core regions, to a certain extent shared DMN hub configuration patterns were observed following acupuncture at either ST36 or NAP. Given that acupuncture is a complex intervention that is intimately intertwined with placebo, patients, and practitioners. Therefore, it is logical that acupuncture may induce both specific and non-specific effects which contribute to its therapeutic effects [6]. That may support the clinical facts that acupuncture at sham points can also provide partial analgesia in chronic pain [91]. Moreover, in our present study, while the locations of these connectivity changes had overlap between verum and sham there were apparent differences as to the specific frequency bands between post-acupuncture modulation and post-sham modulation. Although STG were not among the DMN core regions during the resting state, it began to serve as a hub following both kinds of acupuncture. Nevertheless, it is implicated that sham intervention exerts such effect within only theta and alpha bands, while verum acupuncture produces additional influence for the gamma band. Likewise, the MFG demonstrates as well the acupuncture-evoked impacts on hub configurations within theta band following the verum intervention, in relative to the alpha band for the control group. In addition, the SFG constitutes as a DMN hub within the alpha and beta bands during the resting state. As illustrated in our results, the sham acupuncture seems to exert no effect on its hub configuration, remaining as a hub within the alpha and beta bands. Following verum intervention, however, the SFG served as a hub within not only these two bands, but additionally delta and theta rhythms.

In conclusion, the present study demonstrated differential alterations within 5 conventional frequency bands (delta, theta, alpha, beta and gamma) of DMN hub configurations following acupuncture at ST36 relative to NAP. With the complementary advantage of fMRI and MEG, we are able to explore spatiotemporally the specific biological mechanism underlying acupuncture, especially on the modulation of PCC as a DMN hub within the theta, alpha and beta bands. Overall, though it is a preliminary work, our results may provide additional evidence for the specificity of acupoint. We hope that this article serves as an introduction that will help to explore this fascinating topic in more depth and, as a consequence, shed more light on the specific neurophysiological mechanisms of acupuncture.

Acknowledgments

We would like to thank Fengbing Wang and Ying Jiang for valuable technical assistance in conducting this research.

Author Contributions

Conceived and designed the experiments: RD JT YY. Performed the experiments: YY LB HC. Analyzed the data: YY LB. Contributed reagents/materials/analysis tools: ZL WW. Wrote the paper: JT YY.

References

1. NCDP A (1998) NIH Consensus Conference. Acupuncture. JAMA 280: 1518–1524.
2. Witt CM, Manheimer E, Hammerschlag R, Ludtke R, Lao LX, et al. (2012) How Well Do Randomized Trials Inform Decision Making: Systematic Review Using Comparative Effectiveness Research Measures on Acupuncture for Back Pain. Plos One 7.
3. Bai L, Qin W, Tian J, Liu P, Li LL, et al. (2009) Time-varied characteristics of acupuncture effects in fMRI studies. Human brain mapping 30: 3445–3460.
4. Cho ZH, Chung S, Jones J, Park J, Park H, et al. (1998) New findings of the correlation between acupoints and corresponding brain cortices using functional MRI. Proceedings of the National Academy of Sciences 95: 2670–2673.
5. Bai L, Qin W, Tian J, Dong M, Pan X, et al. (2009) Acupuncture modulates spontaneous activities in the anticorrelated resting brain networks. Brain research 1279: 37–49.
6. Qin W, Tian J, Bai L, Pan X, Yang L, et al. (2008) FMRI connectivity analysis of acupuncture effects on an amygdala-associated brain network. Mol Pain 4: 1–17.
7. Qin W, Bai L, Dai J, Liu P, Dong M, et al. (2011) The temporal-spatial encoding of acupuncture effects in the brain. Mol Pain 11: 19.
8. Melchart D, Streng A, Hoppe A, Brinkhaus B, Witt C, et al. (2005) Acupuncture in patients with tension-type headache: randomised controlled trial. Bmj 331: 376–382.
9. Brinkhaus B, Witt CM, Jena S, Linde K, Streng A, et al. (2006) Acupuncture in patients with chronic low back pain: a randomized controlled trial. Archives of internal medicine 166: 450.
10. Linde K, Streng A, Jürgens S, Hoppe A, Brinkhaus B, et al. (2005) Acupuncture for patients with migraine. JAMA: the journal of the American Medical Association 293: 2118–2125.
11. Mandeville JB, Marota JJA, Ayata C, Zaharchuk G, Moskowitz MA, et al. (1999) Evidence of a cerebrovascular postarteriole windkessel with delayed compliance. Journal of Cerebral Blood Flow & Metabolism 19: 679–689.
12. Buxton RB, Wong EC, Frank LR (2005) Dynamics of blood flow and oxygenation changes during brain activation: the balloon model. Magnetic Resonance in Medicine 39: 855–864.
13. Rosen BR, Buckner RL, Dale AM (1998) Event-related functional MRI: past, present, and future. Proceedings of the National Academy of Sciences 95: 773–780.
14. Ghuman AS, McDaniel JR, Martin A (2011) A wavelet-based method for measuring the oscillatory dynamics of resting-state functional connectivity in MEG. Neuroimage.
15. Rodriguez E, George N, Lachaux JP, Martinerie J, Renault B, et al. (1999) Perception's shadow: long-distance synchronization of human brain activity. nature 397: 430–433.
16. Sarnthein J, Petsche H, Rappelsberger P, Shaw G, Von Stein A (1998) Synchronization between prefrontal and posterior association cortex during human working memory. Proceedings of the National Academy of Sciences 95: 7092–7096.
17. Cohen D (1972) Magnetoencephalography: detection of the brain's electrical activity with a superconducting magnetometer. Science (New York, NY) 175: 664.
18. Hämäläinen M, Hari R, Ilmoniemi RJ, Knuutila J, Lounasmaa OV (1993) Magnetoencephalography – theory, instrumentation, and applications to noninvasive studies of the working human brain. Reviews of modern Physics 65: 413.
19. Baillet S, Mosher JC, Leahy RM (2001) Electromagnetic brain mapping. Signal Processing Magazine, IEEE 18: 14–30.
20. Dale AM, Halgren E (2001) Spatiotemporal mapping of brain activity by integration of multiple imaging modalities. Current opinion in neurobiology 11: 202–208.
21. Dale AM, Sereno MI (1993) Improved localizadon of cortical activity by combining eeg and meg with mri cortical surface reconstruction: A linear approach. Journal of Cognitive Neuroscience 5: 162–176.
22. Liu AK, Belliveau JW, Dale AM (1998) Spatiotemporal imaging of human brain activity using functional MRI constrained magnetoencephalography data: Monte Carlo simulations. Proceedings of the National Academy of Sciences 95: 8945–8950.
23. Bullmore E, Sporns O (2009) Complex brain networks: graph theoretical analysis of structural and functional systems. Nature Reviews Neuroscience 10: 186–198.
24. Achard S, Bullmore E (2007) Efficiency and cost of economical brain functional networks. PLoS computational biology 3: e17.
25. Wang K, Liang M, Wang L, Tian L, Zhang X, et al. (2007) Altered functional connectivity in early Alzheimer's disease: A resting-state fMRI study. Human brain mapping 28: 967–978.
26. Damoiseaux J, Rombouts S, Barkhof F, Scheltens P, Stam C, et al. (2006) Consistent resting-state networks across healthy subjects. Proceedings of the National Academy of Sciences 103: 13848–13853.
27. Raichle ME, MacLeod AM, Snyder AZ, Powers WJ, Gusnard DA, et al. (2001) A default mode of brain function. Proceedings of the National Academy of Sciences 98: 676–682.
28. Buckner RL, Andrews-Hanna JR, Schacter DL (2008) The brain's default network. Annals of the New York Academy of Sciences 1124: 1–38.
29. Tomasi D, Volkow ND (2011) Functional connectivity hubs in the human brain. Neuroimage 57: 908–917.
30. de Pasquale F, Della Penna S, Snyder AZ, Marzetti L, Pizzella V, et al. (2012) A Cortical Core for Dynamic Integration of Functional Networks in the Resting Human Brain. Neuron 74: 753–764.
31. Hahn A, Wadsak W, Windischberger C, Baldinger P, Höflich AS, et al. (2012) Differential modulation of the default mode network via serotonin-1A receptors. Proceedings of the National Academy of Sciences 109: 2619–2624.
32. Miao X, Wu X, Li R, Chen K, Yao L (2011) Altered Connectivity Pattern of Hubs in Default-Mode Network with Alzheimer's Disease: An Granger Causality Modeling Approach. PloS one 6: e25546.
33. Wicker B, Ruby P, Royet JP, Fonlupt P (2003) A relation between rest and the self in the brain? Brain Research Reviews 43: 224–230.
34. Mason MF, Norton MI, Van Horn JD, Wegner DM, Grafton ST, et al. (2007) Wandering minds: the default network and stimulus-independent thought. science 315: 393–395.
35. Gilbert DT, Wilson TD (2007) Prospection: experiencing the future. science 317: 1351–1354.
36. Mayer DJ (2000) Acupuncture: an evidence-based review of the clinical literature. Annual review of medicine 51: 49–63.
37. Liu B, Chen J, Wang J, Liu X, Duan X, et al. (2012) Altered Small-World Efficiency of Brain Functional Networks in Acupuncture at ST36: A Functional MRI Study. PloS one 7: e39342.
38. Hui KKS, Liu J, Marina O, Napadow V, Haselgrove C, et al. (2005) The integrated response of the human cerebro-cerebellar and limbic systems to acupuncture stimulation at ST 36 as evidenced by fMRI. NeuroImage 27: 479–496.
39. Fang J, Jin Z, Wang Y, Li K, Kong J, et al. (2009) The salient characteristics of the central effects of acupuncture needling: Limbic-paralimbic-neocortical network modulation. Human brain mapping 30: 1196–1206.
40. Dhond RP, Yeh C, Park K, Kettner N, Napadow V (2008) Acupuncture modulates resting state connectivity in default and sensorimotor brain networks. Pain 136: 407–418.
41. You Y, Bai L, Dai R, Zhong C, Xue T, et al. (2012) Acupuncture Induces Divergent Alterations of Functional Connectivity within Conventional Frequency Bands: Evidence from MEG Recordings. PloS one 7: e49250.
42. Chen L, Tang J, White P, Sloninsky A, Wender R, et al. (1998) The effect of location of transcutaneous electrical nerve stimulation on postoperative opioid analgesic requirement: acupoint versus nonacupoint stimulation. Anesthesia & Analgesia 87: 1129–1134.
43. Han JS (2011) Acupuncture analgesia: areas of consensus and controversy. Pain 152: S41–48.
44. Hui KKS, Liu J, Makris N, Gollub RL, Chen AJW (2000) Acupuncture modulates the limbic system and subcortical gray structures of the human brain: evidence from fMRI studies in normal subjects. Human brain mapping 9: 13–25.
45. Xing C (1987) Chinese acupuncture and moxibustion. Beijing, China: Foreign Languages Press.
46. Kong J, Gollub R, Huang T, Polich G, Napadow V, et al. (2007) Acupuncture de qi, from qualitative history to quantitative measurement. The Journal of Alternative and Complementary Medicine 13: 1059–1070.
47. Montez T, Poil SS, Jones BF, Manshanden I, Verbunt J, et al. (2009) Altered temporal correlations in parietal alpha and prefrontal theta oscillations in early-stage Alzheimer disease. Proceedings of the National Academy of Sciences 106: 1614.
48. Castelli F, Glaser DE, Butterworth B (2006) Discrete and analogue quantity processing in the parietal lobe: A functional MRI study. Proceedings of the National Academy of Sciences of the United States of America 103: 4693–4698.
49. Friston KJ, Ashburner JT, Kiebel SJ, Nichols TE, Penny WD (2011) Statistical Parametric Mapping: The Analysis of Functional Brain Images: Academic Press.
50. Greicius MD, Krasnow B, Reiss AL, Menon V (2003) Functional connectivity in the resting brain: a network analysis of the default mode hypothesis. Proceedings of the National Academy of Sciences 100: 253.
51. Jiao Q, Lu G, Zhang Z, Zhong Y, Wang Z, et al. (2011) Granger causal influence predicts BOLD activity levels in the default mode network. Human brain mapping 32: 154–161.

52. Greicius MD, Srivastava G, Reiss AL, Menon V (2004) Default-mode network activity distinguishes Alzheimer's disease from healthy aging: evidence from functional MRI. Proceedings of the National Academy of Sciences of the United States of America 101: 4637–4642.
53. Calhoun V, Adali T, Pearlson G, Pekar J (2001) A method for making group inferences from functional MRI data using independent component analysis. Human brain mapping 14: 140–151.
54. Calhoun V, Adali T, Pearlson G, Pekar J (2001) Spatial and temporal independent component analysis of functional MRI data containing a pair of task-related waveforms. Human brain mapping 13: 43–53.
55. Hyvärinen A, Hurri J, Hoyer PO (2009) Independent component analysis. Natural Image Statistics: 151–175.
56. Liao W, Mantini D, Zhang Z, Pan Z, Ding J, et al. (2010) Evaluating the effective connectivity of resting state networks using conditional Granger causality. Biological cybernetics 102: 57–69.
57. Uddin LQ, Clare Kelly A, Biswal BB, Xavier Castellanos F, Milham MP (2009) Functional connectivity of default mode network components: correlation, anticorrelation, and causality. Human brain mapping 30: 625–637.
58. Gusnard DA, Akbudak E, Shulman GL, Raichle ME (2001) Medial prefrontal cortex and self-referential mental activity: relation to a default mode of brain function. Proceedings of the National Academy of Sciences 98: 4259.
59. Meindl T, Teipel S, Elmouden R, Mueller S, Koch W, et al. (2010) Test–retest reproducibility of the default-mode network in healthy individuals. Human brain mapping 31: 237–246.
60. Stoffers D, Bosboom J, Deijen J, Wolters E, Berendse H, et al. (2007) Slowing of oscillatory brain activity is a stable characteristic of Parkinson's disease without dementia. Brain 130: 1847–1860.
61. Douw L, Schoonheim M, Landi D, Van Der Meer M, Geurts J, et al. (2011) Cognition is related to resting-state small-world network topology: an magnetoencephalographic study. Neuroscience 175: 169–177.
62. Stam C, De Haan W, Daffertshofer A, Jones B, Manshanden I, et al. (2009) Graph theoretical analysis of magnetoencephalographic functional connectivity in Alzheimer's disease. Brain 132: 213–224.
63. Scherg M (1992) Functional imaging and localization of electromagnetic brain activity. Brain topography 5: 103–111.
64. Anderson KL, Ding M (2011) Attentional modulation of the somatosensory mu rhythm. Neuroscience.
65. Zhang Y, Ding M (2010) Detection of a weak somatosensory stimulus: Role of the prestimulus mu rhythm and its top–down modulation. Journal of Cognitive Neuroscience 22: 307–322.
66. Del Gratta C, Della Penna S, Ferretti A, Franciotti R, Pizzella V, et al. (2002) Topographic organization of the human primary and secondary somatosensory cortices: comparison of fMRI and MEG findings. Neuroimage 17: 1373–1383.
67. Keil A, Sabatinelli D, Ding M, Lang PJ, Ihssen N, et al. (2009) Re-entrant projections modulate visual cortex in affective perception: Evidence from Granger causality analysis. Human brain mapping 30: 532–540.
68. Nihashi T, Kakigi R, Kawakami O, Hoshiyama M, Itomi K, et al. (2001) Representation of the ear in human primary somatosensory cortex. Neuroimage 13: 295–304.
69. Whittaker J (1990) Graphical models in applied multivariate statistics: Wiley New York.
70. Hampson M, Peterson BS, Skudlarski P, Gatenby JC, Gore JC (2002) Detection of functional connectivity using temporal correlations in MR images. Human brain mapping 15: 247–262.
71. Salvador R, Suckling J, Coleman MR, Pickard JD, Menon D, et al. (2005) Neurophysiological architecture of functional magnetic resonance images of human brain. Cerebral Cortex 15: 1332–1342.
72. Stam CJ (2004) Functional connectivity patterns of human magnetoencephalographic recordings: a'small-world'network? Neuroscience letters 355: 25.
73. Marrelec G, Horwitz B, Kim J, Pélégrini-Issac M, Benali H, et al. (2007) Using partial correlation to enhance structural equation modeling of functional MRI data. Magnetic Resonance Imaging 25: 1181–1189.
74. Marrelec G, Krainik A, Duffau H, Pélégrini-Issac M, Lehéricy S, et al. (2006) Partial correlation for functional brain interactivity investigation in functional MRI. Neuroimage 32: 228–237.
75. Liu P, Zhang Y, Zhou G, Yuan K, Qin W, et al. (2009) Partial correlation investigation on the default mode network involved in acupuncture: an fMRI study. Neuroscience letters 462: 183–187.
76. He BJ, Snyder AZ, Zempel JM, Smyth MD, Raichle ME (2008) Electrophysiological correlates of the brain's intrinsic large-scale functional architecture. Proceedings of the National Academy of Sciences 105: 16039.
77. Benjamini Y, Yekutieli D (2001) The control of the false discovery rate in multiple testing under dependency. Annals of statistics: 1165–1188.
78. Gong G, He Y, Concha L, Lebel C, Gross DW, et al. (2009) Mapping anatomical connectivity patterns of human cerebral cortex using in vivo diffusion tensor imaging tractography. Cerebral Cortex 19: 524–536.
79. Buckner RL, Sepulcre J, Talukdar T, Krienen FM, Liu H, et al. (2009) Cortical hubs revealed by intrinsic functional connectivity: mapping, assessment of stability, and relation to Alzheimer's disease. The Journal of Neuroscience 29: 1860–1873.
80. Fransson P, Marrelec G (2008) The precuneus/posterior cingulate cortex plays a pivotal role in the default mode network: Evidence from a partial correlation network analysis. Neuroimage 42: 1178.
81. Sherman KJ, Hogeboom CJ, Cherkin DC, Deyo RA (2002) Description and validation of a noninvasive placebo acupuncture procedure. The Journal of Alternative & Complementary Medicine 8: 11–19.
82. Streitberger K, Kleinhenz J (1998) Introducing a placebo needle into acupuncture research. Lancet 352: 364–365.
83. Birch S (2003) Controlling for non-specific effects of acupuncture in clinical trials. Clinical acupuncture and oriental medicine 4: 59–70.
84. Hui KKS, Marina O, Claunch JD, Nixon EE, Fang J, et al. (2009) Acupuncture mobilizes the brain's default mode and its anti-correlated network in healthy subjects. Brain research 1287: 84–103.
85. Greicius MD, Menon V (2004) Default-mode activity during a passive sensory task: uncoupled from deactivation but impacting activation. Journal of Cognitive Neuroscience 16: 1484–1492.
86. Kennedy DP, Courchesne E (2008) The intrinsic functional organization of the brain is altered in autism. Neuroimage 39: 1877.
87. Lowe MJ, Phillips MD, Lurito JT, Mattson D, Dzemidzic M, et al. (2002) Multiple Sclerosis: Low-Frequency Temporal Blood Oxygen Level–Dependent Fluctuations Indicate Reduced Functional Connectivity – Initial Results1. Radiology 224: 184–192.
88. Bai L, Tian J, Zhong C, Xue T, You Y, et al. (2010) Acupuncture modulates temporal neural responses in wide brain networks: evidence from fMRI study. Mol Pain 6: 73.
89. Tracey I, Mantyh PW (2007) The cerebral signature for pain perception and its modulation. Neuron 55: 377–392.
90. Lewith GT, White PJ, Pariente J (2005) Investigating acupuncture using brain imaging techniques: the current state of play. Evidence-Based Complementary and Alternative Medicine 2: 315.
91. Richardson P, Vincent C (1986) Acupuncture for the treatment of pain: a review of evaluative research. Pain.

10

In Silico Investigation of Potential Src Kinase Ligands from Traditional Chinese Medicine

Weng Ieong Tou[1,2], Calvin Yu-Chian Chen[2,3,4,5,6]*

1 School of Medicine, China Medical University, Taichung, Taiwan, **2** Laboratory of Computational and Systems Biology, China Medical University, Taichung, Taiwan, **3** Department of Medical Research, China Medical University Hospital, Taichung, Taiwan, **4** Department of Biotechnology, Asia University, Taichung, Taiwan, **5** Department of Biomedical Informatics, Asia University, Taichung, Taiwan, **6** China Medical University Beigang Hospital, Yunlin, Taiwan

Abstract

Src kinase is an attractive target for drug development based on its established relationship with cancer and possible link to hypertension. The suitability of traditional Chinese medicine (TCM) compounds as potential drug ligands for further biological evaluation was investigated using structure-based, ligand-based, and molecular dynamics (MD) analysis. Isopraeroside IV, 9alpha-hydroxyfraxinellone-9-O-beta-D-glucoside (9HFG) and aurantiamide were the top three TCM candidates identified from docking. Hydrogen bonds and hydrophobic interactions were the primary forces governing docking stability. Their stability with Src kinase under a dynamic state was further validated through MD and torsion angle analysis. Complexes formed by TCM candidates have lower total energy estimates than the control Sacaratinib. Four quantitative-structural activity relationship (QSAR) *in silico* verifications consistently suggested that the TCM candidates have bioactive properties. Docking conformations of 9HFG and aurantiamide in the Src kinase ATP binding site suggest potential inhibitor-like characteristics, including competitive binding at the ATP binding site (Lys295) and stabilization of the catalytic cleft integrity. The TCM candidates have significantly lower ligand internal energies and are estimated to form more stable complexes with Src kinase than Saracatinib. Structure-based and ligand-based analysis support the drug-like potential of 9HFG and aurantiamide and binding mechanisms reveal the tendency of these two candidates to compete for the ATP binding site.

Editor: Ramón Campos-Olivas, Spanish National Cancer Center, Spain

Funding: This research was supported by grants from the National Science Council of Taiwan (NSC 100-2325-B-039-001), Committee on Chinese Medicine and Pharmacy (CCMP100-RD-030), China Medical University and Asia University (DMR-101-094). This study is also supported in part by Taiwan Department of Health Clinical Trial and Research Center of Excellence (DOH101-TD-B-111-004) and Taiwan Department of Health Cancer Research Center of Excellence (DOH101-TD-C-111-005). The funders had no role in study design, data collection and analysis, decision to publish, or preparation of the manuscript.

Competing Interests: The authors have declared that no competing interests exist.

* E-mail: ycc929@MIT.EDU

Introduction

Src kinases are nonreceptor tyrosine kinases that are of physiological importance in cell survival, bone metabolism, angiogenesis, proliferation, migration, and invasion [1]. Overexpression of Src kinase has been linked to various cancers and is now a well-established proto-oncogene [2–7]. The physiological pathway involved in hypertension is also associated with Src-dependent signaling pathways, suggesting a potential link between hypertension and Src [8–15].

Figure 1 illustrates the components of Src kinase and its activation mechanism [16,17]. In general terms, the catalytic activity of Src is co-regulated by SH3 and SH2 domains. Src is locked in the closed conformation (inactive) when SH2 binds to the phosphorylated Tyr530, and SH3 binds with prolines on the linker domain (Figure 1A). When Tyr530 is dephosphorylated, Src assumes an open conformation, achieving full activity when Tyr416 within the catalytic domain is autophosphorylated (Figure 1B). This opening of the Src structure frees the SH2 and SH3 domains to interact with surface receptors such as focal adhesion FAK and initiate downstream signaling governing the aforementioned physiological pathways [1]. In this regard, inactivation of Src can be achieved through hindering disassembly of the regulatory SH2 and SH3 Src domains, or by inhibiting ATP binding to the Src catalytic site [16,18].

Many small molecular Src inhibitors have been identified due to the involvement of Src in cancer. Comprehensive reviews on such advancements are detailed elsewhere [16]. Most Src inhibitors discovered to date are Type I inhibitors that compete with ATP for binding at the ATP binding pocket [19,20]. Structures of the three most studied Type I inhibitors Bosutinib, Dasatinib, and Saracatinib and are shown in Figure 2 along with their respective status in clinical trials [21–32]. The varying efficacies of these commercial drugs highlight the need for novel compounds that can exhibit more consistent inhibition of Src.

The goal of this research is to investigate novel small compounds from traditional Chinese medicine (TCM) that may be potential Src kinase ligands. During the past decade, our laboratory has focused on constructing the most comprehensive TCM database (TCM Database@Taiwan, url:) (http://tcm.cmu.edu.tw/) [33]. In addition, we've also developed the first cloud-computing webserver based on TCM Database@Taiwan, url: (http://iscreen.cmu.edu.tw/) [34] and an integrative website combining TCM and systems biology (http://iSMART.cmu.edu.tw/) [35]. Utilizing these TCM computational resources, several novel lead compounds from TCM with application potential for different diseases have been

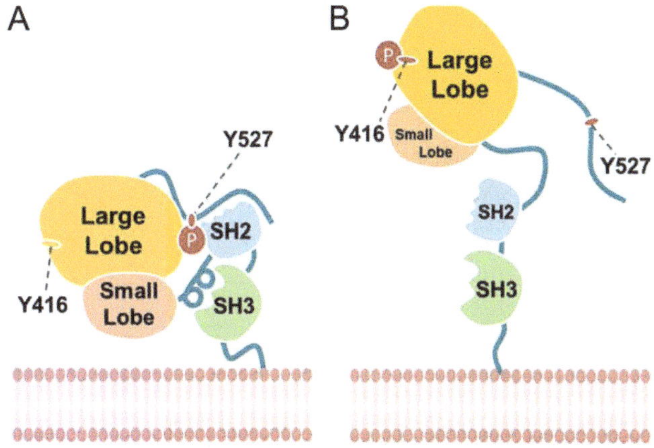

Figure 1. Components of Src and its activation mechanisms. (A) SH2 binds to the phosphorylated Tyr530 and SH3 binds with prolines on the linker domain, effectively locking the Src in an inactive closed conformation. (B) Src is activated when Tyr530 is dephosphorylated and Tyr416 within the catalytic domain is autophosphorylated.

successfully uncovered [36–44]. In the current research, we utilize the newly updated TCM Database@Taiwan to screen for novel, TCM-origin ligands with drug-like properties against Src kinase.

Results and Discussion

Docking

Based on the DockScore, top ranking TCM candidates selected for further investigation were Isopraeroside IV, 9alpha-hydroxy-fraxinellone-9-O-beta-D-glucoside (9HFG), and aurantiamide (Table 1). Isopraeroside IV is a coumarin isolated from the root of *Angelica dahurica* [45]. 9HFG originates from the root of *Dictamnus dasycarpus*, which has been used as a folk remedy for inflammation and skin ailments [46]. Aurantuamide is a composition of *Curcuma wenyujin*, a dried rhizome used for bleeding and menstrual disorders in traditional Chinese medicine. Structural comparisons of the TCM candidates with Saracatinib are illustrated in Figure 3.

DockScore is the negative sum of the ligand/receptor interaction and the ligand internal energy calculated by DS. For clarification purposes, the ligand internal energy consists of a van der Waals (vdW) term computed using a standard 9-6 (unsoftened) potential and an optional electrostatic term. Since TCM candidates and Saracatinib have similar predicted binding energies, differences in DockScore were primarily affected by the respective calculated ligand internal energies of each compound (Table 1). The low DockScore observed for Saracatinib is mainly due to its high calculated ligand internal energy. The positive ligand internal energy value is indicative of a highly strained chemical structure, a phenomenon commonly observed among synthetic compounds. By contrast, low calculated ligand internal energies of the TCM compounds suggest energetically stable structures in which intermolecular atoms are not too close to exhibit replusion and result in high DockScore values. Based on DS2.5 calculations, the TCM candidates have higher DockScores and binding energies comparable to Saracatinib, which may lead to equal if not better binding to the Src kinase binding site compared to Saracatinib.

The ADMET properties of the TCM candidates are summarized in Figure 4 and Table 2. All candidates were estimated to be within the 99% adsorption ellipse (Figure 4) and have good to moderate adsorption (Table 2). The TCM candidates are more highly bound to plasma proteins, and less likely to inhibit cytochrome P4502D6 metabolism.

As our designated binding site overlapped with the Src kinase ATP binding pocket, it is referred to as the latter for clarification purposes. Docking poses of the candidates in the ATP binding pocket are illustrated in Figure 5. The docking model of Saracatinib indicates π-interactions with Leu273 and Lys295, and an H-bond with Met341 within the ATP binding pocket (Figure 5A). Isopraeroside IV formed a total of five H-bonds with Met341, Ser345, Asp348 (Figure 5B), possibly contributing to the high estimated binding energy in Table 1. The three hydroxyl groups on the cyclohexane moiety of 9HFG interacted with Lys295, Met341, and Asp404, forming a total of five H-bonds (Figure 5C) in which three were formed with Lys295. Auraniamide interacted with Leu273, Lys295, Ser345, Asp348, forming two π interactions at the terminal benzenes with Leu273 and Lys295 and H-bonds with Ser345 and Asp 348 (Figure 5D).

Ligplot diagrams illustrating hydrophobic and H-bond interactions are shown in Figure 6. In general, the higher ability of ligands to form hydrophobic interactions with hydrophobic amino acids of the binding site, the higher the binding affinity. As shown in Figure 6, TCM candidates are surrounded by hydrophobic amino acids, therefore are harder to remove from the ATP binding pocket under physiologically dynamic conditions. Less hydrophobic interactions were formed by Saracatinib. Minor variations in H-bond formation were observed in LigPlot diagrams compared to 3D-docking poses generated by DS 2.5 (Figure 5). Additional H-bonds were formed with Tyr340 and Glu399 by Isopraeroside IV (Figure 6B). 9HFG formed two additional H-bonds at Ala390 and Asn391 (Figure 6C). In auraniamide (Figure 6D), the H-bonds at Leu273 and Lys295 were replaced by hydrophobic interactions. These differences may be due to the DS cutoff distance of 2.5 Å or to the HBPLUS program used to calculate H-bonds in LigPlot. The number of H-bonds and hydrophobic interactions determined through LigPlot is summarized in Table 3. These simulation results suggest that TCM candidates have a higher number of stabilizing interactions than Saracatinib.

Key amino acids and important structural moieties can be summarized based on the docking simulation results. Leu273 is important for H-bonds and π-interactions, and ligands form interactions with its nonpolar, aliphatic alkyl group. Saracatinib, 9HFG, and auraniamide interact with Src kinase through Lys295. The importance of Lys295 is reinforced by the three H-bonds and two π-interactions formed by the aforementioned ligands. Other amino acids serving as anchor points in the Src kinase ATP binding pocket include Met341, Ser345, Asp348, and Asp390. The chemical structures of the candidates facilitate hydrophobic interactions with surrounding amino acids, and enable higher ligand-protein affinity and complex stability.

Bioactivity Prediction by SVM and MLR

The 75 descriptors relevant to the training set were determined and GFA further employed to determine the top ten descriptors that could most accurately describe the training set. The descriptors thus determined were: *C_Count* (the amount of carbon atoms within the ligand), *ES_Sum_sCH*$_3$ (sum of the electrotopological state (E-state) values for carbons with single bonds), *E_ADJ_equ* (molecule differentiation based on edge adjacency), *CHI_2* (number of pairs of bonds within a molecule), *CHI_3_P* (number of phosphate molecules with three bonds), *Kappa_2* (shape index of order 2 describing topological descriptors), *Kappa_3* (shape index of order 3 describing topological descriptors), *Jurs_FNSA_1* (sum of negative

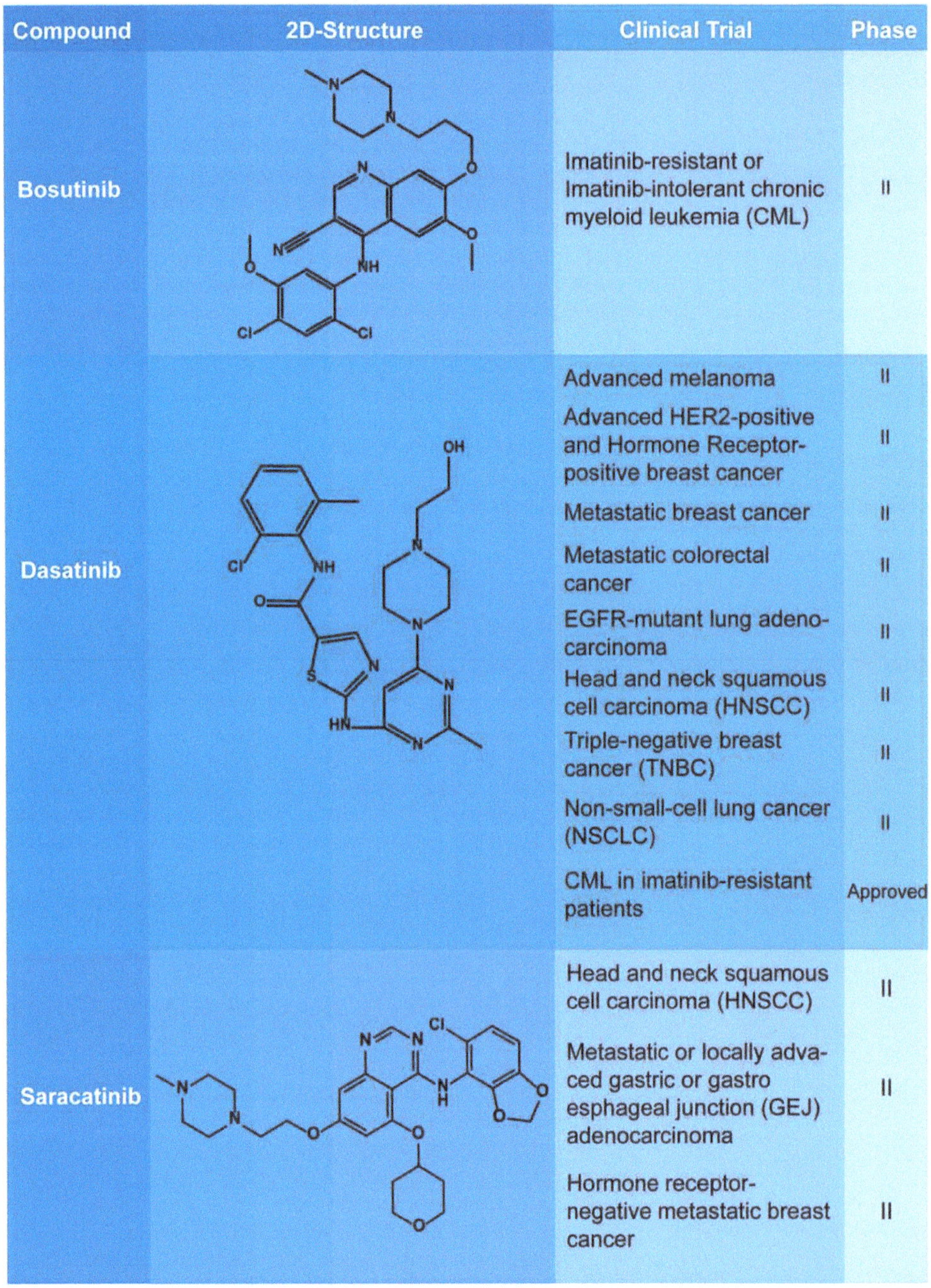

Figure 2. Scaffolds of Bosutinib, Dasatinib, amd Saracatinib, and their respective status in clinical trials.

surface areas divided by total molecular solvent-accessible surface area), *Jurs_PNSA_1* (sum of solvent-accessible surface areas of all negatively charged atoms), *Shadow_nu* (characterizes molecule shape using ratio of largest to smallest dimension).

Using these descriptors, the MLR model generated was:

$$pIC_{50} = -13.037 + 0.67442 * C\_Count - 0.22096 * ES\_Sum\_sCH_3 - 0.18787 * E\_ADJ\_equ + 6.4515 * CHI\_2 + 1.345 * CHI\_3\_P + 1.5976 * Kappa\_2 - 4.0379 * Kappa\_3 - 47.403 * Jurs\_FNSA1 + 0.065128 * Jurs\_PNSA\_1 - 0.50161 * Shadow\_nu$$

As shown in Figure 7, the square correlation coefficients for the MLR and SVM models were 0.837 and 0.7922, respectively, indicating reliable models. Predicted bioactivities (pIC_{50}) of the TCM candidates by the generated MLR and SVM models are listed in Table 2. Both models predicted higher pIC_{50} values for Isopraeroside IV and 9HGF than aurantiamide. The predicted bioactivities for Saracatinib was 4.9410 using MLR and 7.3036 using SVM. These predicted results, when compared to the *in vitro* inhibition concentration of Saracatinib ($pIC_{50} = 8.57$) [47], indicate that values predicted by the SVM model may be closer to actual inhibition concentrations observed *in vitro*. The higher accuracy of the SVM model is expected as its predictions are generated on a non-linear model.

Table 1. DockScore and related attributes of Sacracatinib and top three TCM candidates calculated by Discovery Studio 2.5 (D.S. 2.5).

Name	Ligand Internal Energy	Binding Energy	Dock Score
Isopraeroside IV	−42.52	−63.39	97.28
9HFG	−35.33	−60.24	93.12
Aurantiamide	−37.24	−57.12	83.02
Saracatinib*	34.20	−60.81	27.09

Candidates ranked by Dock Score.
*Control.
9HFG: 9alpha-hydroxyfraxinellone-9-O-beta-D-glucoside.

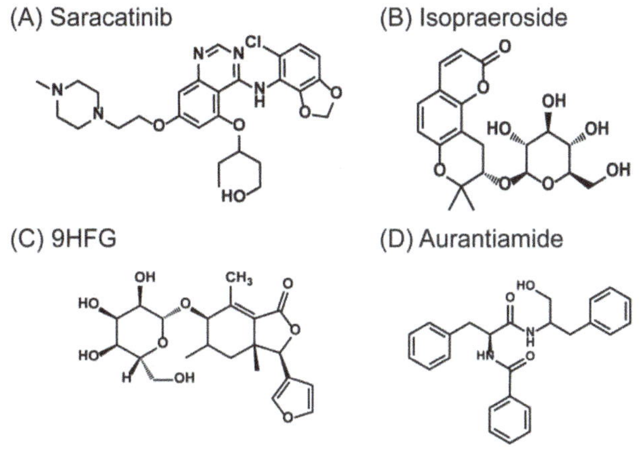

Figure 3. Structural scaffolds of TCM candidates and Saracatinib. (A) Saracatinib, (B) Isopraeroside IV, (C) 9HFG, and (D) aurantiamide.

Bioactivity Prediction by 3D-QSAR

Table 4 summarizes the PLS results of CoMFA and CoMSIA models. Steric fields are the dominant factor in CoMFA. Under an optimal number of components (ONC) of 6, cross-validated correlation coefficient (q^2) and non-cross-validated correlation coefficient (r^2) of 0.430 and 0.920 indicate a reliable model. Multiple CoMSIA models were generated using different factor combinations (Table 4). Models SHD and SEHD were the best overall models with high q^2 (q^2>0.4), high r^2, low SEE, and large F values. However, addition of an electrostatic variable in model SEHD did not significantly increase model correlation or strength (F-value), thus model SHD was selected as the optimum CoMSIA model. Reliability of the selected CoMFA and CoMSIA models are validated by the q^2 and r^2 values (Table 4).

The observed, predicted and calculated residual pIC_{50} values of the training and test set compounds by CoMFA and CoMSIA are summarized in Table S1. Differences between observed and predicted pIC_{50} ranged between −0.667 and 1.066. Residuals using the CoMSIA model ranged from −0.5 to 0.821, indicating high accuracy of the predictions from our generated model with actual biologically verified values. All ratio values calculated through CoMSIA were within 1±0.1 indicating high accuracy. The correlation coefficient between the observed and predicted pIC_{50} using the CoMFA model was 0.8448 (Figure 8A). With the CoMSIA model, the correlation coefficient was 0.9014 (Figure 8B). Both models are highly reliable.

Superimposing CoMFA and CoMSIA contour maps on Saracatinib and the TCM candidates provide insights into the predicted bioactivity of the compounds. Saracatinib (Figure 9A), Isopraeroside IV (Figure 9B), and 9HFG (Figure 9C) contoured well to the CoMFA model. No bulk structures were located in the steric disfavoring (yellow) region. In addition, bulky ring moieties in Saracatinib and 9HFG were located in the steric favoring (green) region. By comparison, a benzene ring of aurantiamide was located within the steric disfavoring region, suggesting a lower biological activity due to its deviation from the CoMFA contour map (Figure 9D). These results agree with the MLR and SVM results in which aurantiamide had the lowest predicted bioactivity

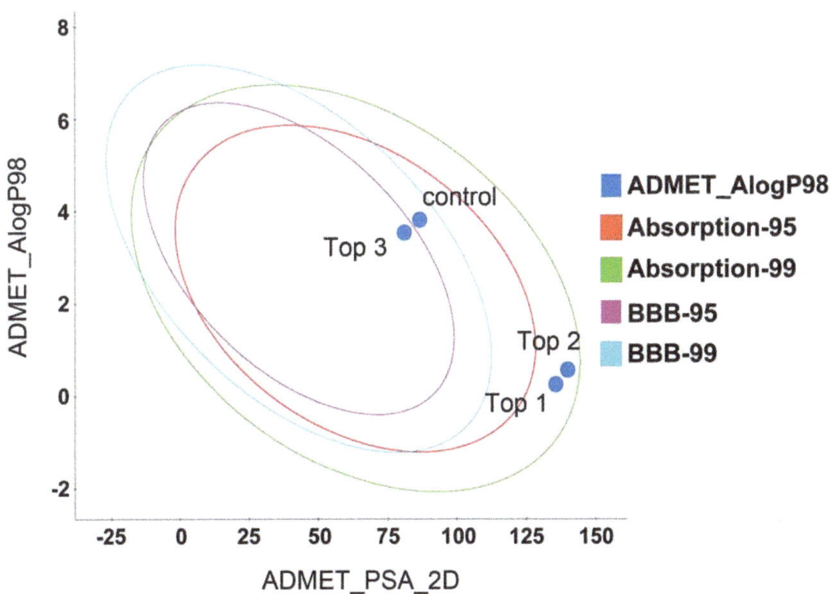

Figure 4. ADMET adsorption model of Saracatinib and the TCM candidates generated by DS 2.5.

Table 2. Adsorption, distribution, metabolism, toxicity properties and predicted pIC_{50} of Saracatinib and the top three TCM compounds.

Name	ADMET Adsorption Level[1]	PPB Level[2]	CYP2D6 Probability[3]	Hepatoxicity[4]	Bioactivity Prediction (pIC_{50})	
					SVM	MLR
Isopraeroside IV	1	2	0.356	0	6.0277	7.7282
9HFG	1	2	0.297	0	6.8590	7.5342
Aurantiamide	0	2	0.475	0	4.6490	4.4080
Saracatinib*	0	0	0.297	0	7.3036	4.9410

*Control.
[1]ADMET Adsorption levels: 0 = Good; 1 = Moderate; 2 = Low; 3 = Very low.
[2]Plasma Protein Binding: 0 = Binding <90% ;1 = Binding >90%; 2 = Binding >95%.
[3]Inhibition probability of Cytochrome P450 2D6 enzyme.
[4]Hepatoxicity: 0 = Nontoxic; 1 = Toxic.

among the tested compounds. With regard to CoMSIA maps, Saracatinib forms H-bonds with Met341 which is located near the region favoring hydrogen bond donors (purple) and hydrophobic interactions (cyan) (Figure 10A). Isopraeroside IV was a smaller compound and its interactions with Src did not fall within the disfavoring regions of the CoMSIA map (Figure 10B). A similar contour was observed in 9HFG (Figure 10C). In aurantiamide, the benzene moieties were in proximity to the steric disfavoring regions, suggesting a lower bioactivity of the ligand (Figure 10D). Results of the ligand-based studies are consistent, and suggest high bioactivity for Saracatinib, moderate to high bioactivity for Isopraeroside and 9HFG, and moderate to low bioactivity for aurantiamide.

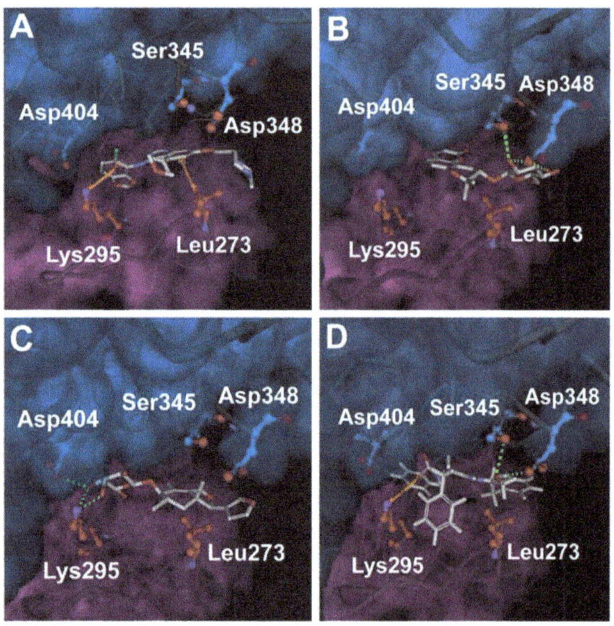

Figure 5. Docking poses of different ligands in Src kinase ATP binding pocket. Shown are snapshots of (A) Saracatinib,(B) Isopraeroside IV, (C) 9HFG, and (D) aurantiamide during docking simulation with Src kinase. Purple and blue surfaces are added to denote the small lobe (267–337) and large lobe (340–520) of Src kinase, respectively. Hydrogen bonds are shown as dotted green lines and pi-interactions are shown in orange. (A) Pi-interactions with Lys273 and Lys295 are critical for Saracatinib. (B) Isopraeroside IV docks to the outer region of the ATP binding pocket via H-bonds at Ser345 and Asp348. (C) 9HFG structure enables docking in the inner regions of the ATP binding pocket, forming H-bonds with Lys295 and Asp404. (D) Similar to Saracatinib, aurantiamide forms pi-interactions with Lys295, in addition to H-bonds with Ser345 and Asp348.

Molecular Dynamics Simulation

More realistic interactions of the candidates with Src kinase in a biological system were simulated through MD. Interaction differences at key residues for each tested compound during docking and MD are summarized in Table 5. H-bond formation and occupancies during and the H-bond distance profiles are presented in Table 6 and Figure 11, respectively. The primary binding residue for Saracatinib was Lys295 where stable π-interactions and a high occupancy H-bond were formed (Figure 11A). The H-bond observed at Met341 during docking was substituted by an H-bond with Thr338 throughout MD. The π interaction with Leu273 during docking was not observed during MD. As illustrated in Figure 12A, the head-on direction of the H atom and the near perpendicular spatial arrangements facilitate the formation of π-sigma interaction between Leu273 and Saracatinib. During MD, angle increase due to ligand and Leu273 fluctuations disrupted the formation of π-sigma interactions (Figure 12A).

Isopraeroside IV formed stable H-bonds with Met341, Lys343, and Ser345 (Table 6). H-bonds formed with Tyr340 (Figure 11B) and Asp348 (Figure 11C) were not stable and could not contribute to stability of Isopraeroside when in complex with Src kinase. Sharp decreases in H-bond distances observed for Lys343 and Ser345 (Figure 11B–C) are likely due to rotations of the residues which bring the ligand into closer proximity for H-bond formation (Figure 13A).

The highest number of H-bonds was formed by 9HFG with Lys295 and Asp404 (Table 5–6) Rhythmic fluctuations of H-bond distances with the key binding residue Lys295 (Figure 11D–F) are likely due to rotations of the amine group on Lys295 (Figure 13B). 9HFG also formed two H-bonds with Asp404, but the H-bond with Ala390 during docking was lost (Figure 11G).

Aurantiamide was primarily bound to the ATP binding pocket through the π interaction at Lys295 and H-bonds with Ser345 and Asp348 (Table 5). Increased distance fluctuations in Ser345 (Figure 11H) could be due to the rotation of benzene moieties (Figure 13C). Similar to Saracatinib, the loss of the π interaction at Leu273 involved torsion of the benzene moiety (Figure 12B). Benzene ring torsion during MD reduced angles between the H

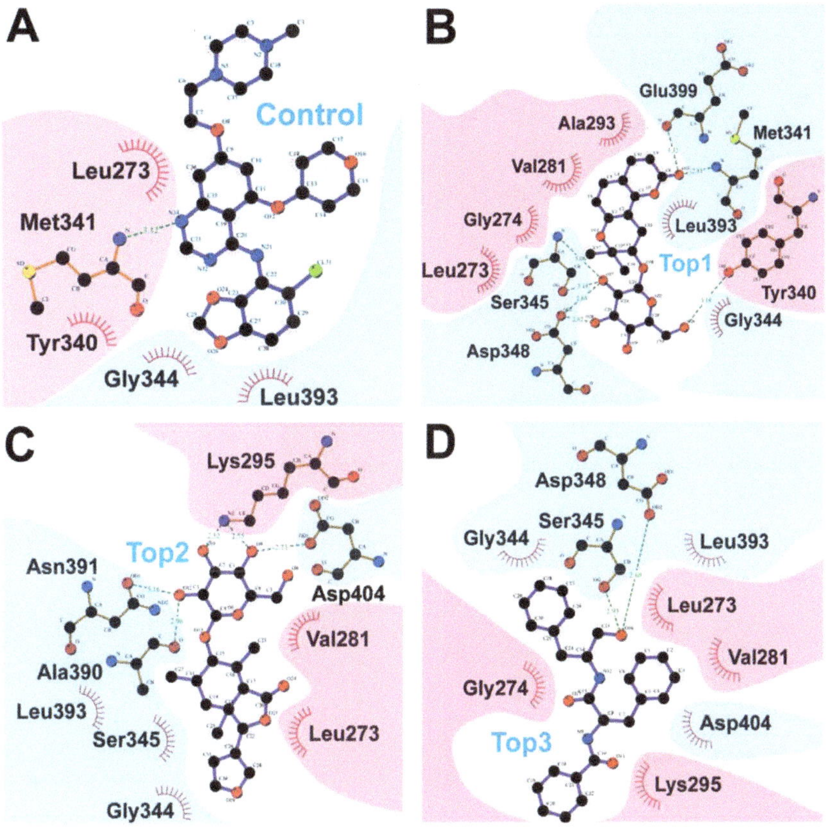

Figure 6. Ligplot diagrams illustrating protein-ligand interactions during docking. (A) Saracatinib, (B) Isopraeroside IV, (C) 9HFG, and (D) aurantiamide. Hydrophobic interactions are represented by red spokes radiating towards the ligand atoms they contact. Ligands are represented in purple. C, N, O, and Cl atoms are represented in black, blue, red, and green, respectively. Pink backgrounds highlight amino acids of the small lobe (267–337), and blue background highlight those belonging to the large lobe (340–520). Hydrophobic interactions shown in this illustration are calculated through the Ligplot algorithm.

Table 3. Ligand-protein interactions determined through LigPlot.

Amino acid in Src kinase	Hydrophobic interactions[1]	Ligand			
		Saracatinib	**Isopraeroside IV**	**9HFG**	**Aurantiamide**
Leu273/Leu393	+	A/A	A/A	A/A	A/A
Gly274/Gly344	+	-/A	A/A	-/A	A/A
Val281	+	-	A	A	A
Ala293/Ala390	+	-	A/-	H1	-
Lys295	+	-	-	H2	A
Tyr340	+	A	H1	-	-
Met341	–	H1	H1	-	-
Ser345	–	-	H2	A	H1
Asp348/Asp404	–	-	H2/-	-/H1	H1/A
Asn391	–	-	-	H1	-
Glu399	–	-	H1	H1	-

[1]Amino acid residues where hydrophobic interactions are observed are denoted by the "+" symbol.
A: hydrophobic interaction.
H1: form one hydrogen bond between ligand and amino acid.
H2: form two hydrogen bond between ligand and amino acid.

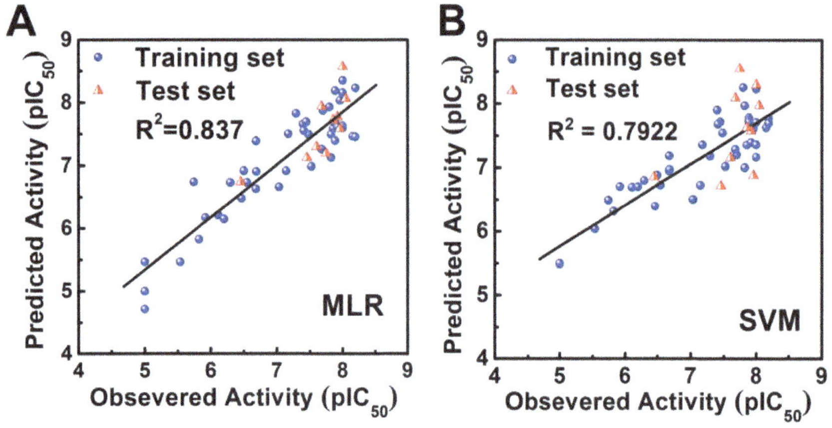

Figure 7. Correlation between observed and predicted activities of 53 Src inhibitors using different prediction models. (A) MLR and (B) SVM. Correlation coefficients (R^2) calculated from the training set were 0.837 and 0.7922 for MLR and SVM models respectively.

Table 4. CoMFA and CoMSIA models constructed from 53 known Src kinase inhibitors[1].

	Cross validation		Non-cross validation			Fraction				
	ONC	q^2cv	r^2	SEE	F	S	E	H	D	A
CoMFA	6	0.430	0.920	0.291	68.862	1	0	-	-	-
CoMSIA										
S	6	0.567	0.879	0.357	43.751	1	-	-	-	-
H	6	0.449	0.922	0.287	70.832	-	-	1	-	-
SA	5	0.370	0.821	0.428	34.018	0.587	-	-	-	0.413
SE	5	0.468	0.845	0.399	40.426	1	0	-	-	-
SH	6	0.486	0.935	0.262	86.523	0.367	-	0.633	-	-
HD	6	0.499	0.929	0.273	78.719	-	-	0.695	0.305	-
SEH	5	0.527	0.914	0.298	78.403	0.368	0	0.632	-	-
SHD*	6	0.519	0.944	0.244	100.517	0.260	-	0.468	0.272	-
SHA	6	0.439	0.936	0.260	87.726	0.293	-	0.492	-	0.215
EHD	6	0.531	0.929	0.273	78.719	-	0	0.695	-	0.305
HDA	5	0.446	0.928	0.275	77.512	-	-	0.550	0.253	0.197
SEHD	6	0.539	0.944	0.244	100.517	0.261	0	0.468	0.272	-
SEHA	5	0.506	0.920	0.286	85.421	0.287	0	0.485	-	0.228
SHDA	6	0.467	0.946	0.238	105.771	0.222	-	0.400	0.219	0.158
EHDA	6	0.464	0.928	0.275	77.512	-	0	0.550	0.253	0.197
SEHDA	6	0.452	0.946	0.238	105.771	0.222	0	0.400	0.219	0.158

[1]: Structures and inhibitory activities adapted from [54].
ONC: Optimal number of components.
S: Steric.
SEE: Standard error of estimate.
E: Electrostatic.
F: F-test value.
H: Hydrophobic.
PLS: partial least squares.
D: Donor.
*: Optimum prediction model.
A: Acceptor.

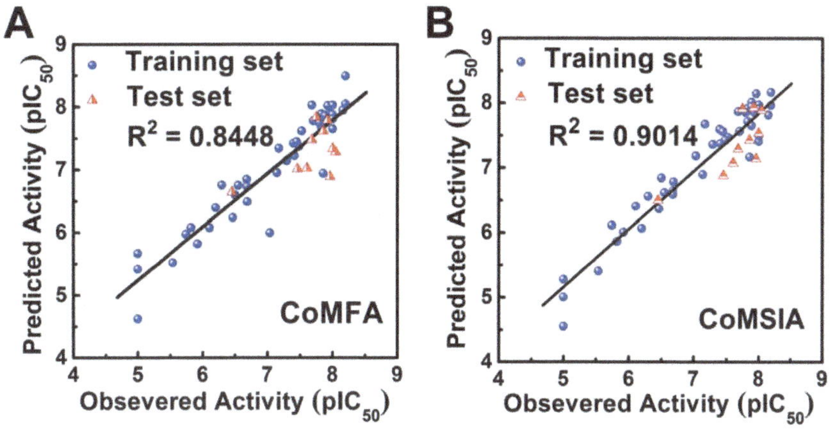

Figure 8. Correlation between observed and predicted activities of 53 Src inhibitors using different 3D-QSAR models. (A) CoMFA and (B) CoMSIA. Correlation coefficients (R^2) calculated from the training set were 0.8448 and 0.9014 for CoMFA and CoMSIA models respectively.

atom and the benzene normal plane to approximately 90 degrees, making the formation of π-interactions unlikely (Figure 12B). In general, MD results were in agreement with docking (Table 5).

Torsion angles also provide molecular insights into ligand stability (Figure 14). Torsion angle fluctuations critical to the stability of Saracatinib were not observed (Figure 14A). Torsion angles recorded for Isopraeroside IV were relatively stable with the exception of **c** and **d** (Figure 14B). Notable torsion angle changes at **c** and **d**, may account for the decrease in H-bond distances observed for Tyr340 (6.34 ns) (Figure 11B). Subsequent increase in bond distance and resulting loss of the Tyr340 H-bond could be due to sharp angle changes of **d** from 17.44 ns to the end of MD simulation. Torsion angles for 9HFG provide supporting evidence for the cause of H-bond fluctuations in Figure 11D–G. Since the stable torsion angles at **c** and **e** (Figure 14C) imply a relatively stable ligand, fluctuations in bond distance (Figure 11D–F) should be due to changes in Lys295. Further evidence is given by torsion angle changes at **f**. As **f** is associated with the binding of O9 with Lys295 and H39 with Asp404, should ligand stability be the cause of fluctuation, bond distances at both locations should be equally affected. However, H39 forms stable H-bond with Asp404, but O9

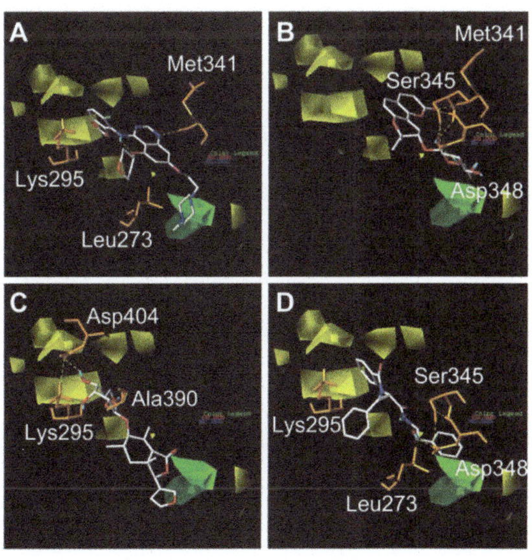

Figure 9. Spatial contour of test ligands to generated CoMFA maps. Map areas favoring and disfavoring steric fields are represented respectively in green and yellow. Saracatinib (A), Isopraeroside IV (B), and 9HGF (C) contoured well to the bioactivity map. A benzene ring of aurantiamide was located within the steric disfavoring region (D), suggesting lower bioactivity than it other tested ligands.

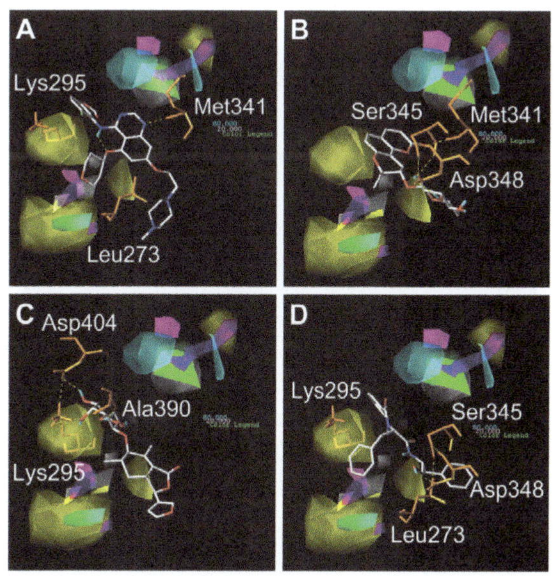

Figure 10. Spatial contour of test ligands to generated CoMSIA maps. Color blocks represent favor/disfavor steric field (green/yellow), favor/disfavor hydrophobic interaction (cyan/white), favor/disfavor hydrogen donor (purple/magenta). Saracatinib (A) forms H-bonds with Met341 which is located near the region favoring hydrogen bond donors and hydrophobic interactions. The compact structures of Isopraeroside IV (B) and 9HGF (C) allowed interactions with Src kinase without defying regions disfavoring interactions. The benzene moieties of aurantiamide (D) were in proximity to the steric disfavoring region, suggesting lower bioactivity.

Table 5. Summary of interaction type, location, and frequency of test ligands following docking and MD simulation.

Ligand	Interaction Location/Type/Frequency*									
	Leu273	**Lys295**	**Thr338**	**Tyr340**	**Met341**	**Lys343**	**Ser345**	**Asp348**	**Ala390**	**Asp404**
Saracatinib-docking	π	π			H					
Saracatinib-MD		πH	H		H					
Isopraeroside IV-docking					H		HH	HH		
Isopraeroside IV-MD				H	H		HHH			
9HFG		HHH							H	H
9HFG-MD		HHHHHH								HH
Aurantiamide	π	π					H	H		
Aurantiamide-MD		π					H	H		

*: each letter denotes one interaction.
π: pi-interaction.
H: H-bond.

Table 6. H-bond distance and occupancies[1] of different ligands during MD.

Ligand	H-bond	Ligand Atom	Amino acid	Distance (Å)			H-bond occupancy
				Max.	**Average**	**Min.**	
Saracatinib	1	O24	LYS295:HN	3.865	2.492	1.863	59.8%
	2	O24	THR338:HG1	3.875	3.198	2.296	0.1%
	3	Cl31	ASP404:HN	5.164	4.193	2.480	0.15%
Isopraeroside IV	1	H50	TYR340:OH	6.354	4.565	1.773	7.75%
	2	O15	MET341:HN	4.145	2.655	1.714	39.45%
	3	H53	LYS343:O	5.479	2.331	1.746	49.25%
	4	H51	SER345:OG	3.933	2.601	1.896	70.55%
	5	O27	SER345:HG	4.195	2.894	2.165	7.85%
	6	O27	SER345:HN	4.094	2.976	1.929	6.7%
	7	H51	ASP348:OD2	5.625	4.741	2.193	15.3%
9HFG	1	O9	LYS295:HZ1	3.92	2.358	1.565	60.2%
	2	O10	LYS295:HZ1	4.099	2.773	1.61	40.6%
	3	O8	LYS295:HZ2	5.772	4.166	2.451	0.05%
	4	O9	LYS295:HZ2	3.31	2.327	1.601	63.95%
	5	O10	LYS295:HZ2	3.741	2.350	1.592	71.15%
	6	O9	LYS295:HZ3	4.354	2.627	1.633	42.85%
	7	O10	LYS295:HZ3	4.102	2.637	1.562	57.55%
	8	H41	ALA390:O	5.284	3.869	2.186	0.05%
	9	H39	ASP404:OD1	4.427	3.246	1.784	14.35%
	10	H39	ASP404:OD2	4.427	3.246	1.784	99.4%
Aurantiamide	1	H40	SER345:OG	3.764	2.431	1.743	61.5%
	2	H44	ASP348:OD1	3.896	3.182	2.151	0.9%

[1]: Occupancy calculated based on the default cut-off distance of 2.5 Å.

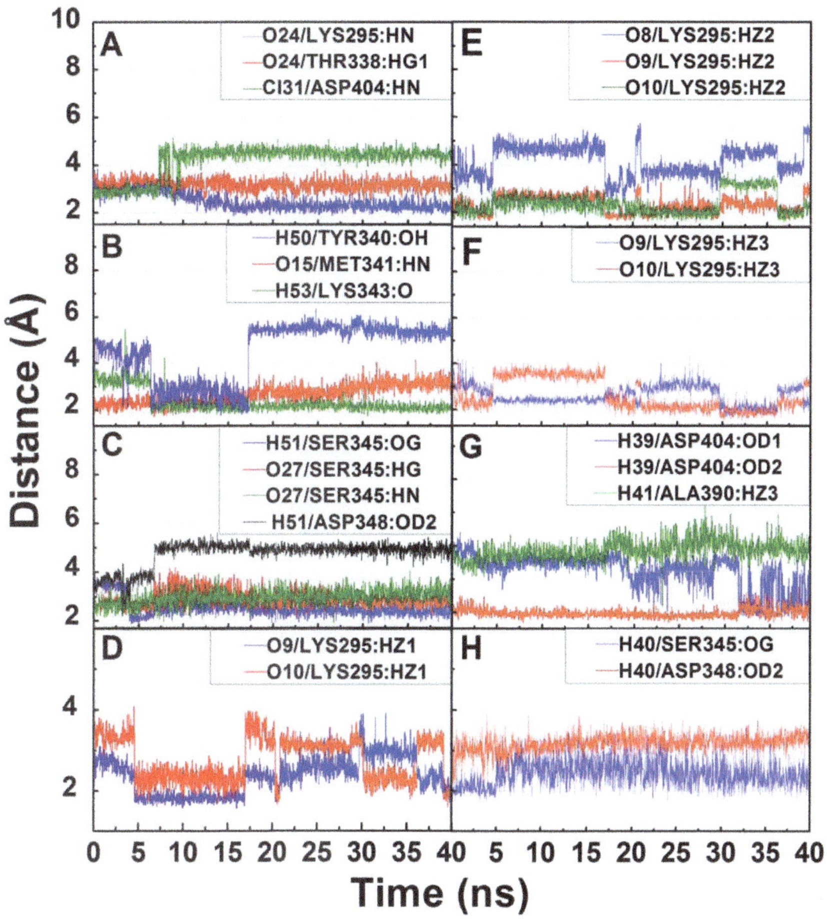

Figure 11. Hydrogen bond distance profiles between Src kinase and TCM candidates during 20 ns MD simulation. Distances (Å) shown are profiles of amino acids implicated as binding residues during docking with (A) Saracatinib, (B,C) Isopraeroside IV, (D–G) 9HFG, and (H) aurantiamide.

does not form stable bonding with Lys295, validating that the primary reason for the lack of stable binding with Lys295 is due to the instability of the amino acid itself. Among the torsion angles recorded for aurantiamide (Figure 14D), only **a**, **d**, and **l** are relatively unstable with angle fluctuations greater than 50 degrees. Stable H-bonds are formed as a result of the stability of the ligand.

Figure 15 summarizes the RMSD and total energy trajectories of the ligands during MD. All compounds, with the exception of 9HFG from 20–24 ns, had relatively stable ligand RMSDs. Whole molecule RMSDs and total energies reached equilibration after 16 ns. Among the four test compounds, Saracatinib had the highest complex RMSD and total energy. The TCM candidates exhibited similar complex RMSDs, but aurantuamide had higher total energy than Isopraeroside IV and 9HFG after stabilization. The higher energy and complex RMSD of Saracatinib may be associated with its high internal ligand energy (Table 1). Once bound, the internal energy is transferred to the complex, causing more fluctuations and higher energy levels. Isopraeroside IV and 9HFG are smaller structures compared to Saracatinib. The lower energy profiles and complex RMSD may be attributed to the compact structures and formation of multiple H-bonds. Flexible moieties in Isopraeroside IV are anchored to the ATP binding pocket through H-bonds, limiting the fluctuations of the complex and increasing stability. By contrast, H-bonds formed by 9HFG stabilizes the phenyl moiety, but the remaining structure is unbound and can freely rotate. This could be the reason for high ligand RMSDs observed for 9HFG (Figure 15B). Aurantuamide is a larger compound that shares similarities with Saracatinib. As previously discussed, aurantuamide interacts with Src kinase ATP binding pocket through a π interaction with Lys295 and an H-bond at Ser345, leaving two benzene moieties free for rotation. The larger ligand RMSD and higher total energy is likely due to these rotations. In summary, all four test compounds formed stable complexes at the ATP binding pocket for the duration of MD. TCM candidates exhibited higher stability than Saracatinib, indicating advantages as substitutes for the commercial drug.

Assessment of TCM candidate mode of action

Despite promising drug-like characteristics, one must consider binding mechanisms of the ligand compounds to objectively speculate their effect on Src kinase. As described previously, most Src inhibitors, including Saracatinib, compete with ATP for binding to Lys295 (Type I inhibitors). Src kinase is activated when interactions between SH2 and SH3 are broken, and when Tyr416 becomes phosphorylated [18] (Figure 1). Among our TCM candidates, 9HFG and aurantiamide show Src Type I inhibitor-like docking characteristics. Aurantiamide interacts primarily with

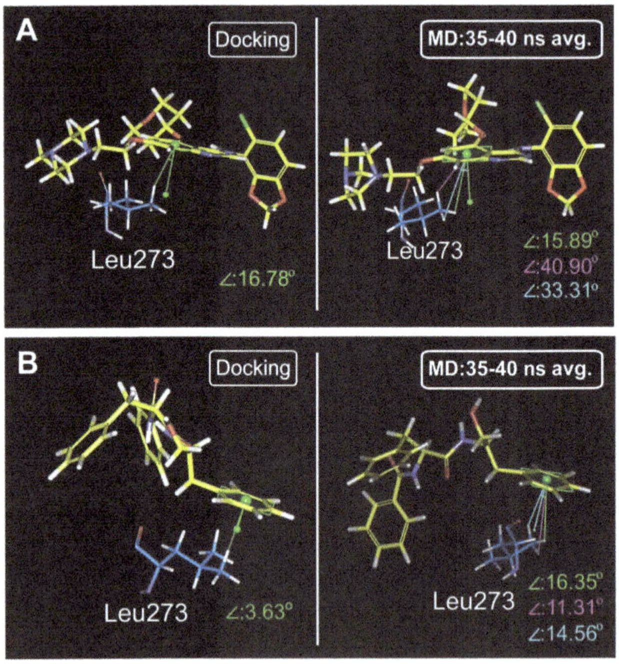

Figure 12. Molecular changes contributing to the disappearance of pi interactions in Saracatinib and aurantiamide during MD. Loss of pi-interaction with Leu273 in both ligands was due to torsion of the benzene ring within the ligand structures.

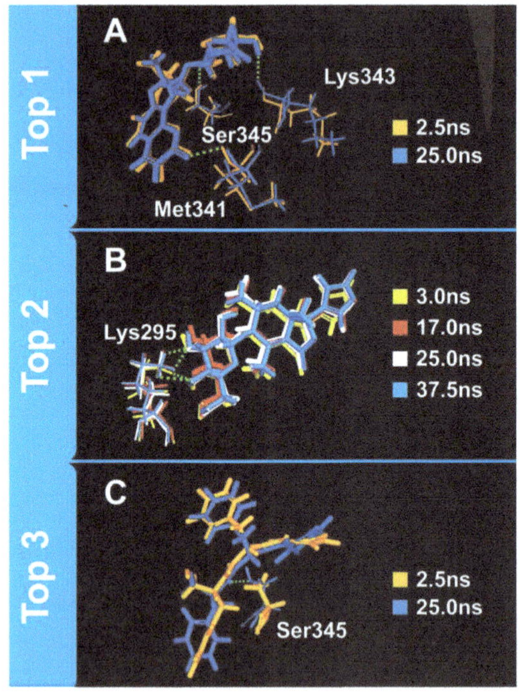

Figure 13. Molecular changes contributing to protein-ligand complex stability during MD. (A) Lys343 and Ser345 amine group rotations bring Isopraeroside IV into proximity for H-bond formation. (B) The rhythmic fluctuations observed in 9HFG can be attributed to the rotations of the NH_3 group on Lys295. (C) Rotation of the benzene moieties led to increased distance fluctuations in Ser345 during MD.

Lys295, and thus its mode of inhibition would also be through competitive binding against ATP for Lys295 (Figure 16A). However, its lower total energy (Figure 15) implies a more stable protein-ligand complex than Saracatinib. Intriguingly, 9HFG is a potential candidate that mimics the natural autoinhibitory mechanisms in Src kinases. Not only does 9HFG bind strongly to Lys295, but it simultaneously binds to Asp404 as well (Figure 16A). This is an important feature as it mimics the bridging function of Mg^{2+} between these two amino acids in native Src kinases and stabilizes the structural integrity of the catalytic cleft (Figure 16B) [18]. The dual function of 9HFG as a binding site competitor and stabilizer of the catalytic cleft suggests good potential for Src kinase inhibition. On the contrary, Isopraeroside IV may not affect Src kinase activity despite its good binding affinity and predicted bioactivities. Isopraeroside IV binds to regions located deeper within the catalytic cleft than Lys295 (Table 3, Table 5) and does not interact directly with Lys295. Though Isopraeroside IV may limit the ability of ATP to bind to Lys295 through steric hindrance, there is no evidence from our structure-based analysis to support such a claim.

Conclusion

The potential of Isopraeroside IV, 9HFG, and aurantiamide as potential leads for Src-kinase was assessed through structure- and ligand-based *in silico* approaches. Docking and MD suggest that Isopraeroside IV, 9HFG, and aurantiamide have higher and more stable binding affinities with Src kinase than Saracatinib. Assessment of biological activity through ligand structures further implied that the TCM candidates were biologically active compounds. Considering the interaction between the TCM candidates and the Src ATP binding region, 9HFG, and aurantiamide may exert inhibition against Src kinase by competitive binding against ATP. Our results may be applicable to drug development in different ways. TCM compounds 9HFG and aurantiamide may be directly used as candidate lead compounds in biological studies based on their high stability and predicted bioactivities. In addition, structural insights such as key amino acids and important moieties which form stable interactions can be utilized for *de novo* synthesis of more stable compounds that interact with Src kinase.

Materials and Methods

Docking

The protein structure of human Src kinase (PDB: 2H8H) was obtained from Protein Data Bank [47]. The binding site used in this study was based on the space occupied by Saracatinib within 2H8H. The binding site was located within the cleft separating the carboxyl-terminal lobe (residues 345–523) and the amino-terminal lobe (residues 270–340), and surrounded by residues Lys295, Trp340, Met341, Lys343, Gly344, Ser345, Leu373, Leu393, and Asp404. Over 20,000 ligands from TCM Database@Taiwan were used for docking in the Src kinase binding site. All ligands were pre-treated with CHARMm [48] to attach missing H-atoms. Saracatinib was used as the control. TCM ligands were docked into the binding site using the LigandFit program [49] within Discovery Studio 2.5 and DockScore selected as the primary scoring function for assessing binding affinities. TCM ligands were further screened with Lipinski's Rule of Five [50,51] and absorption, distribution, metabolism, excretion and toxicity (ADMET) [52] in DS 2.5 to rule out potentially toxic derivatives.

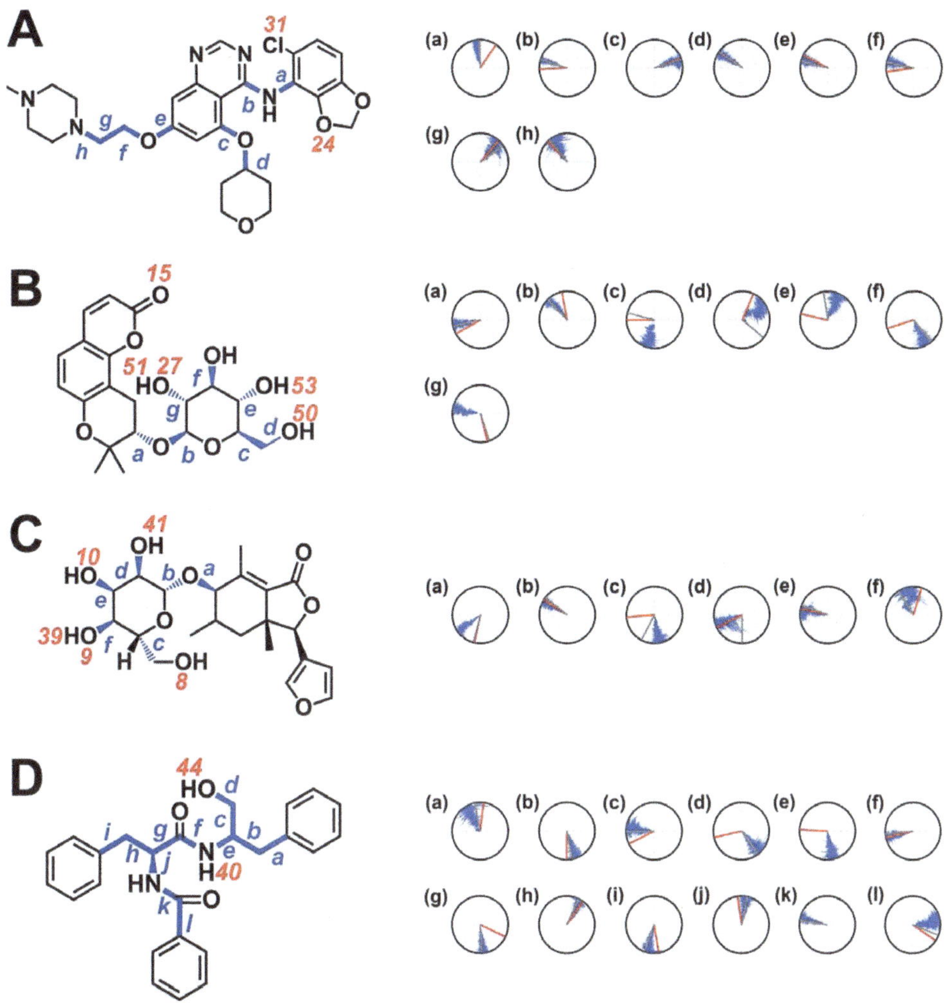

Figure 14. Torsion angles of test candidates during MD simulation. Torsion angle measured is designated by a lower case alphabet which corresponds to the radar chart with the same alphabet. Red numbers indicate the locations where H-bonds are formed. (numbering corresponds to those in Table 5). Blue lines indicate the torsion angles recorded; the red and gray lines indicate the angle during docking and at time 0 of MD, respectively.

Attraction forces (H-bond and hydrophobic interactions) between the ligand and protein were analyzed using LigPlot v.2.2.25 [53]. The 3D protein-ligand complexes generated during docking were flattened to 2D diagrams through the ligplot algorithm.

Bioactivity Prediction by Support Vector Machine (SVM) and Multiple Linear Regression (MLR)

DS 2.5 was used to calculate individual molecular property descriptors of 53 Src inhibitors with known pIC_{50} values [54]. Representative descriptors for the inhibitors were determined from a pool of 552 descriptors through genetic function approximation (GFA) [55,56]. A QSAR models were calculated by GFA and ranked by square correlation coefficient (R^2) corresponding to the fitness of each model. Descriptors from the model with the highest R^2 were used to construct MLR and SVM models for predicting the bioactivity of TCM candidates. The linear MLR model [57] was constructed with the representative descriptors using MATLAB [58].

In addition to the linear MLR model, a non-linear QSAR model utilizing support vector machine (SVM) [59,60] for the regression of continuous bioactivity data (pIC_{50}), also termed support vector regression (SVR), was also constructed. SVR uses the Kernel function to map the input data set into a high-dimensional feature space in order to find the hyperplane that best predicts data distribution. The SVR formulation is

$$\min_{w,b\xi,\xi*} \frac{1}{2}\left\|w^2\right\| + C\sum_{i=1}^{l}(\xi_i + \xi_i^*) \tag{1}$$

$$\text{s.t.}\left\{\begin{array}{l} y_i - \langle w,x_i\rangle - b) \leq \varepsilon + \xi_i \\ \langle w,x_i\rangle + b - y_i \leq \varepsilon + \xi_i^* \\ \xi_i, \xi_i^* \geq 0, i = 1,\ldots,l \end{array}\right\} \tag{2}$$

The parameters (x_1, y_1), …, (x_l, y_l) represent data within a given training set and can also be expressed as $f(x) = <w,x>+b$, $w \in R^d, b \in R$. The parameter w is calculated by performing ε-

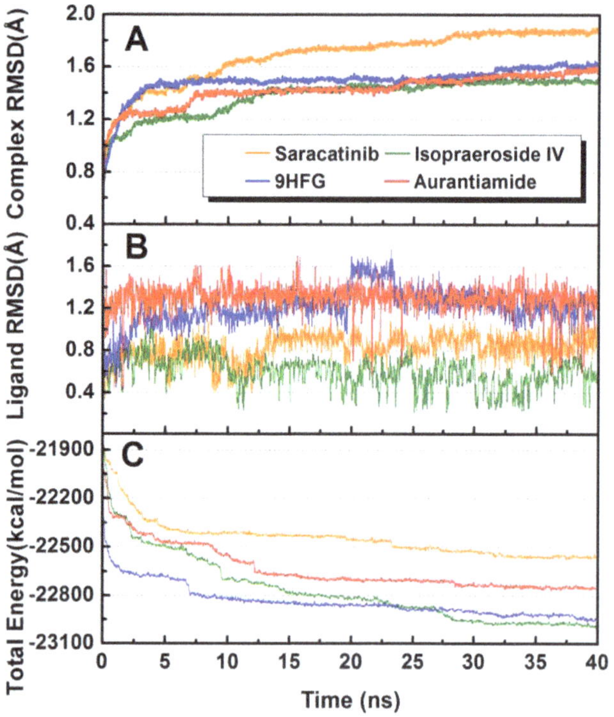

Figure 15. Measured trajectories during MD. (A) Complex, (B) ligand, and (C) total energy during MD. Saracatinib had the highest complex RMSD and total energy. The lower complex RMSDs and total energy of Isopraeroside IV and 9HFG may be attributed to their compact structure and multiple H-bond formations. The higher RMSD and total energy observed in auranruamide is possibly the result of the rotating benzene moieties.

insensitive loss function. The performance of SVR is dependent on parameters C,ε, the kernel function and kernel parameters. To further optimize this to nonlinear functions, Lagrange multipliers and kernel $k(x,x') = \langle \phi(x), \phi(x') \rangle$ are used. The nonlinear functions and predictions are determined by:

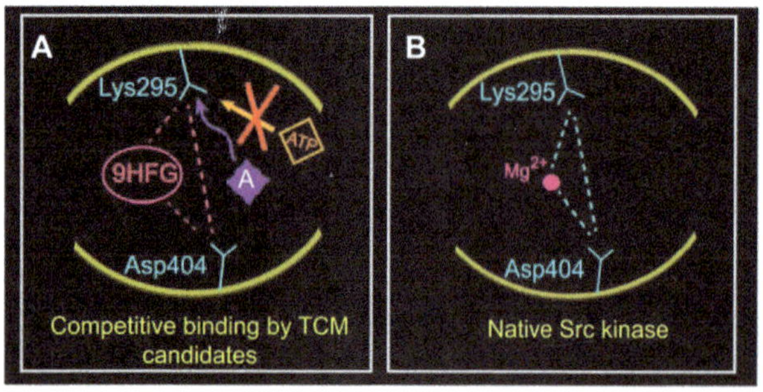

Figure 16. Mechanisms underlying Src kinase inhibition and activation. (A) Based on the molecular interactions observed through MD, TCM candidates 9HFG and aurantiamide (A; violet diamond) may inhibit Src kinase activation through different pathways. Aurantiamide binds directly to Lys295, competing with ATP for the binding site. 9HGF also binds to Lys295, but has additional binding with Asp404, which acts similarly to Mg^{2+} found in native Src kinase. (B) The bridging function of Mg^{2+} between Lys295 and Asp404 in native Src kinase.

$$\max.\left\{\begin{array}{l} -\frac{1}{2}\sum_{i,j=1}^{1}(\alpha_i-\alpha_i^*)(\alpha_j-\alpha_j^*)k(x_i,x_j) \\ -\varepsilon\sum_{i=0}^{1}(\alpha_i-\alpha_i^*)+\sum_{j=0}^{1}y_i(\alpha_j-\alpha_j^*)+ \end{array}\right\} \quad (3)$$

$$\text{s.t.}\sum_{i=0}^{1}(\alpha_i-\alpha_i^*)=0 \text{ and } \alpha_i-\alpha_i^*\in[0,C]$$

$$f(x)=\sum_{i=1}^{l}(\alpha_i-\alpha_i^*)k(x_i,x)+b \text{ s.t. } 0\le\alpha_i^*\le C, 0\le\alpha_i\le C \quad (4)$$

The SVM model was constructed by applying the LibSVM [61] within the gridregression.py program to determine key parameters C cost, epsilon and gamma.

Bioactivity Prediction by 3D Quantitative Structure-Activity Relationship (QSAR) Analysis

The 53 Src kinase inhibitors [54] used in this study were randomly divided into a training set of 43 compounds and a test set of 10 compounds. Alignment of the training set molecules was performed using atom-fit module of SYBYL-X 1.1 [62] Comparative force field analysis (CoMFA) and comparative similarity indices analysis (CoMSIA) models were constructed for 3D-QSAR. The steric and electrostatic field descriptors in CoMFA were calculated using Lennard-Jones potential and Coulombic potential, respectively. For CoMSIA models, the steric, electrostatic, hydrophobic and hydrogen bond donor and acceptors were calculated through Gaussian functions. Partial least squares (PLS) regression was utilized to analyze the 3D-QSAR models with descriptor used as an independent variable. Structural contour to the generated CoMFA and CoMSIA models were used to predict bioactivity of TCM candidates.

Molecular Dynamics (MD) Simulation

Src kinase complexes of the TCM candidates were subjected to molecular dynamics (MD) simulation under the force field of CHARMm [48] using DS 2.5. The energy of each complex was minimized using 500 steps of Steepest Descent and 500 steps of Conjugate Gradient method. The system was heated without constraint from 50 K to 310 K in 50 ps, and equilibrated for 200 ps. The final production was conducted for 40 ns in NVT ensemble with snapshots saved at 2.5 ps intervals. The time step was set to 2 fs. Hydrogen bond frequencies, energy trajectories, and hydrogen bond distances were calculated via DS 2.5 Analyze Trajectory module to analyze molecular interactions within the protein-ligand system.

Supporting Information

Table S1 Predicted and observed activity (pIC_{50}) of 53 known Src kinase inhibitors[1] using generated CoMFA and CoMSIA models.
(DOC)

Acknowledgments

We are grateful to the Asia University cloud-computing facilities and Dr. Su-sen Chang for technical assistance in preparing the manuscript.

Author Contributions

Conceived and designed the experiments: CYCC. Performed the experiments: WIT. Analyzed the data: WIT CYCC. Contributed reagents/materials/analysis tools: CYCC. Wrote the paper: WIT.

References

1. Wheeler DL, Iida M, Dunn EF (2009) The role of Src in solid tumors. Oncologist 14: 667–678.
2. Oneyama C, Morii E, Okuzaki D, Takahashi Y, Ikeda J, et al. (2011) MicroRNA-mediated upregulation of integrin-linked kinase promotes Src-induced tumor progression. Oncogenedoi: 10.1038/onc.2011.367 [Advanced E-pub].
3. Gianni D, Taulet N, DerMardirossian C, Bokoch GM (2010) c-Src-mediated phosphorylation of NoxA1 and Tks4 induces the reactive oxygen species (ROS)-dependent formation of functional invadopodia in human colon cancer cells. Mol Biol Cell 21: 4287–4298.
4. Miyake T, Parsons SJ (2011) Functional interactions between Choline kinase alpha, epidermal growth factor receptor and c-Src in breast cancer cell proliferation. Oncogenedoi: 10.1038/onc.2011.332 [Advanced E-pub].
5. Irwin ME, Bohin N, Boerner JL (2011) Src family kinases mediate epidermal growth factor receptor signaling from lipid rafts in breast cancer cells. Cancer Biol Ther 12: 718–726.
6. Thomas S, Overdevest JB, Nitz MD, Williams PD, Owens CR, et al. (2011) Src and caveolin-1 reciprocally regulate metastasis via a common downstream signaling pathway in bladder cancer. Cancer Res 71: 832–841.
7. Kim HS, Han HD, Armaiz-Pena GN, Stone RL, Nam EJ, et al. (2011) Functional roles of Src and Fgr in ovarian carcinoma. Clin Cancer Res 17: 1713–1721.
8. Ferrandi M, Molinari I, Torielli L, Padoani G, Salardi S, et al. (2010) Adducin- and ouabain-related gene variants predict the antihypertensive activity of rostafuroxin, part 1: experimental studies. Sci Transl Med 2: 59ra86.
9. Ferrari P (2010) Rostafuroxin: an ouabain-inhibitor counteracting specific forms of hypertension. Biochim Biophys Acta 1802: 1254–1258.
10. Manunta P, Ferrandi M, Bianchi G, Hamlyn JM (2009) Endogenous ouabain in cardiovascular function and disease. J Hypertens 27: 9–18.
11. Bianchi G (2005) Genetic variations of tubular sodium reabsorption leading to "primary" hypertension: from gene polymorphism to clinical symptoms. Am J Physiol Regul Integr Comp Physiol 289: R1536–1549.
12. Ferrandi M, Molinari I, Barassi P, Minotti E, Bianchi G, et al. (2004) Organ hypertrophic signaling within caveolae membrane subdomains triggered by ouabain and antagonized by PST 2238. J Biol Chem 279: 33306–33314.
13. Scheiner-Bobis G, Schoner W (2001) A fresh facet for ouabain action. Nat Med 7: 1288–1289.
14. Liu J, Tian J, Haas M, Shapiro JI, Askari A, et al. (2000) Ouabain interaction with cardiac Na+/K+-ATPase initiates signal cascades independent of changes in intracellular Na+ and Ca2+ concentrations. J Biol Chem 275: 27838–27844.
15. Ferrandi M, Salardi S, Tripodi G, Barassi P, Rivera R, et al. (1999) Evidence for an interaction between adducin and Na(+)-K(+)-ATPase: relation to genetic hypertension. Am J Physiol-Heart C 277: H1338–H1349.
16. Aleshin A, Finn RS (2010) SRC: A Century of Science Brought to the Clinic. Neoplasia 12: 599–607.
17. Roskoski R (2004) Src protein-tyrosine kinase structure and regulation. Biochem Biophys Res Commun 324: 1155–1164.
18. Xu W, Doshi A, Lei M, Eck MJ, Harrison SC (1999) Crystal structures of c-Src reveal features of its autoinhibitory mechanism. Mol Cell 3: 629–638.
19. Zhang J, Yang PL, Gray NS (2009) Targeting cancer with small molecule kinase inhibitors. Nat Rev Cancer 9: 28–39.
20. Liu Y, Gray NS (2006) Rational design of inhibitors that bind to inactive kinase conformations. Nat Chem Biol 2: 358–364.
21. Cortes JE, Kantarjian HM, Brummendorf TH, Kim DW, Turkina AG, et al. (2011) Safety and efficacy of bosutinib (SKI-606) in chronic phase Philadelphia chromosome-positive chronic myeloid leukemia patients with resistance or intolerance to imatinib. Blood 118: 4567–4576.
22. Kluger HM, Dudek AZ, McCann C, Ritacco J, Southard N, et al. (2011) A Phase 2 Trial of Dasatinib in Advanced Melanoma. Cancer-Am Cancer Soc 117: 2202–2208.
23. Mayer EL, Baurain JF, Sparano J, Strauss L, Campone M, et al. (2011) A Phase 2 Trial of Dasatinib in Patients with Advanced HER2-Positive and/or Hormone Receptor-Positive Breast Cancer. Clin Cancer Res 17: 6897–6904.
24. Herold CI, Chadaram V, Peterson BL, Marcom PK, Hopkins J, et al. (2011) Phase II Trial of Dasatinib in Patients with Metastatic Breast Cancer Using Real-Time Pharmacodynamic Tissue Biomarkers of Src Inhibition to Escalate Dosing. Clin Cancer Res 17: 6061–6070.
25. Sharma MR, Wroblewski K, Polite BN, Knost JA, Wallace JA, et al. (2011) Dasatinib in previously treated metastatic colorectal cancer: a phase II trial of the University of Chicago Phase II Consortium. Invest New Drugs doi: 10.1007/s10637-011-9681-x [Advanced E-pub].
26. Johnson ML, Riely GJ, Rizvi NA, Azzoli CG, Kris MG, et al. (2011) Phase II trial of dasatinib for patients with acquired resistance to treatment with the epidermal growth factor receptor tyrosine kinase inhibitors erlotinib or gefitinib. J Thorac Oncol 6: 1128–1131.
27. Brooks HD, Glisson BS, Bekele BN, Ginsberg LE, El-Naggar A, et al. (2011) Phase 2 study of dasatinib in the treatment of head and neck squamous cell carcinoma. Cancer-Am Cancer Soc 117: 2112–2119.
28. Finn RS, Bengala C, Ibrahim N, Roche H, Sparano J, et al. (2011) Dasatinib as a Single Agent in Triple-Negative Breast Cancer: Results of an Open-Label Phase 2 Study. Clin Cancer Res 17: 6905–6913.
29. Johnson FM, Bekele BN, Feng L, Wistuba I, Tang XM, et al. (2010) Phase II Study of Dasatinib in Patients With Advanced Non-Small-Cell Lung Cancer. J Clin Oncol 28: 4609–4615.
30. Fury MG, Baxi S, Shen RL, Kelly KW, Lipson BL, et al. (2011) Phase II Study of Saracatinib (AZD0530) for Patients with Recurrent or Metastatic Head and Neck Squamous Cell Carcinoma (HNSCC). Anticancer Res 31: 249–253.
31. Mackay HJ, Au HJ, McWhirter E, Alcindor T, Jarvi A, et al. (2011) A phase II trial of the Src kinase inhibitor saracatinib (AZD0530) in patients with metastatic or locally advanced gastric or gastro esophageal junction (GEJ) adenocarcinoma: a trial of the PMH phase II consortium. Invest New Drugsdoi: 10.1007/s10637-011-9650-4 [Advanced E-pub].
32. Gucalp A, Sparano JA, Caravelli J, Santamauro J, Patil S, et al. (2011) Phase II trial of saracatinib (AZD0530), an oral SRC-inhibitor for the treatment of patients with hormone receptor-negative metastatic breast cancer. Clin Breast Cancer 11: 306–311.
33. Chen CYC (2011) TCM Database@Taiwan: the world's largest traditional Chinese medicine database for drug screening in silico. PLoS One 6: e15939.
34. Tsai TY, Chang KW, Chen CYC (2011) iScreen: world's first cloud-computing web server for virtual screening and de novo drug design based on TCM database@Taiwan. J Comput Aided Mol Des 25: 525–531.
35. Chang KW, Tsai TY, Chen KC, Yang SC, Huang HJ, et al. (2011) iSMART: an integrated cloud computing web server for traditional Chinese medicine for online virtual screening, de novo evolution and drug design. J Biomol Struct Dyn 29: 243–250.
36. Yang SC, Chang SS, Chen CYC (2011) Identifying HER2 Inhibitors from Natural Products Database. PLoS One 6: e28793.
37. Yang SC, Chang SS, Chen HY, Chen CYC (2011) Identification of potent EGFR inhibitors from TCM Database@Taiwan. PLoS Comput Biol 7: e1002189.
38. Sun MF, Chang TT, Chang KW, Huang HJ, Chen HY, et al. (2011) Blocking the DNA repair system by traditional Chinese medicine? J Biomol Struct Dyn 28: 895–906.
39. Chang SS, Huang HJ, Chen CYC (2011) Two Birds with One Stone? Possible Dual-Targeting H1N1 Inhibitors from Traditional Chinese Medicine. PLoS Comput Biol 7: e1002315.
40. Chen KC, Chen CYC (2011) Stroke prevention by traditional Chinese medicine? A genetic algorithm, support vector machine and molecular dynamics approach. Soft Matter 7: 4001–4008.
41. Chang TT, Sun MF, Chen HY, Tsai FJ, Fisher M, et al. (2011) Screening from the world's largest TCM database against H1N1 virus. J Biomol Struct Dyn 28: 773–786.
42. Chang PC, Wang JD, Lee MM, Chang SS, Tsai TY, et al. (2011) Lose weight with traditional Chinese medicine? Potential suppression of fat mass and obesity-associated protein. J Biomol Struct Dyn 29: 471–483.
43. Chen CY, Chen CYC (2010) Insights into designing the dual-targeted HER2/HSP90 inhibitors. J Mol Graph Model 29: 21–31.
44. Chen CY, Chang YH, Bau DT, Huang HJ, Tsai FJ, et al. (2009) Discovery of potent inhibitors for phosphodiesterase 5 by virtual screening and pharmacophore analysis. Acta Pharmacol Sin 30: 1186–1194.
45. Choi SY, Ahn EM, Song MC, Kim DW, Kang JH, et al. (2005) In vitro GABA-transaminase inhibitory compounds from the root of Angelica dahurica. Phytother Res 19: 839–845.
46. Yoon JS, Sung SH, Kim YC (2008) Neuroprotective limonoids of root bark of Dictamnus dasycarpus. J Nat Prod 71: 208–211.
47. Hennequin LF, Allen J, Breed J, Curwen J, Fennell M, et al. (2006) N-(5-chloro-1,3-benzodioxol-4-yl)-7-[2-(4-methylpiperazin-1-yl)ethoxy]-5- (tetrahydro-2H-pyran-4-yloxy)quinazolin-4-amine, a novel, highly selective, orally available, dual-specific c-Src/Abl kinase inhibitor. J Med Chem 49: 6465–6488.
48. Brooks BR, Brooks CL, Mackerell AD, Nilsson L, Petrella RJ, et al. (2009) CHARMM: the biomolecular simulation program. J Comput Chem 30: 1545–1614.
49. Montes M, Miteva MA, Villoutreix BO (2007) Structure-based virtual ligand screening with LigandFit: pose prediction and enrichment of compound collections. Proteins 68: 712–725.
50. Ganesan A (2008) The impact of natural products upon modern drug discovery. Curr Opin Chem Biol 12: 306–317.
51. Keller TH, Pichota A, Yin Z (2006) A practical view of 'druggability'. Curr Opin Chem Biol 10: 357–361.

52. Khan MT (2010) Predictions of the ADMET properties of candidate drug molecules utilizing different QSAR/QSPR modelling approaches. Curr Drug Metab 11: 285–295.
53. Wallace AC, Laskowski RA, Thornton JM (1995) LIGPLOT: a program to generate schematic diagrams of protein-ligand interactions. Protein Eng 8: 127–134.
54. Noronha G, Barrett K, Boccia A, Brodhag T, Cao JG, et al. (2007) Discovery of [7-(2,6-dichlorophenyl)-5-methylbenzo [1,2,4]triazin-3-yl]-[4-(2-pyrrolidin-1-ylethoxy)phenyl]amine - a potent, orally active Src kinase inhibitor with anti-tumor activity in preclinical assays. Bioorg Med Chem Lett 17: 602–608.
55. Kowar TR (1998) Genetic function approximation experimental design (GFAXD): A new method for experimental design. J Chem Inf Comp Sci 38: 858–866.
56. Jamois EA (2004) Analysis of multiple QSAR models from genetic function approximation: A basis for experimental design. Abstr Pap Am Chem S 227: U905–U905.
57. Slinker BK, Glantz SA (2008) Multiple linear regression: accounting for multiple simultaneous determinants of a continuous dependent variable. Circulation 117: 1732–1737.
58. MATrix LABoratory. Natick, MA, US: The MathWorks Inc.
59. Hasegawa K, Funatsu K (2010) Non-linear modeling and chemical interpretation with aid of support vector machine and regression. Curr Comput Aided Drug Des 6: 24–36.
60. Koh IS, Kim JH, Lee J, Oh B, Kimm K (2004) Prediction of phosphorylation sites using SVMs. Bioinformatics 20: 3179–3184.
61. Chang C-C, Lin C-J (2011) LIBSVM: A Library for Support Vector Machines. ACM Transcations on Intelligent Systems and Technology 2: 27:21–27:27.
62. SYBYL-X. 1.1 ed. St Louis, MO, USA: Tripos.

11

Assessing the Quality of Reports about Randomized Controlled Trials of Acupuncture Treatment on Mild Cognitive Impairment

Xiao Lu[1,2], Shang Hongcai[1,2]*, Wang Jiaying[1,3], Hu Jing[4], Xiong Jun[5]

1 Tianjin University of Traditional Chinese Medicine, Tianjin, China, **2** MOE Virtual Research Center of Evidence-Based Medicine, Chengdu, China, **3** Evidence Based Medicine Center in Tianjin, Tianjin, China, **4** Peking University, Beijing, China, **5** Department of Acupuncture, Jiang Xi Hospital of Traditional Chinese Medicine, Jiangxi Province, China

Abstract

Objective: To evaluate the reports' qualities which are about randomized controlled trials (RCTs) of acupuncture treatment on Mild Cognitive Impairment (MIC).

Methods: Nine databases including the Cochrane Central Register of Controlled Trials (CENTRAL,2010), PUBMED (1984-5/2010), EMbase (1984-5/2010), MEDLINE (1984-5/2010), CINAL (1984-5/2010), China National Knowledge Infrastructure (CNKI, 1980-5/2010), China Biomedicine Database disc (CBMdisc, 1980-5/2010), VIP (a full text issues database of China, 1989-5/2010) were searched systematically. Hand search for further references was conducted. Language was limited to Chinese and English. We identified 14 RCTs that used acupuncture as an intervention and assessed the quality of these reports against the Consolidated Standards for Reporting of Trials (CONSORT) statement and Standards for Reporting Interventions in Controlled Trials of Acupuncture (STRICTA).

Results: In regard to the items in the CONSORT statement, 13(92.86%) RCTs described baseline demographic and clinical characteristics in each group. 7 (50.0%) mentioned the method of generating the random sequence, only 2 (14.3%) RCTs had adequate allocation concealment. No RCTs used blinding. RCTs reported the sample size calculation. In regard to the items in STRICTA, 10 (71.43%) mentioned the depths of insertion, 6 (42.86%) reported acupuncture response, 11 (78.57%) mentioned the technique of acupuncture, 12 (85.71%) recorded the time, and only 3 (21.43%) RCTs reported the numbers of needles inserted. No RCTs reported the background of the acupuncture practitioners and professional title of practitioners.

Conclusion: The reporting quality of RCTs of acupuncture for mild cognitive impairment was moderate to low. The CONSORT statement and STRICTA should be used to standardize the reporting of RCTs of acupuncture in future.

Editor: Joseph Ross, Yale University School of Medicine, United States of America

Funding: New Century Excellent Talent Project Grant (No 2009613). The funders had no role in study design, data collection and analysis, decision to publish, or preparation of the manuscript.

Competing Interests: The authors have declared that no competing interests exist.

* E-mail: shanghongcai@foxmail.com

Introduction

Mild Cognitive Impairment (mild cognitive disorder) is a clinical state with disease characteristics between normal aging and mild dementia. Most clinical researches show that 44% of the patients diagnosed as cognitive impairment turn into Alzheimer's transit (AD) within 3 years in follow-up studies at an annual average rate of 15% [1]. Recognizing cognitive impairment and identifying individuals at high risk of dementia have become a hot issue in dementia studies in recent years. Lacking in effective drugs and rehabilitation treatment, many patients with mild cognitive impairment begin to try alternative and complementary medicine therapies which include acupuncture treatment. However, despite the publication of a number of case-based research papers the effectiveness of acupuncture on mild cognitive impairment is to be tested and to do so a reliable scientific method is needed. Some research teams decide to adopt the randomized controlled trials (RCTs). RCTs, also known as randomized clinical trials, is a prospective study to test the efficacy and effectiveness of certain treatment or protective measures after comparing the results of the treatment group with those of the control group, thus the subjects involved in the study being randomized divided into two groups [2]. At present, randomized controlled trials (RCTs) is generally considered as the best design plan to verify the efficacy of intervention measures for it boasts rigorous design and scientific methods. It contributes to ensure high-quality systematic reviews, health technology assessment reports, and a variety of other reports for decision analysis, which meets the top requirements of evidence-based medical research [3]Therefore, we have adopted the internationally recognized standards for trial reporting (the CONSORT statement) [4] and the international standards for clinical trials of acupuncture interventions (STRICTA) [5] to evaluate the quality of reports of randomized controlled trials of acupuncture treatment for mild cognitive impairment in order to shed light on its further improvement.

Methods

Search strategy

The nine databases we have searched include Cochrane Central Register of Controlled Trials(CENTRAL,2010), PUBMED(1984-5/2010), EMbase(1984-5/2010), MEDLINE(1984-5/2010), CINAL(1984-5/2010), China National Knowledge Infrastructure (CNKI, 1980-5/2010), China Biomedicine Database disc (CBMdisc, 1980-5/2010), and VIP(a full text issues database of China,1989-5/2010). The work was done comprehensively and systematically and further references were searched by hand. Our search is featured by a wide coverage of reports and prospective studies in this field to provide enough information for research.

However, our search confined itself to reports written or published either in Chinese or in English. For one thing, it is because a majority of journal papers on acupuncture are published in these two languages and it is apparently impossible for reports written in Chinese to be included in non-Chinese databases. Besides, our team members were unable to read reports in languages other than Chinese and English. It may constitute to a limitation of this study.

We did not limit our search to a specific publication date range at the beginning of this study because we wanted to find as many reports as possible concerning mild cognitive impairment in the above databases. However, the databases themselves have such limitations.

Eligibility of the study

We included original reports in Chinese or English that described acupuncture as an intervention, stated the method, and provided specific data in this study and excluded commercials, speeches, letters and meeting reports.

Selection of reports to be studied

At first, one researcher (XL) picked out duplications of these reports using NoteExpress, and scanned the title and abstract of the citation retrieved by the selection search engine (first scanning). Another researcher (WJY) then viewed the full text of all potentially eligible reports obtained. After that, similar reports were marked "suspicious duplications" and compared. If the similarity rate of these articles was beyond 80% (including 80%), the one with the fullest information was included while the others were omitted. Disagreements between the two researchers were discussed by the whole team and were solved at last. (Figure 1)

Data abstraction

Two researchers (XL and WJY) compiled a table to list the general information of the final included reports. Items of the table include report title, journal name, year of publication, type of control, number of participants and country of publication. Any missed information was coded as "not reported" and disagreements were resolved after getting more information from related references before finalizing the table. Two reviewers scanned the full text of all 14 reports and filled the table.

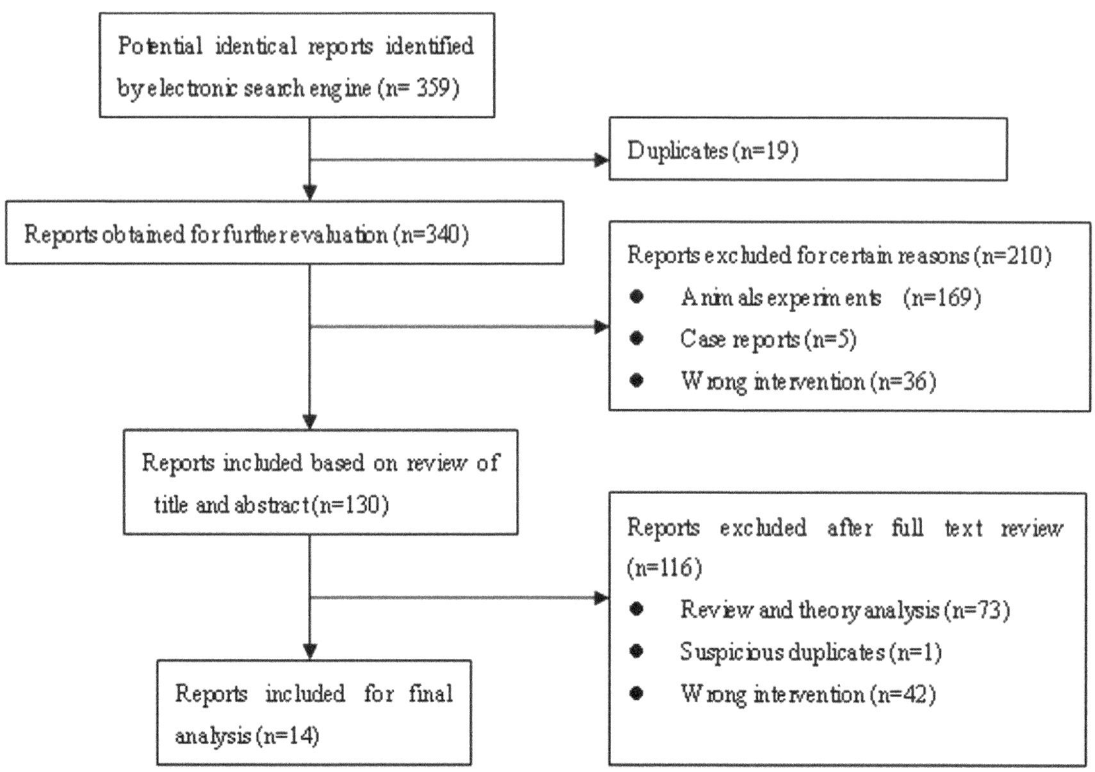

Figure 1. Flow chart of reports selection. This figure shows the process of the selection. The researchers applied the search method to find 359 reports related to the topic. One researcher (XL) picked out 19 duplications of these reports by the software NoteExpress and 169 reports of animals experiments, 5 cases and 36 reports of the wrong intervention by scanning the title and abstract of the citation retrieved by the selection search engine (first scanning). Another researcher (WJY) then viewed the full text of all potentially eligible reports obtained and picked out 73 reviews and theory analyses, one suspicious duplicate and 42 reports of the wrong intervention. At last, 14 reports are included for final analysis.

Assessment methods

We assessed the quality of these reports by CONSORT and STRICTA standards. CONSORT (consolidated standards of reporting trails) was introduced in 1996 [6] in an attempt to alleviate the problems arising from inadequate reporting, and it was revised five years later [7]. STRICTA (standards for reporting interventions in controlled trials of acupuncture) was compiled between late 2001 and early 2002 [8].

The CONSORT statement comprises a 22-item checklist including abstract, background, participants, interventions, objectives, outcome measures, sample size, sequence generation, allocation concealment, implementation, blinding, statistical methods, participant flow, recruitment, demographic data, numbers analyzed, outcomes and estimation, ancillary analyses, adverse events, interpretation and overall evidence.

STRICTA consists of 15 items including acupuncture rationale, points used, number of needle inserted depths of insertion, response elicited, needle stimulation, needle retention time, needle type, treatment regimen, co-interventions, practitioner background, duration of training, length of clinical experience, expertise, control interventions. The above information can also be found in Table 2 and Table 3.

Two researchers were required to study the CONSORT and STRICTA standards before making assessment to ensure correct understanding of every item listed in the two checklists. If they had any difficulties or disagreements in the process, they solved the problem in discussions. The 14 reports were then assessed according to the two standards respectively and each item was marked "M" (mentioned) or "NM" (not mentioned).

Results

Report selection

A total of 359 potentially relevant reports were identified from the databases for review. 229 publications were considered to be unfit for our study after a preliminary review of title and abstract. Another 74 were excluded after full-text review. At last a total of 14 full-text reports [9–22] were regarded eligible for a more systematic analysis.

Characteristics of the Reports

The characteristics of all the included reports are presented in Table 1. All the 14 reports were found in 11 different medical journals published by six different publishing houses. Sample sizes ranged from a small pilot study of 17 subjects to a large scale, and the largest sample included 104 subjects. Only one report was published in America. All the 14 studies included in our assessment were published during the year 2006–2010, while in 2009 the number of reports published reached the peak (43%) (Figure 2).

Use of CONSORT and STRICTA

At first we found that none of the reports included in the assessment explicitly mentioned the CONSORT or STRICTA statement. After referring to the official websites of the 11 journals, we found that only two journals require manuscripts to be submitted to meet the CONSORT or STRICTA standards. However, we found out later that there were 3 reports that included 19 items of CONSORT and 12 items of STRICTA

Table 1. Characteristics of the reports included (N = 14).

Report title	Journal name	Year of publication	Type of control	Number of participants	Country of publication
He 2008	JOURNAL OF PRACTICAL TRADITIONAL CHINESE MEDICINE	2008	aceglutamide	60	China
Yu 2007	SHAANXI JOURNAL OF TRADITIONAL CHINESE MEDICINE	2007	Nimodipine	67	China
Sun 2009	JOURNAL OF CLINICAL ACUPUNTURE AND MOXIBUSTION	2009	duxil tablet	60	China
Hou 2010	WORLD JOURNAL OF INTEGRATED TRADITIONAL AND WESTERN MEDICINE	2010	Sham acupuncture	36	China
Hou 2009	JOURNAL OF BEI JING UNIVERSITY OF TRADITONAL CHINESE MEDICINE	2009	Sham acupuncture	40	China
Sun 2007	Chinese Journal of Traditional Medical Science and Technology	2007	Aricept	62	China
Su 2006	LIAO NING JOURNAL OF TRADITIONAL CHINESE MEDICINE	2006	Nimodipine	100	China
Zhou 2008	SHANGHAI JOURNAL OF ACUPUNTURE AND MOXIBUSTION	2008	Sham acupuncture	60	China
Zhou 2008	GUANGXI JOURNAL OF TRADITIONAL CHINESE MEDICINE	2008	Regular treatment	60	China
Liu 2009	SHANGHAI JOURNAL OF ACUPUNTURE AND MOXIBUSTION	2009	Aricept	17	China
Chen 2008	JOURNAL OF EMERGENCY IN TRADITIONAL CHINESE MEDICINE	2008	Regular treatment	60	China
Chen 2009	Chinese Journal of Traditional Medical Science and Technology	2009	Regular treatment	60	China
Feng 2009	Jilin Journal of Traditional Chinese Medicine	2009	Sham acupuncture	104	China
Pei 2009	THE JOURNAL OF ALTERNATIVE AND COMPLEMENTARY MEDICINE	2009	Conventional rehabilitation	38	America

Table 2. Reporting quality of 14 RCTs based on CONSORT.

Total number of items	Number of reported RCTs (%)	
Abstract	7	50.00
Introduction		
Background	11	78.57
Methods		
Participants	12	85.71
Interventions	13	92.86
Objectives	12	85.71
Outcomes	13	92.86
Sample size	14	100.00
Randomization		
Sequence generation	7	50.00
Allocation concealment	2	14.29
Implementation	1	7.14
Blinding	0	0.00
Statistical methods	12	85.71
Results		
Participant flow	0	0.00
Recruitment	0	0.00
Baseline data	13	92.86
Numbers analyzed	12	85.71
Outcomes and estimation	10	71.43
Ancillary analyses	4	28.57
Adverse events	3	21.43
Discussion		
Interpretation	13	92.86
Overall evidence	7	50.00

checklist, which means that the two statements have actually been employed by more authors.

Reporting Assessment Using CONSORT and STRICTA

The results are presented in Table 2 and Table 3. Not a single report fulfilled either all the 21 items of the CONSORT checklist or the 15 STRICTA items. Above all, the main problem we found was a lack of information concerning method

Table 3. Reporting quality of interventions in 14 RCTs based on STRICTA.

Intervention	Number of reported RCTs (%)	
Acupuncture rationale	13	92.86
Needling details		
Points used	14	100
Number of needles inserted	3	21.43
Depths of insertion	10	71.43
Response elicited	6	42.86
Needle stimulation	11	78.57
Needle retention time	12	85.71
Needle type	7	50.00
Treatment regimen	11	78.57
Co-interventions	3	21.43
Practitioner background	0	0.00
Duration of training	0	0.00
Length of clinical experience	0	0.00
Expertise	0	0.00
Control intervention(s)	11	78.57

of blinding, practitioner background, and participant flow and recruitment.

CONSORT. Seven CONSORT items were mentioned in less than 30% of the total reports. They are methods of blinding, participant flow and recruitment (0%), implementation of randomization (7.14%), description of allocation concealment (14.29%), adverse events of acupuncture (21.43%) and outcomes of ancillary analyses (28.57%).

Another four CONSORT items were included in more than half of all the reports, i.e., abstract, sequence generation and overall evidence in the section of discussion.

STRICTA. None of these studies gave any information about practitioner background which was made up of expertise, duration of training and length of clinical experience. Two STRICTA items, namely, number of needles inserted and co-interventions were explained in 21.43% of the reports. Another two items were made clear in less than half of the reports, i.e., needle type (50%) and response elicited.

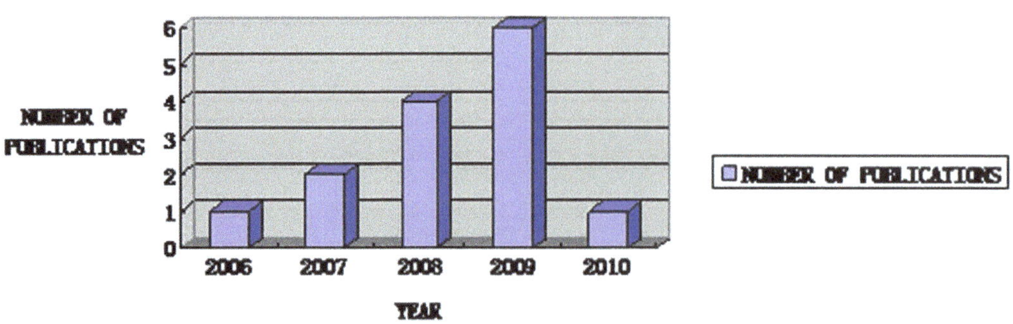

Figure 2. Number of reports published in the recent five years. According to the Table 1, the years of publication of included reports is mainly during these five years, namely from the 2006 to 2010. Figure 2 shows one report is published in 2006, two in 2007, four in 2008, six in 2009, and one in 2010.

Discussion

Summary of the study

The main strength of our study is that we have searched a total of nine databases in order to encompass all the related reports. Moreover, reports selection, data collection, reports assessment and all the other work were carefully conducted by well-trained researchers.

Another important strength of our study is that we use the CONSORT and STRICTA statement to evaluate RCTs of acupuncture. Both of them are the most widely accepted criteria for reporting quality assessment in acupuncture studies. Plain in words and ready for use, the two statements were developed in the aim of alleviating the problems arising from inadequate reporting of randomized controlled trials. They are powerful tools, as has been proved by the fact that the majority of their items were well reported, with a few exceptions (7 CONSORT items and 9 STRICTA ones were poorly reported).

We believe it is high time to call for clinical researchers to follow the two statements in conducting RCTs and in thesis writing. At present, Chinese journals set down no requirements for the author to follow the CONSORT or STRICTA statement in reporting Therefore, we recommend that mainstream Chinese journals make the application of CONSORT or STRCITA a prerequisite, so that transparency and integrity of RCTs can be ensured. More importantly, for policy makers, it is urgent to let more clinical researchers know about the CONSORT and STRICTA statement.

Limitations

Although we have assessed the 14 reports comprehensively and systematically, there are still some limitations. First, the reports included in our study were published exclusively in years between 2006 and 2010 although we didn't make any limitations on the date of publication during sample selection. The fact that the selected reports cover a narrow time span may harm the value of our study. However, it is worth mentioning that the whole concept of mild cognitive impairment was not put forward until 1999 by American scholar Petersen. Apparently it took some time for the diagnostic criteria to be introduced to China and to be widely accepted by Chinese scholars. In addition, it probably cost more time for acupuncture, a complementary and alternative intervention, to be involved in the treatment. Recently, some research groups propose the need to test the efficacy of acupuncture treatment after three or four years' clinical practice in cognitive impairment patients, thus RCTs were conducted. Nevertheless, at the beginning we didn't realize it was impossible for us to find any target report before 1999 if sample selection was conducted with "mild cognitive impairment" as a search word, which means we have done something useless and our search strategy remains to be improved.

According to resources and databases accessible to us, the earliest RCTs were carried out in 2006. However, there might be earlier articles in the database that we didn't find for certain reasons, such as language competence. We limited our search to reports written in Chinese and English, but the English report turned out to be one in number. It seems that our quality review was confined to domestic reports. Results may vary if we were able to include more reports in other languages, but this requires our team members to attain a higher level of language skills, a target we are confident to reach in the future.

Another limitation lies in that we didn't follow the rule of blinding when assessing and allocating the reports. Researches who did the scanning were directly involved in the evaluation process. This is because we believe two researchers are enough to evaluate the whole 14 selected reports and allocation was unnecessary. However, although the two researchers had studied the same version of the checklist items beforehand, they came out with different opinions on certain issues. This shows that assessment bias still exists.

Conclusion

Our study suggests that the reporting quality of recently published reports of RCTs of acupuncture treatment for mild cognitive impairment remains to be improved. However, we have found only one published report had formally appealed for the adoption of CONSORT in future research. With more articles published on this subject, it is necessary to call for the wide application of the CONSORT and STRICTA standards to improve the quality of reporting, and this study should be pursued further with a greater number of reports on this subject assessed and analyzed.

Acknowledgments

Give our thanks to the authors of the cited articles timely reply our questions and SHANG Hongcai professor's for his careful guidance.

Author Contributions

Conceived and designed the experiments: WJY XL SHC. Performed the experiments: XL WJY. Analyzed the data: HJ XL WJY. Contributed reagents/materials/analysis tools: HJ XJ. Wrote the paper: WJY XL. Resolved the disagreement and bias: SHC HJ XJ.

References

1. Gmdman M, Petemen RC, Morris JC, ADSC Cooperative Study, et al. (1996) Rate of dementia of the Alzheimer type in subjects with mild cognitive impairment[J]. Neurology 46: A403.
2. WANG Ying, HAO Guangyue, GAO Bing (2006) introduction of revised edition of CONSORT statement–the reliable standard to improve qualities reporting evaluation [J]. Journal of Baotou medicine college. pp 355–357.
3. ZHANG Xiaoli, LI Jing, ZHANG Mingming, etc (2006) Assessing the Reporting Quality of Randomized Controlled Trials on Acupuncture for Acute Ischemic Stroke Using the CONSORT Statement and STRICTA [J]. Chinese Journal of Evidence Based Medicine 6(8): 586690.
4. Altman DG, Schulz K, Moher D, et al. (2001) The Revised Statement CONSORT for Reporting Randomized Trials Explanation and Elaboration. Ann Intern Med 134(8): 663–694.
5. Mac Pherson H, White A, Cummings M, et al. (2002) STRICTA(Standards for Reporting Interventions in Controlled Trials of Acupunture). Acupunture in Medicine 20(1): 22–25.
6. Begg C, Cho M, Eastwood S, Horton R, Moher D, et al. (1996) Improving the quality of reporting of randomized controlled trials, the CONSORT statement JAMA 276(8): 637–639.
7. Moher D, Schula KF, Altman D, CONSORT Group (Consolidated Standards of Reporting Trials) (2001) The CONSORT statement: Revised recommendations for improving the quality of repors of parallel-group randomized trials JAMA 285(15): 1987–1991.
8. MacPherson H, White A, Cummings M, Jobst K, Rose K, et al. (2001) Standards for reporting invention in controlled trials of acupunture: The STRICTA recommendations. Complement Ther Med (1): 216–249, 20(1):22-25, 8(1):85-89.
9. He Xia (2008) Clinical Research on Mild Cognitive Impairment Treated by Combination of Acupuncture and Medicine. JOURNAL OF PRACTICAL TRADITIONAL CHINESE MEDICINE ZYAO, 2008(11).
10. Yu Tao (2007) Acupunture Treatment of Vascular Cognitive Impairment without Dementia in 31 Cases. SHAANXI JOURNAL OF TRADITIONAL CHINESE MEDICINE SXZY, 2007(06).
11. Sun Yuanzheng, Zhang Ying (2009) Clinical Research on Mild Cognitive Impairment Treated by Combination of Acupunture and Duxil Tablet. JOURNAL OF CLINICAL ACUPUNTURE AND MOXIBUSTION ZJLC, 2009(09).
12. Hou Xiaobing, et al. (2010) The Impact of Acupunture on Mild Cognitive Impairment in Functional Magnetic Resonance Imaging. WORLD JOURNAL OF INTEGRATED TRADITIONAL AND WESTERN MEDICINE SJZX, 2010(02).
13. Hou Xiaobing (2009) Brain Functional Magnetic Resonance Imaging (fMRI) Changes in Leukoaraiosis with Mild Cognitive Impairment before and after Treatment of Acupunture. Beijing University of Traditional Chinese Medicine.

14. Sun Yuanzheng, Zhu Pengyu, Zhang Yan (2007) 30 Cases of of Mild Cognitive Impairment Treated with Acupuncture and Oral Donepezil. Chinese Journal of Traditional Medical Science and Technology. TJYY, (03).
15. Su Zhiwei, Liu Huanrong (2006) 100 Cases of Mild Cognitive Impairment Treated with Yishen Tongdu Method Liaoning Journal of Traditional Chinese Medicine LNZY, 2006(08).
16. Zhou Xiaoping, et al. (2008) Effect of the Acupunture Method of Regulating Mild and Smooth Meridian on Patients with Mild Cognitive Impairment after Cerebral infarction. Shanghai Journal of Acupunture and Moxibustion SHZJ, 2008(05).
17. Zhou Xiaoping, et al. (2008) Effect of the Acupunture Method of Regulating Mild and Smooth Meridian on Patients with Mild Cognitive Impairment. GUANGXI JOURNAL OF TRADITIONAL CHINESE MEDICINE GXZY, 2008(02).
18. Liu Jie, Liu Zhiyan (2009) Clinical Observation on Electro-acupunture Treatment for Mild Cognitive Impairment of Deficiency of Kidney Essence. Shanghai Journal of Acupunture and Moxibustion. SHZJ, 2009(06).
19. Chen Shangjie, et al. (2008) Effects of Different Acupunture Methods on Neurological Deficit Score and Quality of Life of Patients with Mild Cognitive Impairment. Journal of Emergency in Traditional Chinese Medicine ZYJZ, 2008(03).
20. Chen Shangjie, et al. (2009) Effects of Different Acupunture Methods on SMS and MBI of Patients with Mild Cognitive Impairment. Chinese Journal of Traditional Medical Science and Technology. TJYY 2009(01).
21. Feng Chunqing, et al. (2009) Effects observation of "Qi-reinforcing, Blood-regulating and Body resistance-strengthening" Acupunture Method for Treating Mild Cognitive Impairment. Lin Journal of Traditional Chinese Medicine. 2009 29(10).
22. P C, C H, L JG(2009) Effects of electroacupunture treatment on impaired cognition and quality of life in Taiwanese stroke patients. Journal of alternative and complementary medicine (New York, N.Y.), 2009(10).

12

Favorable Circulatory System Outcomes as Adjuvant Traditional Chinese Medicine (TCM) Treatment for Cerebrovascular Diseases in Taiwan

Hsienhsueh Elley Chiu[1,2,4]*, Yu-Chiang Hong[1,4], Ku-Chou Chang[2,4], Chun-Chuan Shih[5], Jen-Wen Hung[3,4], Chia-Wei Liu[2,4], Teng-Yeow Tan[2,4], Chih-Cheng Huang[1]

1 Department of TCM, Chang Gung University College of Medicine, Kaohsiung, Taiwan, **2** Department of Neurology, Chang Gung University College of Medicine, Kaohsiung, Taiwan, **3** Department of Rehabilitation, Chang Gung University College of Medicine, Kaohsiung, Taiwan, **4** Chang Gung Memorial Hospital, Chang Gung University College of Medicine, Kaohsiung, Taiwan, **5** School of Chinese Medicine for Post-Baccalaureate, I-Shou University, Kaohsiung, Taiwan

Abstract

Background: This study searches the National Health Insurance Research Database (NHIRD) used in a previous project, aiming for reconstructing possible cerebrovascular disease-related groups (DRG),and estimating the costs between cerebrovascular disease and related diseases.

Methods and Materials: We conducted a nationwide retrospective cohort study in stroke inpatients, we examined the overall costs in 3 municipalities in Taiwan, by evaluating the possible costs of the expecting diagnosis related group (DRG) by using the international classification of diseases version-9 (ICD-9) system, and the overall analysis of the re-admission population that received traditional Chinese medicine (TCM) treatment and those who did not.

Results: The trend demonstrated that the non-participant costs were consistent with the ICD-9 categories (430 to 437) because similarities existed between years 2006 to 2007. Among the TCM patients, a wide variation and additional costs were found compared to non-TCM patients during these 2 years. The average re-admission duration was significantly shorter for TCM patients, especially those initially diagnosed with ICD 434 during the first admission. In addition, TCM patients demonstrated more severe general symptoms, which incurred high conventional treatment costs, and could result in re-admission for numerous reasons. However, in Disease 7 of ICD-9 category, representing the circulatory system was most prevalent in non-TCM inpatients, which was the leading cause of re-admission.

Conclusion: We concluded that favorable circulatory system outcomes were in adjuvant TCM treatment inpatients, there were less re-admission for circulatory system events and a two-third reduction of re-admission within ICD-9 code 430 to 437, compared to non-TCM ones. However, there were shorter re-admission duration other than circulatory system events by means of unfavorable baseline condition.

Editor: Jinglu Ai, St Michael's Hospital, University of Toronto, Canada

Funding: This study was supported by the Chung Gung Research Project, CMRPG 890961. The corresponding author and the first author had full access to all data in the study and had final responsibility for the decision to submit the paper for publication. The funders had no role in study design, data collection and analysis, decision to publish, or preparation of the manuscript.

Competing Interests: All authors and contributors declared that no conflict of interest exists.

* E-mail: elleychiu@hotmail.com

Introduction

Cerebrovascular diseases pose a critical threat to human health. The prevalence of cerebrovascular diseases in the study population older than 45 years old was 17.5/1000 (95% confidence interval 17.0–18.0) [1]. Cerebrovascular diseases, such as hemorrhage, thrombosis and necrosis, are malignant and can cause death or disability, which has a detrimental effect on individuals, families, and society [2,3]. According to World Health Organization (WHO) reports, cerebrovascular diseases in high income countries were among the world's top 10 leading causes of death in 2005, and were the second highest cause of death overall. Every year, 770 000 people die from cerebrovascular diseases, and in middle-income countries they are the leading cause of death (3.14 million deaths per year). [4]. Taiwan's Health Department reported that cerebrovascular disease has been among the top three leading causes of death for 10 consecutive years, and in 2005 and 2006, it was responsible for the second highest number of deaths (malignant tumors were the leading cause of death). Numerous inpatients survive with appropriate stroke management. However, acute stage patients are in a compromised situation that could easily lead to infections, it could result in a sequel of neurological deficits, such as limb, language, bowel control, vision, and emotional dysfunctions. The health burden of cerebrovascular diseases was measured at an annual population prevalence of 11.7/1000 (95% confidence interval of 11.3 to 12.1), and it is estimated that up to 67% of cerebrovascular disease survivors are unable to be self-supporting [1], and 10% of survivors require

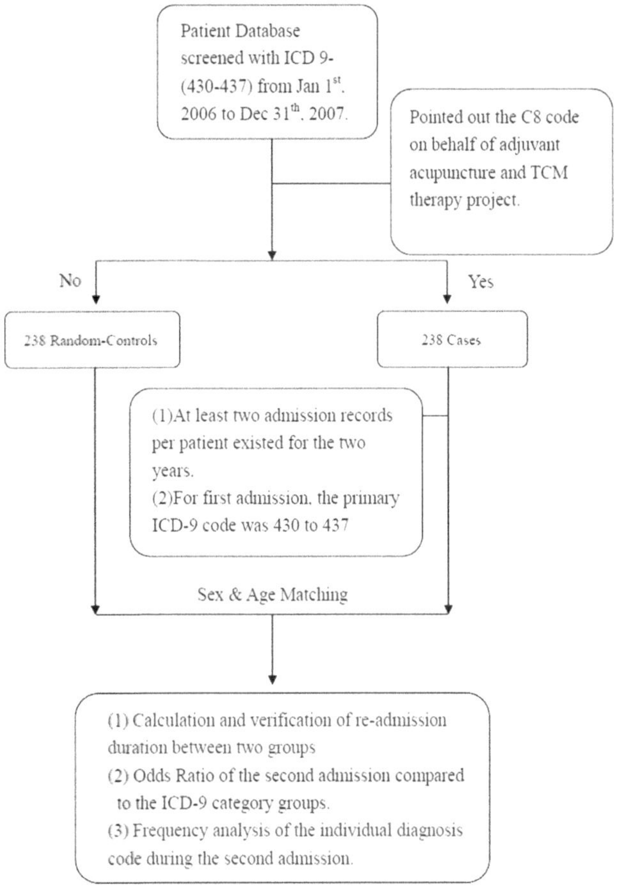

Figure 1. Analysis Strategy (2006–2007).

long-term care in paramedical institutions [5]. Cerebrovascular disease not only causes a great inconvenience for inpatients, but also has a tremendous impact on families. In addition, the cost to the community is high, and effectively managing the medical and social support costs remains a challenge.

Traditional Chinese medicine (TCM) has been used to treat cerebrovascular disease for millenary. Treatments include passive massage and Tai-Chi rehabilitation. Acupuncture and moxibustion have been used for at least two thousand years [6]. Traditional Chinese medicine acupuncturists select specific acupoints on both the healthy and affected side of the body, based on the Zang-Fu thesis for patients who clinically suffer hemiplegia. Most patients experience functional recovery to varying degrees. Numerous animal and human experiments have indicated that acupuncture can lead to improved blood circulation and induces various biochemical reactions. Acupuncture, moxibustion, and electro-acupuncture could cause localized biological reactions through remote response or systemic reactions. These treatments work mainly through the excitement of the central nervous pathway, and consequently influence more than one physical system, including the central and peripheral nervous systems [10–14]. Recently, acupuncture has become widely used around the world, and according to a statement by the National Institutes of Health in the U.S.A., the application of acupuncture has been recognized for cerebrovascular diseases [7,12]. Studies on acupuncture and moxibustion conducting in China and Europe indicated positive results for treating cerebrovascular disease [8]. A double-blinded study, using computed tomography, found that the severity of neuronal damage of patients who accepted acupuncture treatment was half that of patients who did not accept. In addition, acupuncture reduced the severity of motor paralysis [9].

Since 2006, the Pilot Scheme of National Health Policy in Stroke Adjuvant Acupuncture and Traditional Chinese Medicine (TCM) Therapy has been applied. Our previous reports demonstrated that verum acupuncture, in moderate to severe ischemic stroke patients, might play a protective role against comorbidity and mortality during admission, as well as for 6 months after discharge. However, the studies did not find improvements in neurological deficits [15]. Thus, the severe stroke burden contributed to clinical and economic policies. We therefore conducted a nationwide retrospective cohort analysis in stroke inpatients, aiming for reconstructing possible cerebrovascular disease-related groups (DRG),and estimating the costs between cerebrovascular disease and related diseases. we examined the overall costs in three municipals in Taiwan, and estimated the possible costs for the expecting diagnosis related group (DRG) using the ICD-9 system, and an overall analysis of the re-admission population (including inpatients who did and did not receive TCM treatment).

Methods and Materials

We analyzed inpatient costs using the 2006 to 2007 research database. Ambulatory care costs were analyzed using the profiles international classification of diseases version-9 (ICD-9) code 430 to 437 from the research database of the National Health Insurance (NHIRD) to determine attributes such as in-patient

Table 1 Database of Case Groups.

ICD-9 CM_CODE	Number of Cases (First admission)	Number of Re-admissions	Duration (days)	Age
430	40	20	55.90±60.66	52.85±18.49
431	209	93	67.58±86.15	60.56±12.68
432	0	0	-	-
433	8	6	128.50±109.84	66.83±9.93
434	291	114	67.00±88.55	66.46±12.01
435	1	1	30	58
436	3	1	5	74
437	4	3	58.33±60.75	67.33±2.89

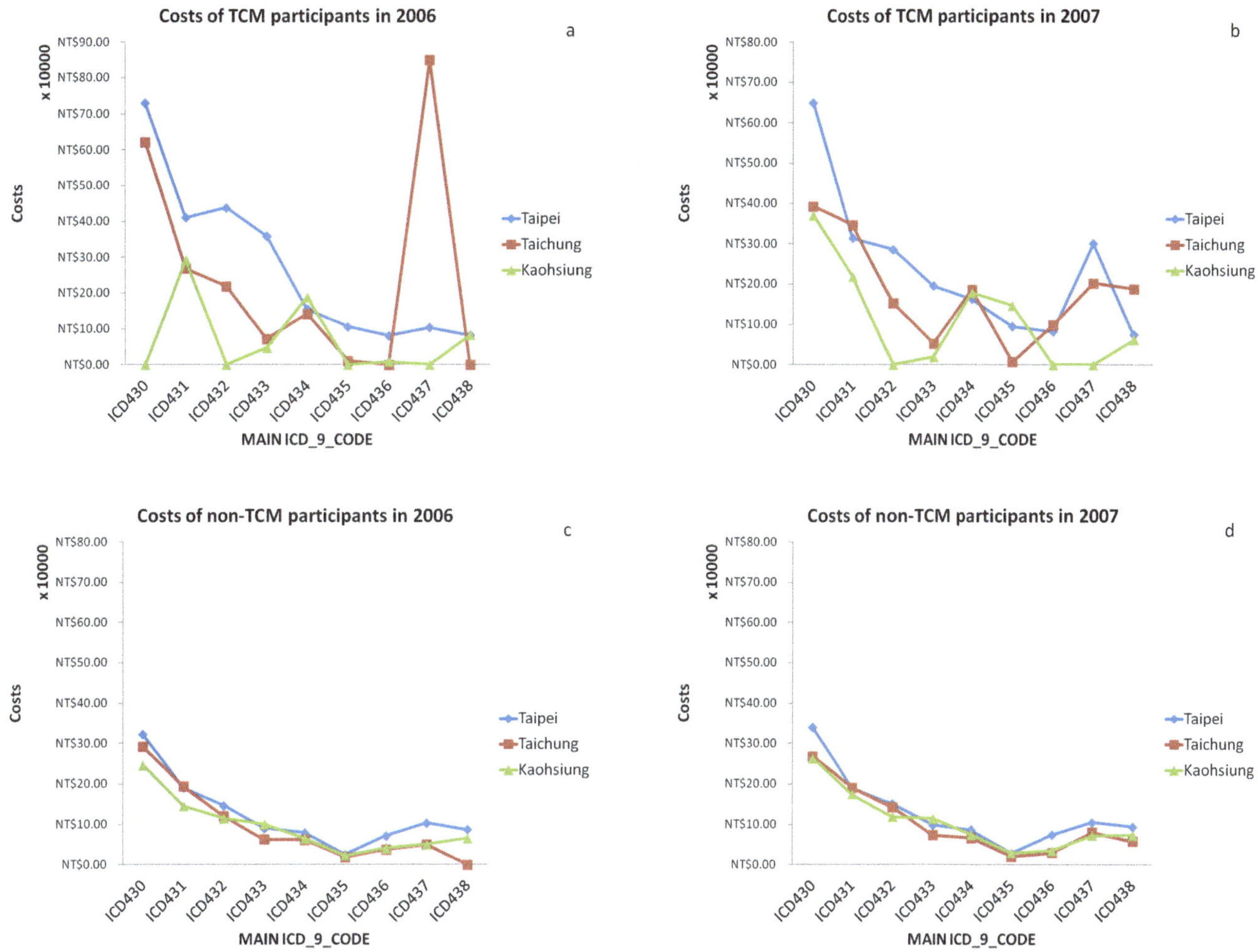

Figure 2. The inpatients expenditures as admission in year 2006 and 2007 (by insurance covered city).

duration-time, age, and sex. The investigation project was approved by the ethical committee of Chang Gung Memorial Hospital (Institution Review Board No.99-1800B). The apriori association rule was used to perform data mining using the primary ICD-9 code to identify cerebrovascular disease-related groups. To analyze expenses, we first combined the identity number (ID) and the first date of admission (IN_DATE) column as an index key to distinguish duplicative data based on a screen of the ICD code (430–437). Second, we classified medical institution types based on column of contract hospital type (HOSP_CONT _TYPE). Third, if the department type for selecting if Chinese Medical Treatment records (FUNC_TYPE) column number 60–69 existed, we considered it as a TCM treatment. In Taiwan, acupuncture and Chinese Traumatology manipulation are classified as one TCM therapeutic method. Finally, to determine whether combined TCM and western medical treatment data existed, we used the ID column to compare the medical records.

Because the detail document (DD document) of the hospital medical costs database is screened under the main diagnosis code bar unit and filtered under a cerebrovascular code from the research database of the Bureau of National Health Insurance, the first time follow-up patient data were analyzed by (1) merging the ID digital number field and the hospital date as the index key, which was differentiated using repeat gender data, (2) distinguishing between medical institution and special category field outpatient data, (3) regarding the column of interview specialty on medical character, if a TCM code (60 to 69) appeared, we defined it as a rational to distinguish between TCM and western medicine patient treatments, (4) finally, comparing ID digital numbers to identify if any duplications existed in the combination of TCM and western medicine treatments. The analysis of outpatient costs included outpatient visits, and character counting, and was scaled to 100,000 inpatients and the details of the drug and diagnosis and treatments, and pharmacy services costs, as well as information on the amount and average amount of costs related to partial cash payments for treatments. A decomposition analysis of medical cost was conducted to investigate cost trends compared to average medical costs per annum per person. All medical causes of the disease were influenced by age. Therefore, high costs are an accepted factor for aging populations, and result in a rise in total costs. In addition, the average age of the population is growing, which influences average costs. Therefore, the first step of the medical treatment cost analysis was to consider the average age of the population and include an analysis of the population structure. We filtered inpatients out using the ICD-9 code (430 to 437), and included all inpatients that received TCM treatments (case group), and also evaluated the re-admission inpatients database for the 2 years covered by this study. The random-control population was selected from inpatients who did not receive TCM treatments. (Figure 1) The multivariate Cox proportional hazard models by

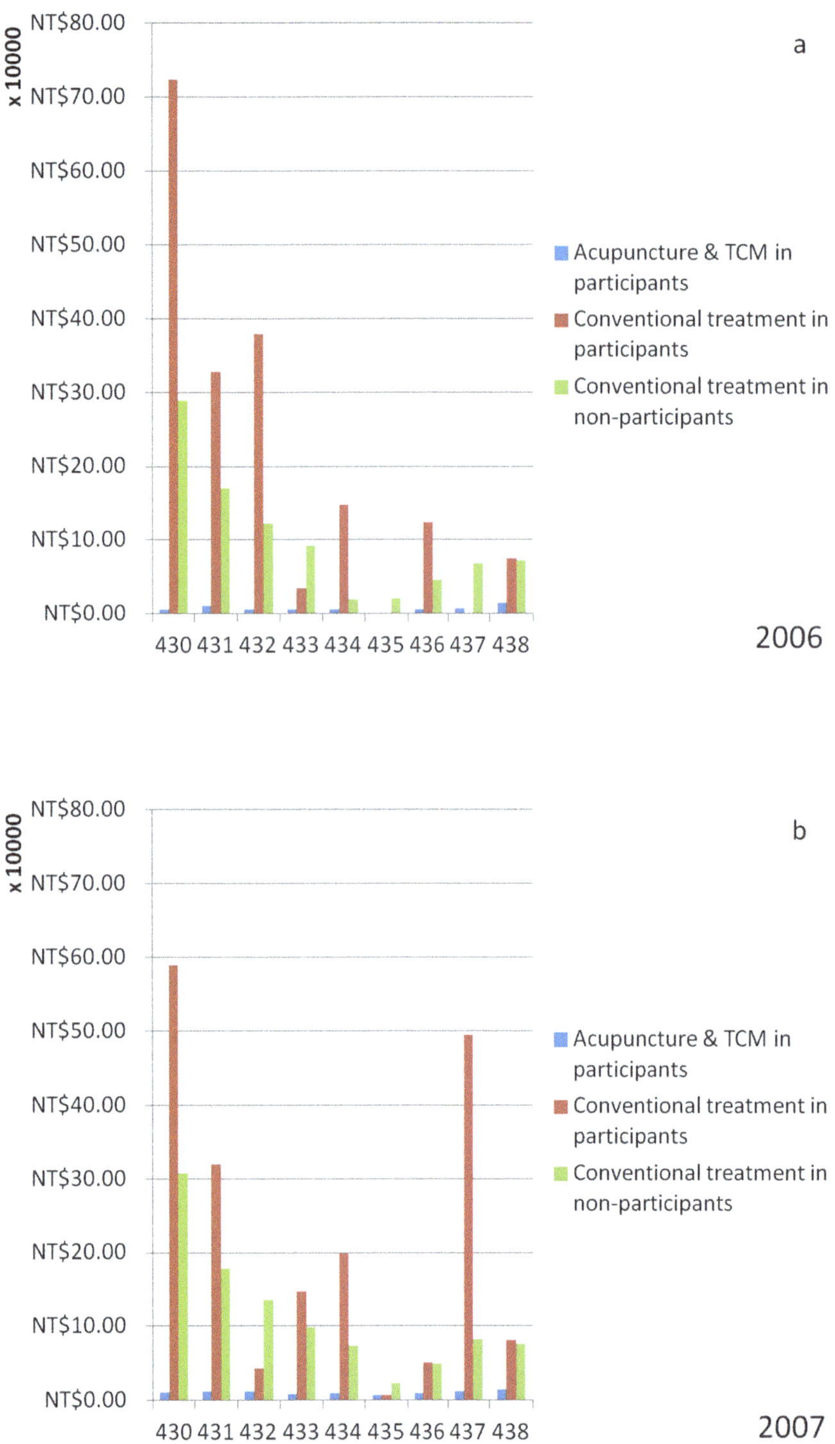

Figure 3. The inpatient expenditures as admissions in each diagnosis related groups (DRG) in year 2006 (3a) and 2007 (3b).

adjusting age, sex, occupation, low income, diabetes, hypertension, hyperlipidemia, mental disorder, anticoagulant medication, anti-platelet medication, and lipid-lowering medication. The odds ratio was calculated by Chi-square test according to 17 disease categories. The 95% confidence interval is analyzed for the significance of OR. Independent T test is used for continuous variable such as age variable. If the sample size violated parametric assumption, we replaced Independent T test with Mann-Whitney U test. Defied as statistical significance if p value is less than 0.05. The impact of adjuvant TCM therapy on the frequency and expenditure of emergency care and hospitalization after the index stroke admission, were analyzed in the general linear regressions by adjusted for age, sex, occupation, low income, coexisting medical conditions, stroke-related medication, medical center, types of stroke, history of stroke, length of stay, and neurosurgery.

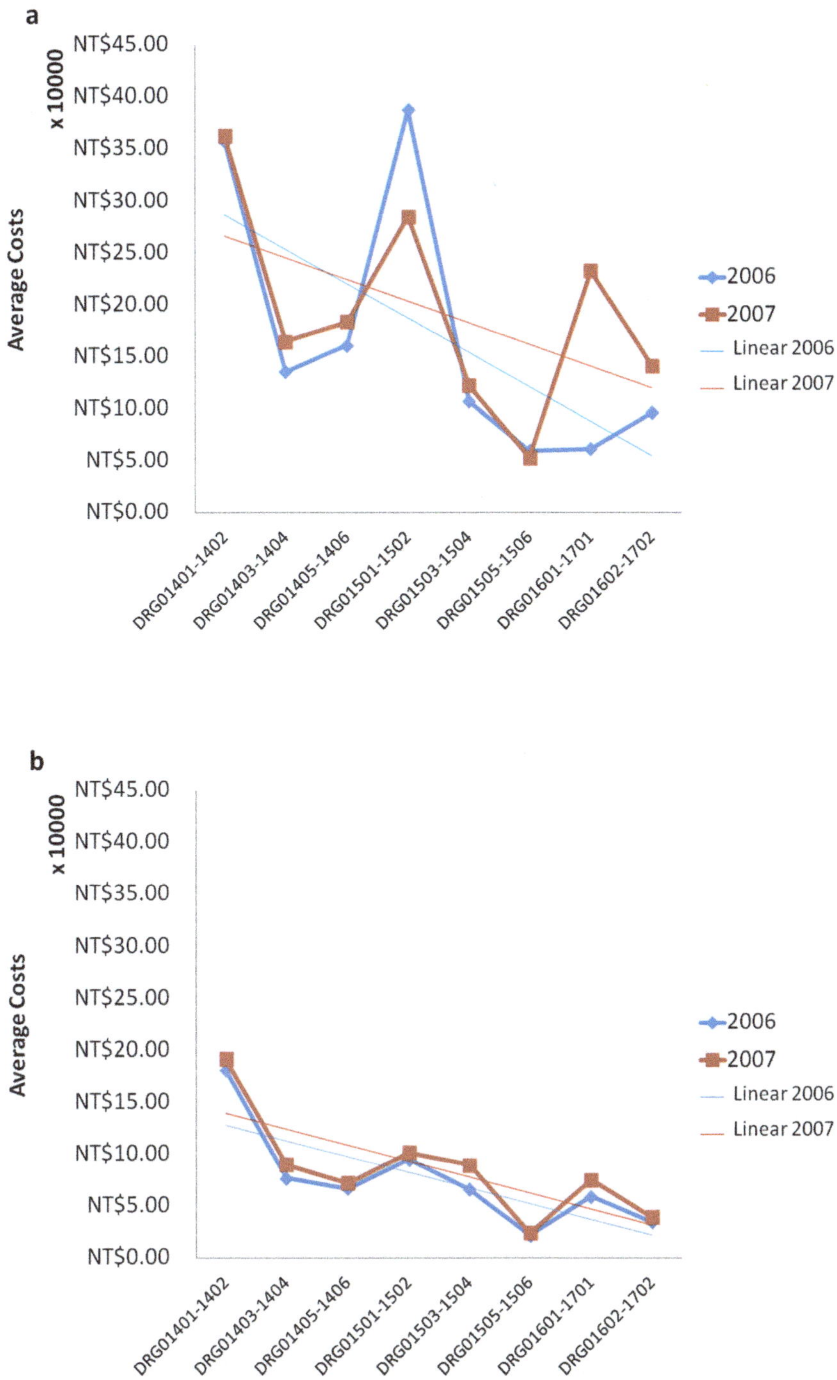

Figure 4. Expected costs of TCM participants (4a) and non-TCM participants (4b) with DRG in year 2006 and 2007.

Results

In 2006, the inpatients' first ICD-9 code between 430–437 as the primary analysis population, random-control group matched for sex, age by propensity score matching procedures. (Table 1) The adjusted hazard ratios (HRs) and 95% confidence intervals (CIs) of post-stroke complications and mortality associated with adjuvant TCM treatments were calculated again in ICD-9 codes. The number of hospitalizations in 2006–2007 was of 3,140,164 people, while the random-control group was 131,789 inpatients (deduction of TCM consultation inpatients within ICD-9 code 430–437). Adjuvant TCM treatment inpatients as the first diagnosis code within 430–437 were 558 inpatients, which including 238 re-admission ones.

Analysis showed that the adjuvant TCM treatment group had less odds (68.4%/31.6% = 2.16) than non-TCM treatment group (87.4%/12.6% = 6.93), favorable odds on non-TCM treatment group by re-admission ICD-9 code 430 ~ 437 (relative risk ratio, 6.93/2.16 = 3.2), 95% confidence interval not containing 1, $P<0.01$. A two-third reduction of re-admission within ICD-9 code 430 ~ 437 favored the adjuvant TCM treatment group, the difference was statistically significant.

Table 2 Duration of Re-admission Cases and Random-Controls.

ICD-9 CM_CODE	Numbers of Re-admissions	Sex	Age	Control Population	Re-admission Duration (days)		*P*
					Cases	Controls	
430	20	M: 12	44.17±16.19	3820	66.58±76.09	55.83±61.79	.707
		F: 8	65.88±13.88		39.88±19.99	115.38±173.07	.258
431	93	M: 63	58.32±12.90	21281	63.40±76.77	89.35±142.98	.219
		F: 30	65.27±10.96		76.37±104.04	127.67±170.26	.165
433	6	M: 4	62.00±7.12	4664	143.75±127.23	283.50±232.20	.331
		F: 2	76.50±7.78		98.00±94.75	103.50±126.57	.965
434	114	M:59	62.56±12.38	73784	63.00±78.05	134.21±149.94	.001
		F: 55	70.65±10.14		71.29±99.14	115.77±129.83	.047
435	1	M:1	58	17852	30	167	-
		F: 0	-		-		-
436	1	M: 0	-	6203	-		-
		F: 1	74		5	381	-
437	3	M:1	69	4185	1	222	
		F: 2	66.50±3.54		87.00±49.49	198.00±142.84	.408

We estimated that overall, only 4% of the annual budget was spent on TCM treatments, and the rest was spent on conventional treatments. We investigated three municipals— Kaohsiung, Taichung and Taipei, they are on behalf of the south, the middle and the north part of Taiwan. The medical expenditure trend indicated that the costs for non-TCM treatment inpatients were consistent in the ICD-9 category (430 to 437), and were similar for both years. However, wide variation and more costs were incurred by TCM participants than non-TCM ones during these 2 years.(Figure 2)

The overall secondary costs to western medicine treatment for all inpatients were more in 2006, as indicated by ICD 430, 432, 434, and 436, than in 2007. In 2007, ICD 433 and 437 reported higher costs than in 2006. In 2007, the trend demonstrated that

Table 3 Odds Ratio of Major Disease Re-admission in Cases/ Random –Controls.

Disease Group	OR			Lower 95% CI			Upper 95% CI		
	total	*men*	*women*	total	*men*	*women*	total	*men*	*women*
Disease 1	0.43	0.40	0.48	0.12	0.07	0.04	1.37	1.81	3.45
Disease 2	0.84	1.97	0.19	0.26	0.41	<0.01	2.72	12.39	1.74
Disease 3	0.48	0.96	-	0.08	0.13	-	2.28	7.32	-
Disease 4	1.95	-	-	0.10	-	-	115.49	-	-
Disease 5	0.48	0.96	-	0.01	0.01	-	9.35	76.23	-
Disease 6	1.47	1.72	0.97	0.46	0.43	0.07	5.11	8.21	13.77
Disease 7	0.27*	0.20*	0.44*	0.17	0.10	0.21	0.44	0.37	0.91
Disease 8	0.93	1.07	0.75	0.54	0.52	0.30	1.62	2.24	1.85
Disease 9	1.47	1.17	2.07	0.70	0.45	0.61	3.13	3.15	8.00
Disease 10	1.94	2.00	1.90	0.87	0.60	0.61	4.55	7.65	6.51
Disease 11	-	-	-	-	-	-	-	-	-
Disease 12	1.22	0.48	2.00	0.26	0.01	0.28	6.22	9.31	22.53
Disease 13	0.41	0.64	0.24	0.07	0.05	<0.01	1.82	5.67	2.47
Disease 14	0.48	-	-	0.01	-	-	9.35	-	-
Disease 15	-	-	-	-	-	-	-	-	-
Disease 16	0.86	1.21	0.57	0.28	0.25	0.09	2.56	6.25	3.06
Disease 17	0.50	0.31	0.63	0.18	0.03	0.17	1.29	1.79	2.08

Disease group means ICD-9 category 1 to 17;
OR means odds ratio.
*means $P < .01$, favors random-controls.

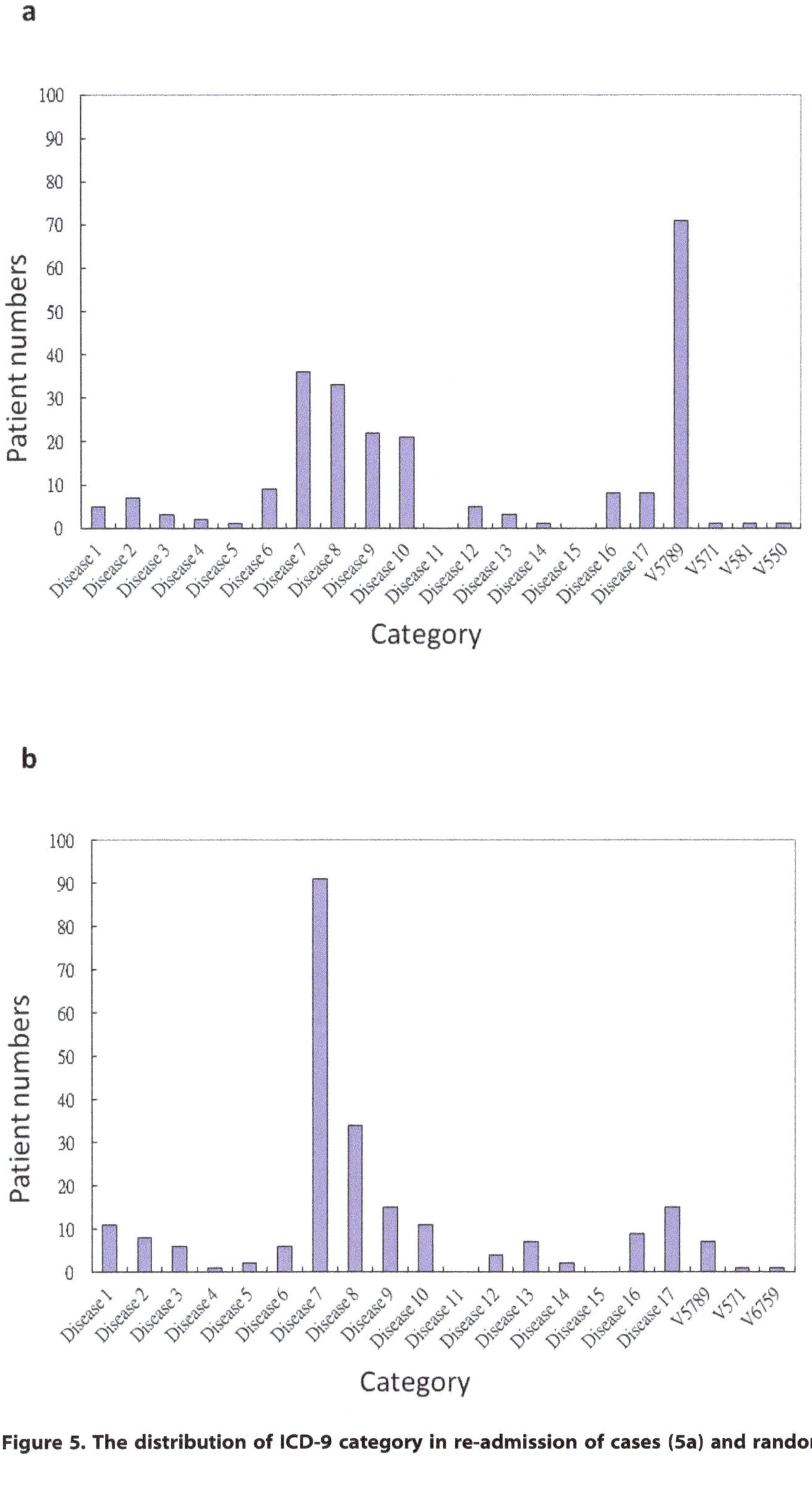

Figure 5. The distribution of ICD-9 category in re-admission of cases (5a) and random-controls (5b) group.

adjuvant TCM treatment inpatients paid less for conventional treatments, with the exception of ICD 437, which appeared to be higher in the first instance.(Figure 3)

This study demonstrated that for inpatients receiving TCM treatments for the DRG1501-02 Project, the annual costs during 2007 were significantly lower than in 2006. By contrast, for DRG1601-1702, if the TCM associated medical costs were excluded, the medical treatment costs for the 2 years were similar.(Figure 4)

During the first hospitalization, the percentage of adjuvant TCM treatments was 0.82% in 2006 and 1.70% in 2007. In addition, the re-admission rate of TCM inpatients was 17.84% in 2006 and 19.04% in 2007. During the first hospitalization, 99.18% (2006) and 98.3% (2007) of the whole population were non-TCM inpatients, and the re-admission rate was 10.56% in 2006 and 9.43% in 2007. The average re-admission duration was significantly shorter for TCM participants, especially for the initial ICD 434 cases.(Table 2) However, during subsequent re-admission episodes, the odds ratio for Disease 7 of ICD-9 category, representing circulatory system diseases, significantly favored non-TCM participants among all potential causes. (Table 3)(Figure 5)

Discussion

Among inpatients who were diagnosed with ICD-9 code (430 to 437) upon first admission, the average re-admission duration was significantly shorter for TCM inpatients. In addition, the inpatients being introduced to TCM demonstrated more severe general symptoms, which were costly to deal with conventional treatments, and the severity of underline diseases might be causative re-admission. However, adjuvant TCM treatment inpatients appeared to have significantly lower circulatory system events while re-admission. However, there were shorter re-admission duration other than circulatory system events by means of unfavorable baseline condition.

The disease diagnosis related group (DRG) measure enforces equal medical fee payments for diagnosis-related groups and helps to reduce unnecessary medical costs that burden the system. Recently, Taiwan has been planning to implement the DRG. However, after numerous meetings, consultations, commissioning of scholars and experts to lead relevant research projects, some public interest-related support measures have been developed for the short-term, but no guarantee exists that public health interests are not negatively influenced by the waste of additional medical resources. Since 2009, DRG measures have focused on the gradual implementation of health payments with a pilot project. This study's design was based on a previous study focusing on data from 2006 and 2007 Taiwanese National Health Insurance Research Database, and included study participants that were diagnosed under the international standard code for diagnosis of disease (ICD-9) in the cerebrovascular disease Group (430 to 437) for analysis. In April 2006, the National Health Council issued a Pilot Scheme of Health Policy in Stroke Adjuvant Acupuncture and TCM Therapy [15], and we used this scheme to investigate the statistics on TCM participation per patient per year for all inpatients hospitalized during 2006 and 2007. We then analyzed the overlapping use of integrative Chinese and Western medicine in hospitals to understand regional differences between inpatients that participated in pilot scheme in three municipals by analyzing the costs of admission and number of outpatients. In addition, we partially launched the DRG project in 2011. The 2006 to 2007 database of the NHIRD was used to perform cost predictions for retrospective classifications. However, the national medical institutions failed to timeously implement the pilot scheme in 2006, and ragged data could not be avoided. Therefore, additional research of the health insurance database is needed.

Conclusion

Among inpatients diagnosed with ICD-9 code 430 to 437 upon first admission, the adjuvant TCM treatment patients appeared to be significantly less re-admission for circulatory system events. A two-third reduction of re-admission within ICD-9 code 430 ~ 437 favored the adjuvant TCM treatment patients.

Supporting Information

File S1 Appendix S1.
(DOCX)

Acknowledgments

The authors give thanks to the Taiwan Traditional Chinese Medicine Association for providing information of HPSAAT. We acknowledge the contribution of Hen-Hong Chang MD/PhD and Sheng-Teng Huang MD/PhD in the administration support of this study, and Jer-Ming Sheen MD, Cheng-Nan Lu MD, Guo-Wei Bi MD, and Wu-Long Hu MD in treating the HPSAAT patients in KCGMH.

Author Contributions

Conceived and designed the experiments: HEC. Performed the experiments: HEC KCC JWH CWL TYT. Analyzed the data: HEC CCS JWH. Contributed reagents/materials/analysis tools: HEC YCH. Wrote the paper: HEC. Critical review of Statisitcs: HEC CCH.

References

1. O'Mahony PG, Thomson RG, Dobon R (1999) The prevalence of stroke and associated disability. J Public Health Med 21:1666–1671.
2. Hackett ML, Duncan JR, Anderson CS, Broad JB, Bonita R (2000) Health-related quality of life among long-term survivors of stroke: results from the Auckland Stroke Study, 1991–1992. Stroke 31:440–447.
3. Murry CJ, Lopez AD (1997) Mortality by cause for eight regions of the world: Global Burden of Disease Study. Lancet 349:1269–1276.
4. World Health Organization (2007) The Top Ten Causes of Death. Fact sheet N° 310. February 2007:5.
5. Southampton and South West Hampshire Health Commission (1994). Annual report. Director of Public Health.
6. Wu JN (1996) A short history of acupuncture. J Altern Complement Med 2:19–21.
7. Han JS, Terenius L (1982) Neurochemical basis of acupuncture analgesia. Annu Rev Pharmacol Toxicol 22:193–220.
8. Jansen G, Lundeberg T, Kjartansson S, Samuelson UE (1989) Acupuncture and sensory neuropeptides increase cutaneous blood flow in rats. Neurosci Let 97:305–309.
9. Magnusson M, Johansson K, Johansson BB (1994) Sensory stimulation promotes normalization of postural control after stroke. Stroke 25:1176–1180.
10. Sun HL, Li XM (2001) Clinical study on treatment of cerebral apoplexy with penetration needling of scalp acupoints. Chin Acupunct Moxi 21:275–278.
11. NIH Consensus Conference (1998) Acupuncture. JAMA 280:1518–1524.
12. Chen ZM, Sandcock P, Xie JX, Collins R, Liu LS (1997) Hospital management of acute ischemic stroke in China. J Stroke Cerebrovasc Dis. 6:361–367.
13. Naeser MA, Alexander MP, Stiassny-Eder D, Galler V, Hobbs J, et al (1994) Acupuncture in the treatment of paralysis in chronic and acute stroke patients--improvement correlated with specific CT scan lesion sites. Acupunct Electrother Res 19:227–249. javascript:PopUpMenu2_Set(Menu7625245);
14. Dean RH (2004) Retrospective Studies and Chart Reviews. Respir Care 49:1171–1174.
15. Wei YC, Sun MF, Chang KC, Chang CJ, Hung YC, et al (2011) Pilot scheme of health policy in stroke adjuvant acupuncture therapy for acute and subacute ischemic stroke in Taiwan. eCAM 2011:689813.

13

HPLC–MS/MS Analysis of a Traditional Chinese Medical Formulation of Bu-Yang-Huan-Wu-Tang and Its Pharmacokinetics after Oral Administration to Rats

Lee-Hsin Shaw[1], Lie-Chwen Lin[1,2], Tung-Hu Tsai[1,3,4*]

1 Institute of Traditional Medicine, National Yang-Ming University, Taipei, Taiwan, **2** National Research Institute of Chinese Medicine, Taipei, Taiwan, **3** Graduate Institute of Acupuncture Science, China Medical University, Taichung, Taiwan, **4** Department of Education and Research, Taipei City Hospital, Taipei, Taiwan

Abstract

Bu-yang-huan-wu-tang (BYHWT) is one of the most popular formulated traditional Chinese medicine prescriptions, and is widely for prevention of ischemic cardio-cerebral vascular diseases and stroke-induced disability. A specific high-performance liquid chromatography-tandem mass spectrometry (HPLC-MS/MS) has been developed and validated for simultaneous quantification of the nine main bioactive components, i.e., astragaloside I, astragaloside II, astragaloside IV, formononetin, ononin, calycosin, calycosin-7-O-β-d-glucoside, ligustilide and paeoniflorin in rat plasma after oral administration of BYHWT extract. This method was applied to investigate the pharmacokinetics in conscious and freely moving rats. No significant matrix effects were observed. The overall analytical procedure was rapid and reproducible, which makes it suitable for quantitative analysis of a large number of samples. Among them, three astragalosides and four isoflavones in A. *membranaceus*, ligustilide in Radix Angelicae Sinensis and Rhizoma Ligustici Chuanxiong and paeoniflorin in Radix Paeoniae Rubra were identified. This developed method was then successfully applied to pharmacokinetic studies of the nine bioactive constituents after oral administration of BYHWT extracts in rats. The pharmacokinetic data demonstrated that astragaloside I, astragaloside II, astragaloside IV and ligustilide presented the phenomenon of double peaks. The other herbal ingredients of formononetin, ononin, calycosin, calycosin-7-O-β-d-glucoside and paeoniflorin appeared together in a single and plateau absorption phase. These phenomenona suggest that these components may have multiple absorption sites, regulation of enterohepatic circulation or the gastric emptying rate, or there is ingredient-ingredient interaction. These pharmacokinetic results provide a constructive contribution to better understand the absorption mechanism of BYHWT and to support additional clinical evaluation.

Editor: William C. S. Cho, Queen Elizabeth Hospital, Hong Kong

Funding: Funding for this study was provided in part by research grants from the National Science Council (NSC99-2113-M-010-001-MY3, NSC99-2628-B-010-008-MY3) Taiwan; Committee on Chinese Medicine and Pharmacy, Department of Health (CCMP99 -RD-024) Taiwan and TCH 96001-62-014; 10001-62-007 from Taipei City Hospital, Taipei, Taiwan.

Competing Interests: The authors have declared that no competing interests exist.

* E-mail: thtsai@ym.edu.tw

Introduction

BYHWT is one of the most popular formulated traditional Chinese medicine (TCM) prescriptions, with wide use in clinical medication for the treatment and prevention of ischemic cardio-cerebral vascular diseases and stroke-induced disability. BYHWT was originally recorded in the traditional herbal text *Yi-Lin-Gai-Cuo* (Chinese mean: corrections of errors among physicians) from the Qing Dynasty, published in 1830. From the viewpoint of traditional Chinese medicine, it was used to invigorate the body, promote blood circulation, and activate energy (*qi*) flow through energy meridians. Considerable clinical evidence has indicated that the ameliorative effects of BYHWT on coronary heart disease with *qi* deficiency and blood stasis syndrome in rats are associated with the inhibition of C-reactive protein and the CD40 gene, as well as the regulation of endothelium-derived vasoactive factors [1]; and mediating by the improvement of hemorheological disorders and energy metabolism [2]. A previous study has found that BYHWT could protect mice against ischemic stroke and extend lifespan, primarily through a significant down-regulation of genes involved in inflammation, apoptosis, angiogenesis and blood coagulation, as well as an up-regulation of genes mediating neurogenesis and nervous system system development [3]. Another recent study showed that the neuroprotective mechanism was associated with the down-regulation of metabotropic glutamate receptor-1 RNA and the inhibition of glutamate release resulting from cerebral ischemia [4].

BYHWT is one of the most classical medicinal prescriptions, comprised of seven commonly used Chinese herbs. According to the *Chinese Pharmacopoeia* (2005), the formula includes the following 7 herbs: (1) Radix Astragali (*huangqi*), the dried roots of *Astragalus membranaceus* (Fisch.) Bge.var. *mongholicus* (Bge.) Hsiao; (2) the carda part of Radix Angelicae Sinensis root (*guiwei*), the dried lateral roots of *Angelica sinensis* (Oliv.) Diels; (3) Radix Paeoniae Rubra (*chishao*), the dried roots of *Paeonia lactiflora* Pall.; (4) Rhizoma Chuanxiong (*chuanxiong*), the dried rhizomes of *Ligusticum chuanxiong* Hort; (5) Flos Carthami (*honghua*), the dried flowers of *Carthamus tinctorius* L.; (6) Semen Persicae (*taoren*), the dried seeds of *Amygdalus persica* L.; and (7) Pheretima (*dilong*), the dried bodies of *Pheretima aspergillum* (E. Perrier), in the ratio of 120:6:4.5:3:3:3:3 on a dry weight basis, respectively. In cases such as this, the combined effects of herbs in a multi-herbal formula may produce a powerful curative action.

Based on the theories of traditional Chinese medicine, a traditional herbal formulation contains more than single Chinese herb. Generally speaking, a traditional herbal formulation such as BYHWT is prescribed according to the principle of monarch, minister, assistant and guide. The monarch of Radix Astragali acts as the chief drug for treating the disease; the minister of Radix Angelicae Sinensis root serves to intensify the effect of the monarch drug; the assistant of Radix Paeoniae Rubra, Rhizoma Chuanxiong, Flos Carthami and Semen Persicae helps to deal with the secondary symptoms or inhibit the toxicity of the monarch drug; and the guide drug of Pheretima leads the other herbs to the diseased parts and balances the effects of all herbs.

According to the ratio of 120:6:4.5:3:3:3:3 on the dry herbal weight of BYHWT, Radix Astragali is the most abundant content of BYHWT and also a frequently used Chinese herb for oriental medicine. Radix astragali mainly contained the components such as saponins, isoflavone, polysaccharide and amino acid [5]. Pharmacological studies and chemical investigations of Radix Astragali have found that flavonoids and saponins are the two main types of beneficial compounds responsible for its pharmacological activities and therapeutic efficacy [6][7]. Both saponins and flavonoids should be considered as marker compounds for the chemical evaluation of Radix Astragali [5]. In the present study, astragaloside IV was the marking compound of Radix astragali for quality identification, and three main astragalosides such as astragaloside I, astragaloside II and astragaloside IV were selected for analysis. Thus, the qualitative and quantitative analysis of astragalosides should be observed.

Major flavonoids in Radix astragali were formononetin, ononin, calycosin and its glycoside [8], which boost energy, strengthen the immune system, promote health activities and promote skin growth [9]. Ligustilide, a phthalide derivative, is the most abundant constituent in the herb and was also the most abundant bioactive ingredient in Radix Paeoniae Rubra and Rhizoma Chuanxiong. Vasodilatation, antiplatelet aggregation, antithrombotic, serotonergic activity, and antiproliferative properties of ligustilide have been well documented [10][11]. Paeoniflorin was the marking compound in Radix Paeoniae Rubra. The effects were inhibited the fluorescent intensity of intracellular Ca2+ and the activities of mitogen-activated protein kinase and protein kinase C [12]. Hypoxanthine was the major marker component in Pheretima aspergillum (Di Long). However, in our preliminary experiments, hypoxanthine could not be observed in rat plasma after oral administration of BYHWT.

We expected that several major compounds of BYHWT extract would be detected in rat plasma after oral administration. Based on a pilot study, we finally detected nine BYHWT-related compounds in rat plasma. It can be observed that astragaloside I, astragaloside II, astragaloside IV, formononetin, ononin, calycosin, calycosin-7-O-β-d-glucoside, ligustilide and paeoniflorin were the main bioactive compounds in rat plasma after oral administration of BYHWT extract.

Several analytical methods have been developed for quantification of the target components in BYHWT, such as HPLC-DAD-ELSD coupled with HPLC-TOF/MS [13][14]. However, there are few reports available regarding pharmacokinetic studies of BYHWT. One report has previously described the analysis of multiple components of BYHWT in a pharmacokinetic study, with the determination of formononetin, ononin, calycosin, calycosin-7-O-β-d-glucoside and paeoniflorin by LC-MS [15]. However, dealing with just five constituents from one or two medicinal herbs is not corresponding with the characteristics of exhibiting effects on multiple targets. The multicomponent analysis of BYHWT, however, is not easy due to the complexity of its components.

To the best of our knowledge, no LC-MS/MS method has been reported for the simultaneous estimation of multiple constituents (i.e., flavonoids and saponins) in a single run of a conscious and freely moving rat for pharmacokinetic investigation. As a common analytical tool for various compounds, LC–MS/MS provides several advantages over LC-MS in terms of sensitivity, selectivity, etc. In this study we describe an HPLC-MS/MS assay with multiple reaction monitoring (MRM) for the measurement of nine compounds in rat plasma. This analytical method using MRM was expected to be more specific and sensitive than single-ion monitoring (SIM). Therefore, in order to simultaneously characterize and identify astragaloside I, astragaloside II, astragaloside IV, formononetin, ononin, calycosin, calycosin-7-O-β-d-glucoside from Radix Astragalis; ligustilide from Radix Angelicae Sinensis and Rhizoma Ligustici Chuanxiong and paeoniflorin from Radix Paeoniae Rubra, an LC-MS/MS experiment was employed to examine the specific fragmentation patterns. The applicability of these methods in assessing plasma bioactive compound following oral administration of BYHWT extract to the pharmacokinetic study in rat is also described. The pharmacokinetic study of the above components could help to elucidate the absorption mechanism of BYHWT for additional interpretation of traditional Chinese medicine. It also could help to evaluate the effectiveness of this prescription and provide comprehensive quantification to ensure accuracy in clinical application.

Materials and Methods

Reagents

The authentic standards of astragaloside I, astragaloside II, formononetin, calycosin, and calycosin-7-O-β-d-glucoside were purchased from the Shanghai Tauto Biotech Co. LTD. (China) and stored at 4°C. The standard for ononin was obtained from Extrasynthese (France). Ligustilide was supplied by ChromaDex. Inc. USA (10 mg/mL in acetonitrile). Paeoniflorin was from Nacalai tesque, Inc. (Kyoto, japan). Astragaloside IV, digoxin (internal standard), pentobarbital and heparin were provided by Sigma-Aldrich Chemicals (St. Louis, MO, USA). Ammonium acetate, formic acid, acetonitrile, and methanol were of HPLC grade for analysis grade from E. Merck (Darmstadt, Germany). Triply deionized water from Millipore (Bedford, MA, USA) was prepared for all aqueous solutions.

Herbal preparation of bu-yang-huan-wu-tang

The crushed herbs of Radix Astragali (1800 g), Radix Angelicae sinensis (90 g), Radix Paeoniae rubra (90 g), Rhizoma Chuanxiong (45 g), Semen Persicae (45 g), Flos Carthami (45 g), and Phizoma Chuanziong (45 g) were purchased from a Chinese traditional herbal medicine store in Taipei and prepared in the National Research Institute of Chinese Medicine, Taipei, Taiwan. The herbal admixture was decocted with 50% ethanol in a water bath (70°C, 18 L, 3 times) for 9 h and the least volume of solvent was added to the given aliquot. The extracted solution was evaporated under vacuum and partitioned. Water was removed by freeze drying. The yield of the crude extract of BYHWT was 366 g. The lyophilized powder of BYHWT was used for the following experiment.

Content of astragaloside I, astragaloside II, astragaloside IV, formononetin, ononin, caycosin, calycosin-7-O-β-d-glucoside, ligustilide and paeoniflorin in BYHWT To calculate the administration dosage, the contents of astragaloside I, astragaloside II, astragaloside IV, formononetin, ononin, caycosin, calycosin-7-O-β-d-glucoside, ligustilide and paeoniflorin in BYHWT were determined by HPLC external standard method with the analytical method (section 2.5) used in this study. The results demonstrated that the content of the constituents were quantitated in BYHWT as follows (mg/g): astragaloside I 2.46 mg/g, astragaloside II 0.69 mg/g, astragaloside IV 0.54 mg/g, formononetin 2.44 mg/g, ononin 0.63 mg/g, caycosin 0.68 mg/g, calycosin-7-O-β-d-glucoside 2.56 mg/g, ligustilide 1.08 mg/g and paeoniflorin 3.11 mg/g. The structures of astragaloside I, astragaloside II, astragaloside IV, formononetin, ononin, caycosin, calycosin-7-O-β-d-glucoside, ligustilide and paeoniflorin were shown in Fig. 1.

Freely-moving rat model

The protocol listed below has been reviewed and approved by the Institutional Animal Care and Use Committee (IACUC; approval number 1010409) by the Institutional Animal Experimentation Committee of the National Yang-Ming University. Male pathogen-free Sprague-Dawley rats (250±50 g body weight) were obtained from the Laboratory Animal Center of National Yang Ming University. The animals had free access to food (Laboratory rodent diet 5P14, PMI Feeds, Richmond, IN, USA) and water was allowed at all times. All animal experiments followed the National Yang-Ming University guidelines and procedures for the care of laboratory animals.

A freely-moving rat model was applied to minimize the stress caused by restraint or anesthesia [16]. Experimental rats were initially anesthetized with pentobarbital (50 mg/kg, i.p.), and polyethylene tubing was implanted in the right jugular vein for blood sampling. The tube crossed the subcutaneous tissue and was fixed at its exit from the dorsal neck region. The patency tubing was maintained by filling with heparinized saline (20 units/mL). After surgery, the rats were placed in experimental cages and allowed to recuperate for one day. The rats were kept fasted for 12 h and water were available ad libitum before the BYHWT administration.

Oral administration and sample preparation

BYHWT extract was dissolved in normal saline at doses of 10 g/kg for oral administration and fed by gavages to rats, respectively. The dosage of BYHWT was selected by the indication of concentrated herbal extracts (powdered) for clinical application which was 3.5 g each time and 3–4 times daily in adults. According to the dose translation from animal to human studies [17], we used the body surface area (BSA) normalization method to convert the dose of nine active compounds for translation from humans to rat. In our study, the dose of BYHWT (10 g/kg) was appropriate for oral administration in rats. An aliquot of 100–120 μL blood sample was withdrawn from the jugular vein into a heparin-rinsed vial with a fraction collector according to a programmed schedule at 5, 15, 30, 45, 60, 90, 120, 150, 180, 240, 300, 360, 480, 600 and 720 min. The condensed

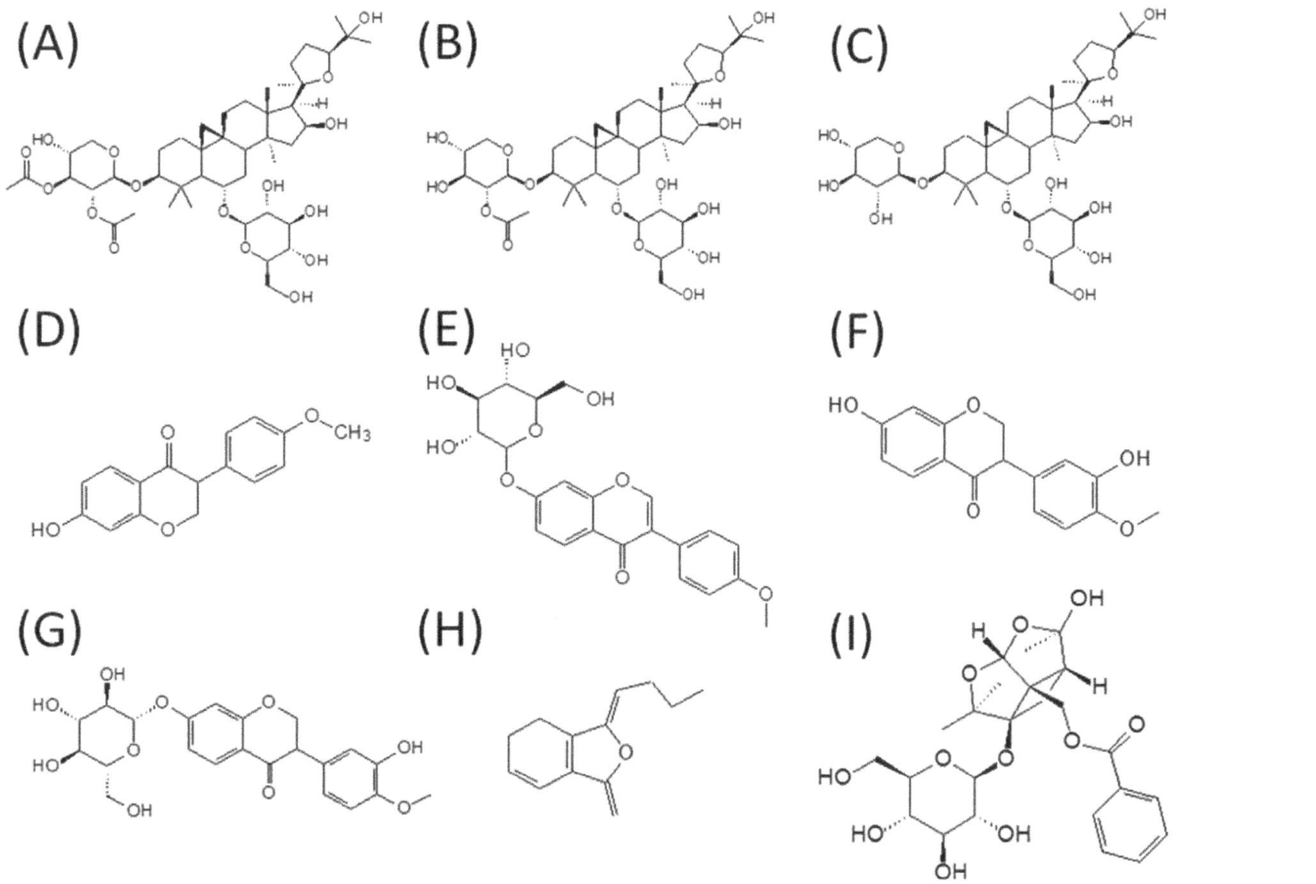

Figure 1. Structure formula of 9 components in bu-yang-huan-wu-tang extract of astragaloside I (A), astragaloside II (B), astragaloside IV (C), formononetin (D), ononin (E), calycosin (F), calycosin-7-O-β-D-glucoside (G), ligustilide (H) and paeoniflorin (I).

blood collection in the absorption phase is to figure out the maximum concentration and the time when it reaches the maximum concentration. The time points in the elimination phase are not close. This strategy is commonly used in the pharmacokinetic studies but the total blood consumption should not be over 20% of body blood. In these experimental rats, the total blood sampling volume is within 20% during 12 h [18]. Plasma was separated by centrifuging the blood sample at 6000 rpm for 10 min at 4°C. The plasma samples (50 μL) were vortex-mixed with double volume (100 μL) of acetonitrile containing digoxin (100 ng/mL) as the internal standard for protein precipitation. The samples were vortexed and centrifuged at 16,100×g for 10 min. In our micro-analysis, less than 200 μL is needed. Actually, the collected blood volume is around 120–150 μL for each time point. After centrifugation, the plasma samples (50 μL) were vortex-mixed with 100 μL of acetonitrile. The supernatants were collected and filtered. Around 20 μL aliquot of the supernatants was transferred into the vial for analysis by HPLC-MS/MS system. The acetonitrile but not the real sample was used in the needle pre-wash standard procedure [18][19].

Liquid chromatography–tandem mass spectrometry

The LC–MS/MS system consisted of an Agilent 1100 series LC with automatic liquid chromatographic sampler, injector, bi-pump and degasser; and Applied Biosystems/MDS Sciex API 3000 tandem quadrupole mass spectrometry equipped with electrospray ionization (ESI) interface using the following parameters: nebulizer gas (NEB):10, curtain gas (CUR): 7, collisionally activated dissociation gas (CAD): 12, ionspray voltage (IS): 5000 V, turbo ionspray temperature (TEM): 450°C. Nitrogen was used in all cases. The mass spectrometer was operated in the positive ion detection mode. Analytes were quantified by multiple-reaction monitoring (MRM) mode performing the following precursor-to-product ion pairs of the transitions m/z: m/z 886.6 $[M+NH_4]^+$→m/z 143.2 for astragaloside I (declustering potential 55 V, focusing potential 290 V, entrance potential 12 V, collision energy 23 V, collision cell exit potential 13 V); m/z 844.5 $[M+NH_4]^+$→m/z 143.2 for astragaloside II (DP 62 V, FP 330 V, EP 13 V, CE 25 V, CXP 13 V); m/z 802.6 $[M+NH_4]^+$→m/z 143.2 for astragaloside IV (DP 65 V, FP 370 V, EP 14 V, CE 28 V, CXP 10 V); m/z 269.2 $[M+H]^+$→m/z 253.2 for formononetin (DP 190 V, FP 380 V, EP 14 V, CE 37 V, CXP 16 V); m/z 431.3 $[M+H]^+$→m/z 269.2 for ononin (DP 80 V, FP 380 V, EP 13 V, CE 20 V, CXP 18 V); m/z 285.2 $[M+H]^+$→m/z 270.2 for calycosin (DP 190 V, FP 380 V, EP 13 V, CE 33 V, CXP 17 V); m/z 447.2 $[M+H]^+$→m/z 285.1 for Calycosin-7-O-β-D-glucoside (DP 80 V, FP 380 V, EP 12 V, CE 23 V, CXP 19 V); m/z 208.1 $[M+NH_4]^+$→m/z 173.2 for ligustilide (DP 70 V, FP 380 V, EP 14 V, CE 25 V, CXP 12 V); m/z 498.3 $[M+NH_4]^+$→m/z 179.2 for paeoniflorin (DP 76 V, FP 390 V, EP 14 V, CE 25 V, CXP 12 V) and m/z 798.6 $[M+NH_4]^+$→m/z 651.6 for digoxin (DP 20 V, FP 160 V, EP 10 V, CE 18 V, CXP 11 V, internal standard). Nine active constituents and the internal standard were separated by using a Phenomenex® Gemini C18 (150 mm×2.0 mm I.D, 5 μm particles) column maintained at ambient temperature. The following linear gradient program was applied to the analyte with the mobile phase consisting of methanol (0.1% formic acid, solvent A) and NH_4OAc (0.1% formic acid, solvent B): 0–1 min: 30–70% A; 1–2 min 70–90%; 2–8 min: 90–90%; 8–9 min: 90–30%, 9–18 min: 30–30%, v/v. The sample injection volume was 10 μL. The flow rate was maintained at 0.2 μL/min.

Preparation of calibration standards

The stock standard solution containing astragaloside I (1 mg/mL), astragaloside II (1 mg/mL), formononetin (1 mg/mL), ononin (1 mg/mL), calycosin (1 mg/mL), calycosin-7-O-β-d-glucoside (1 mg/mL) and paeoniflorin (1 mg/mL) was prepared in methanol. The standard powder of astragaloside IV was dissolved in 50% (v/v) acetonitrile to make a 1 mg/mL stock solution, and ligustilide was prepared in 100% acetonitrile for a 10 mg/mL stock solution. The internal standard stock solution of 1 mg/mL was also dissolved in 50% (v/v) acetonitrile. All solutions were stored at −20°C before use. These solutions were further diluted to give a serial of working standard solutions and samples for calibration in plasma were prepared by spiking aliquots of the stock solutions into drug-free plasma samples to obtain final concentrations in the range of 0.5–100 ng/mL for astragaloside I, astragaloside II, astragalosdie IV, ononin; 5–1000 ng/mL for formononetin; 5–100 ng/mL for calycosin; 1–100 ng/mL for calycosin-7-O-β-d-glucoside, ligustilide and 0.5–1000 ng/mL for paeoniflorin, and then processed according to the procedures described in Section 2.4.2. The validation samples were also prepared in the same way (1, 10, 100 ng/mL for astragaloside I, astragaloside II, astragalosdie IV, ononin calycosin-7-O-β-d-glucoside, ligustilide; 10, 100, 1000 ng/mL for formononetin, calycosin, paeoniflorin) at low, middle and high concentrations.

Method validation

Full validation of the analytical method evaluated in this study was according to the US Food and Drug Administration guidelines for validation of bioanalytical methods [20]. Full validation was performed for determination of analyte samples in this study. Specificity, sensitivity, linearity, precision, accuracy, recovery, matrix effect, and stability were evaluated during the method validation.

The specificity was assessed by confirming the blank plasma extract for the presence or absence of interference as well as the lot-to-lot variation regarding interference. Sensitivity of analytes was determined by calculating the signal-to-noise ratio of lowest limit of quantitation (LLOQ) samples. The limits of detection (LOD) and quantification (LOQ) were determined at S/N (the ratio of signal to noise) of 3 and 10 under the present chromatographic conditions. The calibration standard curves were obtained by least-squares linear regression of the peak area versus the concentrations. All calibration curves were required to have a correlation value of at least 0.995. The concentration of each sample was derived from the calibration curve and corrected by the respective dilution volume. For a standard curve, the ratios of the chromatographic peaks area (analytes/internal standard) as ordinate variables were plotted versus the concentration of these drugs as abscissa. The samples in six replicates on the same day (intra-day) and on six successive days (inter-day) were prepared in the same manner to verify the precision and accuracy of the analytical method. The accuracy was calculated from the nominal concentration (Cnom) and the mean value of observed concentration (Cobs) as follows: accuracy (bias, %) = [(Cnom − Cobs)/Cnom] × 100. The precision (relative standard deviation, RSD) was calculated from the standard deviation and observed concentration as follows: precision (RSD, %) = [standard deviation (SD)/Cobs] × 100. The inter-day and intra-day accuracy and precision value for the lowest acceptable reproducibility concentrations were defined as being within ±15%.The LLOQ was defined as which the signal/noise ratio was ≥10 and the accuracy and precision were within 80–120%.

The matrix effect was determined at low, medium and high concentrations using three replicates as the ratio of the mean peak area of an analyte spiked post-extraction (set 2) to the mean peak area of the same analyte standards (set 1)×100%. The extraction recovery of analytes were determined at three concentrations by calculating as the ratio of the mean peak area of an analyte spiked before extraction (set 3) to the mean peak area of an analyte spiked post- extraction (set 2)×100%.

Stability was also assessed using the low, medium and high concentrations of analytes. Freeze-thaw stability was assessed over three freeze-thaw cycles. Short-term stability was determined by placing the samples at room temperature for 6 h. Long-term stability was evaluated by analyzing samples kept at −20°C for 14 days. Autosampler stability was determined by maintaining the samples at the autosampler temperature (8°C) for 12 h. All stabilities were calculating as the ratio of average concentration and freshly prepared samples.

Pharmacokinetic application

Pharmacokinetic parameters including maximum plasma concentration (Cmax), time to reach the maximum concentrations (Tmax), half-life ($t_{1/2}$), area under concentration–time curve (AUC) and oral clearance (CL) were estimated by a non-compartmental analysis using the pharmacokinetic program, WinNonlin Standard Edition Version 1.1 (Scientific Consulting, Apex, NC, USA). All results were expressed as average mean ± standard deviation (S.D.). ANOVA was used to evaluate differences, and a value of $P<0.05$ was taken as statistically significant.

Results and Discussion

Chromatographic and tandem mass spectrometric condition

Owing to the complexity of traditional Chinese medicine, many analogues may be co-eluted during analyses. In order to develop a sensitive and accurate LC-MS/MS method for the determination of BYHWT active compounds in rat plasma, a triple quadruple mass spectrometer equipped with electrospray ionization (ESI) source is currently one of the most useful tools available for simultaneous quantification of herbal compounds because of its high sensitivity and selectivity. Qualification analysis was performed using an MRM system consisting of two parts: selecting the precursor ion (MS 1) and selecting a specific fragment of precursor ion (MS 2). These two devices generate a very specific and sensitive response for the selected analyte. Thus the integrated peak for the target compound could be monitored in a sample after a simple one dimensional chromatographic separation. The determination of nine active compounds and internal standard were performed by positive mode ESI-MS/MS since higher ion intensities were observed using positive relative to negative mode. To characterize the fragment ions of the investigated compounds, an electrospray interface with good sensitivity, fragmentation and linearity was optimized.

The astragaloside profiles of astragaloside I, astragaloside II and astragaloside IV in the Radix Astragali could be observed. However, due to the complexity of the extract and the similar structures of astragalosides, it has been noted that these peaks require careful identification and separation [21]. Astragaloside I produced a positive ion of m/s 886.6, corresponding to the $[M+NH_4]^+$ precursor ions. The succeeding product ion of the precursor ion produced a fragmentation pattern lead to an ion at m/z 143.2. in addition, the mass transit ion patterns m/z 844.5→143.2 and m/z 802.6→143.2 were selected to monitor astragaloside II and astragaloside IV, respectively.

For isoflavonoids, the chemical structure of formononetin is similar to that of calycosin, differing in the substituent group located on a ring with a hydroxyl group [22]. The behavior of calycosin fragmentation could be extended to other isoflavones; and the protonated isoflavone aglycones reveal that the loss of a methyl radical was the predominant fragmentation for the aglycones, due to the formation of very stable cation radical structures. The major product ion of m/z 253.2 for formononetin may be due to the loss of a hydroxyl group. The compounds ononin and calycosin-7-*O*-β-d-glucoside are *O*-glycosides. In positive ion mode, the glycosidic bond of *O*-glycosidies were easily cleaved to produce daughter ions of $[M+H-162]^+$ at 269.2 and 285.1 by the facile neutral loss of a glycoside residue from the corresponding protonated molecule ions at 431.3 and 447.2, respectiviely. The major product ions of ligustilide in Radix Angelicae Sinensis and Rhizoma Ligustici Chuanxiong at 173.2 corresponded to one hydroxyl group loss from the precursor ion. The major product ion of m/z 179.2 for paeoniflorin in Radix Paeoniae Rubra may be due to the loss of a glucose molecule, a benzoic acid molecule and a hydrone molecule [23]. The main fragments of the BYHWT active compoment are listed in Table 1. The MS/MS parameters manually obtained the highest response for each of the precursor and product ion combinations.

In this developed method, the degree of interference was assessed by inspection of MRM mode. No significant interfering peaks from the plasma were found at the retention time and the ion channel of either the analytes or internal standard. Hence the development of the chromatographic system was concentrated on short retention times substituted for chromatographic separation. As shown in Fig. 2, the 9 selected marker compounds with IS cover a broad polarized range. The gradient elution, proper column and flow rate were pivotal influences on separation for multi-compounds. The chromatographic conditions achieved good resolution and appropriate ionization in the presence of endogenous species and co-elution. The chemical structures of astragalosides and internal standard have been noted as being relatively stable to acids [24]. To improve the sensitivity, adding acid to the mobile phase to enhance the ionization of astragalosides has also been suggested. It was also discovered that addition of 0.1% formic acid in the mobile phase provided a higher response and better peak sensitivity. In the course of the current study, several mobile phase systems, such as acetonitrile-water and methanol-water, in different ratios were examined. The acetonitrile-water system provides good separation for the investigated compounds, but the ligustilide peak had serious interference in the chromatogram. Finally, methanol- NH_4OAc with 0.1% formic acid was employed, providing an appropriate retention time and low background noise, and was thus selected as the mobile phase system.

Ideally, a compound with similar physical-chemical properties should be used as the internal standard for analysis. Digoxin, which has a chemical structure similar to astragaloside I, astragaloside II and astragaloside IV, was chosen as the internal standard in the quantitative method in plasma. This compound was consistent with investigated analytes in chromatographic recovery and ionization properties. With extensive separation and optimization, the conditions established for reference compounds could be eluted with baseline separation in approximately 18 min. Under the proposed conditions, the electrospray ion mass spectrometer was used for quantitative analysis

Table 1. The analytical condition of LC-MS/MS for the identification of the nine compounds and internal standard.

Compounds	Molecular weight	RT (min)	Mass fragments	
			Q1 Mass (amu)	Q3 Mass (amu)
Astragaloside I	869.04	11.21	886.6 $[M+NH_4]^+$	143.2
Astragaloside II	827.01	10.73	844.5 $[M+NH_4]^+$	143.2
Astragaloside IV	784.97	11.18	802.6 $[M+NH_4]^+$	143.2
Formononetin	268.26	8.32	269.2 $[M+H]^+$	253.2
Ononin	430	8.23	431.3 $[M+H]^+$	269.2
Calycosin	284.2	8.72	285.2 $[M+H]^+$	270.2
Calycosin-7-O-β-D-glucoside	446.4	7.68	447.2 $[M+H]^+$	285.1
Ligustilide	190.24	10.05	208.1 $[M+NH_4]^+$	173.2
Paeoniflorin	480.47	7.37	498.3 $[M+NH_4]^+$	179.2
Digoxin (IS)	780.94	9.12	798.6 $[M+NH_4]^+$	651.6

Linearity, limit of determination (LOD) and limit of quantification (LOQ)

The linearity of calibration curves were demonstrated by the good determination of coefficients (r^2) obtained for the regression line. Good linearity was achieved over the calibration range, with all coefficients of correlation greater than 0.995. All samples were freshly prepared from the same stock solution, except for the standard solution. All the linear regressions of astragaloside I, astragaloside II, astragaloside IV, formononetin, ononin, calycosin, calycosin-7-O-β-d-glucoside, ligustilide and paeoniflorin in rat plasma displayed good linear relationships over the range mentioned in section 2.6. The mean values of regression equation of the analytes in rat plasma were: $y = 0.0027x - 0.0003$ ($r2 = 0.998$, astragaloside I), $y = 0.0039x + 0.0002$ ($r2 = 0.999$, astragaloside II), $y = 0.0044x - 0.0012$ ($r2 = 0.999$, astragaloside IV), $y = 0.0046x + 0.0271$ ($r2 = 0.998$, formononetin), $y = 0.1458x - 0.0001$ ($r2 = 0.999$, ononin), $y = 0.0059x + 0.0196$ ($r2 = 0.998$, calycosin), $y = 0.0671x - 0.0461$ ($r2 = 0.999$, calycosin-7-O-β-D-glucoside), $y = 0.0251x - 0.0006$ ($r2 = 0.999$, ligustilide) and $y = 0.0278x + 0.0054$ ($r2 = 0.9972$, paeoniflorin).

The data showed that the LOD for the herbal ingredients in rat plasma were astragaloside I (0.1 ng/mL), astragaloside II (0.1 ng/mL), astragaloside IV (0.1 ng/mL), formononetin (1 ng/mL), ononin (0.1 ng/mL), calycosin (1 ng/mL), calycosin-7-O-β-D-glucoside (0.5 ng/mL), ligustilide (0.5 ng/mL) and paeoniflorin (0.1 ng/mL). Peak areas in chromatograms for the spiked plasma samples containing the above lowest concentrations were compared with the signal-to-noise ratio ≥3. Sensitivity was evaluated by the LOQ determinations, which are defined as the lowest concentration that can be reliably and reproducibly measured in at least three replicates. The data showed that the LOQ for the herbal ingredients in rat plasma were astragaloside I (0.5 ng/mL), astragaloside II (0.5 ng/mL), astragaloside IV (0.5 ng/mL), formononetin (5 ng/mL), ononin (0.5 ng/mL), calycosin (5 ng/mL), calycosin-7-O-β-D-glucoside (1 ng/mL), ligustilide (1 ng/mL) and paeoniflorin (0.5 ng/mL). Peak areas in chromatograms for the spiked plasma samples containing the above lowest concentrations was compared with the signal-to-noise ratio ≥10.

Precision and accuracy

The precision and accuracy of the method were assessed in plasma by performing replicate analyses of spiked samples against calibration standards. The procedures were repeated on the same day and between six different days on the spiked samples with low, middle and high concentrations. The intra-day and inter-day precision and accuracy of the method are shown in Table 2. The precisions (relative standard deviation; RSD) were all less than 10%. The data indicated that the precision and accuracy of this method were acceptable.

Matrix effect and recovery

The extraction recoveries and matrix effect from rat plasma are shown in Table 3. The one-step extraction procedure was fairly rapid. The protein precipitation by the organic solvent, acetonitrile (0.1% formic acid) was used to prepare the plasma samples for LC–MS/MS. Co-eluting compounds may enhance or suppress the ionization of the analytes. Owing to the sample preparation of the biological matrix (protein precipitation), matrix effects were expected. In order to avoid these matrix effects, good separation of the analytes was pursued. To measure the matrix effect, it was determined at three different concentrations for all analytes. An absolute matrix effect was observed for some of the analytes at some of the low, middle and high concentrations. Nevertheless, no relative matrix effects were seen, since the coefficients of variation (CV %) at each concentration level were <15% for all compounds. The extraction recoveries were also determined for three replicates from rat plasma spiked with low, middle and high concentrations of the nine analytes and internal standard. The mean recoveries of most samples were within 80–120%, except for astragaloside II. The recoveries of astragaloside II were 79.9±12% and 76.3±5.7% at concentration of 10 ng/mL and 100 ng/mL. Even it was slightly out of range, the extraction recovery of astragaloside II was stable and there was no other significant interference over the range.

Stability

To estimate the stability of extracted samples during the experiments, storage, and sample preparation processes were designed and conducted under different conditions, including freeze-thaw cycle analysis, short-term stability, long-term stability and autosampler stability by analysis using biological samples. Deviation of the mean measured concentrations of the samples from the nominal concentration was within 15%. All established stabilities for nine active compounds are shown in Table 4. The

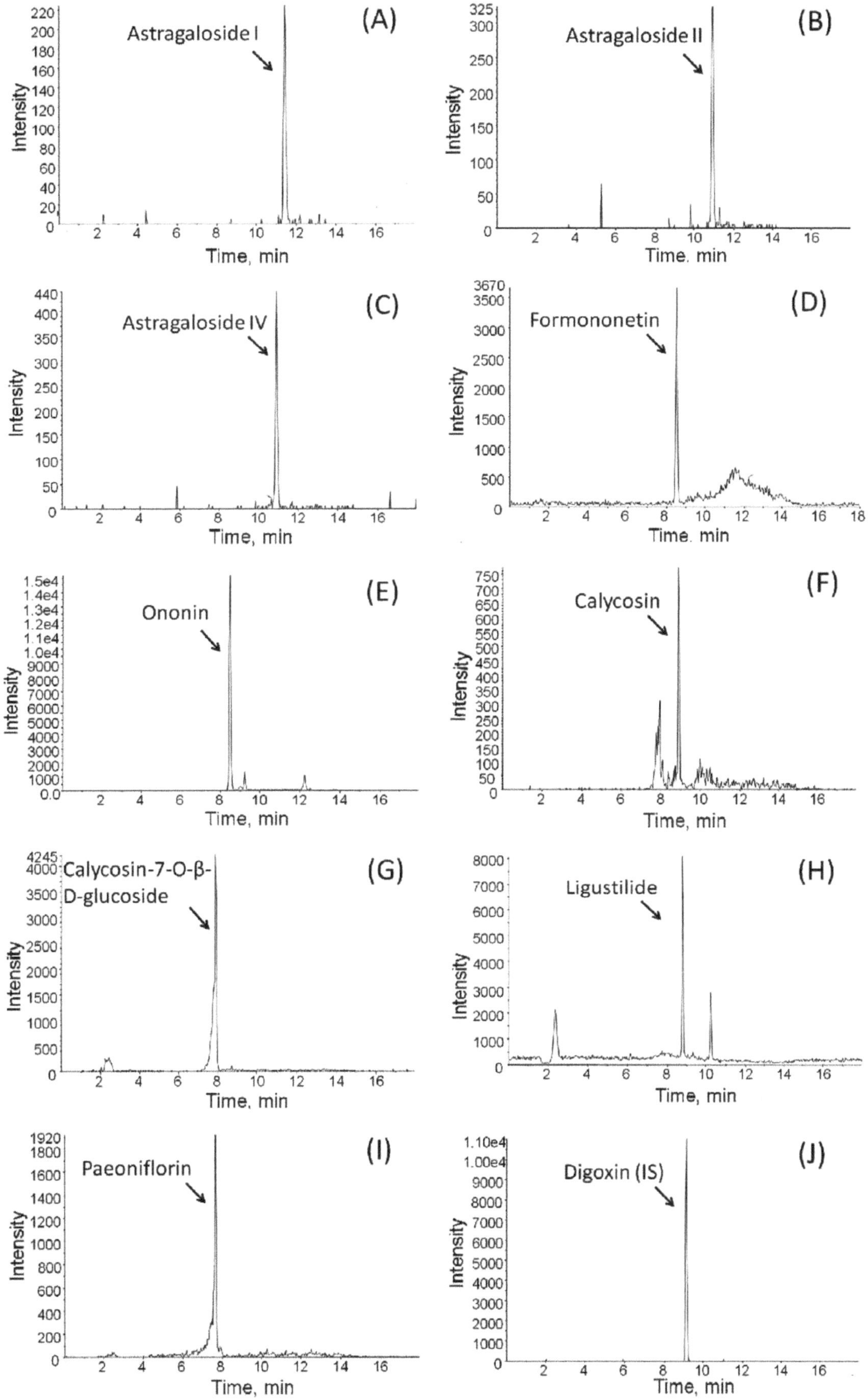
(A)
Astragaloside I
Intensity
Time, min
(B)
Astragaloside II
Intensity
Time, min
(C)
Astragaloside IV
Intensity
Time, min
(D)
Formononetin
Intensity
Time, min
(E)
Ononin
Intensity
Time, min
(F)
Calycosin
Intensity
Time, min
(G)
Calycosin-7-O-β-D-glucoside
Intensity
Time, min
(H)
Ligustilide
Intensity
Time, min
(I)
Paeoniflorin
Intensity
Time, min
(J)
Digoxin (IS)
Intensity
Time, min

Figure 2. Typical MRM chromatograms of rat plasma sample after administration of bu-yang-huan-wu-tang extract: (A) Astragaloside I; (B) Astragaloside II; (C) Astragaloside IV; (D) Formononetin; (E) Ononin; (F) Calycosin; (G) Calycosin-7-O-β-D-glucoside; (H) Ligustilide; (I) Paeoniflorin and (J) Digoxin (IS).

stability of freeze-thaw cycle analysis, short-term and autosampler remained generally stable under the analyte storage and analytical process conditions. The long-term tests showed little variation compared to the initial concentration in astragaloside I (100 ng/mL), calycosin (100, 1000 ng/mL), Calycosin-7-O-β-D-glucoside (10, 100 ng/mL), ligustilide (100 ng/mL) and paoniflorin (10, 1000 ng/mL). These observations indicate that testing must be executed after the sample extraction. Based on the above method validation, the processes for the analysis of these herbal ingredients were acceptable.

Table 2. Intra-day and inter-day precision and accuracy for the determination for nine compounds from the assay samples (n = 6).

Nominal concentration (ng/mL)	Intra-day			Inter-day		
	Observed concentration (ng/mL)	Precision (%)	Accuracy (%)	Observed concentration (ng/mL)	Precision (%)	Accuracy (%)
Astragaloside I						
1	1.14±0.1	5.3	4.2	0.92±0.2	6.1	1.1
10	11.2±2.7	4.2	−1.9	11.1±2.9	4.3	−1.3
100	99.4±6.8	4.1	−3.3	99.8±7.1	4.6	0.8
Astragaloside II						
1	1.22±0.3	7.2	2.2	1.1±0.8	5.5	1.3
10	10.3±3.0	5.5	−1.8	11.0±3.1	3.2	−1.2
100	102±6.4	4.9	1.5	101±5.4	2.8	0.2
Astragaloside IV						
1	1.31±0.3	3.9	1.4	9.91±0.3	7.9	1.9
10	11.0±2.3	4.1	2.8	11.2±2.1	3.0	0.2
100	98.4±4.4	2.5	1.9	102±4.6	1.7	1.8
Formononetin						
10	11.0±2.3	5.6	2.7	9.37±1.9	2.8	3.2
100	99.1±4.2	4.9	1.3	98.6±5.5	4.3	−1.1
1000	998±18.2	2.9	1.8	1002±16.2	3.1	0.4
Ononin						
1	0.95±0.4	3.6	2.7	0.93±1.7	4.9	0.9
10	10.5±2.8	2.8	−1.1	10.5±2.1	3.4	−0.2
100	98.8±3.2	2.9	0.4	99.2±2.7	2.9	1.3
Calycosin						
10	10.2±1.1	6.4	2.5	9.67±1.3	5.4	4.8
100	101±5.2	4.1	1.0	99.3±4.6	2.1	2.1
1000	1005±7.1	4.8	0.9	1004±9.8	3.7	1.9
Calycosin-7-O-β-D-glucoside						
1	1.11±0.7	5.2	2.3	0.96±0.4	2.6	1.8
10	10.8±2.1	3.3	−1.1	10.2±1.6	3.3	−0.7
100	98.4±5.7	2.8	2.8	101.4±43.3	1.2	0.3
Ligustilide						
1	0.92±0.4	4.9	0.3	1.03±0.2	3.8	2.1
10	10.2±2.1	0.5	2.4	9.43±1.7	4.1	−0.9
100	97.3±5.5	3.6	−0.4	98.3±5.6	1.7	1.1
Paeoniflorin						
10	9.60±0.77	5.7	−1.1	11.3±0.4	0.9	1.1
100	97.3±7.64	7.4	0.2	10.8±3.9	−0.6	−0.3
1000	1008±42.5	4.7	0.3	1006±16	0.1	−3.6

Table 3. Extraction recovery and matrix effect of nine compounds and internal standard in rat plasma.

Compounds	Set 1[a]	Set 2[b]	Set 3[c]	Matrix effect (%)[d]	Recovery (%)[e]
Astragaloside I					
1	1.08±0.1	1.03±0.4	1.08±0.4	95.5±12	105±6.2
10	10.2±1.2	8.67±2.8	7.62±1.2	85.0±7.6	87.9±12
100	99.7±5.3	74.3±7.5	77.3±5.8	74.5±1.5	104±14
Astragaloside II					
1	1.24±0.2	1.00±0.1	0.88±0.3	80.9±7.4	87.4±6.0
10	10.8±0.6	9.63±1.5	7.70±2.0	89.2±6.8	79.9±12
100	101±3.2	80.9±6.3	61.7±4.9	80.1±13	76.3±5.7
Astragaloside IV					
1	1.28±0.2	1.16±0.5	1.12±0.3	90.4±1.4	96.5±2.6
10	9.81±1.3	11.1±2.4	10.8±3.2	113±4.3	97.7±9.4
100	98.2±5.8	105±4.2	99.4±3.9	107±8.1	94.6±9.4
Formononetin					
10	11.4±2.3	12.0±1.2	10.5±2.1	105±6.9	87.9±12
100	101±4.2	99.1±5.3	92.1±6.0	98.1±5.6	92.9±9.5
1000	995±11	918±14	898±20	92.3±5.9	97.8±0.2
Ononin					
1	0.98±0.2	0.93±0.3	0.86±0.1	94.8±7.5	92.2±6.0
10	11.2±1.3	10.6±2.9	10.6±2.2	94.9±9.5	100±2.6
100	97.9±5.2	96.4±6.3	90.8±3.9	98.5±8.2	94.2±8.7
Calycosin					
10	11.1±2.2	12.3±2.3	11.7±1.8	111±3.3	95.1±3.3
100	97.8±4.4	105±5.8	97.9±6.3	107±8.0	93.5±2.3
1000	997±8.8	1056±20	1056±23	106±10.1	100±0.2
Calycosin-7-O-β-D-glucoside					
1	1.19±0.3	0.95±0.4	0.83±0.2	80.0±8.7	87.6±8.3
10	9.86±1.3	9.69±2.1	9.39±1.4	98.3±8.2	96.9±0.9
100	98.7±4.3	97.9±6.7	93.8±8.2	99.2±4.4	95.8±7.1
Ligustilide					
1	0.97±0.5	0.93±0.1	0.90±0.3	95.7±10	97.3±3.1
10	11.4±1.1	11.8±2.7	11.3±0.4	103.8±5.7	95.5±9.9
100	99.3±7.1	98.8±9.3	95.1±6.2	99.5±7.5	96.2±1.9
Paeoniflorin					
10	10.2±1.7	10.4±2.3	11.0±2.9	102±9.0	106±5.2
100	98.8±3.9	98.8±6.2	94.7±4.6	100±7.7	95.8±4.2
1000	995±17	991±11	966±15	99.6±1.4	97.5±3.8
Digoxin (IS)					
66.7	64.3±4.4	65.5±5.3	65.6±4.7	102±5.2	100±4.2

Data are expressed as means ± S.D. (n = 3).
[a]Neat is the standard in injection solvent.
[b]Post-spiked is the standard spiked in the prepared control plasma.
[c]Pre-spiked is the standard spiked into control plasma before prepared.
[d]Matrix effect (%) calculated as [(b/a)×100]%.
[e]Recovery (%) calculated as [(c/b)×100]%.

Application of the analytical system in pharmacokinetics study

The validated HPLC-MS/MS method was successfully applied for the simultaneous determination of nine active constituents for 12 h after BYHWT extract administration (10 g/kg, p.o.) in the rat. The mean plasma concentration-time profiles are illustrated in Fig. 3 and the pharmacokinetic parameters are presented in Table 5.

The concentration-time curves of astragaloside I, astragaloside II, astragaloside IV and ligustilide presented the phenomenon of a double-peak absorption phase in the plasma profile, and the other analytes seemed to have the same tendency. However, the other herbal ingredients of formononetin, ononin, calycosin, calycosin-7-

Table 4. Stability of the nine compounds in rat plasma samples.

Concentration (μg/mL)	Stability (%)			
	Freeze-thaw stability	Short-term stability	Long-term stability	Autosampler stability
Astragaloside I				
1	4.6±3.6	−3.6±8.0	−14±17	−5.3±7.9
10	3.8±2.7	−4.1±10	−8.3±2.3	4.3±6.6
100	−1.8±5.4	−6.4±6.4	−27±12	−4.9±7.0
Astragaloside II				
1	4.4±3.6	2.4±12	8.7±10	13±10
10	−2.3±0.8	−1.3±1.9	−0.8±16	−0.3±11
100	0.4±1.2	−6.8±5.7	1.7±21	−5.4±13
Astragaloside IV				
1	−3.2±5.0	12±15	−17±5.3	3.8±9.8
10	−4.1±3.4	4.7±6.2	−6.3±8.8	3.3
100	6.1±0.4	1.6±9.1	2.1±13.5	−8.6±12
Formononetin				
10	−4.9±3.8	−3.4±12	−13±5.5	−13±4.1
100	5.8±10	1.1±10	−12±7.5	−4.6±11
1000	−3.5±6.0	1.5±10.4	1.0±6.4	0.8±12
Ononin				
1	3.9±6.4	12±6.3	−7.2±10	4.7±7.7
10	−2.5±7.3	−12±4.6	−6.2±2.9	−7.0±1.4
100	4.2±1.3	6.7±2.1	3.2±3.9	8.1±3.8
Calycosin				
10	9.6±4.7	1.4±11	2.5±5.7	−3.5±11
100	8.6±3.8	14±12	17±5.2	−2.2±3.5
1000	2.9±4.5	13±7.3	21±12	7.1±4.9
Calycosin-7-O-β-D-glucoside				
1	5.8±6.1	2.5±11	6.4±12	−8.4±12
10	4.9±3.5	7.3±12	23±13	2.1±9.1
100	7.0±1.2	−0.1±0.9	20±12	3.5±7.9
Ligustilide				
1	8.7±5.9	14±11	6.7±10	2.0±10
10	2.7±2.2	11±10	5.0±14	13±7.2
100	6.5±1.4	12±7.5	23±12	−1.6±10
Paeoniflorin				
10	7.3±4.6	7.7±10	21±15	−3.3±7.3
100	2.1±1.8	−1.8±9.4	10±7.3	−1.6±8.2
1000	9.5±0.2	11±8.4	27±9.9	8.5±5.1

Data are expressed as means ± S.D. (n = 3).

O-β-d-glucoside and paeoniflorin presented a single and plateau absorption phase, consistent with a previous report [15]. By means of plateau absorption or multiple-peak absorption phase, these phenomenona were similar to another report on Chinese herbal compounds [25]. There were many possible explanations that attempt to explain the phenomenon of multiple-peak behavior. Similar multiple peak phenomena have been observed for a number of other oral drugs [26][27]. Several mechanisms have been proposed for the phenomenon: 1) enterohepatic recycling, the cycle in which bile salts and drugs excreted by the liver are absorbed by the intestinal mucosa and returned to the liver via the portal circulation [28]. 2) the presence of absorption sites along the stomach and different gastrointestinal segments [29]. 3) variable gastric emptying; a previous report suggests that the drug may cause increased gastric pH which in turn increases the gastric emptying rate [30]. After increasing the gastric emptying rate, a substantial amount of drug emptied into the duodenum soon after the administration can cause a rapid increase in plasma concentrations, resulting in the disappearance of double peaks [31].

Herbal preparation is a complex formulation which contains several herbs and ingredients. It is possible that the different characteristics of physical-chemical properties for individual ingredients may affect each other. In an in vitro herbal analysis,

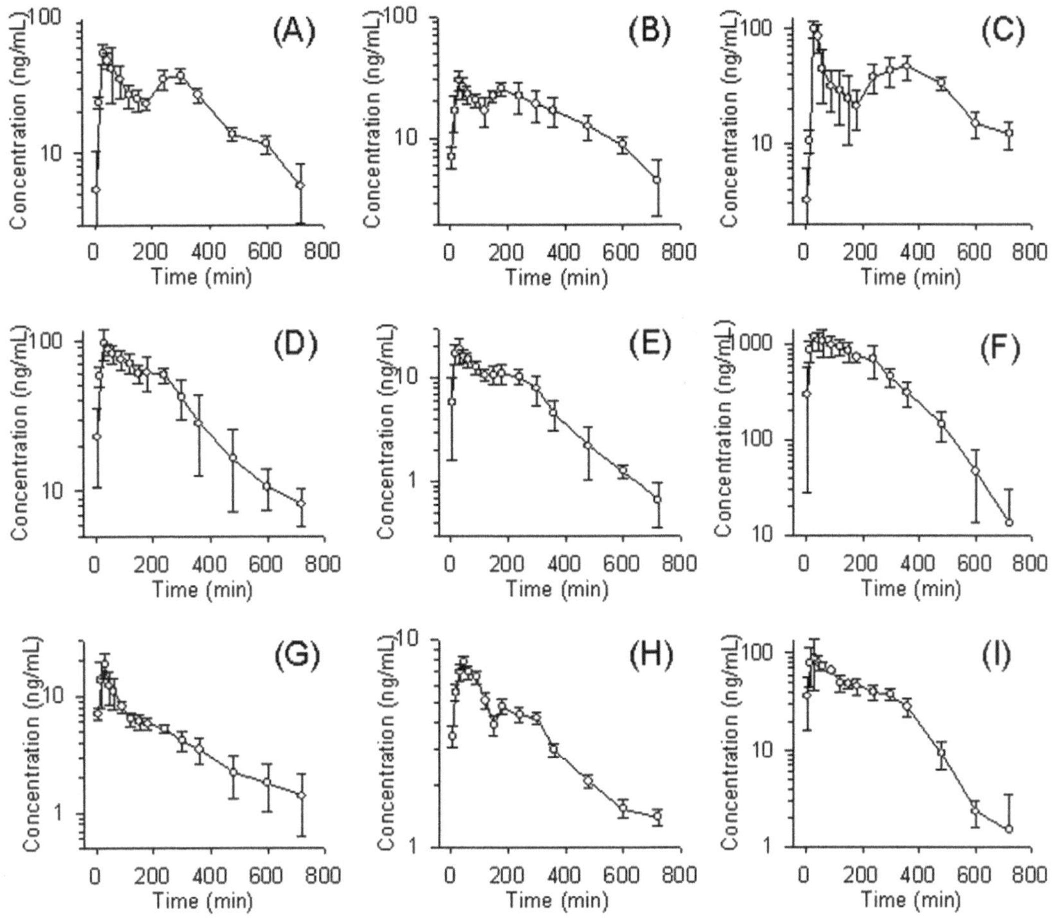

Figure 3. Mean plasma concentration–time profile in rat plasma after oral administration of bu-yang-huan-wu-tang extract for astragaloside I (A), astragaloside II (B), astragaloside IV (C), formononetin (D), ononin (E), calycosin (F), calycosin-7-O-β-D-glucoside (G), ligustilide (H) and paeoniflorin (I).

it is indicated that the berberine content in herbal preparation of Huang-Lian-Jiee-Dwu-Tang (8.15±0.39 mg/g) was less in the single herb Coptidis Radix (53.63+2.45 mg/g) but higher in Phellodendri Cortex (3.02+0.22 mg/g) when extracted with water, which suggest that herbal matrix effects were involved in the multiple compositions of the herbal preparation [32]. Another in vivo experiment discussed the pharmacokinetic of single herbal ingredient, single herbal extract and herbal preparation. Rutaecarpine (25 mg/kg/day, p.o.) (the herbal ingredient of Evodia rutaecarpa), the ethanol extract of Evodia rutaecarpa (1 g/kg/day,

Table 5. Pharmacokinetic parameters of the nine compounds in rat after oral administration of bu-yang-huan-wu-tang.

Parameter	C_{max} (ng/mL)	T_{max} (min)	$t_{1/2}$ (min)	AUC (min mg/mL)	Cl (mL/min/kg)
Astragaloside I	55±7.8	40±16	166±28	16.6±2.6	90.5±14
Astragaloside II	30±4.9	37±6.8	212±14	11.4±2.3	129±15
Astragaloside IV	100±16	35±7.7	170±8.3	23.0±5.7	64.3±13
Formononetin	98±17	38±8.2	175±13	26.7±6.0	57.4±14
Ononin	19±4.5	35±7.7	134±9.6	4.6±1.0	351±47
Calycosin	1231±171[a]	40±16	75±11	308±73[b]	5.4±1.3
Calycosin-7-O-β-D-glucoside	18±4.1	32±6.1	338±132	3.25±0.7	428±143
Ligustilide	7.8±0.2	45±0.0	267±1.2	2.43±0.06	532±11
Paeoniflorin	97±33	35±7.7	93±32	21.0±3.9	76.5±15

Data expressed as mean ± standard error. (n = 6) Cmax: the maximum plasma concentration, $t_{1/2}$: half-life, AUC: area under the concentration-time curve, Cl: clearance.
[a]Significantly different ($p<0.05$) from the other active compounds in C_{max}.
[b]Significantly different ($p<0.05$) from the other active compounds in AUC.

p.o.) and multiple herbal preparation of Evodia rutaecarpa (Wu-Chu-Yu-Tang; 1 g/kg/day, p.o.) were individually pretreated daily for three consecutive days in rats and caffeine was administered (2 mg/kg, i.v.) on the fourth day. The results indicate that the rutaecarpine (single ingredient), extract of Evodia rutaecarpa, and herbal preparation (Wu-Chu-Yu-Tang) provide significant interaction for the pharmacokinetics of caffeine [33].

Rat is anatomically lack of gall bladder and the bile juice is directly excreted into duodenum. A previous biliary excretion report indicates that the gastrodin (an active substance isolated from *Gastrodia elata* Blume) and its metabolite have been detected in the bile duct [34]. Another pair-rats experimental model is designed to investigate the enterohepatic circulation of colchicine [35]. The results show that the AUC of colchicine was 847.7±141.0 and 55.5±29.2 min μg/mL in the donor and recipient rats, respectively. The biliary excretion and enterohepatic circulation may have significant effects on the pharmacokinetics of a number of drugs. Our data demonstrate that the double-peak phenomenon in the pharmacokinetic curve may be caused by the biliary excretion and enterohepatic circulation. However, this is the first reported case of double peaks for BYHWT absorption. The double-peak phenomenon caused by the hypothesized mechanism may have important therapeutic and drug interaction implications, especially because traditional medicines are commonly coadministered with other drugs. Furthermore, studies are needed to investigate the mechanism underlying the double-peak phenomenon for BYHWT with its active components in the future.

The cycloartane-type triterpene glycosides group in Radix Astragali of astragaloside I, astragaloside II and astragaloside IV, which were comprised of the same aglycone cycloastragenol and only differ in number and position of glucosyls, but their pharmacokinetic behaviors were significant different. The contents of astragaloside I, astragaloside II and astragaloside IV in the herbal preparation of BYHWT were 2.46, 0.69 and 0.54 mg/g, respectively. However, the values of C_{max} and AUC of astragaloside I and astragaloside II were much lower than astragaloside IV. This phenomenon might be referred to the biotransformation of astragaloside I to astragaloside IV about intestinal bacteria and enzymatic reaction, arising from great increase of astragaloside IV in vivo. Moreover, the constituents in herbal preparations may be the substrates of inhibitors, or inducers of Cytochromal enzymes, and hence had individual or combination effects on the pharmacokinetics of each other [36].

Calycosin displayed rapid and sustained absorption, with the largest C_{max} at 1231±171 ng/mL ($p<0.05$) and AUC at 308±73 min mg/mL ($p<0.05$); and at 5±11, calycosin had the shortest elimination half-life min among nine tested compounds of BYHWT. Formononetin had second largest amount of AUC value, perhaps due to its structural similarity to calycosin. Ononin and calycosin-7-O-β-d-glucoside had identical pharmacokinetic parameters in organisms, with their C_{max} and T_{max} being similar and both of them having low AUC. However, the BYHWT contents of ononin and calycosin-7-O-β-d-glucoside in were 0.63 and 2.56 mg/g, respectively, since the ononin content in plasma was higher. This might be ascribed to the relatively weak polarity of ononin.

Ligustilide is one of the most important bioactive components of Radix Angelicae Sinensis and Rhizoma Ligustici Chuanxiong, and paeoniflorin is the major bioactive ingredient in Radix Paeoniae Rubra in BYHWT. Significantly, the amounts of crude drug of Radix Angelicae Sinensis and Rhizoma Ligustici Chuanxiong in BYHWT were much higher than that of Radix Paeoniae Rubra. But there was less ligustilide than paeoniflorin found in the quantitative results, and our findings indicated that the C_{max} and AUC of ligustilide were much lower than paeoniflorin in a living organism. Moreover, the extent and rate of drug uptakes into the systemic circulation of AUC and C_{max} for ligustilide were the lowest in BYHWT. However, the previous report did not monitor ligustilide as one of their target components [15]. In this study, we provide more detailed information to enable better understanding for the pharmacokinetic profiles of the herbal preparation BYHWT. Moreover, based on the interpretation of pharmacokinetic profiles for the individual herbal ingredients, the pharmacokinetic characteristics of this complicated traditional Chinese herbal preparation might be gradually revealed.

Conclusion

In present study, reliable high-performance liquid chromatography coupled with tandem mass spectrometry was successfully used for the quantitation of bioactive compounds of astragaloside I, astragaloside II, astragaloside IV, formononetin, ononin, calycosin, calycosin-7-O-β-d-glucoside, ligustilide and paeoniflorin in rat plasma after oral administration of BYHWT. These pharmacokinetic studies were performed through an experimental model of freely moving rats. The assay provided adequate recovery and matrix effect with good precision and accuracy. These pharmacokinetic results provide a constructive contribution to better understand the extensive action mechanism of absorption, distribution, metabolism and excretion, and to prepare for future clinical evaluation.

Author Contributions

Conceived and designed the experiments: LHS THT. Performed the experiments: LHS LCL THT. Analyzed the data: LHS THT. Contributed reagents/materials/analysis tools: LHS LCL THT. Wrote the paper: LHS THT. Herbal preparation: LHS LCL.

References

1. Zhang H, Wang WR, Lin R, Zhang JY, Ji QL, et al. (2010) Buyang Huanwu decoction ameliorates coronary heart disease with Qi deficiency and blood stasis syndrome by reducing CRP and CD40 in rats. J Ethnopharmacol 130: 98–102.
2. Wang WR, Lin R, Zhang H, Lin QQ, Yang LN, et al. (2011) The effects of Buyang Huanwu Decoction on hemorheological disorders and energy metabolism in rats with coronary heart disease. J Ethnopharmacol 137: 214–220.
3. Wang HW, Liou KT, Wang YH, Lu CK, Lin YL, et al. (2011) Deciphering the neuroprotective mechanisms of Bu-yang Huan-wu decoction by an integrative neurofunctional and genomic approach in ischemic stroke mice. J Ethnopharmacol 138: 22–33.
4. Zhao LD, Wang JH, Jin GR, Zhao Y, Zhang HJ (2012) Neuroprotective effect of Buyang Huanwu decoction against focal cerebral ischemia/reperfusion injury in rats–time window and mechanism. J Ethnopharmacol 140: 339–344.
5. Qi LW, Yu QT, Yi L, Ren MT, Wen XD, et al. (2008) Simultaneous determination of 15 marker constituents in various radix Astragali preparations by solid-phase extraction and high-performance liquid chromatography. J Sep Sci 31: 97–106.
6. Yesilada E, Bedir E, Calis I, Takaishi Y, Ohmoto Y (2005) Effects of triterpene saponins from Astragalus species on in vitro cytokine release. J Ethnopharmacol 96: 71–77.
7. Ma X, Tu P, Chen Y, Zhang T, Wei Y, et al. (2004) Preparative isolation and purification of isoflavan and pterocarpan glucosides from Astragalus membranaceus Bge. var. mongholicus (Bge.) Hsiao by high-speed counter-current chromatography. J Chromatogr A 1023: 311–315.
8. Xiao HB, Krucker M, Albert K, Liang XM (2004) Determination and identification of isoflavonoids in Radix astragali by matrix solid-phase dispersion extraction and high-performance liquid chromatography with photodiode array and mass spectrometric detection. J Chromatogr A 1032: 117–124.
9. Zhang D, Wang D, Yu Y (2011) [Effects and mechanisms of total flavonoids of astragali radix and calycosin on inhibiting human erythroleukemia cell line K562]. Zhongguo Zhong Yao Za Zhi 36: 3502–3505.

10. Yan R, Ko NL, Li SL, Tam YK, Lin G (2008) Pharmacokinetics and metabolism of ligustilide, a major bioactive component in Rhizoma Chuanxiong, in the rat. Drug Metab Dispos 36: 400–408
11. Lu Q, Qiu TQ, Yang H (2006) Ligustilide inhibits vascular smooth muscle cells proliferation. Eur J Pharmacol 542: 136–140.
12. Ji B, Geng P, Liu JG, Shi DZ, Wang YY (2006) [Effects of active components extracted from Qixue Bingzhi Recipe on proliferation of vascular smooth muscle cells and expressions of platelet-derived growth factor and its receptor genes]. Zhong Xi Yi Jie He Xue Bao 4: 30–34.
13. Liu EH, Qi LW, Cheng XL, Peng YB, Li P (2010) Simultaneous determination of twelve bioactive constituents in Buyang Huanwu decoction by HPLC-DAD-ELSD and HPLC-TOF/MS. Biomed Chromatogr 24: 125–131.
14. Liu EH, Qi LW, Peng YB, Cheng XL, Wu Q, et al. (2009) Rapid separation and identification of 54 major constituents in Buyang Huanwu decoction by ultra-fast HPLC system coupled with DAD-TOF/MS. Biomed Chromatogr 23: 828–842.
15. Zhang J, Yang G, Lin R, Hu Z (2011) Determination of paeoniflorin, calycosin-7-O-beta-D-glucoside, ononin, calycosin and formononetin in rat plasma after oral administration of Buyang Huanwu decoction for their pharmacokinetic study by liquid chromatography-mass spectrometry. Biomed Chromatogr 25: 450–457.
16. Wu YT, Wu MT, Lin CC, Chien CF, Tsai TH, et al. (2011) Pharmacokinetic studies of Chinese medicinal herbs using an automated blood sampling system and liquid chromatography-mass Spectrometry. J Tradition Complement Med 2: 30–40.
17. Reagan-Shaw S, Nihal M, Ahmad N (2008) Dose translation from animal to human studies revisited. FASEB J 22: 659–661.
18. Wu YT, Huang CM, Lin CC, Ho WA, Lin LC, et al. (2010) Oral bioavailability, urinary excretion and organ distribution of melamine in Sprague-Dawley rats by high-performance liquid chromatography with tandem mass spectrometry. J Agric Food Chem 58: 108–111
19. Hsieh YJ, Lin LC, Tsai TH (2006) Measurement and pharmacokinetic study of plumbagin in a conscious freely moving rat using liquid chromatography/tandem mass spectrometry. J Chromatogr B Analyt Technol Biomed Life Sci 844: 1–5.
20. Guidance for Industry. Available: http://www.fda.gov/downloads/Drugs/GuidanceComplianceRegulatoryInformation/Guidances/ucm070107.pdf. Accessed 2001 May.
21. Zu Y, Yan M, Fu Y, Liu W, Zhang L, et al. (2009) Determination and quantification of astragalosides in Radix Astragali and its medicinal products using LC-MS. J Sep Sci 32: 517–525.
22. Wen XD, Qi LW, Li B, Li P, Yi L, et al. (2009) Microsomal metabolism of calycosin, formononetin and drug-drug interactions by dynamic microdialysis sampling and HPLC-DAD-MS analysis. J Pharm Biomed Anal 50: 100–105.
23. Tong L, Wan M, Zhou D, Gao J, Zhu Y, et al. (2010) LC-MS/MS determination and pharmacokinetic study of albiflorin and paeoniflorin in rat plasma after oral administration of Radix Paeoniae Alba extract and Tang-Min-Ling-Wan. Biomed Chromatogr 24: 1324–1331.
24. Wang D, Song Y, Li SL, Bian YY, Guan J, et al. (2006) Simultaneous analysis of seven astragalosides in Radix Astragali and related preparations by liquid chromatography coupled with electrospray ionization time-of-flight mass spectrometry. J Sep Sci 29: 2012–2022.
25. Lu T, Song J, Huang F, Deng Y, Xie L, et al. (2007) Comparative pharmacokinetics of baicalin after oral administration of pure baicalin, Radix scutellariae extract and Huang-Lian-Jie-Du-Tang to rats. J Ethnopharmacol 110: 412–418.
26. Li P, Zhang Y, Xiao L, Jin X, Yang K (2007) Simultaneous determination of harpagoside and cinnamic acid in rat plasma by high-performance liquid chromatography: application to a pharmacokinetic study. Anal Bioanal Chem 389: 2259–2264.
27. Huang Y, Bai Y, Zhao L, Hu T, Hu B, et al. (2007) Pharmacokinetics and metabolism of neferine in rats after a single oral administration. Biopharm Drug Dispos 28: 361–372.
28. Zhu Z, Zhao L, Liu X, Chen J, Zhang H, et al. (2010) Comparative pharmacokinetics of baicalin and wogonoside by liquid chromatography-mass spectrometry after oral administration of Xiaochaihu Tang and Radix scutellariae extract to rats. J Chromatogr B Analyt Technol Biomed Life Sci 878: 2184–2190.
29. Yin OQ, Tomlinson B, Chow AH, Chow MS (2003) A modified two-portion absorption model to describe double-peak absorption profiles of ranitidine. Clin Pharmacokinet 42: 179–192.
30. Mummaneni V, Amidon GL, Dressman JB (1995) Gastric pH influences the appearance of double peaks in the plasma concentration-time profiles of cimetidine after oral administration in dogs. Pharm Res 12: 780–786.
31. Mostafavi SA, Foster RT (2003) Influence of cimetidine co-administration on the pharmacokinetics of acebutolol enantiomers and its metabolite diacetolol in a rat model: the effect of gastric pH on double-peak phenomena. Int J Pharm 255: 81–86.
32. Tsai PL, Tsai TH (2002) High-performance liquid chromatographic determination of berberine contained in medicinal herbs and a related traditional Chinese medicine. Anal Let 35:2459–2470.
33. Tsai TH, Chang CH, Lin LC (2005) Effects of Evodia rutaecarpa and rutaecarpine on the pharmacokinetics of caffeine in rats. Planta Med 71: 640–645.
34. Lin LC, Chen YF, Lee WC, Wu YT, Tsai TH (2008) Pharmacokinetics of gastrodin and its metabolite p-hydroxybenzyl alcohol in rat blood, brain and bile by microdialysis coupled to LC-MS/MS. J Pharm Biomed Anal 48: 909–917.
35. Chen YJ, Huang SM, Liu CY, Yeh PH, Tsai TH (2008) Hepatobiliary excretion and enterohepatic circulation of colchicine in rats. Int J Pharm 350: 230–239.
36. Zhou S, Koh HL, Gao Y, Gong ZY, Lee EJ (2004) Herbal bioactivation: the good, the bad and the ugly. Life Sci 74: 935–968.

14

Epidemiology, Quality and Reporting Characteristics of Systematic Reviews of Traditional Chinese Medicine Interventions Published in Chinese Journals

Bin Ma[1], Jiwu Guo[1,2], Guoqing Qi[1], Haimin Li[1], Jiye Peng[3], Yulong Zhang[1,2], Yanqin Ding[1], Kehu Yang[1]*

1 Evidence-Based Medicine Center, Institute of Traditional Chinese and Western Medicine, School of Basic Medical Sciences, Lanzhou University, Lanzhou, Gansu, China, **2** Second School of Clinical Medicine of Lanzhou University, Lanzhou, Gansu, China, **3** The Library of Lanzhou University, Lanzhou, Gansu, China

Abstract

Background: Systematic reviews (SRs) of TCM have become increasingly popular in China and have been published in large numbers. This review provides the first examination of epidemiological characteristics of these SRs as well as compliance with the PRISMA and AMSTAR guidelines.

Objectives: To examine epidemiological and reporting characteristics as well as methodological quality of SRs of TCM published in Chinese journals.

Methods: Four Chinese databases were searched (CBM, CSJD, CJFD and Wanfang Database) for SRs of TCM, from inception through Dec 2009. Data were extracted into Excel spreadsheets. The PRISMA and AMSTAR checklists were used to assess reporting characteristics and methodological quality, respectively.

Results: A total of 369 SRs were identified, most (97.6%) of which used the terms systematic review or meta-analysis in the title. None of the reviews had been updated. Half (49.8%) were written by clinicians and nearly half (47.7%) were reported in specialty journals. The impact factors of 45.8% of the journals published in were zero. The most commonly treated conditions were diseases of the circulatory and digestive disease. Funding sources were not reported for any reviews. Most (68.8%) reported information about quality assessment, while less than half (43.6%) reported assessing for publication bias. Statistical mistakes appeared in one-third (29.3%) of reviews and most (91.9%) did not report on conflict of interest.

Conclusions: While many SRs of TCM interventions have been published in Chinese journals, the quality of these reviews is troubling. As a potential key source of information for clinicians and researchers, not only were many of these reviews incomplete, some contained mistakes or were misleading. Focusing on improving the quality of SRs of TCM, rather than continuing to publish them in great quantity, is urgently needed in order to increase the value of these studies.

Editor: Lisa Hartling, Alberta Research Centre for Health Evidence, University of Alberta, Canada

Funding: The authors have no support or funding to report.

Competing Interests: The authors have declared that no competing interests exist.

* E-mail: kehuyangebm2006@126.com

Introduction

The first systematic review addressing the effect of traditional Chinese medicine (TCM) that was published in a Chinese journal may be sourced back to Chen et al. in 1999 [1]. Since then, systematic reviews of TCM have become been increasingly published in China, and now with a large number. Given the implications of systematic reviews to policy making and clinical practice, achieving highest possible quality in design, conduct, analysis, and reporting is of paramount importance [2].

In the last decade, a few studies have examined the reporting of systematic reviews, and found that the quality of reporting was generally poor [3,4,5]. Three studies, using the Quality of Reporting of Meta-analyses (QUOROM) checklist, examined the quality of reporting of reviews of traditional Chinese medicine, and concluded with similar findings [6,7,8] Nevertheless, they were inherent with limitations, including the failure to report details about epidemiological characteristics of included reviews, and the failure to address methodological quality of those reviews.

In 2009, the newer standard of reporting systematic review, the Preferred Reporting Items for Systematic Reviews and Meta-Analyses (PRISMA) was released to replace the QUOROM for guiding the review reporting [9]. Earlier than that, an instrument, assisting the assessment of methodological quality of systematic reviews, Assessment of Multiple Systematic Reviews (AMSTAR) [10] was published in 2007. This instrument, developed on the biasis of the Oxman-Guyatt Overview Quality Assessment Questionnaire (OQAQ) [11] and Sack's Quality Assessment Checklist [12] is considered a validated tool in assessing the methodological quality of systematic reviews, and receives recognition from international agencies, including The Canadian Agency for Drugs and Technologies in Health (CADTH) [13].

Our study therefore aims to address the limitations of published studies, by assessing epidemiological and reporting characteristics, and methodological quality of systematic reviews of traditional Chinese medicine. We will particularly employ the new instruments for assessing the quality of reporting and methodological quality of those reviews.

Methods

Inclusion Criteria

We included all systematic reviews about TCM published in Chinese Journals. TCM interventions may have included herbal medicine, acupuncture/acupressure, moxibustion, Tuina massage, food therapy, and physical exercise such as tai chi and shadow boxing. TCM interventions may have been administered alone or in combination with conventional western medicine. We included publications described as systematic reviews or those that provided an overview of evidence from multiple studies and where authors described their methods in explicit detail.

Search Strategy(Text S1)

Four Chinese databases (Chinese Biomedicine Literature Database (CBM), Chinese Scientific Journal Full-text Database (CSJD), Chinese Journal Full-text Database (CJFD), and Wanfang Database) were searched from inception through Dec 2009. The search terms included "Systematic Review", "Meta-analysis", "Traditional Chinese Medicine" and "Chinese herbs" etc.

Screening

Two researchers independently screened the titles and abstracts of identified studies. One reviewer subsequently screened the full text articles of potentially included studies (Jiwu GUO) while a second reviewer independently screened a 20% random sample (Bin MA). Disagreement was resolved by discussion.

Data Collection and Analysis

Variables extracted included publication and reporting characteristics as well as items from the PRISMA and AMSTAR checklists. Reviews were classified according to their TCM focus as Herbal (e.g. bulk herbs, decoctions, pills) or Non-herbal (e.g. acupuncture, Tuina). Conditions studied were classified using the International Classification of Diseases (ICD-10). Data was collected using a standardized form and summarized using descriptive statistics (frequency, median, interquartile range (IQR)). Analyses were performed using Excel (version Microsoft Excel 2003; http://office.microsoft.com/zh-cn/) and SPSS (version 13.0; http://www.spss.com).

Results

Search

The searches identified 10,001 records. Screening excluded 9,621 reviews due to duplication, focus on non-TCM interventions, or for not being a SR. After examination of the full texts of 380 article, a further 11 reviews were excluded because they were quality assessments of systematic reviews and meta-analyses. A total of 369 publications were included (Figure 1, Text S2).

Epidemiological Characteristics (Table 1)

The 369 reviews were all written in Chinese and were published in 145 different Chinese Journals. Frequency of citation of each review ranged from 0 to 79; nearly half (46.1%) had not been cited and only 2.4% had been cited more than 15 times. Almost half (49.9%) of the reviews were written by clinicians. The reviews were classified as either Herbal interventions (84.3%) or Non-Herbal interventions. Non-herbal interventions included acupuncture (14.6%) and Tuina (1.1%). The most common conditions studied were diseases of the circulatory system (6.5%) and digestive system (5.7%).

Descriptive Characteristics (Table 2)

The reviews included a median of three authors (IQR: 2.0–5.0). Almost half the reviews (47.7%) were published in specialty journals although this differed significantly between reviews of herbal and non-herbal interventions (79.0% versus 21.0%,

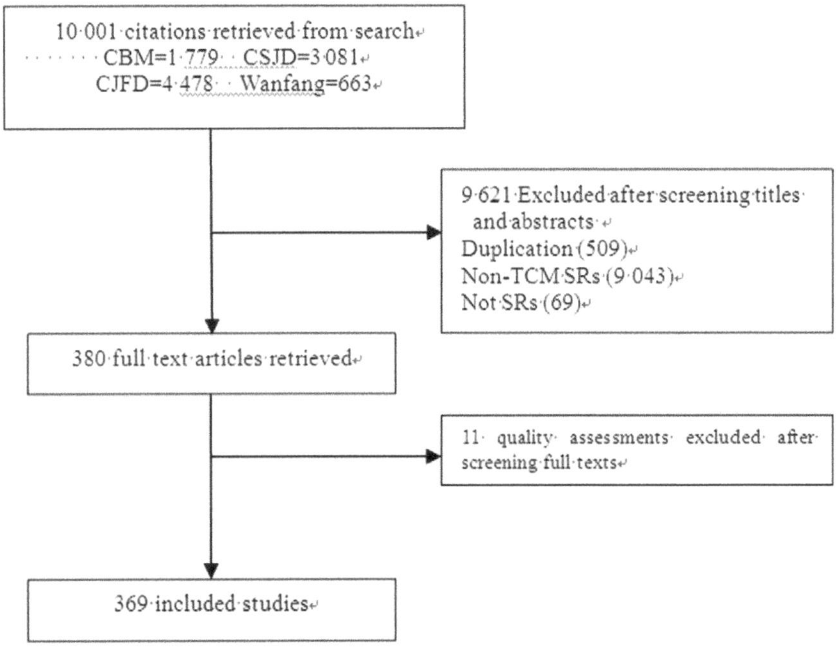

Figure 1. Flow chart of articles identified, included and excluded. SRs, Systematic Review.

Table 1. Epidemiology of Systematic Reviews.

Category	Characteristic	Number (%) of n = 369
Number of times cited	0	170 (46.1)
	1–5	137 (37.1)
	6–10	41 (11.1)
	11–15	12 (3.3)
	>15	9 (2.4)
Role of first author	Clinician	184 (49.9)
	Researcher	82 (22.2)
	Graduate student	54 (14.6)
	Other	49 (13.3)
Focus of reviews	Chinese Herbal Interventions[a]	314 (84.3)
	Non-Herbal Interventions[b]	55 (15.7)
Condition focused on in review (Common ICD-10[c])	Diseases of the circulatory system	24 (6.5)
	Diseases of the digestive system	21 (5.7)
	Diseases of the nervous system	18 (4.9)
	Diseases of the genitourinary system	17 (4.5)
	Diseases of the respiratory system	11 (3.0)
	Diseases of the blood and blood-forming organs and immune mechanism	14 (3.8)
	Diseases of the musculoskeletal system and connective tissue	9 (2.4)
	Mental and behavioural disorders	9 (2.4)
	Diseases of the skin and subcutaneous tissue	5 (1.4)
	Endocrine, nutritional and metabolic diseases	5 (1.4)
	Neoplasms	5 (1.4)
	Infectious and parasitic diseases	3 (0.8)
	Pregnancy, childbirth and the puerperium	2 (0.5)
	Diseases of the ear and mastoid process	1 (0.3)
	Diseases of the eye and adnexa	1 (0.3)
	Symptoms, signs and abnormal clinical and laboratory findings, not classified elsewhere	1 (0.3)

[a]Herbal interventions included bulk herbs, decoctions, pills;
[b]Non-herbal interventions included acupuncture and Tuina;
[c]Common ICD-10: International Classification of Diseases 10.

Table 2. Descriptive Characteristics of Included Systematic Reviews.

Category		All SRs n = 369	Herbal SRs[a] n = 314	Non-herbal SRs[b] n = 55
Number of authors, Median (IQR)		3 (2–5)	3.0 (2–4)	4 (3–5)
Journal type*	General, n (%)	193 (52)	175 (91)	18 (9)
	Specialty, n (%)	176 (48)	139 (79)	37 (21)
Indexed in CSCD[c] Yes n (%)*		120 (33)	91 (76)	29 (24)
Number of included studies Median (IQR)*		10 (7–17)	11 (7–19)	8 (6–13)
Number of participants in included studies	Median (IQR)	952 (562–1596)	1004 (583–1789)	890 (534–1273)
Meta-analysis Yes (%)		343 (93)	292 (93)	51 (93)
Update of a previous review n (%)		0 (0)	0 (0)	0 (0)

[a]Herbal interventions included bulk herbs, decoctions, pills;
[b]Non-herbal interventions included acupuncture and Tuina;
[c]CSCD: Chinese Science Citation Database;
*indicates $p<0.05$.

respectively ($p<0.05$). Only one-third (32.5%) were published in journals cited by Chinese Science Citation Database (CSCD), which again varied significantly between herbal and non-herbal interventions ($p<0.05$). The reviews included a median of 10.0 studies each, involving 951.5 participants. Non-herbal SRs included significantly fewer studies ($p<0.05$) and participants compared to herbal SRs. Meta-analysis was conducted in almost all the reviews (93.0%) and did not differ significantly between groups. None of the reviews had been updated from a previous review.

PRISMA Checklist Assessment (Table 3)

Compliance with PRISMA checklist items ranged from 0–97.6%. Almost all reviews (97.6%) described themselves using the terms "systematic review" or "meta analysis". Most reviews were compliant with the following checklist items: included a clear rationale, described information sources, described method used for assessing risk of bias of individual studies, stated the principle of summary measures, described the results of individual studies, discussed limitations at study and outcome level, provided a general interpretation of results, and presented an available conclusion. More than half of reviews were compliant with the following checklist items: reported eligibility criteria, presented search strategy, stated the process for selecting studies, specified any assessment of risk of bias that may affect the cumulative evidence, described characteristics of included studies, or described risk of bias within studies. Less than half of reviews were compliant with the following checklist items: described data collection process, described synthesis of results, described additional analysis, described how the studies were selected, presented synthesis of results (although this varied across reviews category), presented results of any assessment of risk of bias across studies, or described sources of funding and other support. Few studies provided a description of objectives or purpose, lists of data items, or gave results of additional analysis. None of the studies provided a structured summary, protocol or registration information, or provided a summary of results in the discussion.

AMSTAR Checklist Assessment (Table 4)

Compliance with AMSTAR checklist items ranged from 0–70.2%. More than half of reviews were compliant with the following checklist items: reported that a comprehensive literature

Table 3. PRISMA Assessment of Reporting Characteristics.

Category	Item (Yes)	Overall, n=369 n (%)	Herbs[a] n=314 n (%)	Non-herbs[b] n=55 n (%)
TITLE	1. Title	360 (97.6)	308 (98.1)	52 (94.6)
ABSTRACT	2. Structured summary	0 (0.0)	0 (0.0)	0 (0.0)
INTRODUCTION	3. Rationale	344 (93.2)	292 (93.0)	52 (94.6)
	4. Objectives	74 (20.1)	61 (19.4)	13 (23.6)
METHODS	5. Protocol and registration	0 (0.0)	0 (0.0)	0 (0.0)
	6. Eligibility criteria	214 (58.0)	185 (58.9)	29 (52.7)
	7. Information sources*	363 (72.1)	217 (69.1)	49 (89.1)
	8. Search*	208 (56.4)	165 (52.6)	43 (78.2)
	9. Study selection*	244 (66.1)	215 (68.5)	29 (52.7)
	10. Data collection process*	160 (43.4)	127 (40.5)	33 (60.0)
	11. Data items*	52 (14.1)	35 (11.2)	17 (30.9)
	12. Risk of bias in individual studies*	265 (71.8)	212 (67.5)	43 (78.2)
	13. Summary measures*	275 (74.5)	228 (72.6)	47 (85.5)
	14. Synthesis of results	143 (38.8)	126 (40.1)	17 (30.9)
	15. Risk of bias across studies	196 (53.1)	173 (55.1)	23 (41.8)
	16. Additional analyses	137 (37.1)	121 (38.5)	16 (29.1)
RESULTS	17. Study selection*	166 (45.0)	149 (47.5)	17 (30.9)
	18. Study characteristics	224 (60.7)	189 (60.2)	35 (63.6)
	19. Risk of bias within studies	227 (61.5)	187 (59.6)	40 (72.7)
	20. Results of individual studies	295 (80.0)	251 (79.9)	44 (80.0)
	21. Synthesis of results*	171 (46.3)	153 (48.7)	18 (32.7)
	22. Risk of bias across studies	151 (40.9)	133 (42.4)	18 (32.7)
	23. Additional analysis	78 (21.1)	71 (22.6)	7 (12.7)
DISCUSSION	24. Summary of evidence	0 (0.0)	0 (0.0)	0 (0.0)
	25. Limitations	346 (93.8)	296 (94.3)	50 (90.9)
	26. Conclusions	339 (91.9)	288 (91.7)	51 (92.7)
FUNDING	27. Funding	144 (39.0)	119 (37.9)	25 (45.5)

[a]Herbal interventions included bulk herbs, decoctions, pills;
[b]Non-herbal interventions included acupuncture and Tuina;
*indicates $p<0.05$.

Table 4. AMSTAR Assessment of Methodological Characteristics.

Category (Yes)	Overall, n = 369 n (%)	Herbs, n = 314 n (%)	Non- herbal interventions, n = 55 n (%)
1. Was an 'a priori' design provided?	19 (5.2)	17 (5.4)	2 (3.6)
2. Was there duplicate study selection and data extraction? *	152 (41.2)	120 (38.2)	32 (58.2)
3. Was a comprehensive literature search performed? *	203 (55.0)	159 (50.6)	44 (80.0)
4. Was the status of publication (i.e. grey literature) used as an inclusion criterion?	10 (2.7)	9 (2.9)	1 (1.8)
5. Was a list of studies (included and excluded) provided?	13 (3.5)	10 (3.2)	3 (5.5)
6. Were the characteristics of the included studies provided?	221 (59.9)	182 (58.0)	39 (70.9)
7. Was the scientific quality of the included studies assessed and documented?	259 (70.2)	219 (69.8)	42 (76.4)
8. Was the scientific quality of the included studies used appropriately in formulating conclusions?	254 (68.8)	212 (67.5)	40 (72.7)
9. Were the methods used to combine the findings of studies appropriate? *	108 (29.3)	100 (31.9)	8 (14.6)
10. Was the likelihood of publication bias assessed? *	161 (43.6)	147 (46.8)	14 (25.5)
11. Was the conflict of interest stated?	30 (8.1)	27 (8.6)	3 (5.5)

a Herbal interventions included bulk herbs, decoctions, pills;
b Non-herbal interventions included acupuncture and Tuina;
*indicates $p<0.05$.

search was performed, provided the characteristics of included studies, assessed and documented the scientific quality of the included studies, or appropriately addressed the quality of included studies in formulating conclusions. Less than half of reviews were compliant with the following checklist items: reported that there were duplicated study selection and data extraction, used appropriate methods to combine the findings of studies (although this varied across reviews category), or assessed the likelihood of publication bias. Few studies provided an 'a priori' design, reported the status of publication used as an inclusion criterion, provided a list of studies, or stated if there was a conflict of interest or not. .

Discussion

Our study identified 369 systematic reviews of TCM interventions published since 1999, most of which evaluated herbal interventions. This study updates previous reviews of this topic [6,7,8] by including an additional 258 SRs. This review is also the first to examine compliance of Chinese SR authors with the PRISMA reporting guideline and AMSTAR tool for assessing methodological quality.

Our review examined some of the same variables described in Moher et al.'s investigation of SRs written in English and indexed in Medline [5]. In that study, the authors reported that the 300 SRs they included were published in 132 journals, including the Cochrane Library. In contrast to our review, only 8% of their included SRs were of complementary and alternative medicine (CAM) interventions. While most (91%) of their SRs were published in specialty journals, 45% of all 132 journals did not have an impact factor. Most (93%) of our SRs included a meta-analysis compared to 54% of the English studies and while 44% of our studies assessed for publication bias, only 23% of the English studies reporting doing so. Funding sources were reported in 39% of our studies compared to 59% of the English studies.

The range of diseases addressed in our reviews are similar with those in the three reviews [6,7,8] focusing on the Chinese literature. The three reviews, however, failed to report details about the epidemiological and study characteristics of systematic reviews, including number of times cited, journal type, number of studies included, number of participants, and whether it is an update of a published review. Moreover, one study [6] did not report the prevalence of reviews meeting each individual item of QUOROM. In addition we found that, despite the increasing use of the terms "systematic review" and "meta-analysis" in the title and subsequent manuscript sections, the quality of reporting remains poor.

While many deficits in reporting were evident in the Chinese SRs, we identified areas of particular concern. These included evidence that suggested that the SRs were not highly referenced by other researchers working in the same field. This may be due, in part, to the overall poor quality of this body of work, which may also be a reason that less than one third were indexed in the Chinese Science Citation Database (CSCD), which is similar to the Science Citation Index, in that indexed journals are considered of higher quality than non-indexed journals.

There is also evidence that even though SRs have become an increasingly popular source of up-to-date knowledge, they are under utilized by Chinese clinicians. Because although the Chinese Cochrane Center was established in 1997 by the Ministry of Health of the people's republic of China, recent studies reported that most clinicians and nurses had not heard of or did not understand the meaning of evidence-based medicine (EBM) [14,15]. In addition, not all medical schools have introduced EBM curricula in China.

Although it is well known that results from reviews are most useful when they are up-to-date [16], none of the reviews included in our SR reported being an update of a previous review. This may be due to lack of policies in China to encourage updates and reluctance of Chinese journals to publish updated reviews that are not substantially different from previous publications. The review by Moher et al. reported that 18% of the English SRs were updates, however, only those SRs published in the Cochrane Library had been updated [5], suggesting that this problem is not restricted to Chinese journals.

We have demonstrated that compliance with PRISMA reporting guidelines is low for many Chinese SRs. Items of particular concern included lack of appropriate abstracts or structured summaries and details of protocols or summaries of evidence. In order to improve the quality of reporting, we strongly recommend the use of reporting guidelines by authors. We also recommend that editors of medical journals recognize and promote use of reporting guidelines in their publications. Lastly, medical schools should introduce reporting guidelines into medical education as early as possible.

Reviews of numerous medical specialties, as well as comprehensive reviews, have concluded that the quality of SR and meta-analysis (MA) reporting is generally poor [6,7,17]. Examination of changes in reporting quality of MAs published in Medline, Embase and the Cochrane Database of Systematic Reviews, suggested that quality had improved after the release of the QUORUM reporting guidelines [18,19]. We anticipate that increased use of PRISMA by Chinese authors will be helpful in increasing the reporting quality of SRs published in Chinese journals.

Our study has also shown that the methodological quality of Chinese SRs of TCM is poor. Areas of particular concern include lack of report of an 'a priori' design, description of status of publication used as an inclusion criterion, as well as statement of conflict of interest, all factors which may be associated with biased results. In addition, statistical mistakes appeared in one-third (29.3%) of reviews. For instance, many reviews did not explore reasons for statistical heterogeneity but simply pooled results using a random effects model to account for heterogeneity. Where heterogeneity is substantial, an overall pooling of results may be inappropriate and may lead to the incorrect interpretation of results.

One explanation for limited compliance with methodological guidelines may be that AMSTAR has not been published or promoted in Chinese journals outside of a brief abstract published in the Chinese Journal of Evidence-based Medicine in September 2010 [20]. Broader promotion of methodological quality guidelines is a necessary step in enhancing dissemination and implementation of AMSTAR.

However, our study has limitations. First, the majority of articles failed to follow the PRISMA guideline. This is likely due to the fact that the PRISMA guideline had not yet been released at the time these studies were published. Second, our study included systematic reviews published only in Chinese journals, whereas Chinese investigators increasingly publish articles in international journals. Third, we have found differential results between systematic reviews addressing herbal versus non-herbal medicines. This is possibly because reviews addressing non-herbal medicines would have studies with fewer events, resulting in absence of statistical difference of comparisons. Last, in our search, we included the terms "systematic review" and "meta-analysis". Some potentially eligible systematic review (i.e., systematic reviews needs to be plural) may, however, not use these terms in their publications.

Our purpose was to provide readers with a broad overview of the reporting and methodological characteristics of SRs of TCM published in Chinese journals. Although many such SRs have been published, the quality of these reviews is troubling. As a potential key source of information for clinicians and researchers, not only were many of these reviews incomplete, some contained mistakes or were misleading. Focusing on improving the quality of SRs of TCM, rather than continuing to publish them in great quantity, is urgently needed in order to increase the value of these studies.

Supporting Information

Text S1 Four Chinese databases search strategy and hyperlink address.
(DOC)

Text S2 Three hundred and sixty-nine systematic review of traditional chinese medicine interventions published in Chinese journals
(DOC)

Acknowledgments

We thank Dr. Denise Adams (CARE Program, Department of Pediatrics, Faculty of Medicine, University of Alberta, Edmonton, Alberta, Canada.) and Prof. Xin Sun (Center for Health Research, Northwest, Portland, Oregon, United States) for providing assistance with editing the final manuscript. We thank the library of Lanzhou University for database access and acquiring full texts.

Author Contributions

Conceived and designed the experiments: BM KY J-WG G-QQ H-ML. Analyzed the data: J-WG BM J-YP Y-LZ Y-QD. Wrote the paper: BM J-WG. Extracted data from trials: J-WG BM. Final approval of manuscript: BM J-WG G-QQ H-ML J-YP Y-LZ Y-QD K-HY.

References

1. Chen ZH, Zhang JH (1999) Troditional Chinese herbs for precancerous lesion of esophagus: a meta analysis. TCM Res 12: 20–21.
2. Petticrew M (2000) Systematic reviews from astronomy to zoology: myths and misconceptions. BMJ 322: 98–101.
3. Jadad AR, McQuay HJ (1996) Meta-analyses to evaluate analgesic interventions: a systematic qualitative review of their methodology. J Clin Epidemiol 49: 235–2343.
4. Shea B, Moher D, Graham I, Pham B, Tugwell P (2002) A comparison of the quality of Cochrane reviews and systematic reviews published in paper-based journals. Eval Health Prof 25: 116–129.
5. Moher D, Tetzlaff J, Tricco AC, Sampson M, Altman DG (2007) Epidemiology and reporting characteristics of systematic reviews. PLoS Med 4: e78.
6. Li TQ, Liu XM, Zhang MM, Ma JX, Du L, et al. (2007) Assessment of Systematic Reviews and Meta-analyses on Traditional Chinese Medicine Published in Chinese Journals. Chin J Evid-based Med 7: 180–188.
7. Liu JP, Xia Y (2007) Quality appraisal of systematic reviews or meta-analysis on traditional Chinese medicine published in Chinese journals. Zhongguo Zhong Xi Yi Jie He Za Zhi 4: 306–311.
8. ZHZANGJuhua, SHANGHongcai, GAOXiumei, et al. (2007) Methodology and reporting quality of systematic review/meta-analysis of traditional Chinese medicine. J Altern Complement Med 13: 797–805.
9. Moher D, Liberati A, Tetzlaff J, Altman DG, PRISMA Group (2010) Preferred reporting items for systematic reviews and meta-analyses: the PRISMA statement. Int J Surg 8: 336–341.
10. Shea BJ, Grimshaw JM, Wells GA, Boers M, Andersson N, et al. (2007) Development of AMSTAR: a measurement tool to assess the methodological quality of systematic reviews. BMC Med Res Methodol 7: 10.
11. Oxman AD (1994) Checklists for review articles. BMJ 309: 648–651.
12. Sacks H, Berrier J, Reitman D, Berk A, Chalmers T (1987) Meta-analyses of randomized controlled trials. N Engl J Med 316: 450–455.
13. Bessa-Nogueira RV, Vasconcelos BC, Niederman R (2008) The methodological quality of systematic reviews comparing temporomandibular joint disorder surgical and non-surgical treatment. BMC Oral Health 8: 27.
14. Wang XP, Fan GH (2010) Investigation cognition about Evidence-based Medicine. Medical information 8: 2537–2539.
15. Liu K, Guo L, Zhang L (2010) Investigation into Nursing Staff's Cognition Status of Evidence- based Medicine. Journal of Liao ning Medical University 3: 259–262.
16. Moher D, Tsertsvadze A (2006) Systematic reviews: When is an update an update? Lancet 367: 881–883.
17. Moher D, Liberati A, Tetzlaff J, Altman DG, PRISMA Group (2009) Preferred reporting items for systematic reviews and meta-analyses: the PRISMA statement. BMJ 339: b2535.
18. Moher D, Cook DJ, Eastwood S, Olkin I, Rennie D, et al. (1999) Improving the quality of reports of meta-analyses of randomised controlled trials: the QUOROM statement. Quality of Reporting of Meta-analyses. Lancet 354: 1896–1900.
19. Delaney A, Bagshaw SM, Ferland A, Manns B, Laupland KB, et al. (2005) A systematic evaluation of the quality of meta-analyses in the critical care literature. Crit Care 9: R575–R582.
20. Xiong J, Du YH (2010) Assessing tool of methodology quality for systematic reviews and meta analysis: introduction of AMSTAR. Chin J Evid-based Med 9: 44–44.

Electroacupuncture for Moderate and Severe Benign Prostatic Hyperplasia: A Randomized Controlled Trial

Yang Wang[1], Baoyan Liu[2], Jinna Yu[1], Jiani Wu[1], Jing Wang[1], Zhishun Liu[1]*

1 Guang'anmen Hospital, China Academy of Chinese Medical Sciences, Beijing, China, **2** China Academy of Chinese Medical Sciences, Beijing, China

Abstract

Purpose: To evaluate the effects of electroacupuncture (EA) on the International Prostate Symptom Score (IPSS), postvoid residual urine (PVR), and maximum urinary flow rate (Qmax), and explore the difference between EA at acupoints and non-acupoints in patients with moderate to severe benign prostate hyperplasia (BPH).

Subjects and Methods: Men with BPH and IPSS ≥8 were enrolled. Participants were randomly allocated to receive EA at acupoint (treatment group, n = 50) and EA at non-acupoint (control group, n = 50). The primary outcome measure includes the change of IPSS at the 6th week and the secondary outcome measures include changes of PVR and Qmax at the 6th week and change of IPSS at the 18th week.

Results: 100/192 patients were included. At the 6th week, treatment group patients had a 4.51 ($p<0.001$) and 4.12 ($p<0.001$) points greater decline in IPSS than the control group in the intention to treat (ITT) and per-protocol (PP) populations. At the 18th week, a 3.2 points ($p = 0.001$) greater decline was found in IPSS for the treatment. No significant differences were found between the two groups in Qmax at the 6th week ($p = 0.819$). No significant difference was observed in PVR ($P = 0.35$).

Conclusion: Acupoint EA at BL 33 had better effects on IPSS, but no difference on PVR and Qmax as compared with non-acupoint EA. The results indicate that EA is effective in improving patient's quality of life and acupoint may have better therapeutic effects than non-acupoints in acupuncture treatments of BPH.

Trial Registration: ClinicalTrials.gov NCT01218243.

Editor: Praveen Thumbikat, Northwestern University, United States of America

Funding: This study is supported by a grant from the "Twelfth Five-Year Plan" of National Science and Technology Support Program (Project Number: 2012BAI24B01) and Guang'anmen Hospital (2009S208). No other potential conflict of interest related to this trial. The funders had no role in study design, data collection and analysis, decision to publish, or preparation of the manuscript.

Competing Interests: The authors have declared that no competing interests exist.

* E-mail: liuzhishun@yahoo.com.cn

Introduction

Benign prostate hyperplasia (BPH) is an enlargement of the prostate gland due to progressive hyperplasia of the stromal and glandular cells of the prostate. The prevalence of BPH is as high as 40% in men in their fifties and 90% in men in their eighties [1]. BPH is one of the most common causes of lower urinary tract symptoms (LUTS) which include frequent urination, urgent urination, nocturia, urinary stream hesitancy, straining to void, and dribbling [1]. Although the pathophysiology of BPH is characterized by non-neoplastic histological changes, urine storage and voiding problems increase patients' risk of urinary tract infection and chronic kidney diseases and adversely affect patients' quality of life [2,3]. Current treatment options for BPH include watchful waiting, lifestyle modifications, alpha blockers, 5 alpha-reductase inhibitors, phytochemicals, and BPH-related surgery [4]. Although most of the aforementioned therapies have various degrees of documented effectiveness in the management of BPH, the use of these interventions are limited to specific patient populations or have certain side effects that interfere with patient's quality of life [5].

Acupuncture is a traditional Chinese medicine treatment which has been commonly used in the management of LUTS in China for thousands of years. The effects of acupuncture on LUTS were well documented in Chinese medicine textbooks and are well-supported by modern research studies [6]. Ricci et al [7] found that electroacupuncture (EA) had better effects in decreasing number of voiding times of urinary urgency that persisted after transurethral resection of the prostate. Kubista et al [8] found that EA could significantly increase the closing pressure in women with stress incontinence as compared with placebo, and Philp et al [9] found that acupuncture increased the bladder capacity in patients with bladder instability. Besides effects on urinary storage problems, acupuncture was also found effective in the prevention of recurrent lower urinary tract infections in adult women [10,11], in improving the quality of life in patients with chronic prostatis [12], in primary monosymptomatic nocturnal enuresis [13].

BPH is clinically characterized by various LUTS which may include or be similar to urinary urgency, stress incontinence,

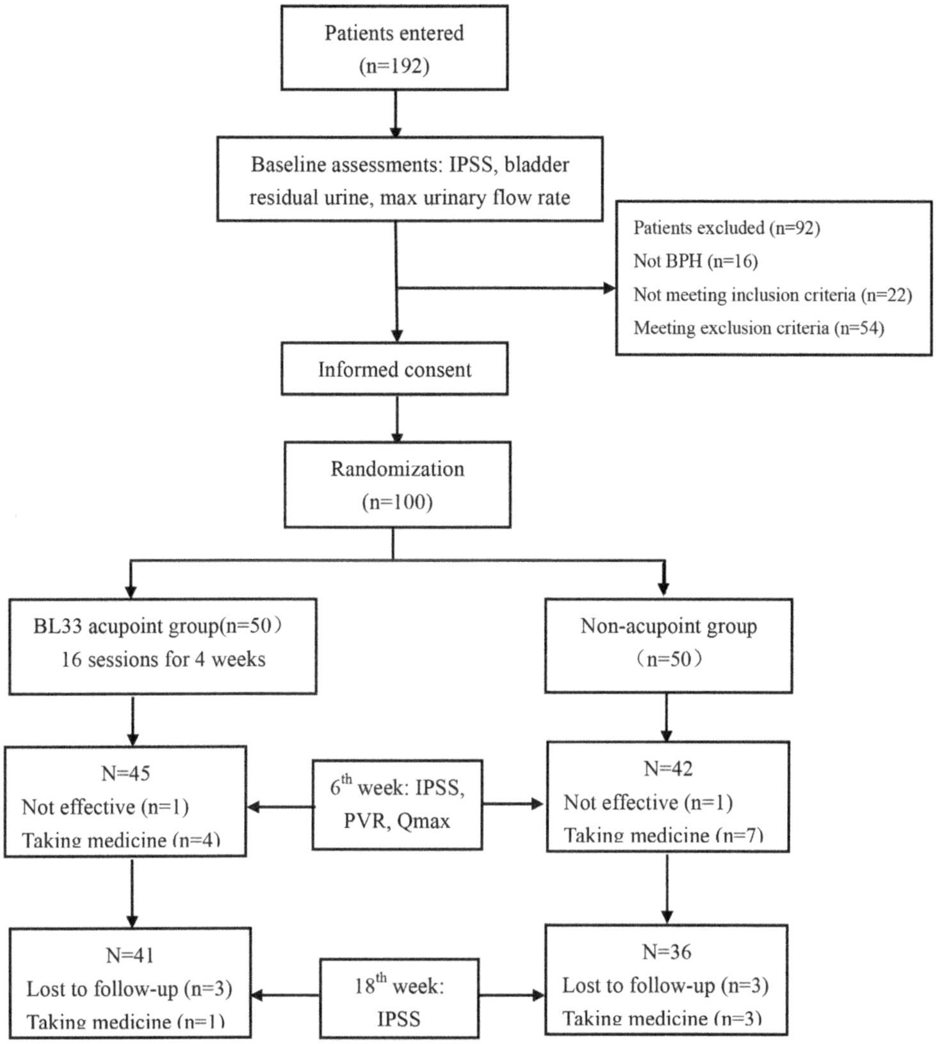

Figure 1. The flowchart of study participation.

bladder instability, and UTIs; therefore, we hypothesize that acupuncture may be effective in the management of BPH.

This hypothesis is supported by our previous studies in which we found that acupuncture at BL33 had better effects than terazosin in improving International Prostate Symptom Score (IPSS), post-void residual urine (PVR), and maximum urinary flow rate (Qmax) on patients diagnosed with mild to moderate BPH [14,15]. In addition, we also compared the therapeutic effectiveness of EA at bilateral acupoints of BL33 with EA at non-acupoints (2 cun [around 6.7 cm] lateral to BL33s) in a randomized controlled pilot study; the results demonstrated acupoint EA was more effective than non-acupoint EA in reducing IPSS [16]. However, terazosin is not necessarily the standardized treatment option for patients with BPH and the pilot study related to effects of acupoint on the EA treatment of BPH has a relative small sample size with efficacy measurements of IPSS only [14–16].

Theories of traditional Chinese medicine and results from modern studies indicate that acupoints of the fourteen meridians have specific functional regulatory effect on zang-fu organs [17–19]; however, studies in western countries found that dry needling, an acupuncture procedure at trigger points (including non-acupoints that do not belong to the meridian system), were effective in the management of various diseases [20–21]. Both dry needling and traditional acupuncture treat diseases via inserting stainless needles into the human body. However, differences between acupuncture at acupoints and acupuncture at non-acupoints have not been fully investigated. In the present study, we aimed to evaluate the effects of EA on IPSS, PVR, and Qmax, and explore the difference between EA at acupoints and non-acupoints in patients with moderate to severe BPH.

Methods

The protocol for this trial and supporting CONSORT checklist are available as supporting information; see Checklist S1 and Protocol S1.

Study Design

This was a randomized control trial which was performed at the Acupuncture Department of Guang An Men Hospital, China Academy of Chinese Medical Sciences. The study protocol was registered with ClinicalTrials. gov (Identifier: NCT01218243) and was previously published [22]. In the original study protocol, patients with IPSS score higher than 20 (including 20) were

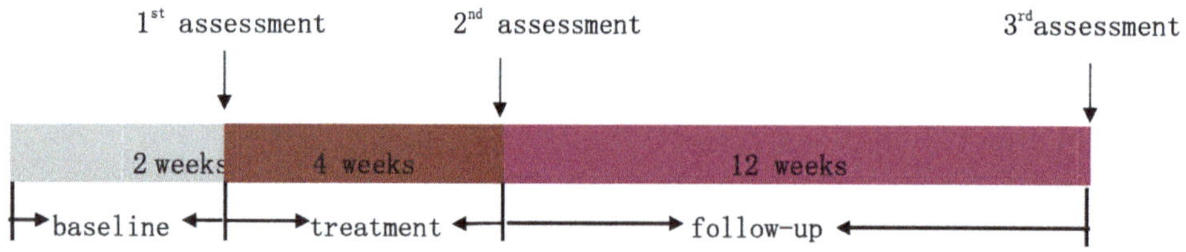

Figure 2. Time frame of each period. Figure 2 shows the time frame of baseline period, treatment period and follow-up period.

proposed to be excluded; however, we changed the inclusion criteria to patients with IPSS≥8 during the actual study, as most patients who visited the acupuncture department and were willing to participate in the study had moderate to severe BPH. The study design complies with the Consolidated Standards of Reporting Trials (CONSORT) and was approved by the hospital ethics committee. Participants were recruited through advertisements on local newspapers and posters and signed informed consent before study participation.

Sequentially numbered, opaque, sealed envelopes were distributed to patients by an investigator who was not involved in acupuncture procedures and data analyses. Based on odd or even numbers assigned in the envelope, participants were randomly allocated to receive EA at acupoint (treatment group, n = 50) and EA at non-acupoint(control group, n = 50).

Based on the results of our pilot study, the reduction of IPSS of the EA at acupointgroup was seven [16]. Therefore, in conjunction with methods and results of the studies by Chapple et al [23] and Yu et al [24], 50 patients will be needed for each group (1:1 allocation) in the present study to detect a seven point reduction in IPSS with a two-tailed significance level of 5% and a power of 90% while allowing for a 20% dropout rate. Sample size was calculated with a standard deviation (SD) of 2.30 as per reports in the epidemiology monograph by Wang [25].

Participants

For inclusion, the following criteria were fulfilled: 1) 50–70 years old; 2) mild to moderate BPH evaluated by I-PSS; 3) patients having urinary dysfunction more than 3 months; 4) patients with stable life signs; 5) not on any α1 receptor blocker, 5α-reductase inhibitor or traditional Chinese medicine for over 1 week; 6) volunteer to join this research and give informed consent prior to receiving treatment. For safety reasons, patients were instructed of possible emergency conditions and were told to seek appropriate medical help if happens.

The exclusion criteria included 1) urinary dysfunction caused by gonorrhea or urinary tract infection; 2) oliguria and anuria caused by urinary calculi, prostate cancer, bladder tumor and acute/chronic renal failure; 3) urinary dysfunction caused by neurogenic bladder, bladder neck fibrosis and urethral stricture; 4) failure of invasive therapy for prostatic obstruction; 5) injured local organs, muscle and nerve caused by pelvic operation or trauma; 6) upper urinary obstruction and hydrocoele combined with damaged renal function due to BPH diagnosed by B-ultrasound; 7) Patients unable to commit to treatment because of commuting problems to the hospital.

Initial diagnosis and assessment were made by an urologist who was not involved in the study. Patients on LUTS medications were requested to stop medications one week before baseline assessment. The baseline assessments included IPSS, PVR and Qmax.

Table 1. Demographic Information and Baseline Characteristics.

	Acupoint group (n = 50)	Non-point group (n = 50)	P-value (two-tailed)
Age	64.80±7.05	65.94±6.74	0.411
Course of disease	76.08±57.59	73.66±57.72	0.834
IPSS	20.10±6.52	18.76±6.06	0.289
Qmax	13.04±6.73	15.93±7.33	0.051
PVR (ml)	20 (0,128)	16 (0,128)	0.260

Table 2. Descriptive Statistics of ITT Population.

		Acupoint group (n = 50)	Non-point group (n = 50)
IPSS	baseline	20.10±6.52	18.76±6.06
	6th week	12.84±5.87	16.42±6.80
	Change in IPSS	7.26±5.12	2.34±4.85
	18th week	14.62±5.76	16.96±6.47
	Change in IPSS	5.48±5.16	1.8±5.06
PVR (ml)	Baseline	20 (0,128)	16 (0,128)
	6th week	20 (0,300)	15(0,180)
	Change in PVR	0 (−172,84)	0 (−120,80)
Qmax,	Baseline	13.04±6.73	15.93±7.33
	6th week	12.63±6.11	15.00±6.50
	Change in Qmax	0.36±4.51	0.98±4.05

Acupuncture protocol

Huatuo brand needles (size 0.30 mm×100 mm, manufactured by Suzhou Medical Appliance, Suzhou, Jiangsu Province, China) together with GB6805-2 Electro-Acu Stimulators (HuayiMedical Supply &Equipment Co., Ltd, Shanghai, China) were used. In traditional Chinese medicine, acupuncture at Baliao points (BL31-34) are commonly used as treatment options for LUTS, lumbodynia, and reproductive disorders [6]; our previous study confirmed the effects of acupuncture at BL33 on LUTS [14–16]. In the present study, BL33s were used in the acupoint treatment group; whereas the two points which are 2 cun (around 6.7 cm) lateral to BL33s were used in the non-acupoint control group. Localization of BL33 which corresponds with the third sacral foramen was reported previously [26]. In order to accuratelylocalize bilateral BL33, a line is drawn between the two posterior superior iliac spines (PSIS) which cross over at point A of the spinal column. Then, each PSIS and point A are connected to construct two separate lines. Finally, two different equilateral triangles are drawn inferiorly and the apexes B and C of these two equilateral triangles are the two BL33 acupoints. The acupuncturists inserted acupuncture needles at BL33obliquely at an angle of about 45° for about 6 cm–8 cm until the patient felt heaviness and numbness locally or even with radiation sensation to the genitalia. Acupuncture procedures were performed bilaterally at two BL33 acupoints and electrodes of the electric stimulator were attached to the handle of the needle bilaterally. Disperse-dense wave, 20 Hz electric current was used in the present study. The intensity of electric current was increased to the patients' maximum tolerance and then slightly reduced to a bearable level. Acupuncture treatment protocol and electric stimulator parameters were the same for non-acupoint acupuncture procedures in the control group, except for the genitalial radiating sensation upon acupuncture.

Patients received a total of 16 sessions of acupuncture treatment which include five sessions in the 1st and 2nd week, acupuncture once a day; three sessions in the 3rd and 4th week, acupuncture every other day. Acupuncture procedures were implemented by an acupuncturist with more than 10 years' clinical experience. Data management and analysis were performed by researchers who were blinded to the acupuncture procedures.

Outcome Assessment

All patients were evaluated during the first week for baseline values which include IPSS, PVR, and Qmax. The primary outcome involves the change of IPSS at the 6th week; secondary outcomes include the changes of PVR, Qmax at the 6th week and change of IPSS at the 18th week. Safety evaluation includes hematoma, fainting, severe pain, and local infection during and after acupuncture. In addition, emergency conditions which require catheterization were also recorded if any.

Statistical analysis

The statistical analysis was performed by a statistician blinded to treatment allocation in the Clinical Evaluation Center of China Academy of Chinese Medical Sciences. SPSS statistical package program (ver.16.0) was used and a significance level was set at $\alpha<0.05$. Data analysis of baseline characteristics was based on the intention-to-treat (ITT) population which included all participants who were randomized. Primary and secondary outcomes were mainly based on the data of the ITT population; however, primary outcome was also analyzed based on per-protocol (PP) population as an extra supportive analysis. Quantitative data of IPSS and Qmax were expressed with mean±SD; PVR was expresses as Range (Median) as the data was not normally distributed. For primary and secondary outcome measures, analysis of covariance was used to investigate the differences between acupoint acupuncture and non-acupoint acupuncture on IPSS and Qmax. Changes of the IPSS and Qmax after treatment were the dependent variable, the group was the fixed factor and the baseline data were the covariate. The Mann Whitney U test was used for the analysis of PVR.

Table 3. Descriptive statistics of PP population.

		Acupoint group (n=45)	Non-point group (n=42)
IPSS	Baseline	19.84±6.46	18.83±6.00
	6th week	12.60±5.85	16.05±6.83
	Change in IPSS	7.24±5.23	2.79±5.17

Results

From September, 2010 to May, 2012, a total of 192 patients with LUTS visited the Acupuncture Department at Guang'anmen Hospital in Beijing. 92 patients were excluded from the present study for the following reasons: 16 did not have BPH; 22 did not meet the inclusion criteria; 54 met the exclusion criteria. 100 of them were included and equally randomized to receive acupoint acupuncture and non-acupoint acupuncture treatments (Figure 1). Figure 2 details the time frames of recruitment, treatment and follow-up periods.

Demographic characteristics and baseline information of the 100 participants are shown in Table 1. 25 patients in the acupoint acupuncture group and 23 in the non-acupoint control group were diagnosed as severe BPH (IPSS≥20). No statistically significant differences were found between the two groups in age, gender, and baseline values. The mean age of all participants was 65.37±6.89 years old.

IPSS

Analyses of IPSS at the 6th week were based on both of ITT population and PP population (See Table 2 and Table 3). At the 6th week, the ITT analysis indicated that IPSS reduced from 20.10±6.52 at baseline to 12.84±5.87 for the acupoint treatment group, and from 18.76±6.06 at baseline to 16.42±6.80 for non-point control group. With the PP analysis, IPSS of the two groups reduced to 12.60±5.85 and 16.05±6.83 respectively. At the 6th week, acupoint group patients had a 4.51 ($p<0.001$) and 4.12 ($p<0.001$) points greater decline than the non-acupoint control group in the ITT and PP populations respectively (Table 4). At the 18th week, a 3.2 points ($p=0.001$) greater decline was found for the acupoint treatment group as compared with the non-acupoint control group.

Qmax and PVR

No significant differences were found between the two groups in Qmax at the 6th week ($p=0.819$, Table 4). PVR data followed a non-normal distribution and no significant difference was found ($P=0.35$).

Adverse Events

No serious adverse events happened in eithergroups. Two cases of mild hematoma were reported in the non-acupoint control group during study. The patients were told to apply ice and compression within 24 hours and heat compression after 24 hours to the acupuncture treatment areas. Hematoma disappeared in about two weeks.

Discussion

The results of this trial showed that greater decrease in IPSS in the BL33 group than in the non-acupoint group, but no significant difference was found in Qmax and PVR. The change of IPSS indicates that EA at acupoints significantly improved the quality of life in patients diagnosed with BPH. The IPSS change matched the results of our previous studies and added further credence in the use of acupuncture for patients with BPH [14–16]. The IPSS was decreased by 7.26 (from20.10 to 12.84, $P=0.000$) and 2.34 (from 18.76 to 16.42, $P=0.001$) in BL33 acupoint EA group and

Table 4. ANCOVA estimation of outcomes.

		Treatment effect estimate (Mean difference)	Standard error	P-value
IPSS (ITT)	6th week	4.51	0.93	0.000
	18th week	3.20	0.93	0.001
IPSS (PP)	6th week	4.12	1.03	0.000
Qmax(ITT)	6th week	0.18	0.80	0.819

ANCOVA: Analysis of Covariance.

the non-point EA group respectively. Compared to the non-point control group, the acupoint group was associated with a 4.51-point greater decline in IPSS at the 6th week ($P<0.01$). The difference of IPSS decrease indicates that EA at acupoints had significantly better effects than EA at non-acupoint on the quality of life in patients diagnosed with BPH. As EA procedures at both acupoint and non-acupoint share the same electric stimulation parameters and same EA protocol, the specificity of needling site at BL33 acupoint may be accountable for the difference in IPSS in the present study. This echoed the results of our pilot study stating that acupoints have better effects than non-acupoints [16]. The results of the present study also increases the credibility of results of other related studies indicating that the acupoint of the meridian system seem to have specific functional regulatory effects compared to non-acupoints [17–19].

In a similar trial comparing EA with sham EA (shallow needle insertion of 2 mm) for BPH, greater increase of Qmax was found in the EA group than the sham EA group; whereas IPSS was similar in both groups [27]. With a close analysis, acupoints use, manipulation methods, parameters of EA and number, frequency and duration of treatment sessions could all cause the differences between the two studies. Nonetheless, both studies demonstrated that standard EA at acupoint had better effects than EA with shallow needle insertion of 2 mm or EA at non-acupoints on at least certain clinical parameter(s). In addition, IPSS improve in the present study is also supported by results from the study by Johnstone et al [28] in which some difference in IPSS ($p = 0.063$) was found between acupuncture and blank control. As only 20 out of 30 patients were treated with acupuncture in the study by Johnstone et al [28], the p value is likely to drop to lower than 0.05 if the sample size is increased. Consequently, we should believe the specificity of acupoints in acupuncture treatment even though the mechanism of acupuncture at acupoints has not been fully elucidated.

Studies demonstrate that sacral neuromodulation could improve symptoms of overactive bladder [29–30]. As BL33 is actually the third sacral nerve which travels through the 3rd sacral foramen, we should believe that EA at BL33 is actually one type of sacral neuromodulation. Sacral acupuncture was found to be effective in improving symptoms of acetic acid-induced bladder irritation in rats through inhibition of capsaicin-sensitive C-fiber activation [31]. Therefore, EA for BPH may be related to acupuncture sacral neuromododulation.

Although the exact mechanism of EA treatment for BPH has yet to be clarified, researchers believe that the effects of acupuncture are less likely to be related to histological changes of the prostate, as no difference was found in PSA levels, between sham and vera EA and between acupuncture and blank control [27,28]. As results of acupuncture fMRI studies showed a significant connection between brain activities and acupuncture procedures, and the human brain is closely involved in the sensation and control of the lower urinary system [32–34], we should also believe that brain modulation by acupuncture may also play a role in the effects of EA on BPH. This was confirmed by in-vivo animal study in which Chung et al [35] found that expression of c-Fos expression in the pontine micturition center (PMC), ventrolateral periaqueductal gray (vlPAG), and medial preoptic nucleus (MPA) was increased in stress urinary incontinence, and acupuncture significantly decreased c-Fos expression in these areas. Nonetheless, further studies are needed to explore the mechanism of acupuncture on BPH.

Limitations

As blinding is difficult in acupuncture studies, real randomized placebo controlled trials seem impossible. Although non-acupoint EA procedures were used as control in the present study, they are still acupuncture procedures; thus we could not rule out the confounding factor of needling and placebo effects in the present study. Patients in the present study were only treated for 4 weeks and followed up till the 18th week, long term effects and optimal treatment regimens of EA for BPH remain to be established. In addition, this RCT was performed in only one hospital rather than multi-centers; therefore, the results of the present study may not well-characterize the general response of patients with BPH in the world. To further test the therapeutic effects of EA on BPH, further large scale, multi-center, international cooperative studies are warranted.

Conclusion

In the present study, acupoint EA at BL 33 had better effects on IPSS, but no difference on PVR and Qmax as compared with non-acupoint EA. The results indicate that EA is effective in improving patient's quality of life and acupoint may have better therapeutic effects than non-acupoints in acupuncture treatments of BPH.

Supporting Information

Checklist S1 CONSORT Checklist.
(PDF)

Protocol S1 Trial Protocol.
(PDF)

Author Contributions

Conceived and designed the trial: ZL. Contributed materials: BL. Performed the trial: JY J. Wu. Analyzed the data: J. Wang. Wrote the paper: YW.

References

1. Nickel JC (2006) The overlapping lower urinary tract symptoms of benign prostatic hyperplasia and prostatitis. CurrOpinUrol 16: 5–10.
2. Hong SK, Lee ST, Jeong SJ, Byun SS, Hong YK, et al (2010) Chronic kidney disease among men with lower urinary tract symptoms due to benign prostatic hyperplasia. BJU Int 105(10): 1424–8.
3. Bruskewitz RC (2003) Quality of Life and Sexual Function in Patients with Benign Prostatic Hyperplasia. Rev Urol 5: 72–80.
4. Tanguay S, Awde M, Brock G, Casey R, Kozak J, et al (2009) Diagnosis and management of benign prostatic hyperplasia in primary care. Can UrolAssoc J 3(3 Suppl 2): S92–S100.
5. American Urology Association (2012) Guideline on the Management of Benign Prostatic Hyperplasia. http://www.auanet.org/content/guidelines-and-quality-care/clinical-guidelines/main-reports/bph-management/chap_1_GuidelineManagementof(BPH). pdf (accessed 1/31/2013).
6. Wang QC (2003) Acupuncture therapeutics. Beijing: China Traditional Chinese Medicine Publishing.
7. Ricci L, Minardi D, Romoli M, Galosi AB, Muzzonigro G (2004) Acupuncture reflexotherapy in the treatment of sensory urgency that persists after transurethral resection of the prostate: a preliminary report. NeurourolUrodyn 23(1): 58–62.
8. Kubista E, Altmann P, Kucera H, Rudelstorfer B (1976) Electro-acupuncture's influence on the closure mechanism of the female urethra in incontinence. Am J Chin Med (Gard City N Y) 4(2): 177–81.
9. Philp T, Shah PJ, Worth PH (1988) Acupuncture in the treatment of bladder instability. Br J Urol 61(6): 490–3.
10. Aune A, Alraek T, LiHua H, Baerheim A (1998) Acupuncture in the prophylaxis of recurrent lower urinary tract infection in adult women. Scand J Prim Health Care 16(1): 37–9.
11. Alraek T, Soedal LI, Fagerheim SU, Digranes A, Baerheim A (2002) Acupuncture treatment in the prevention of uncomplicated recurrent lower urinary tract infections in adult women. Am J Public Health 92(10): 1609–11.
12. Capodice JL, Jin Z, Bemis DL, Samadi D, Stone BA, et al (2007) A pilot study on acupuncture for lower urinary tract symptoms related to chronic prostatitis/chronic pelvic pain. Chin Med 6;2: 1.
13. Karaman MI, Koca O, Küçük EV, Öztürk M, Güneş M (2010) Laser acupuncture therapy for primary monosymptomatic nocturnal enuresis. J Urol 185(5): 1852–6.
14. Yang T, Zhang XQ, Feng YW, Xu HR, Liu ZS, et al (2008) Efficacy of Electroacupuncture in Treating 93 Patients with Benign Prostatic Hyperplasia. Chinese Journal of Integrated Traditional and Western Medicine 28(11): 998–1000.
15. Yang T, Liu ZS, Zhang XQ, Feng YW, Xu HR, et al (2008) Evaluation on therapeutic effects of electroacupuncture for benign prostatic hyperplasia: A prospective randomized controlled study. Chinese Journal of Rehabilitation Medicine 23(11): 1028–1031.
16. Ding Y, Yu J, Liu Z (2011) A pilot trial of point speciality using electroacupuncture at Zhongliao point for benign prostatic hyperplasia. Journal of Clinical Acupuncture and Moxibustion 27(7): 1–4.
17. Shuran J, Zhongsuan H (1987) Specific effect of acupuncture at ST36 for visceral pain. Acupuncture Reaearch 1: 73–76.
18. Cheng K, Han Y (2004) Study on the Specificity of Effects of Acupuncture of Different Acupoints in Reducing Gentamycin Induced Ototoxicity in Guinea-pigs. Acupuncture Reaearch 29(3): 204–208.
19. Xu B, Yu XC, Chen CY, Wang LL, Liu JL, et al (2010) Relationship Between Efficacy of Electroacupuncture and Electroacupuncture Stimulation of Different Acupoints and Different Tissue Layers of Acupoint Area in Hypotension plus Bradycardia Rats. Acupuncture Reaearch 35(6): 422–428.
20. Dıraçoğlu D, Vural M, Karan A, Aksoy C (2012) Effectiveness of dry needling for the treatment of temporomandibularmyofascial pain: a double-blind, randomized, placebo controlled study. J Back MusculoskeletRehabil 25(4): 285–90.
21. Kalichman L, VulfsonsS (2010) Dry needling in the management of musculoskeletal pain. J Am Board Fam Med 23(5): 640–6.
22. Wang Y, Liu ZS, Yu JN, Ding TL, Liu X (2011) Efficacy of electroacupuncture at Zhongliao point (BL33) for mild and moderate benign prostatci hyperplasia: study protocol for a randomized controlled trial. Trials 12: 211.
23. Chapple RC, Montorsi F, Teuvo LJT, Wirth M, Koldewijn E, et al (2011) Silodosin therapy for lower urinary tract symptoms in men with Suspected Benign Prostatic Hyperplasia: Results of an International, Randomized, Double-Blind, Placebo- and Active-Controlled Clinical Trial Performed in Europe. European Urology 59: 342–352.
24. Yu HJ, Lin AT, Yang SS, Tsui KH, Wu HC, et al (2011) Non-inferiority of silodosin to tamsulosin in treating patients with lower urinary tract symptoms (LUTS) associated with benign prostatic hyperplasia (BPH). BJU INTERNATIONAL 108(11): 1843–1848.
25. Wang J (2001) Clinical Epidemiology-design, measurement and evaluation. Shanghai: Shanghai Science and Technology Press: 41–142.
26. Liu ZS, Zhou KH, Wang Y, Pan YX(2011)Electroacupuncture improves voiding function in patients with neurogenic urinary retention secondary to caudaequina injury: results from a prospective observational study. Acupunct Med 29(3): 188–192.
27. Yu JS, Shen KH, Chen WC, Her JS, Hsieh CL (2011) Effects of Electroacupuncture on Benign Prostate Hyperplasia Patients with Lower Urinary Tract Symptoms: A Single-Blinded, Randomized Controlled Trial. Evidence-Based Complementary and Alternative Medicine 20: 303198.
28. Johnstone PA, Bloom TL, Niemtzow RC, Crain D, Riffenburgh RH, et al (2003) A prospective, randomized pilot trial of acupuncture of the kidney-bladder distinct meridian for lower urinary tract symptoms. J Urol 169(3): 1037–9.
29. Wendy WL, Michael BC (2005) How does Nerve Stimulation Neuromodulation Works. UrolClin N Am 32: 11–18.
30. Vignes JR, De Seze M, Dobremez E (2005) Sacralneuromodulaiton in lower urinary tract dysfunction. Adv Tech Stand Neurosurg 30: 177–224.
31. Hino K, Honjo H, Nakao M, Kitakoji H (2010) The Effects of Sacral Acupuncture on Acetic Acid-induced Bladder Irritation in Conscious Rats. Urology 75: 730–734.
32. Fang J, Jin Z, Wang Y, Li K, Kong J, et al (2009). The salient characteristics of the central effects of acupuncture needling: limbic-paralimbic-neocortical network modulation. Hum Brain Mapp 30(4): 1196–206.
33. Fang J, Wang X, Liu H, Wang Y, Zhou K, et al (2012) The Limbic-Prefrontal Network Modulated by Electroacupuncture at CV4 and CV12. Evid Based Complement Alternat Med 2012: 515893.
34. Napadow V, Lee J, Kim J, Cina S, Maeda Y, et al (2012). Brain correlates of phasic autonomic response to acupuncture stimulation: An event-related fMRI study. Hum Brain Mapp 000: 00–00.
35. Chung IM, Kim YS, Sung YH, Kim SE, Ko IG, et al (2008) Effects of acupuncture on abdominal leak point pressure and c-Fos expression in the brain of rats with stress urinary incontinence. NeurosciLett 439(1): 18–23.

16

Sub-Typing of Rheumatic Diseases Based on a Systems Diagnosis Questionnaire

Herman A. van Wietmarschen[1,2]*, Theo H. Reijmers[1,3], Anita J. van der Kooij[4], Jan Schroën[2,5], Heng Wei[2,6], Thomas Hankemeier[1,2,3], Jacqueline J. Meulman[4], Jan van der Greef[1,2,6]

1 Division of Analytical Biosciences, LACDR, Leiden University, Leiden, The Netherlands, 2 Sino-Dutch Centre for Preventive and Personalized Medicine, Zeist, The Netherlands, 3 Netherlands Metabolomics Centre, Leiden University, Leiden, The Netherlands, 4 Mathematical Institute, Leiden University, Leiden, The Netherlands, 5 Oxrider, Education and Research, Nieuwegein, The Netherlands, 6 TNO, Zeist, The Netherlands

Abstract

Background: The future of personalized medicine depends on advanced diagnostic tools to characterize responders and non-responders to treatment. Systems diagnosis is a new approach which aims to capture a large amount of symptom information from patients to characterize relevant sub-groups.

Methodology: 49 patients with a rheumatic disease were characterized using a systems diagnosis questionnaire containing 106 questions based on Chinese and Western medicine symptoms. Categorical principal component analysis (CATPCA) was used to discover differences in symptom patterns between the patients. Two Chinese medicine experts where subsequently asked to rank the Cold and Heat status of all the patients based on the questionnaires. These rankings were used to study the Cold and Heat symptoms used by these practitioners.

Findings: The CATPCA analysis results in three dimensions. The first dimension is a general factor (40.2% explained variance). In the second dimension (12.5% explained variance) 'anxious', 'worrying', 'uneasy feeling' and 'distressed' were interpreted as the Internal disease stage, and 'aggravate in wind', 'fear of wind' and 'aversion to cold' as the External disease stage. In the third dimension (10.4% explained variance) 'panting s', 'superficial breathing', 'shortness of breath s', 'shortness of breath f' and 'aversion to cold' were interpreted as Cold and 'restless', 'nervous', 'warm feeling', 'dry mouth s' and 'thirst' as Heat related. 'Aversion to cold', 'fear of wind' and 'pain aggravates with cold' are most related to the experts Cold rankings and 'aversion to heat', 'fullness of chest' and 'dry mouth' to the Heat rankings.

Conclusions: This study shows that the presented systems diagnosis questionnaire is able to identify groups of symptoms that are relevant for sub-typing patients with a rheumatic disease.

Editor: Vladimir Brusic, Dana-Farber Cancer Institute, United States of America

Funding: This work was sponsored by the Netherlands Genomics Initiative, Chinese Academy of Sciences, Ministry of Science and Technology (China) (Grant No.: 2009DFA41250, 2007DFA31060, 2006BAI11B07), TNO (NL), Netherlands Metabolomics Center, The Sino-Dutch Centre for Preventive and Personalized Medicine, the National Genomics Initiative and the Osteo- and Rheumatoid Arthritis Foundation (NL). The funders had no role in study design, data collection and analysis, decision to publish, or preparation of the manuscript.

Competing Interests: The authors have declared that no competing interests exist.

* E-mail: h.vanwietmarschen@lacdr.leidenuniv.nl

Introduction

Pharmacological disease management strategies for rheumatoid arthritis (RA) are for an important part based on trial and error. In general less than 53% of RA patients with a disease duration of less than one year show a positive ACR20 response to treatment [1]. This number goes down to 38% for patients with 5–10 years of RA. Even 30% of RA patients initiating the most effective and expensive treatment option available, anti-TNF therapy, fail to respond [2]. Non-responders are switched to other drugs until one is found that gives the desired effect [3]. A similar trial and error approach is often used for the treatment of osteoarthritis and fibromyalgia as well. The result is that a considerable number of patients experience no benefits from a treatment but just the side effects.

Rheumatoid arthritis patients as well as patients with other rheumatic diseases could benefit substantially from a shift towards a personalized medicine approach which aims to get the right treatment to the right patient, in the right dose, at the right time and via the right route [4,5]. In the traditional approach, patients are classified as according to criteria specified by the American College of Rheumatology (ACR). A single disease management strategy that is specifically developed for treating the particular type of rheumatic disease will then be applied. A more personalized approach will go beyond the ACR classification and will require much more information about the patient and his or her environment [6]. Specific individual patient situations require specific types of treatment, which can consist of specific drugs, life-style changes, psychological support and other interactions depending on the wish of the patient [7].

The challenge for personalized medicine is to characterize groups of patients and relate these groups to certain treatment options. Modern systems biology technologies such as genomics, proteomics and metabolomics [8–10] are currently able to generate an enormous amount of data, which can be seen as signs defined as manifestations that are measured. Several clinical features and molecular markers have been identified for example to sub-type RA patients [11,12]. Anti-citrullinated protein antibodies positive or negative status is found to be related to distinctive RA risk profiles [13]. More inflamed joints and a higher level of joint destruction was reported in Anti-citrullinated protein antibodies positive RA patients [14]. A large dissimilarity has been found in gene expression profiles of INF-1 high and low sub-types of RA patients, but this is not very clear in the clinical features of patients [15]. Unfortunately, this knowledge has not resulted in personalized health strategies in clinical practice yet, which illustrates that searching for clinically relevant subtypes without clear indications of what to look for and based mostly on signs is difficult.

Symptoms, manifestations that are observed by the patient himself, are on the other hand a subjective type of information which is actually much closer to the phenotype of the patient than signs. Symptoms therefore provide an extra dimension of information. A wide variety of symptoms can be collected related to physical manifestations but also to the psychology, the family, the environment, and worldview of the patient which is well known to play a large role in arthritis [16–19].

Diagnosis is the key process in which symptoms and signs are used by a medical practitioner to distinguish the state of a person as different from the 'normal' situation. It is used to differentiate one disease from another and it is used to base treatment on. A move towards personalized medicine needs an optimization and refinement of this diagnostic process. One way is to expand it by including more symptoms than currently in use [20].

Chinese medicine diagnosis is a systems diagnosis approach that takes into account a broad spectrum of symptoms (as reported by the patient) as well as signs observed by the practitioner by listening to the body, feeling the body and observation of the patient [21]. Constitutional, behavioral and social aspects are also considered in the diagnosis and the choice of treatment. In Chinese medicine, rheumatoid arthritis as well as other rheumatic diseases fall into a group of diseases termed Bi-syndromes. A Bi-syndrome is characterized by the presence or absence of over 100 symptoms [22].

Symptoms are related to one or more symptom patterns which are called syndromes in Chinese medicine. These patterns or syndromes lead to treatment principles on which particular treatments are based. Recently two particular patterns of symptoms have been studied more closely [23]. These patterns are called Cold and Heat and are general patterns of symptoms much used in Chinese medicine [21,24]. The Cold pattern can be described as severe pain in a joint or muscle that limits the range of comfortable movement, the pain does not move to other locations. The pain is relieved by applying warmth to the affected area, but increases with exposure to cold. Loose stools are characteristic also, as well as an absence of thirst and clear profuse urine. A thin white tongue coating is seen, combined with a wiry and tight pulse. In contrast, the Heat pattern is characterized by severe pain with hot, red, swollen and inflamed joints. Pain is generally relieved by applying cold to the joints. Other symptoms include fever, thirst, a flushed face, irritability, restlessness, constipation and deep-colored urine. The tongue may be red with a yellow coating and the pulse may be rapid [25].

In a recent study [26] differences have been found between RA Cold and Heat patients when looking at symptoms, gene expression, and metabolomics profiles. Interestingly, the differences turned out to be related to apoptosis, an important biological process. The RA Heat group showed more activity of apoptosis related genes than the RA Cold group. Lu and others found that RA patients with the Cold pattern responded better to biomedical combination therapy (diclofenac, methotrexate, sulfasalazine) than did patients with RA with a Heat pattern, at 12 weeks and 24 weeks of treatment [27]. These findings show that sub-grouping of RA patients using knowledge from Chinese medicine diagnosis can lead to more personalized treatment in RA. Especially the Cold and Heat groups are promising for optimizing treatment.

The objective of the study is to analyze similarities and differences between patients with a rheumatic disease with respect to their symptoms. A questionnaire was therefore designed to establish a systems diagnosis of patients with a rheumatic disease based on a range of symptoms that are used in Chinese and Western medicine. A second objective is to analyze the Cold and Heat status of these patients based on the questionnaire results and an evaluation of the questionnaires by Chinese medicine experts.

Network analysis concepts were used to visualize the relationships between the symptoms and the corresponding syndromes according to Chinese medicine theory, as well as the relationships observed in patients. Categorical principal component analysis was used to find similarities and differences between the patients. The results were interpreted using theoretical and expert knowledge about symptoms and syndromes.

The following part of the analysis focused on the absence and presence of Cold and Heat related symptoms in the patients. Two Chinese medicine experts were asked to rank the Cold and Heat status of each patient on a seven point scale, based on the questionnaire results. These Cold and Heat rankings were introduced as an extra source of information in the categorical principal component analysis. The results were interpreted using Western and Chinese perspectives on arthritis-like diseases. Finally, several suggestions for creating diagnostic tools using the presented systems diagnosis approach will be discussed, which can lead to new opportunities to advance personalized medicine for rheumatic diseases.

Materials and Methods

Design of the questionnaire

The questionnaire was designed to establish a systems diagnosis of patients with rheumatic diseases (see Text S1). Symptoms described as related to Bi-syndromes [28] and reviewed by two Chinese medicine experts were used to create a list of 106 questions related to these symptoms divided into nine areas: location of the symptoms, breathing, climate, digestion, emotions & behaviour, quality of the symptoms, changes in the symptoms, pain, and urination. For most of these questions the 7-point Likert scale [29], was used to assess the frequency or the strength of a symptom. A score of 1 means never or not present, while a score of 7 would mean very frequent or very strongly present. Some of the questions were in binary, yes or no, format.

The questionnaire also represents a number of symptoms used in Western medicine to assess disease activity and the response to treatment, for example 'stiff joints', 'joint pain' and 'swollen joints' [30]. In addition to the questions related to symptoms, some general questions were included concerning disease history, medication, and arthritis related blood factors. The full questionnaire is added as supplementary information.

The questionnaire was designed to reflect Chinese thinking and diagnosis by extensive discussions with two Chinese medicine experts. Additionally, the questionnaire was reviewed by the scientific committee of the two Dutch professional organizations for Chinese medicine practitioners in the field of acupuncture

(Nederlandse Vereniging voor Acupuntuur) and Nederlandse Artsen Acupunctuur Vereniging).

The medical ethical committee of the Leiden University Medical Center was notified of the study before the questionnaire was send out to patients and waived the need for further approval of the study by the medical ethical committee. All participants were informed about the study the data was going to be used for either by e-mail or verbal communication. All participants gave an informed consent in an e-mail or verbally to this use of the data.

Study sample

People with one or more rheumatic diseases were invited to participate in this study by completing a questionnaire. A small invitation text was published on the website of the Osteo- and Rheumatoid Arthritis Foundation in Amsterdam, the Netherlands, http://www.reuma-stichting.nl. The invitation was also published in one of the newsletters of the foundation. Additionally, the questionnaire accompanied with an explanation of the purpose of the study was send to all members of the Netherlands Acupuncture Society.

A total of 91 people requested to participate in the study. A questionnaire was send of which 52 were returned. Three questionnaires could not be used for the analysis: one was missing a full page of answers, of another one only the first page was completed and a third questionnaire contained 11 incorrectly filled answers. Table 1 summarizes the types of rheumatic diseases most prevalent in the respondents and the most used medication.

Data screening and recoding

Before data analysis, the consistency of the data was checked. Inconsistent answers to follow-up questions or to questions requiring a severity and frequency score for the same symptom were converted to missing. For example, if the answer to the question 'Do you feel cold?' is no, the answer to the follow-up question 'Is this cold located mostly in the feet or legs?' should only be no, which is not always the case. The question labeled 'sighing' was removed because multiple interpretations were possible and 'affected parts heavy' was completely covered by 'heavy feeling' and therefore also removed.

Table 1. Characteristics of the respondents.

Rheumatic disease*		**Medication**	
Osteoarthritis	24	Diclofenac	11
Rheumatoid arthritis	11	Ibuprofen	7
Fibromyalgia	5	Paracetamol	6
Systemic lupus erythematosus	2	Prednison	6
Missing entry	4	Methotrexate	5
Other rheumatic disease	10	Hydroxychloroquine	4
		Tramadol	4
		Etoricoxib	3
		Naproxen	2
		Celecoxib	2
		Other medication	15
		No medication	6
		No entry	5

*10 respondents have a combination of two rheumatic diseases.

Most questions contain categories in which only a few patients had a score, which is unfavorable in CATPCA because it may lead to unstable results [31]. Therefore, we merged categories with a frequency less than 7 (the square root of the number of patients) with an adjacent category. This resulted in 10 variables with only a single category which were therefore removed: 'vomiting', 'nightmares', 'joints bend', 'joints stretch', 'tired with slight exertion', 'symptoms wander', 'upper part affected', 'symptoms appear suddenly', 'pain appears slowly', 'pain with redness and swelling'. The variable 'joint pain' was removed because one of the two categories had only four observations. The final dataset used for the CATPCA analysis contained 93 variables.

Network analysis

In Chinese medicine the focus is more on relationships between symptoms than on the symptoms themselves. The symptoms involved in the Bi-syndromes form a network of relationships. Network theory [32–34] therefore offers a perfect set of concepts to visualize and analyze the network properties of the Bi-syndromes. Cytoscape version 2.6.3 [35], an open source network visualization and annotation package, was used to create a network (graph) of the questionnaire. The position of the nodes was calculated using an algorithm [36] implemented in Cytoscape which minimizes the total length of the edges in the graph. An example is given of how the symptom scores of a patient can be mapped on the network. The questionnaire scores are represented in the graph as the weights of the relationships (edges) between symptoms and the corresponding syndromes. Such a symptom fingerprint can be used by a practitioner to get an overview of the symptom patterns for a particular patient.

Categorical principal component analysis

To explore the similarities and differences between the patients with respect to the set of 93 variables, Principal Component Analysis (PCA) would be the appropriate method. However, since our data are categorical, standard PCA is not suitable. Nonlinear Principal Component Analysis (NLPCA) is a method that can deal with categorical data and is therefore the method of choice. NLPCA finds the parameters of the PCA model in an iterative process in which "Optimal Scaling" is incorporated. Optimal Scaling is a technique that finds optimal quantifications for categorical variables. The quantifications are optimal in the sense that the percentage of variance of the *quantified* variables accounted for by the principal components is maximal. NLPCA is available in SAS [37] as PRINQUAL [38,39], and in SPSS [40] as CATPCA [41,42]. In this study we have used CATPCA in SPSS version 17.0.

The number of principal components was determined using parallel analysis [43,44] with permuted data [45]. We used 100 data sets with random permutation within all variables. Because CATPCA maximizes the eigenvalues of the first P components (with P the number of components specified by the user), solutions with different numbers of components are not nested. For instance, the two components in a two-component solution are not equal to the first two components of a three-component solution. Therefore, multiple parallel analyses might be required: If the parallel analysis for the one-component solution shows a significant eigenvalue (greater than the 95th percentile of the random eigenvalues) for the second component, the parallel analysis is repeated for the two-component solution. Then the significance of the third eigenvalue is checked, etc., until the $(P+1)^{th}$ eigenvalue of a P-component solution is not significant, then P is the chosen number of components.

After determining the number of principal components, variables with a total variance accounted for (VAF) ≥50% and another set of variables with a total VAF ≥60% were selected for further analysis. With these two sets of variables the procedure of determining the number of components as described above was repeated (Figure 1).

The loadings resulting from the two CATPCA models were compared with the theoretical relationships between symptoms and syndromes. The two resulting models were interpreted by a Chinese medicine expert. The interpretability determined which of the two sets of variables were the most appropriate for further analysis.

The next part of the analysis focused on the Cold and Heat status of patients and the ability of the questionnaire to provide information on this status. Two Chinese medicine experts (expert 1 and expert 2) were asked which symptoms they deemed most important for Cold and Heat. The two Chinese medicine experts were also asked to determine the Cold and Heat status of each patient based on the questionnaire scores. In the subsequent analysis therefore there are four sources of information: 1) the

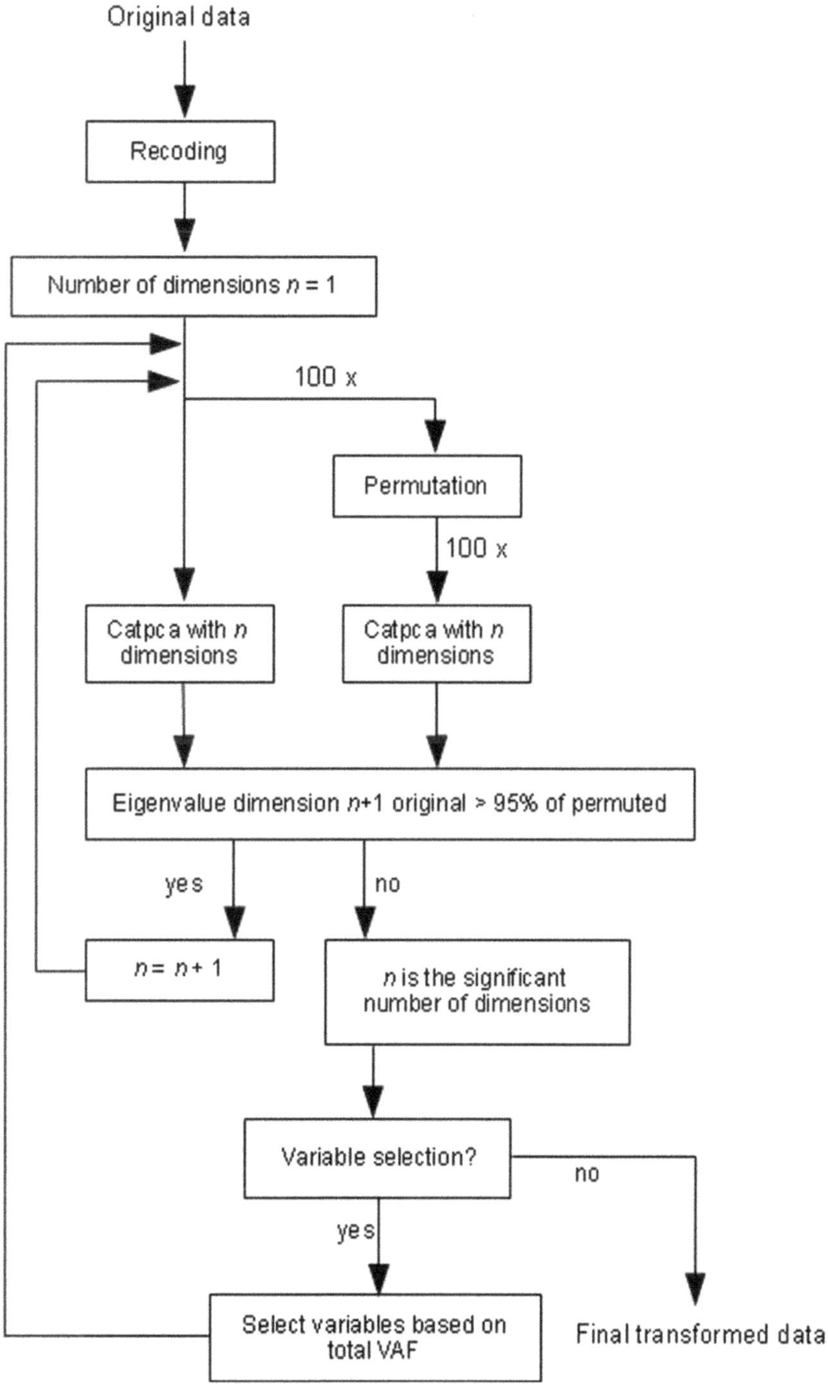

Figure 1. CATPCA data analysis strategy flowchart.

patient scores on the questionnaire, 2) theoretical Cold and Heat related symptoms, 3) Cold and Heat related symptoms according to experts and 4) Cold and Heat ranking of each patient questionnaire by two experts.

The symptoms that the experts used to rank the Cold and Heat status of the patients were compared with the symptoms connected with Cold and Heat according to theory. Furthermore, to examine the relationship between the symptoms and the Cold and Heat ranking by the experts, these rankings were plotted as ordinally scaled supplementary variables in the CATPCA solution [46]. Supplementary treatment of variables implies that they are projected into the component space, but do not participate in defining the component space. The locations of the Cold and Heat rankings of both experts were then examined respective to each other and the other variables.

To find out which symptoms are most related to the experts Cold and Heat ranking, a semi-supervised analysis was performed. In this analysis the Cold and Heat rankings of the two experts did participate in the model building with a large weight (the ranking variables were included a large number of times in the model) [46]. For this analysis the number of principal components was also determined using the permutation testing approach described above. Due to the large weight of the four ranking variables, they almost completely determine the solution, causing the VAF of the other variables to decrease compared to the unsupervised solution. Questionnaire variables with a total VAF ≥25% in one of both dimensions were selected to build a final model.

Results and Discussion

Similarities and differences between patients with a rheumatic disease

The theoretical relationships between symptoms used in the systems diagnosis questionnaire and syndromes were visualized as a graph (Figure 2) [20]. The resulting Bi-syndrome network is a bipartite graph consisting of two types of nodes, the syndromes (red hexagons) and the symptoms (yellow circles). This graph visualizes the relationships between symptoms and syndromes according to Chinese medicine theory. Some symptoms are related to more than one syndrome which might in some instances be referred to as bridge symptoms or bifurcation points. The appearance of such a bridge symptom can indicate a strengthening of the pattern itself,

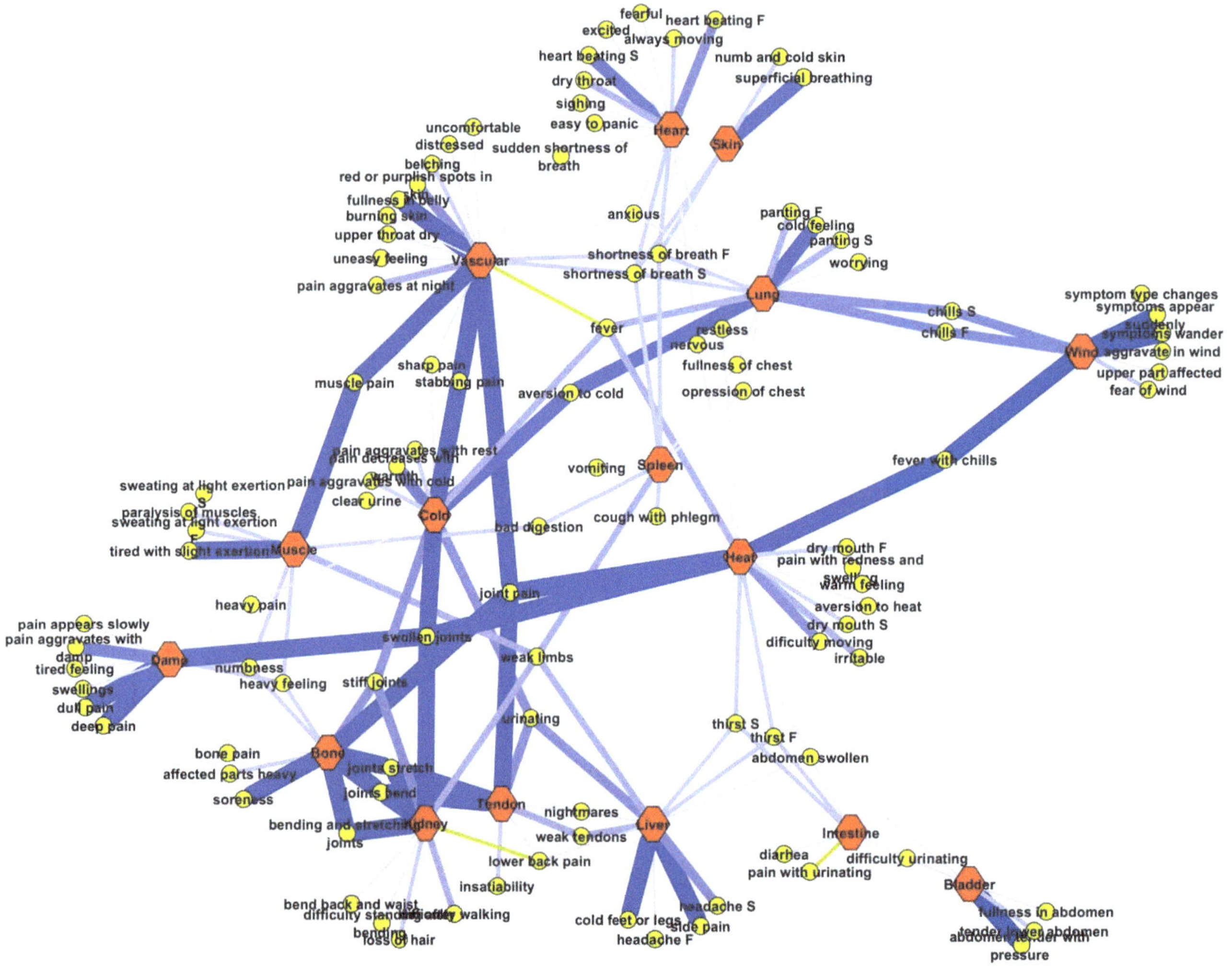

Figure 2. Example of a personalized Bi-syndromes network based on Vangermeersch 1994. The red hexagonal nodes represent the Bi-syndromes (Bi prefix was omitted for brevity), and the yellow circles represent the symptoms and signs related to the Bi-syndromes. The blue lines (edges) represent the relationships between symptoms and syndromes according to theory while the thickness of the lines represent the symptom scores of one patient. Thicker and darker colored edges denote a higher score and thinner, lighter edges denote a lower score.

an upcoming change towards another pattern or a complication of the pattern. Many other symptoms are unique for particular syndromes. Certain related syndromes according Chinese medicine theory are positioned close together in the graph. For example prolonged Bone Bi develops into Kidney Bi, two syndromes which are closely related in theory and thus close together in the network. Heart Bi can develop after a long period of Vascular Bi. Intestine and Bladder Bi are two late stages of the disease related to the Hollow Organs [28].

To visually explore the symptom pattern of a patient, the scores on the questionnaire can be mapped on the network. An example of one patient is shown in Figure 2. Edges that are thicker and darker blue denote high scores while light and thin edges represent low scores.

The results of the CATPCA analyses are as follows. Parallel analysis showed four significant principal components for the model containing all the variables. Two sets of variables were selected, one set consisting of 44 variables with a total VAF >50% and another set consisting of 30 variables with a VAF >60% (see Table S1 and Table S2 for the total VAF tables of both sets of variables). Parallel analysis revealed four significant components for the first set of variables and three significant components for the second set. After discussing both models with the Chinese medicine experts the model with fewer variables and components was retained for further analysis.

In the component score plots (not shown) no clear groups of patients could be observed. The location of the objects in the score plots was compared with the type of arthritis the patients suffered from. No grouping of patients with a similar type of arthritis could be found. The loadings of the first two components of the CATPCA model are shown in Figure 3A. The length of a loading indicates the amount of variance explained by that loading and the distance between two loadings indicates their similarity. All the loadings are positive in the first dimension (40.2% explained variance) indicating a general factor for which no clear interpretation was found. When the loadings in the second dimension (12.5% explained variance) are compared with the theoretical relationships between symptoms and the corresponding syndromes, two groups of loadings stand out. Five variables are theoretically related to the external pathogens Wind ('aggravate in wind', 'fear of wind'), Cold ('aversion to cold') and Heat ('thirst', 'dry mouth s'). Three of these symptoms, 'aggravate in wind', 'fear of wind' and 'aversion to cold', have a fairly high negative loading in the second dimension. Nine variables are related to Chinese Organ concepts such as Heart ('anxious', 'restless', 'excited', 'nervous'), Vascular ('anxious', 'uncomfortable', 'distressed', 'uneasy feeling') and Lung ('panting s', 'worrying'). Four of these symptoms, 'anxious', 'worrying', 'uneasy feeling' and 'distressed', have a fairly high positive loading in the second dimension. Two symptoms which are related to Damp, 'heavy feeling' and 'tired feeling', have a very low loading in the second dimension.

Looking at the distribution of symptoms from a Western medicine perspective reveals that the most common symptoms for rheumatoid arthritis (RA) 'joint pain', 'swollen joints' and 'stiff joints' do not contribute to the variation between the patients. On the other hand two other RA symptoms 'tired feeling' and 'weak limbs' are present but close together. The main osteoarthritis symptoms 'pain' and 'stiffness' are not present. Fibromyalgia is characterized by pain and stiffness as well, but also by 'anxious' and 'distressed', which have a high loading in the second dimension.

According to the Chinese medicine experts the second dimension is related to the Internal or External stage of the disease, one of the key diagnostic concepts used in Chinese medicine [21]. In the Internal stage the organs are affected while in the External stage the skin, muscles and channels are affected.

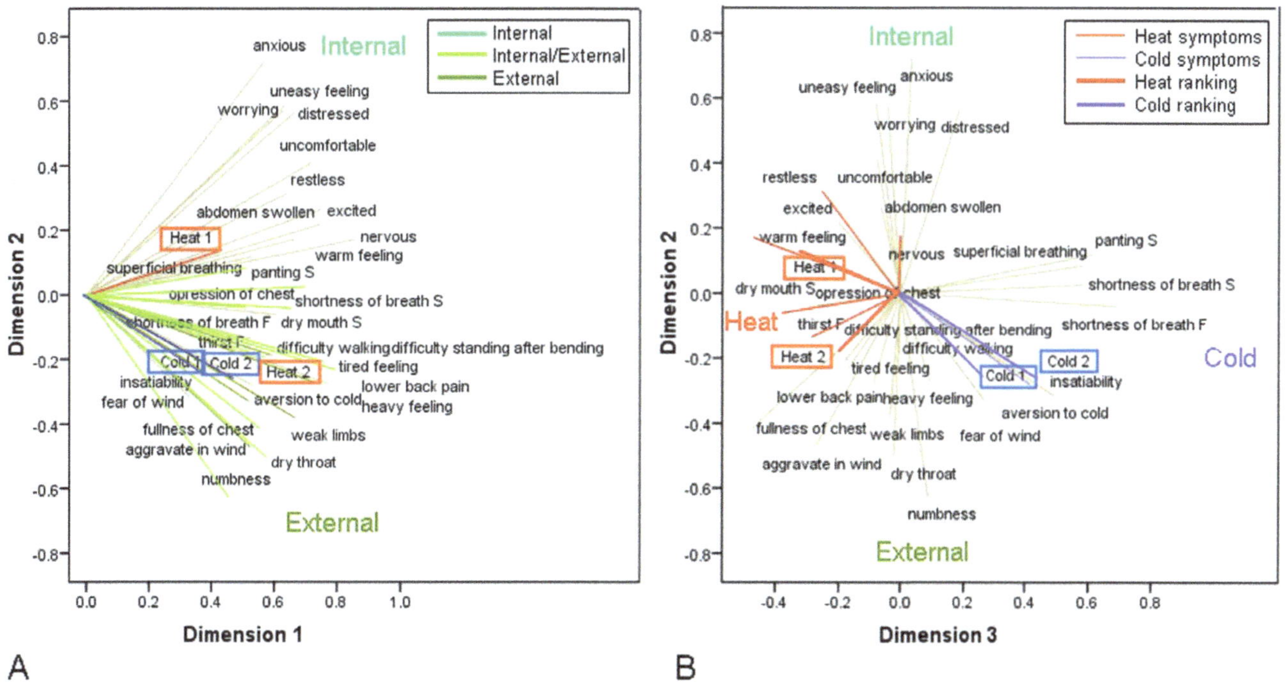

Figure 3. Loading plot of the first two dimensions (panel A) and the second and third dimension (panel B) of the CATPCA model for the 30-variables set. In Panel A, the loading vectors of the symptoms are colored according to their contribution (as indicated by one of the experts) to the Internal or External nature of the disease state. In Panel B, the loading vectors of symptoms which are theoretically related to Cold or Heat are pictured as thin blue or red lines. The supplementary Cold and Heat rankings of the two experts are plotted as thick blue or red lines.

The reaction of the body to the external pathogens Wind, Cold, and Damp that cause the arthritis is expressed by the symptoms that can be observed in the lower right part of Figure 3A. This indicates the first, external stage of the disease when the body defends itself against the invasion of the external pathogens. The appearance of Heat ('dry mouth s' and 'thirst') and Damp ('heavy feeling' and 'tired feeling') symptoms, indicates a transformation of Cold into Heat via Damp. Patients in this stage of the disease will have a low score in the second dimension. A high positive loading in the second dimension indicates a more chronic stage of the disease, in which patients will present Organ symptoms. If the position of the objects in the component score plots is compared to the loadings, it is possible to get an indication of the stage of the disease according to Chinese medicine theory for each patient. The Internal versus External interpretation of the second dimension is in agreement with the distribution of the symptoms that are in theory related to the External or Internal stage of the disease as marked with different colors in Figure 3.

The Cold and Heat status of rheumatic patients

Figure 3B shows the second and third dimension of the CATPCA model. While the second dimension is mostly related to the Internal and External stage of the disease, the third dimension (10.4% explained variance) is related to the Cold or Heat status of the patients. Symptoms related to Heat and Cold according to theory are colored red and blue respectively in Figure 3 and are indicated in Figure 4. Five symptoms that are theoretically related to Heat have a negative loading in the third dimension ('restless', 'nervous', 'warm feeling', 'dry mouth s' and 'thirst'). The group of symptoms with the highest positive loadings in the third dimension ('panting s', 'superficial breathing', 'shortness of breath s' and 'shortness of breath f') are related to Qi deficiency. One symptom ('aversion to cold') theoretically related to Cold also has a fairly high positive loading in the third dimension.

The Cold and Heat rankings of the experts, plotted as supplementary variables in Figure 3, have fairly high loadings in the third dimension indicating that this dimension is related to the Cold and Heat rankings. The Cold rankings are related to the other high positive loadings in the third dimension ('panting s', 'superficial breathing', 'shortness of breath s' and 'shortness of breath f'). One expert indicated to have used these symptoms to rank the Cold status of the patients (Figure 4). The Cold rankings are much closer together than the Heat rankings indicating that the two experts agree more on the Cold status of the patients than on the Heat status.

The experts were asked to indicate which symptoms they used for the ranking of the Cold and Heat status of the patients. In Figure 4 the symptoms reported by the two experts are given. Additionally, the symptoms theoretically related to Cold and Heat are indicated by the red and blue color in the center column. In the figure the overlap in symptom use between theory and the experts is visualized, as well as the overlap between the two experts. The Cold symptom 'aversion to cold' with a large loading in dimension three shown in Figure 3B was indeed indicated by both experts as important, although one expert assigned this symptom a lower status. Of the Heat symptoms with a large loading in dimension three 'warm feeling' was deemed important by both experts. 'Dry mouth s', 'nervous' and 'restless' were important for one expert, while 'thirst f' was mentioned by neither expert. Figure 4 also shows that both experts used a larger set of symptoms to rank Cold and Heat than indicated by theory. Furthermore, both experts indicated to have used symptoms that are not related to Cold and Heat according to theory. This might be due to differences between various Chinese medicine schools and to experience with using symptoms in daily practice.

In the following analysis the Cold and Heat rankings are introduced into the model with a large weight to find the symptoms that are most closely related to the expert rankings, based on the patients scores. Figure 5A is a bi-plot in which the patients scores and Cold and Heat ranking loadings are both plotted in the component space. The position of a patient point relative to the Cold and Heat loadings indicates the Cold and Heat ranking of the patient. Patients in the upper part of the figure for example have a high Cold ranking while patients in the right part of the figure have a high Heat ranking. Figure 5A shows that the distances between the various ranking categories is not equal. Additionally the distance between category 3 in Heat 1 and Heat 2 is large indicating that a Heat ranking of 3 for expert 1 should be interpreted very different from a Heat ranking of 3 for expert 2. To see whether the Cold or Heat ranking has any relationship with the type of arthritis the patients suffer from the outline of the largest groups of patients, the rheumatoid arthritis (RA) and osteoarthritis (OA) patients, are marked by lines. Clearly, the scores of the OA and RA patients are overlapping and is therefore unrelated to the Cold and Heat rankings.

In Figure 5B shows the loadings resulting from the forced classification analysis. The Heat rankings have a high positive loading in the first dimension and the Cold rankings have a high positive loading in the second dimension. This loadings plot reveals which symptoms, and related questions, are most related to the Cold and Heat rankings. 'Aversion to cold', 'fear of wind' and 'pain aggravates with cold' are most related to the Cold rankings and 'aversion to heat', 'fullness of chest' and 'dry mouth' to the Heat rankings. 'Aversion to cold' and 'fear of wind' also have a fairly high positive loading in the third dimension (indicating Cold) of the unsupervised approach (Figure 3B). 'Fullness of chest' and 'dry mouth' have a fairly high negative loading in the third dimension (indicating Heat) of the unsupervised approach.

The results of this study are summarized in Figure 4. First of all the symptoms used in theory to determine the Cold and Heat status of patients are indicated with a blue and red background respectively. 'Fever' and 'swollen joints' have a brown background since they are bridge symptoms between Heat and Cold. Secondly, the figure shows that both experts reported they used most of the theoretical symptoms. Seven symptoms that were not used by either expert are placed at the bottom of the list. Thirdly, the figure shows the agreement and disagreement between the experts on symptom use. In the fourth place, the symptoms resulting from the forced classification analysis are marked by bold type face.

Of the Western symptoms for rheumatoid arthritis 'joint pain' is indicated as a Heat symptom in Chinese diagnosis, 'stiff joints' is indicated as a Cold symptom and 'swollen joints' is indicating both Cold and Heat. However neither expert used 'swollen joints' and 'joint pain' to rank the Cold or Heat status of the patients. 'Weak limbs', another RA symptom showed up in the forced classification as an important indicator for Heat. Some pain related symptoms which can be present in various rheumatic diseases appear to be relevant for Cold and Heat ranking. 'Pain with redness and swelling' is indicated by both experts and theory as an important Heat symptom. 'Stabbing pain' on the other hand is indicated by one expert as a Cold symptom. 'Heavy pain' was not mentioned by the experts, but according to theory it is a Cold symptom. Additionally the results of the analysis show that emotional symptoms more prevalent in fibromyalgia patients are more related to Heat, especially the symptom 'nervous' is mentioned in theory as a Heat symptom and is also an important Heat indicator in the forced classification results.

Expert 1	Symptoms	Expert 2
Cold 3	cold feeling	Cold 3
Cold 3	pain aggravates with cold	Cold 3
Cold 3	pain decreases with warmth	Cold 3
Cold 3	aversion to cold	Cold 2
Cold 3	urinating	
Cold 3	clear urine	
Cold 3	sharp pain	
Cold 2	cold feet or legs	Cold 3
Cold 2	chills S	Cold 3
Cold 2	red or purplish spots in skin	Cold 2
Cold 2	numb and cold skin	Cold 2
Cold 2 & Heat 1	fever with chills	
Cold 2	stabbing pain	
Cold 1	stiff joints	Cold 1
Cold 1 & Heat 3	fever	Heat 3
Cold 1 & Heat 1	pain with urinating	
Cold 1	fear of wind	
Cold 1	joints stretch	
Cold 1	bending and stretching joints	
Cold 1	difficulty walking	
Heat 2	pain aggravates at night	Cold 2
	numbness	Cold 2
	pain aggravates with damp	Cold 2
	superficial breathing	Cold 1
	panting S	Cold 1
	shortness of breath S	Cold 1
	sudden shortness of breath	Cold 1
	sweating at light exertion S	Cold 1
	tired with slight exertion	Cold 1
	weak limbs	Cold 1
	weak tendons	Cold 1
	pain aggravates with rest	Cold 1
	diarhea	Cold 0.5
Heat 3	aversion to heat	Heat 3
Heat 3	pain with redness and swelling	Heat 3
Heat 2	burning skin	Heat 3
Heat 2	dry mouth S	
Heat 2	dry throat	Heat 2
Heat 2	upper throat dry	Heat 2
Heat 2	thirst S	
Heat 2	warm feeling	Heat 3
Heat 1	heart beating S	
Heat 1	insatiability	
Heat 1	always moving	
Heat 1	irritable	
Heat 1	uncomfortable	
Heat 1	distressed	
Heat 1	nervous	
Heat 1	restless	
Heat 1	nightmares	
Heat 1	excited	
Heat 1	difficulty urinating	
	abdomen swollen	Heat 1
	swollen joints	Heat 2
	swellings	Heat 2
	pain aggravates with rest	
	swollen joints	
	heavy pain	
	joint pain	
	thirst F	
	dry mouth F	
	difficulty moving	
	fullness of chest	
	fullness in belly	
	oppression of chest	
	difficulty standing after bending	

Figure 4. Cold and Heat related symptoms. In the first and third column the symptoms used by the experts for the Cold (blue) and Heat (red) ranking are marked. The importance is shown as a number behind the Cold and Heat label and by the color, dark blue or red is more important. The second column shows the names of the symptoms. Symptoms with a blue background are related to Cold according to theory, the red background ones are related to Heat according to theory. Symptoms with a brown background are related to both Cold and Heat. The table also shows which symptoms are important for the Cold and Heat ranking according to the forced classification model in bold type face and in red or blue.

The combination of the patient questionnaire scores information with the analysis and expert rankings resulted in a set of symptoms that are most qualified to develop into a tool to determine the Cold and Heat status of patients in a clinical setting.

Conclusions

This study introduced a systems diagnosis approach, the collection of a large number of symptoms that are usually not used in clinical diagnosis in Western medicine, as an additional dimension of looking at patients with a rheumatic disease. Individual patient scores on this questionnaire can be visually presented in a graph to help the interpretation of the relationships between the symptoms occurring in that patient (Figure 2). This new method of 'symptom fingerprinting' is comparable to other systems biology fingerprinting tools to determine disease state, risk for a disease, and chances of treatment effect [47–49].

The systems diagnosis questionnaire results of 49 patients with a rheumatic disease in this study reveal two interesting and significant dimensions of information. One dimension is related to the stage of the disease with the key symptoms 'anxious', 'worrying', 'uneasy feeling' and 'distressed' for the Internal stage, and 'aggravate in wind', 'fear of wind' and 'aversion to cold' for the External stage. The concept of Internal and External is widely used in Chinese medicine to choose the right treatment option. The fact that this concept explains 12.5% of the total variation in the data shows that it might be a relevant difference in other patients with rheumatic diseases as well.

The second interesting dimension is related to the Cold and Heat status of the patients, explaining 10.4% of the variation in the data. The key symptoms are 'panting s', 'superficial breathing', 'shortness of breath s', 'shortness of breath f' and 'aversion to cold' for the Cold status and 'restless', 'nervous', 'warm feeling', 'dry mouth s' and 'thirst' for the Heat status. A forced classification approach revealed that 'Aversion to cold', 'fear of wind' and 'pain aggravates with cold' are related to the Cold rankings and 'aversion to heat', 'fullness of chest' and 'dry mouth' are related to the Heat rankings by two Chinese medicine experts in these 49 patients. The characterization of the Cold and Heat status in this study is limited by the patient reported symptoms and might be improved by including observations of an expert of the patient.

We believe that the future of medicine lies in an integration of perspectives on disease, health, prevention and medicine. Looking in more detail and at the same time more comprehensively at patients is the way forward towards personalized medicine [5,50]. One step in that direction is finding new sub-groups of patients and optimizing treatment for these sub-groups. For Chinese medicine practitioners it is standard to take the Internal or External status as well as the Cold or Heat status into account for choosing the best treatment option. This study characterizes the symptoms related to these subgroups which might be used to

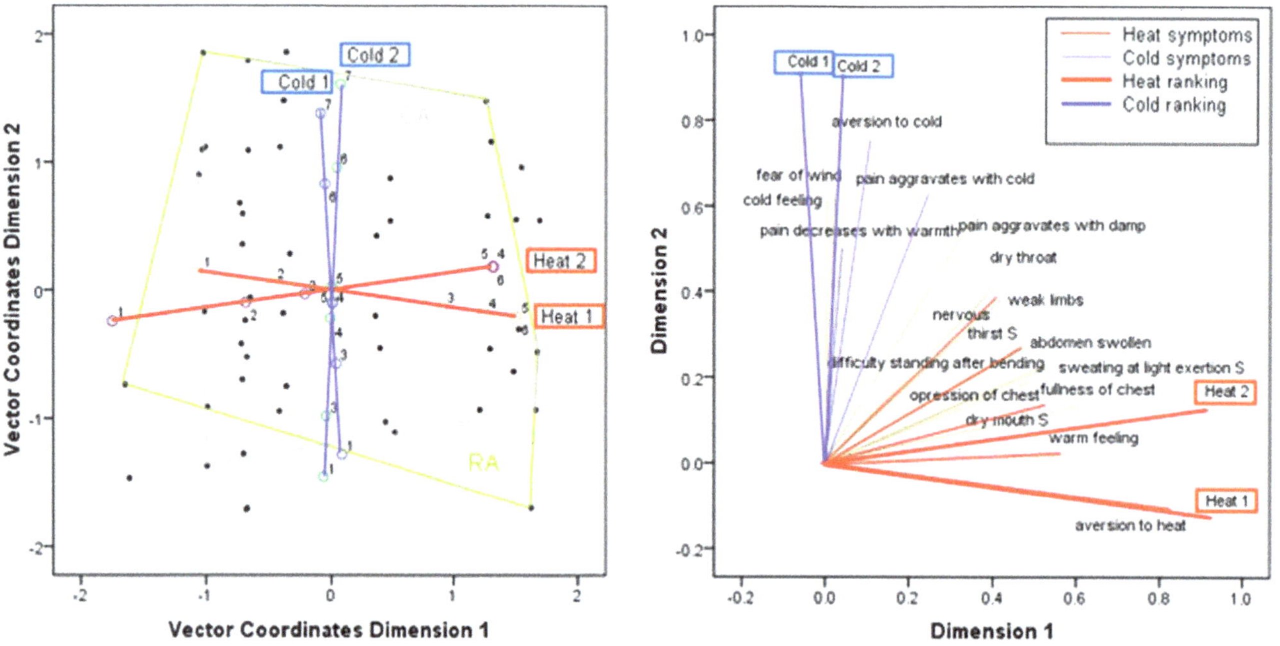

A B

Figure 5. Panel A shows a bi-plot based on a semi-supervised CATPCA model including 19 variables and the 4 expert ranking variables. The four expert rankings are shown on which the categories after transformation are marked by circles. The outline of the group of rheumatoid arthritis (RA) patients is shown as well as the outline of the group of osteoarthritis patients (OA). In Panel B the loadings are shown. The loadings corresponding to symptoms which are related to Cold or Heat according to theory are represented by thin blue or red lines respectively. The Cold and Heat expert rankings are the thick blue en red lines respectively.

develop a diagnostic tool to diagnose these subgroups in clinical practice. Further studies are needed to examine differences in response to medication by Cold and Heat sub-groups of arthritis patients. In this way the combination of Chinese medicine concepts with Western therapeutic options offers exciting opportunities for more personalized treatment and eventually personalized health.

Supporting Information

Text S1 Systems diagnosis questionnaire (in Dutch). (DOC)

Table S1 VAF table for the analysis presented in Figure 3. (DOC)

Table S2 VAF table for the analysis presented in Figure 5. (DOC)

Acknowledgments

The authors would like to thank all the patients and practitioners who kindly contributed their time to participate in the study.

Author Contributions

Conceived and designed the experiments: HAvW THR AJvdK JJM JS. Performed the experiments: HAvW AJvdK. Analyzed the data: HAvW THR AJvdK JS HW TH JJM JvdG. Contributed reagents/materials/analysis tools: THR. Wrote the paper: HAvW AJvdK.

References

1. Anderson JJ, Wells G, Verhoeven AC, Felson DT (2000) Factors predicting response to treatment in rheumatoid arthritis: the importance of disease duration. Arthritis Rheum 43(1): 22–29.
2. Smolen JS, Aletaha D (2005) Challenges of predicting treatment response in patients with rheumatoid arthritis. Nat Clin Pract Rheumatol 1(2): 62–63.
3. Rindfleisch JA, Muller D (2005) Diagnosis and management of rheumatoid arthritis. Am Fam Physician 72(6): 1037–47.
4. Van der Greef J, McBurney RN (2005) Innovation: Rescuing drug discovery: in vivo systems pathology and systems pharmacology. Nat Rev Drug Discov 4: 961–7.
5. Glocker MO, Guthke R, Kekow J, Thiesen H (2006) Rheumatoid arthritis, a complex multifactorial disease: on the way toward individualized medicine. Med Res Rev 26(1): 63–87.
6. Arnett FC, Edworthy SM, Bloch DA, McShane DJ, Fries JF, et al. (1988) The American Rheumatism Association 1987 revised criteria for the classification of rheumatoid arthritis. Arthritis Rheum 31(3): 315–24.
7. Lindström B, Eriksson M (2005) Salutogenesis. J Epidemiol Community Health 59(6): 440–2.
8. van der Greef J, Martin S, Juhasz P, Adourian A, Plasterer T, et al. (2007) The art and practice of systems biology in medicine: mapping patterns of relationships. J Proteome Res 6(4): 1540–59.
9. Verhoeckx KCM, Bijlsma S, Jespersen S, Ramaker R, Verheij E, et al. (2004) Characterization of anti-inflammatory compounds using transcriptomics, proteomics, and metabolomics in combination with multivariate data analysis. Int Immunopharmacol 4(12): 1499–514.
10. van der Greef J, Stroobant P, van der Heijden R (2004) The role of analytical sciences in medical systems biology. Curr Opin Chem Biol 8(5): 559–65.
11. Gaston JSH (2008) Cytokines in arthritis–the 'big numbers' move centre stage. Rheumatology (Oxford) 47: 8–12.
12. Lundy SK, Sarkar S, Tesmer LA, Fox DA (2007) Cells of the synovium in rheumatoid arthritis. T lymphocytes. Arthritis Res Ther 9: 202.
13. van der Helm-van Mil AHM, Huizinga TWJ, de Vries RRP, Toes REM (2007) Emerging patterns of risk factor make-up enable subclassification of rheumatoid arthritis. Arthritis Rheum 56(6): 1728–35.
14. Van der Helm-van Mil AHM, Verpoort KN, Breedveld FC, Toes REM, Huizinga TWJ (2005) Antibodies to citrullinated proteins and differences in clinical progression of rheumatoid arthritis. Arthritis Res Ther 7(5): R949–58.
15. van der Pouw Kraan TCTM, Wijbrandts CA, van Baarsen LGM, Voskuyl AE, Rustenburg F, et al. (2007) Rheumatoid arthritis subtypes identified by genomic profiling of peripheral blood cells: assignment of a type I interferon signature in a subpopulation of patients. Ann Rheum Dis 66(8): 1008–14.
16. van Middendorp H, Geenen R, Sorbi MJ, van Doornen LJP, Bijlsma JWJ (2009) Health and physiological effects of an emotional disclosure intervention adapted for application at home: a randomized clinical trial in rheumatoid arthritis. Psychother Psychosom 78(3): 145–151.
17. van Hoogmoed D, Fransen J, Bleijenberg G, van Riel P (2010) Physical and psychosocial correlates of severe fatigue in rheumatoid arthritis. Rheumatology (Oxford) 49(7): 1294–302.
18. Wells GA (2009) Patient-driven outcomes in rheumatoid arthritis. J Rheumatol Suppl 82: 33–38.
19. Treharne GJ, Lyons AC, Booth DA, Kitas GD (2007) Psychological well-being across 1 year with rheumatoid arthritis: coping resources as buffers of perceived stress. Br J Health Psychol 12(Pt 3): 323–345.
20. van der Greef J, van Wietmarschen H, Schroën J, Wang M, Hankemeier T, et al. (2010) Systems biology-based diagnostic principles as pillars of the bridge between Chinese and Western medicine. Planta Med 76(17): 2036–2047.
21. Maciocia G (2005) The Foundations of Chinese Medicine: A Comprehensive Text for Acupuncturists and Herbalists. Second Edition Churchill Livingstone.
22. Vandeginste BGM, Massart DL, Buydens LMC, De Jong S, Lewi PJ, et al. (1998) Handbook of Chemometrics and Qualimetrics Part B. Elsevier, Amsterdam.
23. Li S, Zhang ZQ, Wu LJ, Zhang XG, Li YD, et al. (2007) Understanding ZHENG in traditional Chinese medicine in the context of neuro-endocrine-immune network. IET Syst Biol 1(1): 51–60.
24. Ni M (1995) The Yellow Emperor's Classic of Medicine: A New Translation of the Neijing Suwen with Commentary. 1st ed Shambhala.
25. Jiang W (2005) Therapeutic wisdom in traditional Chinese medicine: a perspective from modern science. Trends Pharmacol Sci 26: 558–63.
26. van Wietmarschen HA, Yuan K, Lu C, Gao P, Wang JS, et al. (2009) Systems biology guided by Chinese Medicine reveals new markers for sub-typing rheumatoid arthritis patients. Journal of Clinical Rheumatology 15(7): 330–337.
27. Lu C, Zha Q, Chang A, He Y, Lu A (2009) Pattern Differentiation in Traditional Chinese Medicine Can Help Define Specific Indications for Biomedical Therapy in the Treatment of Rheumatoid Arthritis. J Altern Complement Med 15(9): 1021–1025.
28. Vangermeersch L (1994) Bi-syndromes. Brussels: Satas.
29. Likert R (1932) A Technique for the Measurement of Attitudes. Archives of Psychology 140: 1–55.
30. Felson DT, Anderson JJ, Boers M, Bombardier C, Chernoff M, et al. (1993) The American College of Rheumatology preliminary core set of disease activity measures for rheumatoid arthritis clinical trials. The Committee on Outcome Measures in Rheumatoid Arthritis Clinical Trials. Arthritis Rheum 36(6): 729–40.
31. Markus MT (1994) Bootstrap confidence regions in nonlinear multivariate analysis. Leiden, The Netherlands: DSWO Press.
32. Borgatti SP, Everett MG (1997) Network analysis of 2-mode data. Social Networks 19(3): 243–269.
33. Borgatti S, Mehra A, Brass D, Labianca G (2009) Network Analysis in the Social Sciences. Science 323(5916): 892–895.
34. Strogatz SH (2001) Exploring complex networks. Nature 410(6825): 268–76.
35. Cline MS, Smoot M, Cerami E, Kuchinsky A, Landys N, et al. (2007) Integration of biological networks and gene expression data using Cytoscape. Nat Protoc 2(10): 2366–82.
36. Kamada T, Kawai S (1989) An algorithm for drawing general undirected graphs. Information Processing Letters 31(1): 7–15.
37. SAS Institute Inc (2009) SAS/ STAT Software. Cary, N.C.: Sas Institute Inc.
38. SAS Institute Inc (2009) SAS/ STAT 9.2 User's guide. Cary, N.C.: Sas Institute Inc.
39. Young F, Takane Y, de Leeuw J (1978) The principal components of mixed measurement level multivariate data: An alternating least squares method with optimal scaling. Psychometrika 43: 279–281.
40. SPSS Inc (2009) PASW Statistics 17.0. Chicago, Il.: SPSS Inc.
41. Gifi A (1990) Nonlinear multivariate analysis. Chichester, England: Wiley.
42. Meulman JM, Heiser WJ, SPSS Inc (2009) SPSS Categories 17.0. Chicago, Il.: SPSS Inc.
43. Horn J (1965) A rationale and test for the number of factors in factor-analysis. Psychometrika 30(2): 179–185.
44. Zwick WR, Velicer WF (1986) Comparison of five rules for determining the number of components to retain. Psychological Bulletin 99(3): 432–442.
45. Buja A, Eyuboglu N (1992) Remarks on parallel analysis. Multivariate behavioral research 27(4): 509–540.
46. Meulman in: Kaplan D. The Sage handbook of quantitative methodology for the social sciences. SAGE; 2004, Chapter 3.
47. Hendriks MMWB, Smit S, Akkermans WLMW, Reijmers TH, Eilers PHC, et al. (2007) How to distinguish healthy from diseased? Classification strategy for mass spectrometry-based clinical proteomics. Proteomics 7(20): 3672–3680.
48. Ganter B, Zidek N, Hewitt PR, Müller D, Vladimirova A (2008) Pathway analysis tools and toxicogenomics reference databases for risk assessment. Pharmacogenomics 9(1): 35–54.
49. Calvano SE, Xiao W, Richards DR, Felciano RM, Baker HV, et al. (2005) A network-based analysis of systemic inflammation in humans. Nature 437(7061): 1032–7.
50. Zhou X, Liu B, Wu Z, Feng Y (2007) Integrative mining of traditional Chinese medicine literature and MEDLINE for functional gene networks. Artif Intell Med 41(2): 87–104.

17

Assessment of the Reporting Quality of Randomized Controlled Trials on Treatment of Coronary Heart Disease with Traditional Chinese Medicine from the Chinese Journal of Integrated Traditional and Western Medicine: A Systematic Review

Fang-fang Fan[1], Qin Xu[2], Qi Sun[2]*, Sheng-jun Zhao[1]*, Ping Wang[1], Xue-rui Guo[3]

1 Department of Pharmacy, The Affiliated Traditional Medical Hospital, Xinjiang Medical University, Urumqi, Xinjiang Uygur Autonomous Region, China, **2** Medical Research Design and Data Analysis Center, The Affiliated Traditional Medical Hospital, Xinjiang Medical University, Urumqi, Xinjiang Uygur Autonomous Region, China, **3** Department of Pediatrics, The Affiliated Traditional Medical Hospital, Xinjiang Medical University, Urumqi, Xinjiang Uygur Autonomous Region, China

Abstract

Background: Due to language limitations, little is known about the reporting quality of randomized clinical trials (RCTs) on the treatment of coronary heart disease (CHD) with traditional Chinese medicine (TCM) in Chinese Journal of Integrated Traditional and Western Medicine (CJITWM).

Objective: In this study, we utilized the CONSORT 2010 statement to understand the reporting quality of RCTs on CHD with TCM from the CJITWM.

Methods: The China National Knowledge Infrastructure (CNKI) electronic database was searched for CJITWM RCTs on the treatment of CHD with TCM, published between Janurary 1, 2006 and December 31, 2011. We excluded articles reported as "animal studies," "topic review," "diagnostic test," "editorials," or "others." The CONSORT checklist was applied to evaluate the reporting quality of all eligible articles by two independent authors after extensive discussion. Each item was graded as either "yes" or "no" depending on whether the authors had reported it or not.

Results: We identified 21 articles meeting our inclusion criteria. The percentage of 11 of the 37 items was 4.8~95.2%, 14 of the 37 items were reported in all included articles, while 12 items were not mentioned at all. The average reporting percentage for the "title and abstract" section was 52.4%, for the "introduction" section 100.0%, for the "methods" section 45.4%, for the "results" section 57.1%, for the "discussion" section 79.4%, and for the "other information" section 17.5%.

Conclusion: In general, the reviewed RCTs were not consistent with the CONSORT 2010 statement. Authors should adhere to the CONSORT statement in reporting RCTs; editorial departments may consider the CONSORT statement as a guideline and should instruct authors to write manuscripts, and reviewers to judge them according to CONSORT statutes.

Editor: Hua Zhou, Macau University of Science and Technology, Macau

Funding: The authors have no support or funding to report.

Competing Interests: The authors have declared that no competing interests exist.

* E-mail: cums6140@hotmail.com (QS); zyyzsj0707@126.com (SZ)

Introduction

Overwhelming evidence shows that the current reporting quality of randomized controlled trials (RCTs) is suboptimal. Without transparent reporting, readers cannot judge the reliability and validity of trial findings nor extract information for systematic reviews. Recent methodological analyses indicate that inadequate reporting and design are associated with biased estimates of treatment effects. Such systematic error is damaging to RCTs, which are considered the gold standard for evaluating interventions because of their ability to minimize or avoid bias [1]. At present, RCTs accounted for over half of all clinical trials [2], highlighting their importance. This also reflects the standards of the Consolidated Standards of Reporting Trials (CONSORT) statement published in JAMA in 1996 [3] and the CONSORT 2010 statement published in BMJ in 2010 [1]. These guidelines consist of a checklist and flow diagram that authors can use for reporting a RCT. Many leading medical journals and major international editorial groups have endorsed the CONSORT statement, which facilitates critical appraisal and interpretation of RCTs.

Coronary heart disease (CHD) is a leading cause of death in many countries [4]. As the main treatment of CHD, modern medicine has improved dramatically in recent years. Although research of Traditional Chinese Medicine (TCM) on CHD are encouraging in many respects, the role of TCM in the prevention and treatment of CHD has been challenged due to the rapid development of modern medicine. With traditional medicinal opinions and natural medicines originating in herbs, TCM is in widespread clinical use and demonstrates a bright future in CHD treatment.

TCM, or traditional Chinese medicine, is a science of researching human physiology, pathology, diagnosis, prevention, and cure of diseases. Treatment of coronary heart disease (CHD) and preparations of Chinese medicines have more clinical applications, including Compound Salvia Pellet (CSP) for Angina Pectoris. The components of CSP are included salvia miltiorrhiza, notoginseng, and borneol, and they possess expansion of coronary artery atherosclerosis, resisting thrombosis and fall hematic fat action. CSP is the first preparation appoved by the FDA in China for the treatment of cardiovascular disease [5].

In recent years, as evidence-based medicine (EBM) has expanded, a number of multicenter RCTs with large sample sizes that focus on the prevention and treatment of CHD have been carried out in both Chinese and integrative medicine; for example, the randomized, double-blind, placebo-controlled trial on the effect of Xuezhikang (XZK) for regulating serum lipids and for the secondary prevention of CHD [6]. The XZK-treated group decreased the recurrence of nonfatal myocardial infarction in patients with CHD by 62% compared with placebo, and coronary death, coronary events, and total mortality were reduced by 45%, 30%, and 33.0%, respectively. This data filled the gap for information on the regulation of serum lipids in Oriental populations. Furthermore, proprietary Chinese medicine preparations have been used for a long time to treat CHD, with many controlled trials performed to investigate their efficacy [7–8].

The Chinese Journal of Integrated Traditional and Western Medicine (CJITWM) is a peer-review journal in that reflects the latest TCM research in China. However, due to language limitations, little was known about the reporting quality of this journal abroad. Although the quality of reporting in RCTs in medical sciences has been discussed, the quality of reporting in RCTs on the treatment of CHD with TCM published in the Chinese Journal of Integrated Traditional and Western Medicine (CJITWM) has not yet been assessed after publication of the CONSORT 2010 Statement. We aimed to assess the completeness of reporting of RCTs evaluating TCM in the treatment of CHD published in CJITWM from January 1, 2006 to December 31, 2011 based on the CONSORT 2010 checklist [1], and to provide recommendations for improving them in the future.

Methods

This systematic review was performed in accordance with a protocol that prescribed search strategy, eligibility criteria, data extraction, and statistical analysis.

Search strategy

The China National Knowledge Infrastructure (CNKI) electronic database was used to search all articles published between 2006 and 2011 that reported an RCT in which the assignment of participants to interventions was described by the words random, randomly, randomized, or randomization in the full text. We only obtained the full text of RCTs on the treatment of CHD with TCM published between 2006 and 2011. The following search strategy was used: "random, randomly, randomized, or randomization" (in full text) AND "coronary heart disease" or "angina" (in MeSH) AND "Jan. 1, 2006 to Dec. 31, 2011" AND "Chinese Journal of Integrated Traditional and Western Medicine" (in journal search tab).

Eligibility criteria

Two reviewers independently searched the journal and selected potentially relevant articles after screening the titles and abstracts. In case of uncertain eligibility, the full text was screened. RCTs on CHD treated with TCM interventions were selected. We included RCTs in which the allocation of participants to intervention was described by the words random (randomly allocate, randomized, or randomization). We excluded trials reported as "animal studies," "topic review," "diagnostic test," "editorials," or "others."

Data extraction

According to the 25 items (refined to 37 items, 25 primary and 12 secondary) in the CONSORT 2010 checklist of information to include when reporting a randomized trial, we created an evaluation form for each, and for each of the 25 items in the CONSORT 2010 checklist, a "yes" (Y, scored as 1) or "no" (N, scored as 0) option was assigned depending on whether the author had reported it. Two reviewers (Fan FF, Wang P) underwent training and studying for three months on data extraction from the CONSORT 2010 statement. Two independent reviewers analyzed the data and disagreements were resolved by engaging a third expert (Xu Q or Sun Q). The data extraction items included the 25 items in the CONSORT 2010 checklist (Tables 1 and 2).

Table 1. The reporting number and percentage for each article of the CONSORT checklist in CJITWM.

Author	Year	Number(n)	Percentage(%)
		Yes	Yes
Guo ZB [4]	2006	14	37.8
Liu P [5]	2006	11	29.7
Lu XY [6]	2006	21	56.8
Jing L [7]	2007	17	45.9
Wei ZT [8]	2007	16	43.2
Hao Xu [9]	2007	21	56.8
Zhang Y [10]	2007	16	43.2
Wang LJ [11]	2008	19	51.4
Zhang Q [12]	2008	16	43.2
Zhang Q [13]	2008	18	48.6
Cheng WL [14]	2009	19	51.4
Hu YH [15]	2009	13	35.1
LI AM [16]	2009	13	35.1
Yan LY [17]	2009	13	35.1
Cui XY [18]	2009	18	48.6
Wu QT [19]	2009	13	35.1
Yin CH [20]	2010	15	40.5
Zhu H [21]	2010	19	51.4
Zhu HJ [22]	2010	15	40.5
Peng W [23]	2011	18	48.6
Xin L [24]	2011	19	51.4

CJITWM: Chinese Journal of Integrated Traditional and Western Medicine, Yes: Number of trials in which the item was reported.

Table 2. The reporting number and percentage for each item of the CONSORT checklist in CJITWM.

Section/Topic	Item No	Checklist item	Number(n)	Percentage(%)
			Yes	Yes
Title and abstract	1a	Identification as a randomised trial in the title	1 [24]	4.8
	1b	Structured summary of trial design, methods, results, and conclusions (for specific guidance see CONSORT for abstracts)	21 [4–24]	100.0
Introduction				
Background and objectives	2a	Scientific background and explanation of rationale	21 [4–24]	100.0
	2b	Specific objectives or hypotheses	21 [4–24]	100.0
Methods				
Trial design	3a	Description of trial design (such as parallel, factorial) including allocation ratio	9 [6,7,9,11,13,14,21,23,24]	42.9
	3b	Important changes to methods after trial commencement (such as eligibility criteria), with reasons)	0	0
Participants	4a	Eligibility criteria for participants	21 [4–24]	100.0
	4b	Settings and locations where the data were collected	21 [4–24]	100.0
Interventions	5	The interventions for each group with sufficient details to allow replication, including how and when they were actually administered	21 [4–24]	100.0
Outcomes	6a	Completely defined pre-specified primary and secondary outcome measures, including how and when they were assessed	21 [4–24]	100.0
	6b	Any changes to trial outcomes after the trial commenced, with reasons	0	0
Sample size	7a	How sample size was determined	0	0
	7b	When applicable, explanation of any interim analyses and stopping guidelines	0	0
Randomisation				
Sequence generation	8a	Method used to generate the random allocation sequence	20 [4–11,13–24]	95.2
	8b	Type of randomisation; details of any restriction (such as blocking and block size)	21 [4–24]	100.0
Allocation concealment mechanism	9	Mechanism used to implement the random allocation sequence (such as sequentially numbered containers), describing any steps taken to conceal the sequence until interventions were assigned	0	0
Implementation	10	Who generated the random allocation sequence, who enrolled participants, and who assigned participants to interventions	0	0
Blinding	11a	If done, who was blinded after assignment to interventions (for example, participants, care providers, those assessing outcomes) and how	1 [6]	4.8
	11b	If relevant, description of the similarity of interventions	6 [6,7,13,14,23,24]	28.5
Statistical methods	12a	Statistical methods used to compare groups for primary and secondary outcomes	21 [4–24]	100.0
	12b	Methods for additional analyses, such as subgroup analyses and adjusted analyses	0	0
Results				
Participant flow	13a	For each, the numbers of participants who were randomly assigned, received intended treatment, and were analysed for the primary outcome group	21 [4–24]	100.0
	13b	For each group, losses and exclusions after randomisation, together with reasons	8 [9,11,12–14,18,21,23]	38.1
Recruitment	14a	Dates defining the periods of recruitment and follow-up	19 [4,6–18,20–24]	90.5
	14b	Why the trial ended or was stopped	0	0
Baseline data	15	A table showing baseline demographic and clinical characteristics for each group	6 [6,9,12,14,18,24]	28.6

Table 2. Cont.

Section/Topic	Item No	Checklist item	Number(n)	Percentage(%)
			Yes	Yes
Numbers analysed	16	For each group, number of participants (denominator) included in each analysis and whether the analysis was by original assigned groups	21 [4–24]	100.0
Outcomes and estimation	17a	For each primary and secondary outcome, results for each group, and the estimated effect size and its precision (such as 95% confidence interval)	21 [4–24]	100.0
	17b	For binary outcomes, presentation of both absolute and relative effect sizes is recommended)	0	0
Ancillary analyses	18	Results of any other analyses performed, including subgroup analyses and adjusted analyses, distinguishing pre-specified from exploratory	0	0
Harms	19	All important harms or unintended effects in each group (for specific guidance see CONSORT for harms	12 [4,6,9,11–14, 18,20,21,23,24]	57.1
Discussion				
Limitations	20	Trial limitations, addressing sources of potential bias, imprecision, and, if relevant, multiplicity of analyses	8 [6,7,9–11,14,18,21]	38.1
Generalisability	21	Generalisability (external validity, applicability) of the trial findings	21 [4–24]	100.0
Interpretation	22	Interpretation consistent with results, balancing benefits and harms, and considering other relevant evidence	21 [4–24]	100.0
Other information				
Registration	23	Registration number and name of trial registry	0	0
Protocol	24	Where the full trial protocol can be accessed, if available	0	0
Funding	25	Sources of funding and other support (such as supply of drugs), role of funders	11 [4,6–10,14,18,19,21,22]	52.4

CJITWM: Chinese Journal of Integrated Traditional and Western Medicine,
Yes: Number of trials in which the item was reported.

Prior to data extraction, all authors independently evaluated two RCTs reports that were not included into this study. The main content includes "CONSORT 2010 explanation and elaboration: updated guidelines for reporting parallel group randomized trials" [9], the PRISMA statement [10], and medical methodology.

Primary and Secondary Outcomes

The primary outcome of the study was the number and percentage of applicable items on the CONSORT checklist that were reported between 2006 and 2011 in the CJITWM. The number and percentage of articles reporting each applicable section and the percentage value for each article on the checklist was the secondary outcomes.

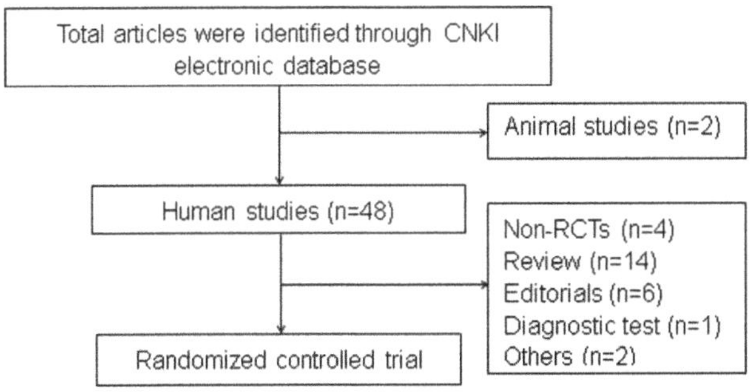

Figure 1. Flow diagram for the selection of articles for inclusion in systematic review.

Statistical analyses

Data were analyzed using Microsoft Excel 2010 and SPSS software (version 19.0, IBM SPSS). In order to assess adherence to CONSORT checklist items, we calculated the number and proportion of articles describing each of the 37 items. The sum of the scores was converted to a percentage value for each article

Table 3. The average reporting percentage for each section and the total of the CONSORT checklist in CJITWM.

Section	Number(n)	Percentage(%)
	Yes	Yes
Title and abstract	11.0	52.4
Introduction	21.0	100.0
Methods	9.5	45.4
Results	10.8	57.1
Discussion	16.7	79.4
Other information	3.7	17.5

CJITWM: Chinese Journal of Integrated Traditional and Western Medicine,
Yes: Number of trials in which the item was reported.

(proportion of each article = the number of reported item/37 items), each item (proportion of each item = the number of reported article/total articles), and each section (proportion of each section = the sum of items percentage of each section/total items of each section).

Results

The initial CNKI database search identified 50 records on CHD or angina published between January 1, 2006 and December 31, 2011. Of these, 2 animal studies, 14 reviews, 1 diagnostic test, 6 editorials, and 2 others were excluded. In total, 21 RCTs [11–31] were selected for analysis by screening the abstract and full text article. Figure 1 presents a flow chart of studies considered for inclusion.

Among the 21 included articles, according to the 37 items in CONSORT 2010 checklist, the reporting percentage in each of the articles was 29.7–56.8% (Table 1).

Among the 21 included articles, according to the 37 items in CONSORT 2010 checklist, only 4.8% (1/21) mentioned "randomization" in the title and blinding to interventions, 95.2% (20/21) reported the method used to generate the random allocation sequence, 42.9% (9/21) reported description of trial design, 28.6% (6/21) reported the similarity of interventions and baseline data with a table, 90.5% (19/21) reported dates defining the periods of recruitment and follow-up, 38.1% (8/21) reported trial limitations, losses, and exclusions after randomization, 57.1% (12/21) reported side effects, and 52.4% (11/21) reported the source of funding (Table 2). 14 of the 37 items (1b, 2a, 2b, 4a, 4b, 5, 6a, 8b, 12a, 13a, 16, 17a, 21, and 22) were reported in all included articles, while 12 items (3b, 6b, 7a, 7b, 9, 10, 12b, 14b, 17b, 18, 23, and 24) were not mentioned at all.

Table 3 summarizes the total mean number and percentages of the breakdown of scores for each section of the CONSORT checklist of the included trials. The average reporting percentage for the "title and abstract" section of the trials published in 2006 and 2011 was 52.4%: for the "introduction" section 100.0%, for the "methods" section 45.4%, for the "results" section 57.1%, for the "discussion" section 79.4%, and for the "other information" section 17.5%.

Discussion

TCM has been widely applied for CHD in China. There have been a large number of controlled clinical studies published in Chinese literature, yet no systematic searching and analysis has been done in the CJITWM. In order to present these trials in an open and transparent manner, all authors need to follow widely accepted CONSORT guidelines. It is important to address this issue for many reasons. First, poorly reported clinical trials make it difficult for other researchers to assess the validity of the results, to replicate the study, and to identify gaps that need to be addressed in the design and reporting of future treatment innovations. In addition, inadequate reporting may mislead healthcare providers in their treatment decisions for patients. Lastly, policy makers depend on information provided in clinical trials to decide whether they should promote CHD with TCM to a larger population.

Although studies similar to the present study have previously been conducted, to our knowledge, this study is the first to investigate the quality of reporting of RCTs, with particular reference to CONSORT 2010 guidelines in the CJITWM following the revised CONSORT Statement (2010 version). Fan et al. [32] carried out a review on treatment of CHD with Compound Salvia Pellet (CSP) reported in 115 RCTs (up to Dec 2005) in published articles both in China and abroad. This study, which assessed the quality of the reporting of clinical trials in CHD, concluded that "the overall quality of reporting of RCTs with CSP evaluated with a revised CONSORT (2001 version) checklist was poor" [32].

Based on the CONSORT 2010 checklist, the reporting quality of RCTs on CHD in this journal was inconsistent in terminologies of the CONSORT 2010 statement. Unfortunately, despite an increasing number of RCTs assessing CHD with TCM in the past two decades, the reporting quality we reviewed is suboptimal and substantial improvement is required to meet CONSORT guidelines. Almost 50% of the trials we reviewed did not satisfy more than half of the criteria in the modified CONSORT checklist. Each of these potentially problematic areas, including title and abstract, introduction, methods, results, discussion, and other information is discussed below to help scientific readers recognize them when reviewing studies of CHD with TCM in the CJITWM and other journals.

Title and abstract

The average reporting percentage for the "title and abstract" section of the trials published in 2006 and 2011 was 52.4%. The ability to identify a report of a randomized trial in an electronic database depends to a large extent on how it was indexed. Indexers may not classify a report as a randomized trial if the authors do not explicitly report this information [33]. A structured summary consists of trial design, methods, results, and conclusions sections. Clear, transparent, and sufficiently detailed abstracts are important because readers often assess a trial in the light of such information. Some readers use an abstract as a screening tool to decide whether to read the full article; thus, the author should adopt a structured summary to accurately report the contents of the full article. Unfortunately, we found only one article identified as a randomized trial in the title with a structured summary as well. To help ensure that a study is appropriately indexed and easily identified, authors should use the word "randomized" in the title to indicate that the participants were randomly assigned to their comparison groups.

Introduction

The average reporting percentage for the "introduction" section was 100.0%. In practice, objectives and hypotheses are not always easily differentiated. Most reports of RCTs provide adequate information about trial objectives and hypotheses [34]. All articles reported scientific background, explanation of rationale, and specific objectives, but all introduced the study objectives without combining hypotheses, because hypotheses are more specific than objectives and are amenable to explicit statistical evaluation.

Methods

9 articles described trial design, such as a parallel controlled trial, while others only described the trial with the word "randomized." The word "design" is often used to refer to all aspects of how a trial is planned; it is important that researchers clearly describe these aspects of the trial, including the unit of randomization. Here we sought information on the type of trial, such as parallel group or factorial, and the conceptual framework, such as superiority or non-inferiority. All articles did not report item 3b, which may be due to the possibility that no important changes were made to the methods after trial commencement. Changes from protocols are not currently well reported. A review of comparisons with protocols showed that approximately half of journal articles describing RCTs had an unexplained discrepancy in primary outcomes [35]. All articles described eligibility criteria for participants, settings and locations where the data were

collected; however, all did not introduce scale of hospitals or research institutions, such as participants recruited from primary, secondary, or tertiary health care facilities or from the community. The information on the settings and locations is crucial to judge the applicability and generalization of a trial. Thus, authors should report the number and type of settings and describe the care providers involved.

All articles described the interventions for each group with sufficient detail. Item 5 emphasized "sufficient details;" the author should describe each intervention thoroughly, including control interventions. The description should allow a clinician to use the intervention in order to know exactly when and how to apply the intervention evaluated in the trial [36].

All articles listed outcome measures, including how and when they were assessed, but most did not completely specify which were or and secondary outcome measures. The primary outcome measure is the pre-specified outcome considered to be of greatest importance and is usually the one used for sample size calculation. This item was not reported in all articles, possibly due to the lack of changes made to outcomes measures after trial commencement.

All articles did not describe how sample size was determined. Item 7a emphasized "how," thus authors should indicate the process of sample size calculation, such as the variation of parameters, the primary outcome, and the formula of calculation or software. Sample size requires careful planning, to ensure a balance between medical and statistical considerations. Reports of studies with small sample sizes may come to an erroneous conclusion that the intervention groups do not differ, when in fact too few patients were studied to make such a claim [37]. Reviews of published trials have consistently found that a high proportion of trials have low power to detect clinically meaningful treatment effects [38–39]. In reality, small but clinically meaningful actual differences are much more likely than large differences but large trials are required to detect them [40]. All articles did not report this item, which may be due to no interim analyses and stopping guidelines during the trial.

20 articles described the method used to generate the allocation sequence, such as "random-number table" and "computerized random number generator," with only 1 article reporting "randomly divided into two groups." Item 8a emphasized "methods," and that "randomly divided into two groups" should not substitute for "methods." Therefore, authors should provide enough information to assess the method of sequence generation and the possibility of bias in the process of dividing into groups. All articles described the sample size of each group, but only 3 reported type of randomization and details of any restriction, such as participants allocated (1:1). Item 8b emphasized "type," where authors should describe restricted randomization when reporting the random method.

All articles did not describe their allocation concealment mechanism. Item 9 emphasizes "mechanism and steps to be implemented," such as "third-party" assignment, the numbered containers, and sealed opaque envelopes. Trials in which the allocation sequence had been inadequately or unclearly concealed yielded larger estimates of treatment effects than did trials in which authors reported adequate allocation concealment. In representative samples of all randomized trials indexed on PubMed, only 18% reported any allocation concealment mechanism, but some of those that reported mechanisms were inadequate [41]. Therefore, the mechanism and steps of random allocation was a critical aspect of high quality RCTs. All articles did not describe "who generated the allocation sequence, who enrolled participants, and who assigned participants to interventions." Item 10 emphasized "who," i.e. who was involved the design and implement of the randomization protocol. The allocation sequence is often performed by a third-party organization without their participation in the actual clinical trials. Health workers who enrolled participants and who assigned participants to interventions did not know the random allocation sequence. Therefore, investigators must then ensure that the assignment schedule is unpredictable and locked away. Only 1 article reported who was blinded to interventions, and how this blinding was ensured. Item 11a emphasized "who" and "how," and that authors should instead explicitly report the blinding status of people involved, for whom this may influence the validity of a trial, rather than merely describing the terms "double blind," "single blind" or "triple blind." A study of 200 RCTs reported as double blind found 18 different combinations of groups actually blinded when the authors of these trials were surveyed; and about one in every five of these trials—reported as double blind—did not blind participants, healthcare providers, or data collectors [42]. 6 articles described the similarity of interventions. Item 11b emphasized "similarity," i.e., that authors should state the similarity of the characteristics of the interventions (such as appearance, taste, smell, and method of administration) so that participants and healthcare providers could not distinguish between the study drug and placebo.

All articles described statistical methods, but most used a simple description of the particular tests and analytic software used. Item 12a emphasized statistical methods of outcome measures; we suggested that authors should adopt a more structured description, for example: X1 was the primary outcome, X1 was used to analyze method A, X2 and X3 were the secondary outcomes, X2 was used to analyze method B, and X3 was used to analyze method C. Data can be analyzed in many ways, and all statistical methods may not be appropriate for all situations. It is essential to specify which statistical procedure was used for each analysis, with further clarification necessary in the results section of the report.

All articles did not describe methods for additional analyses. Some were multicenter studies with data sources and different participant demographics, so that authors should implement additional analyses. A study evaluating the reporting quality of 142 RCT full-text articles published in five leading Chinese medical journals found that only 27% described the method to generate the randomized sequence, 4% had adequate allocation concealment, and only 17% mentioned blinding [43]; these findings are supported by others in the field of TCM [44–45].

Results

All articles described participant flow in some sentences, but all did not adopt a diagram to describe participant flow. 14 articles only described the numbers of participants who were randomly assigned and did not describe the numbers of participants who received the intended treatment and were analyzed for primary outcome. But from the full text, the numbers of last two phases seemed to equal the numbers of randomly assigned participants. Item 13a told authors that the numbers of participants may change in the three stages, including design, study, and analysis. Although CONSORT strongly recommends using this graphical device to communicate participant flow throughout the study, there is no specific, prescribed format. Participant flow was not necessary for some RCTs, if design and execution were straightforward, particularly if there were no losses to follow up or exclusions. However, in more complex studies, authors should adopt the flow for readers to discern whether and why some participants did not receive the allocated treatment, were lost to follow-up, or were excluded from the analysis. 8 articles described losses and exclusions after randomization with reasons for each group. Item 13b emphasized "numbers and reasons." Authors should have described the numbers of design phase, and the numbers and reasons for excluding participants from the analysis. Only in that way, some protocol deviations may be reported, such as participants who did not receive the intended intervention. 19 articles described "dates defining the periods of recruitment and follow-up." Knowing when a study took place and over what period participants were recruited places the study in historical context. The length of follow-up is not always a fixed period after randomization. In many RCTs in which the outcome is time to an event, follow-up of all participants is ended on a specific date. All articles did not describe why the trial ended or was stopped, which may be because there was no such situation. If so, authors should indicate why the trial came to an end and also disclose extrinsic factors that affected the decision to stop the trial, and who made the decision to stop the trial, including reporting the role the funding agency in the deliberations and decision to stop the trial [46]. All articles described baseline data to some degree, while only 6 articles showed baseline data with a table. Although the eligibility criteria indicated who was eligible for the trial, it is also important to know the characteristics of the participants who were actually included. This information allows readers, especially clinicians, to judge how relevant the results of a trial might be to an individual patient. Thus, author should describe this baseline information in a table.

All articles described number of participants (denominator) included in each analysis, but only 2 articles mentioned intention-to-treat (ITT) analysis. The meaning of the ITT analysis was that we should include all randomized participants in the analysis, and all retained in the group to which they were allocated in order to fully preserve the benefit of randomization. The conditions defined an ITT analysis, which was widely recommended as the preferred analysis strategy [47–48]. ITT analysis is generally favored because it avoids bias associated with non-random loss of participants [49–51]. Regardless of whether authors use the term "ITT," they should clarify which and how many participants are included in each analysis. Non-compliance with assigned therapy may mean that the intention-to-treat analysis underestimates the potential benefit of the treatment, so that additional analyses, such as a per-protocol analysis, may be considered [52–53]. It should be noted, however, that such analyses are often considerably flawed [54].

All articles described results for each group, but only 1 article reported the 95% confidence interval. For each outcome, study results should be reported as a summary of the outcome in each group, together with the contrast between the groups, known as the effect size. Furthermore, for all outcomes, authors should provide a confidence interval to indicate the precision (uncertainty) of the estimate. Many journals require or strongly encourage the use of confidence intervals [55]. They are especially valuable in relation to differences that do not meet conventional statistical significance, for which they often indicate that the result does not rule out an important clinical difference. The use of confidence intervals has increased markedly in recent years, although not in all medical specialties [56]. All articles did not mention binary outcome, which may be due to their unavailability. If so, both the relative effect (risk ratio [relative risk] or odds ratio) and the absolute effect should be reported (with confidence intervals), as neither the relative measure nor the absolute measure alone gives a complete picture of the effect and its implications. The common absolute effect included the numerator, denominator, and effect difference. The common relative effect included the risk ratio or risk difference. For survival time data, it could be the hazard ratio or difference in median survival time.

All articles did not describe subgroup analyses and adjusted analyses. Some of the 21 RCTs were multicenter studies with large differences in data sources and participant demographic data. It would be inappropriate to statistically analyze hospitals or research institutions together. In fact, researchers should pre-specify subgroup analyses of other hospital or research institutions, because it may influence the calculation of sample size.

12 articles described adverse effects. The implication of reporting adverse effects is that it easily enables the reader to understand information about the risks and benefits of interventions to make rational and balanced decisions. A review of trials published in six general medical journals in 2006 to 2007 found that, although 89% of 133 reports mentioned adverse events, no information on severe adverse events and withdrawal of patients due to an adverse event was given in 27% and 48% of articles, respectively [57].

Discussion

8 articles described trial limitations, but were superficial and incomplete. Common limitations included: not reporting how sample size was determined, allocation concealment mechanism and implementation, and ITT analysis. These reasons indicated that internal validity was unreliable. While all articles did not report external validity of the trial findings in the discussion section, all described eligibility criteria for participants, settings and locations where the data were collected, interventions, and outcomes, in the materials and methods sections. External validity, also called generalization or applicability, is the extent to which the results of a study can be generalized to other circumstances [58]. Internal validity, the extent to which the design and conduct of the trial eliminate the possibility of bias, is a prerequisite for external validity; the results of a flawed trial are invalid and the question of its external validity becomes irrelevant. All articles described interpretation consistent with results and compared with other articles. Readers will want to know how the present trial's results relate to those of other RCTs. This can best be achieved by including a formal systematic review in the results or discussion section of the report [59–60].

Other information

All articles did not describe registration number and name of trial registry. The World Health Organization states that "the registration of all interventional trials is a scientific, ethical, and moral responsibility." By registering a randomized trial, authors typically report a minimal set of information and obtain a unique trial registration number. If authors had not registered their trial they should explicitly state this and give the reason. All articles did not describe "where the full trial protocol can be accessed, if available." A protocol for the complete trial is important because it pre-specifies the methods of the randomized trial, such as primary outcome. Having a protocol can help to restrict the likelihood of undeclared *post hoc* changes to the trial methods and selective outcome reporting.

There were several ways to obtain the trial protocol. Journals reporting a trial's primary results can make the trial protocol available on their web site. Accessibility to the trial results and protocol is enhanced when the journal is open access. Some journals (such as trials) publish trial protocols, and such a publication can be referenced when reporting the trial's principal results. Trial registration will also ensure that many trial protocol details are available. Trial investigators may also be able to post their trial protocol on a website through their employer. The issue is that most investigators were not aware of publicizing the trial protocol. Certainly, it cannot exclude someone with no complete trial protocol.

11 articles described sources of funding, but all did not introduce the role of funders. Authors should report the sources of funding for the trial, as this is important information for readers assessing it. The level of involvement by a funder and their influence on the design, conduct, analysis, and reporting of a trial varies. If the funder had no such involvement, the authors should state this fact.

Study Limitations

Our study has several limitations. First, we did not contact authors when items were not reported because authors may not have adhered to CONSORT 2010 for reporting RCTs, with some items performed in their studies not reported in the articles. Second, we assessed each item with a "yes" or "no" response according to whether the author had reported all the contents listed in the refined items. A better way to show integrity and accuracy of RCTs would have been to have used a quantitative score approach to assess each article. A study adopted the visual analogue scale (VAS) approach to evaluate the overall quality of the report, "Clinical study of efficacy of GnRH-α combined with add back therapy in treatment of endometriosis" [61]. A study adopted five levels (adequately standardized, relatively standardized, inadequately standardized, not standardized, and not reported) to evaluate the overall quality of the report "Evaluation of the paper titled "Application of Tumor Type M2 Pyruvate Kinase in Diagnosis of Lung Cancer" based on the STARD statement"[62]. This method also can assess reporting quality of RCTs with the CONSORT 2010 statement. Third, we did not use the CONSORT for TCM to evaluate the reporting quality of RCTs on CHD in the journal. CONSORT for TCM is based on the CONSORT 2010 statement [63], with some items (background, objective, participants, intervention and outcomes, baseline, ancillary analyses, interpretation) adding related content of TCM. We selected the CONSORT 2010 statement instead of CONSORT for TCM to assess these articles of TCM because CONSORT for the TCM checklist did not include limitations, registration, protocol, funding, and secondary items. These items also reported the integrity and accuracy of RCTs. Fourth, we did not calculate the Kappa statistic to quantitatively measure inter-observer agreement.

Despite these, our study has some strengths. We conducted an objective data extraction process, with the domains that were included in RCTs marked as "yes" and those not reported as "no" based on standard checklist items recommended by the CONSORT 2010 statement without reviewer inference. Thus, this study's methodology is reproducible.

Conclusion

We demonstrated that the reviewed RCTs were generally not consistent with the CONSORT 2010 statement. Many studies proved that the use of the CONSORT statement has demonstrable benefits in improving the reporting quality of RCTs [64]. Thus, we suggest that authors should adhere to the CONSORT 2010 statement in reporting RCTs, and that editorial departments may consider the CONSORT statement as a guideline and instruct authors to draft manuscripts, and reviewers to judge manuscripts, according to the CONSORT statement, in order to further improve the reporting quality of RCTs.

Supporting Information

Checklist S1 PRISMA checklist. PRISMA 2009 checklist of information to include when reporting a systematic review. (DOC)

Author Contributions

Conceived and designed the experiments: FF QX QS. Performed the experiments: FF SZ PW. Analyzed the data: FF XG SZ. Contributed reagents/materials/analysis tools: FF SZ PW XG. Wrote the paper: FF.

References

1. Schulz KF, Altman DG, Moher D, Group C(2010) CONSORT 2010 statement: updated guidelines for reporting parallel group randomised trials. BMJ 340: c332.
2. Chan AW, Altman DG (2005) Epidemiology and reporting of randomised trials published in PubMed journals. Lancet 365: 1159–1162.
3. Begg C, Cho M, Eastwood S, Horton R, Moher D, et al. (1996) Improving the quality of reporting of randomized controlled trials. The CONSORT statement. JAMA 276: 637–639.
4. Diverse Populations Collaborative Group (2002) Prediction of mortality from coronary heart disease among diverse populations: is there a common predictive function. Heart 88 : 222–228.
5. Zhou DZ (2000) Open the gate to the world for traditional Chinese medicine. Chinese Traditional Patent Medicine,22: 578–580.
6. Lu Z, Kou W, Du B, Wu Y, Zhao S, et al. (2008) Effect of Xuezhikang, an extract from red yeast Chinese rice, on coronary events in a Chinese population with previous myocardial infarction. Am J Cardiol 101: 1689–1693.
7. Zhu XF, Zhang RH, Wang TC, Han L, Wang PP, et al. (2012) Multi-center randomized controlled clinical study of Saffron Yellow Sterile Powder for Injection for the treatment of stable angina pectoris with heart-blood stagnation syndrome in patients. Chinese Traditional Patent Medicine 34:596–601.
8. Zhao S, Song YQ, Yue W, Mao XR, Ju CX, et al. (2007) Multicentric randominzed double blinede clinical study of Yiqi Tongmai Oral Liquid against angina pectoris in patients with coronary heart disease. Zhong Xi Yi Jie He Xue Bao (Journal of Chinese Integrative Medicine) 5(4):383–391.
9. Moher D, Hopewell S, Schulz KF, Montori V, Gotzsche PC, et al. (2010) CONSORT 2010 explanation and elaboration: updated guidelines for reporting parallel group randomised trials. BMJ 340:c869.
10. Moher D, Liberati A, Tetzlaff J, Altman DG (2009) referred reporting items for systematic reviews and meta-analyses: the PRISMA statement. J Clin Epidemiol 62(10):1006–1012.
11. Guo ZB, Fu JG, Zhao Y, Liu MS, Li Q (2006)Therapeutic Efficacy of oxymatrine On Arrhythmia and Heart Rate Variability in Patients with Coronary Heart Disease. Zhongguo Zhong Xi Yi Jie He Za Zhi (Chinese Journal of integrated Traditional and Western Medicine) 26:311–315.
12. Liu P, Zhao YX, Zhang Y, Wang SJ, Jing XW, et al (2006) Clinical Observation of Daidzein Intervention on Serum Inflammatory Factors in Senile Patients with Coronary Heart Disease. Zhongguo Zhong Xi Yi Jie He Za Zhi (Chinese Journal of integrated Traditional and Western Medicine) 26:42–45.
13. Lu XY, Shi DX, Xu H, Chen KJ, Lv SZ (2006) Clinical Study on Effect of Xiongshao Capsule on Restenosis after Percutaneous Coronary Intervention. Zhongguo Zhong Xi Yi Jie He Za Zhi (Chinese Journal of integrated Traditional and Western Medicine) 26:13–17.
14. Jing L, Wang J, Wang T (2007) Valuation on Effects of Disassembled Formulas of Xuefu Zhuyu Decoctiont for Treatment of Angina Pectoris Using Seattle Angina Questionnaire. Zhongguo Zhong Xi Yi Jie He Za Zhi (Chinese Journal of integrated Traditional and Western Medicine) 27:18–23.
15. Wei ZT, Zhao JX (2007) Clinical observation on Effects of Fuzheng Jiedu Granule in treating Coronary Heart Disease in Long Term Contact with Nickel. Zhongguo Zhong Xi Yi Jie He Za Zhi (Chinese Journal of integrated Traditional and Western Medicine) 27:418–421.
16. Xu H, Lu XY, Chen KJ, Shi DZ (2007)Study on correlation of Blood-stasis Syndrome and Its Accompanied Syndromes with Pathological Changes Showed in Coronary Angiography and Restenosis after Percutaneous Coronary Intervention. Zhongguo Zhong Xi Yi Jie He Za Zhi (Chinese Journal of integrated Traditional and Western Medicine) 27:8–12.
17. Zhang Y, Lu S, Liu YY, Song XX, Chen KJ, et al. (2007) Effect of Panax Quinquefolius Saponin on Insulin Sensitivity in Patients of Coronary Heart Disease with Blood Glucose Abnormality. Zhongguo Zhong Xi Yi Jie He Za Zhi (Chinese Journal of integrated Traditional and Western Medicine) 27:1066–1070.
18. Wang LJ, Luo XP, Wang Y, Chen WM, Lu Y, et al..(2008) Evaluation on Tolerability and Safety of Long-term Administration with Shexiang Baoxin Pill in Patients with Coronary Heart Disease of Stable Angina Pectoris. Zhongguo Zhong Xi Yi Jie He Za Zhi (Chinese Journal of integrated Traditional and Western Medicine) 28:399–402.

19. Zhang Q, Zhou JY, Sun NL(2008) Effect of XinkeshuTablet on Heart Rate Variability in Patients with Coronary Heart Disease. Zhongguo Zhong Xi Yi Jie He Za Zhi (Chinese Journal of integrated Traditional and Western Medicine) 28:402–405.
20. Zhang Q, Zhou MX, Huang YS, Hou JR (2008) Effect of Fulu Baoxinping Oral Liquid in Treatment of Coronary Heart Disease Patients with Premature Ventricular Beat. Zhongguo Zhong Xi Yi Jie He Za Zhi (Chinese Journal of integrated Traditional and Western Medicine) 28:509–512.
21. Cheng WL, Wang Y, Cai Z, Ke YN, Liu XF, et al (2009) Effect of Qingre Quyu Granule on the Vulnerable Atherosclerotic Plaque of Carotid Artery in Patients With Stable Coronary Artery Disease. Zhongguo Zhong Xi Yi Jie He Za Zhi (Chinese Journal of integrated Traditional and Western Medicine) 29:1055–1059.
22. Hu YH, Wu HQ, Qi X, Wu H, Zhou YP, et al. (2009) Influence of Shenfu Injection on Heart Function and Bone Marrow Stem Cell Mobilization in Patients with Chronic Heart Failure of Coronary Heart Disease. Zhongguo Zhong Xi Yi Jie He Za Zhi (Chinese Journal of integrated Traditional and Western Medicine) 29:309–312.
23. Li AM, Zhao S (2009) Effect of Renshen Jianxin Capsule for Alleviating Insulin Resistance in Patients with Coronary Heart Disease and Glucose Tolerance Impairment. Zhongguo Zhong Xi Yi Jie He Za Zhi (Chinese Journal of integrated Traditional and Western Medicine) 29:830–833.
24. Yan LY, Zhang YQ, Wang XM, Zhang XP, Li XK (2009) Effect of Buxu Huayu Qutan Decoction on Anti-oxidative Capacity in Aged Patients with Stable Angina Pectoris of Coronary Heart Disease. Zhongguo Zhong Xi Yi Jie He Za Zhi (Chinese Journal of integrated Traditional and Western Medicine) 29:695–698.
25. Cui XY, WY, Nong YB, Wang X, Guo ZQ, et al. (2010) Effect of Liangxue Shengji Recipe on Incidence of Post-percutaneous Coronary Intervention Restenosis and Adverse Cardiovascular Events. Zhongguo Zhong Xi Yi Jie He Za Zhi (Chinese Journal of integrated Traditional and Western Medicine) 30:30–33.
26. Wu TQ, Gu N, Wang FF, Wang J, Pang JH (2010) Effect of Ningxintong Granule in Treating Patients of Coronary Heart Disease with Left Ventricular Diastolic Dysfunction and Qi-deflclency Blood-stasis Syndrome. Zhongguo Zhong Xi Yi Jie He Za Zhi (Chinese Journal of integrated Traditional and Western Medicine) 30:357–360.
27. Yin CH, Bi DP, Du M (2010) Effect of Tongxinluo Capsule on Platelet Aggregation Function in Patients with Aspirin Resistance. Zhongguo Zhong Xi Yi Jie He Za Zhi (Chinese Journal of integrated Traditional and Western Medicine) 30:380–383.
28. Zhu H, Luo XP, Wang LJ, Li Y, Shi HM, et al. (2010) Evaluation on Clinical Effect of Long-term Shexiang Baoxin pill Administration for Treatment of Coronary Heart Disease. Zhongguo Zhong Xi Yi Jie He Za Zhi (Chinese Journal of integrated Traditional and Western Medicine) 30:474–477.
29. Zhu HJ, Lu S, Su W, Gong SY, Zhang ZB, et al. (2010) Effect of Liandou Qingmai Recipe on Atherogenic Indices of Plasma and High-sensitivity C-reactive Protein In Patients with Coronary Heart Disease. Zhongguo Zhong Xi Yi Jie He Za Zhi (Chinese Journal of integrated Traditional and Western Medicine) 30:361–364.
30. Peng W, Shi DZ, Xue YT, Gao HC, Zhang FR (2011) Effect of Xiongshao Capsule in Treating 112 patients with Coronary Heart Disease Angina Pectoris of Xin-blood Stasis Syndrome. Zhongguo Zhong Xi Yi Jie He Za Zhi (Chinese Journal of integrated Traditional and Western Medicine) 31:191–193.
31. Xin L, Xu FQ, Gao R, Gao GD, Sun LJ, et al. (2011) Effects of Xinluotong Tablet on Stable Coronary Heart Disease AnginaÐ A Randomised Controlled Trial. Zhongguo Zhong Xi Yi Jie He Za Zhi (Chinese Journal of integrated Traditional and Western Medicine) 31:1191–1195.
32. Fan T, Wang G, Wang L, Xiong ZY, Mao B (2007) Quality Assessment of Clinical Studies on Compound Salvia Pellet (CSP) for Angina Pectoris[J]. Chin J Evid-based Med,7(6):461–471
33. Dickersin K, Manheimer E, Wieland S, Robinson KA, Lefebvre C, et al. (2002) Development of the Cochrane Collaboration's CENTRAL Register of controlled clinical trials. Eval Health Prof 25:38–64.
34. Bath FJ, Owen VE, Bath PM (1998) Quality of full and final publications reporting acute stroke trials: a systematic review. Stroke 29: 2203–2210.
35. Dwan K, Altman DG, Arnaiz JA, Bloom J, Chan AW, et al. (2008) Systematic review of the empirical evidence of study publication bias and outcome reporting bias. PLoS ONE 3:e3081.
36. Glasziou P, Meats E, Heneghan C, Shepperd S (2008) What is missing from descriptions of treatment in trials and reviews? BMJ 336:1472–4.
37. Altman DG, Bland JM (1995) Absence of evidence is not evidence of absence. BMJ 311: 485.
38. Moher D, Dulberg CS, Wells GA (1994) Statistical power, sample size, and their reporting in randomised controlled trials. JAMA 272:122–4.
39. Charles P, Giraudeau B, Dechartres A, Baron G, Ravaud P (2009) Reporting of sample size calculation in randomised controlled trials: review. BMJ 338:b1732.
40. Yusuf S, Collins R, Peto R. (1984) Why do we need some large, simple randomised trials? Stat Med 3:409–22.
41. Chan AW, Altman DG (2005) Epidemiology and reporting of randomised trials published in PubMed journals. Lancet 365:1159–62.
42. Haahr MT, Hróbjartsson A (2006) Who is blinded in randomised clinical trials? A study of 200 trials and a survey of authors. Clin Trials 3:360–5.
43. Xu L, Li J, Zhang M, Ai C, Wang L (2008) Chinese authors do need CONSORT: Reporting quality assessment for five leading Chinese medical journals. Contemporary Clinical Trials 29:727–731.
44. Mao B, Wang G, Fan T, Chen X, Liu J, et al. (2007) Assessing the Quality of Reporting of Randomised Controlled Trials in Traditional Chinese Medicine. Chinese Journal of Evidece-based Medicine 7:880–887.
45. Zhang XL, Jing L, Zhang MM, Yuan WM (2006) Assessing the Reporting Quality of Randomised Controlled Trials on Acupuncture for Acute Ischemic Stroke Using the CONSORT Statement and STRICTA. Chinese Journal of Evidence-Based Medicine 6: 586–590.
46. Montori VM, Devereaux PJ, Adhikari NK, Burns KE, Eggert CH, et al. (2005) Randomised trials stopped early for benefit: a systematic review. JAMA 294:2203–9.
47. Hollis S, Campbell F (1999) What is meant by intention to treat analysis. Survey of published randomised controlled trials. BMJ 319: 670–674.
48. Herman A, Botser IB, Tenenbaum S, Chechick A. (2009) Intention-to-treat analysis and accounting for missing data in orthopedic randomised clinical trials. J Bone Joint Surg Am 91 : 2137–2143.
49. Lee YJ, Ellenberg JH, Hirtz DG, Nelson KB (1991) Analysis of clinical trials by treatment actually received: is it really an option? Stat Med 10:1595–605.
50. Lewis JA, Machin D (1993) Intention to treat—who should use ITT? Br J Cancer 68:647–50.
51. Lachin JL (2000) Statistical considerations in the intent-to-treat principle. Control Clin Trials 21:526.
52. Sheiner LB, Rubin DB (1995) Intention-to-treat analysis and the goals of clinical trials. Clin Pharmacol Ther 57:6–15.
53. Nagelkerke N, Fidler V, Bernsen R, Borgdorff M (2000) Estimating treatment effects in randomised clinical trials in the presence of non-compliance. Stat Med 19:1849–64.
54. Melander H, Ahlqvist-Rastad J, Meijer G, Beermann B (2003) Evidence b(i)ased medicine–selective reporting from studies sponsored by pharmaceutical industry: review of studies in new drug applications. BMJ 326:1171–3.
55. International Committee of Medical Journal Editors (1997) Uniform requirements for manuscripts submitted to biomedical journals: Ann Intern Med. 126: 36–47.
56. Altman DG (2000) Confidence intervals in practice. In: Altman DG, Machin D, Bryant TN, Gardner MJ, eds. Statistics with confidence. 2nd ed. BMJ Books 6–14.
57. Pitrou I, Boutron I, Ahmad N, Ravaud P (2009) Reporting of safety results in published reports of randomised controlled trials. Arch Intern Med 169: 1756–1761.
58. CAMPBELL DT (1957) Factors relevant to the validity of experiments in social settings. Psychol Bull 54: 297–312.
59. Sadler LC, Davison T, McCowan L (2000) A randomised controlled trial and meta-analysis of active management of labour. BJOG 107:909–15.
60. First International Study of Infarct Survival Collaborative Group (1986) Randomised trial of intravenous atenolol among 16 027 cases of suspected acute myocardial infarction: ISIS-1. Lancet 2:57–66.
61. Xu H, Qin W, Gan W, Sun Q, et al. (2012) Analysis of the quality of reports of randomised controlled trials using CONSORT statement. Chinese General Practice 15: 2304–2310.
62. Bian ZX, Liu BY, David Moher, Wu TX, Shang HC, et al. (2011) Consolidated Standards of Reporting Trials (CONSORT) for Traditional Chinese Medicine: current situation and future development. Front Med 5: 171–177.
63. Xu Q, Sun Q (2009) Evaluation of the paper titled "Application of Tumor Type M2 Pyruvate Kinase in Diagnosis of Lung Cancer"based on the STARD statement. Chinese Journal of Evidece-based Medicine 9:113–118.
64. Moher D, Jones A, LePage L (2001) Use of the CONSORT Statement and quality of reports of randomised trials: a comparative before and after evaluation. JAMA 285:1992–1995.

18

Study on the Main Components Interaction from *Flos Lonicerae* and *Fructus Forsythiae* and Their Dissolution In Vitro and Intestinal Absorption in Rats

Wei Zhou[1,2,3], Xiaobin Tan[4], Jinjun Shan[5], Shouchuan Wang[5], Ailing Yin[1], Baochang Cai[1], Liuqing Di[1,2,3]*

1 College of Pharmacy, Nan'jing University of Chinese Medicine, Nan'jing, People's Republic of China, **2** Jiang'su Engineering Research Center for Efficient Delivery System of TCM, Nan'jing, People's Republic of China, **3** Nan'jing Engineering Research Center for Industrialization of Chinese Medicine Pellets, Nan'jing, People's Republic of China, **4** Laboratory of New Drug Delivery System of Chinese Meteria Medica, Jiang'su Provinical Academy of Chinese Medicine, Nan'jing, People's Republic of China, **5** Jiangsu Key Laboratory of Pediatric Respiratory Disease, Institute of Paediatrics, Nan'jing University of Chinese Medicine, Nan'jing, People's Republic of China

Abstract

The *Flos Lonicerae-Fructus Forsythiae* herb couple is the basic components of Chinese herbal preparations (Shuang-Huang-Lian tablet, Yin-Qiao-Jie-Du tablet and Fufang Qin-Lan oral liquid), and its pharmacological effects were significantly higher than that in *Flos Lonicerae* or *Fructus Forsythiae*, but the reasons remained unknown. In the present study, pattern recognition analysis (hierarchical cluster analysis (HCA) and principal component analysis (PCA)) combined with UHPLC-ESI/LTQ-Orbitrap MS system were performed to study the chemical constitution difference between co-decoction and mixed decoction in the term of chemistry. Besides, the pharmacokinetics *in vivo* and intestinal absorption *in vitro* combined with pattern recognition analysis were used to reveal the discrepancy between herb couple and single herbs in the view of biology. The observation from the chemical view *in vitro* showed that there was significant difference in quantity between co-decoction and mixed decoction by HCA, and the exposure level of isoforsythoside and 3, 5-dicaffeoylquinic acid in co-decoction, higher than that in mixed decoction, directly resulted in the discrepancy between co-decoction and mixed decoction using both PCA and HCA. The observation from the pharmacokinetics displayed that the exposure level *in vivo* of neochlorogenic acid, 3, 4-dicaffeoylquinic acid, isoforsythoside and forsythoside A, higher than that in single herbs, was the main factor contributing to the difference by both PCA and HCA, interestingly consistent with the results obtained from Caco-2 cells *in vitro*, which indicated that it was because of intestinal absorption improvement of neochlorogenic acid, 3, 4-dicaffeoylquinic acid, isoforsythoside and forsythoside A that resulted in a better efficacy of herb couple than that of single herbs from the perspective of biology. The results above illustrated that caffeic acid derivatives in *Flos Lonicerae-Fructus Forsythiae* herb couple could be considered as chemical markers for quality control of its preparations.

Editor: Hua Zhou, Macau University of Science and Technology, Macao

Funding: The present study is supported financially by the National Natural Science Foundation of China (81001499), the Jiangsu Natural Science Foundation (BK2010560), "Qing Lan" Project from Jiangsu Provincial Technology Innovation Team Support Scheme, the priority Academic Program Development of Jiangsu Higher Education Institution (No. ysxk-2010), and 2012 program sponsored for scientific innovation research of college graduate in Jiangsu province (623). The funders had no role in study design, data collection and analysis, decision to publish, or preparation of the manuscript.

Competing Interests: The authors have declared that no competing interests exist.

* Email: diliuqing@hotmail.com

Introduction

Herbs used together in couples (Yaodui in Chinese) are the basic composition units of Chinese herbal formulas and have special clinical significance in Traditional Chinese Medicine (TCM). The herb couples are much simpler than other complicated formulas yet retain the basic therapeutic features. It is important to elucidate the compatibility foundation of TCM formulas by investigating the law and effective substance of herb couples, which are the major areas of research supported by Chinese government [1]. There are magnitudes of methods to study the compatibility rule and principles of herb couples to some extent including literature research [2], extraction and separation [3], pharmacological effects [4–6], pharmacokinetics *in vivo* of active components [7] and serum pharmaco-chemistry methods [8], *etc*. However, up to now, few studies were performed to explain the reasonability of herb couples based on the systemic biopharmaceutics both *in vivo* and *in vitro*.

Flos Lonicerae (FLJ) possesses wide pharmacological actions, such as antibacteria, anti-inflammation, antivirus, antiendotoxin, blood fat reduction, *etc* [9], and *Fructus Forsythiae* (FF) has antibacterial, antiviral, antioxidant, anti-inflammatory, anti-obesic effects, *etc* [10]. The two herbs are the basic components of Chinese herbal preparations such as Shuang-Huang-Lian oral liquid, Yin-Qiao-Jie-Du tablet, Qin-Re-Jie-Du oral liquid and Fufang Qin-Lan oral liquid, which are extensively used in clinical practice [11], and it was shown by Lin (2008) [12] that the pharmacological effects such as anti-inflammatory and antipyretic effects in FLJ-FF herb couples were significantly stronger than that in FLJ or FF, but the reasons were unknown. Thus, it was presumed that the dissolution *in vitro* of main ingredients was significantly higher than that of FLJ and FF or the intestinal absorptions of active components were improved combined with FLJ or FF.

In short, the current study aims to demonstrate the optimal efficacy of FLJ-FF herb couple based on thoughts we provided above analyzed by both hierarchical cluster analysis (HCA) and principal component analysis (PCA) for the further development of herb couples preparations. The specific objectives of the current study include: (1) To study the difference between co-decoction and mixed decoction based on the dissolution *in vitro*. (2) To research the discrepancy between herb couple and single herbs based on the pharmacokinetics *in vivo*. (3) To illustrate the difference via *in vitro* Caco-2 cells between herb couple and single herbs.

Materials and Methods

Ethics statement

All procedures had the approval of the Animal Ethics Committee of the Nanjing University of Chinese Medicine.

Reagents and chemicals

FLJ (bud of *Lonicera japonica* Thunb.) and FF (fruit of *Forsythia suspense*) were purchased from Yi-Feng drug store (Nanjing, China) and authenticated by Prof. Wu (Department of Pharmacognosy, Nanjing University of Chinese Medicine). All voucher specimens were deposited in our laboratory for future reference. Chlorogenic acid, luteoloside, pillyrin, forsythoside A and tinidazole (using as internal standard, IS) were purchased from National Institute for the Control of Pharmaceutical and Biological Products (Beijing, China). Neochlorogenic acid, cryptochlorogenic acid, 3, 4-dicaffeoylquinic acid, 3, 5-dicaffeoylquinic acid and forsythoside B (98% pure) were purchased from Sichuan Weikeqi Bio-tech Co., Ltd. (Sichuan, China). Isoforsythoside, caffeic acid, quinic acid, genistein, luteolin, quercetin, arctigenin, genistin, astragalin, hyperoside, isoquercitrin, pinoresinol-β-D-glucoside, arctiin, rutin, dipsacoside B and loganin (98% pure) were purchased from Chengdu Herbpurify Co., Ltd. (Sichuan, China). Heparin sodium injection was purchased from Changzhou Qianhong Bio-pharma Co., Ltd. (Changzhou, China). Methanol and acetonitrile (HPLC grade) were purchased from Merck (Merck, Germany), and water was purified by a Milli-Q water purification system (Millipore, Bedford, MA, USA). All other chemicals and reagents were of analytical grade.

Trifluoroacetic acid, Lucifer yellow (LY) and DMSO were purchased from Sigma Chemical Co. (St. Louis, MO). Phosphoric acid, acetic acid, formic acid, methanol and acetonitrile (HPLC grade) were purchased from Merck (Merck, Germany), and water was purified by a Milli-Q water purification system (Millipore, Bedford, MA, USA). All other chemicals and reagents were of analytical grade.

Dulbecco's modified Eagle's medium (DMEM), fetal bovine serum (FBS), 0.05% trypsin-EDTA, penicillin-streptomycin and non-essential amino acids were obtained from GibcoBRI, Life and Technologies, USA. Collagen type I, sodium pyruvate, MTT (3-(4, 5-dimethylthiazole-2-yl)-2, 5-diphenyl tetrazolium bromide) and trypsin_TPCK (Tosylamide Phenylethyl Chloromethyl Keton-treated Trypsin) were purchased from Sigma Chemical Co. (St. Louis, MO, USA). HBSS (Hank's balanced salt solution) and PBS (Phosphate Buffered Saline) were purchased from Sigma Chemical Co. (St. Louis, MO, USA). Culture cell inserts for 6 well plates (CCI, 137435) were purchase from Nalge Nunc International. (Roskilde, Denmark).

The human colorectal cancer cell lines (Caco-2, HCT116) were bought from cell bank (Chinese Academy of Sciences).

Male Sprague-Dawley (SD) rats (~250 g) were supplied by the Experimental Animal Center of Nanjing University of Chinese Medicine (Certificate No. SCXK2008-0033). The experimental procedures were in compliance with the animal ethics committee of the Nanjing University of Chinese Medicine.

Preparation of mixed decoction and co-decoction

FLJ (30.0 g, 40 meshes) and FF powders (30.0 g, 40 meshes) were decocted with boiling water (1:10, *w/v*) for 60 min by heating reflux, respectively. The two extracted solutions were filtered through 5 layer gauzes with the concentrations of 100 mg raw medicine per milliliter, respectively. The mixed decoction was prepared by mixing the two extracted solutions (1:1, *v/v*).

FLJ (15.0 g, 40 meshes) combined with FF powders (15.0 g, 40 meshes) (1:1(*w/w*)) as co-decoction were decocted with boiling water (1:10, *w/v*) for 60 min by heating reflux. The extracted solution was filtered through 5 layer gauzes with the concentrations of 100 mg raw medicine per milliliter.

Preparations of FLJ and FF concentrated extracts

FLJ (1000 g) and FF (1000 g) were decocted twice with boiling water (1:10, *w/v*) for 45 min, respectively. The two extracted solutions were filtered through 5 layer gauzes, and concentrated to

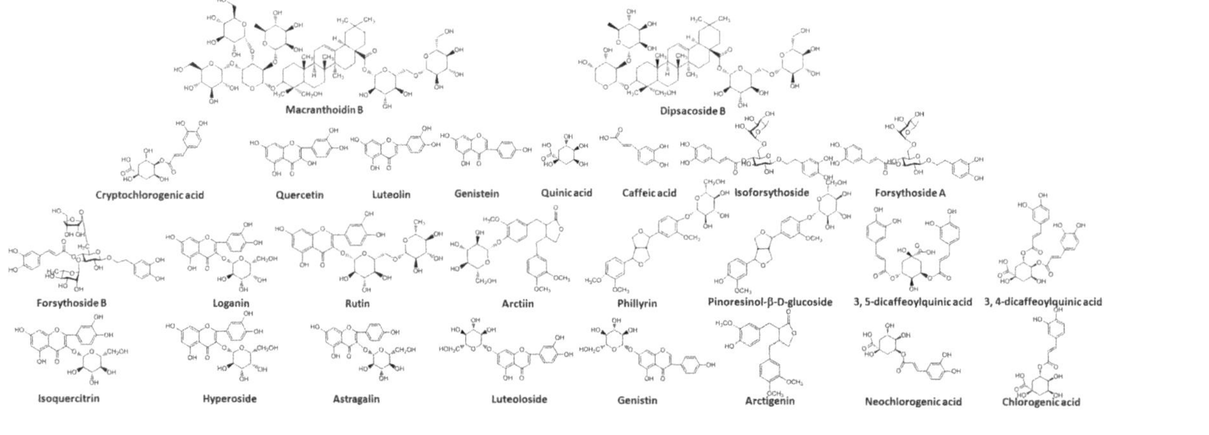

Figure 1. Structural formulae of analyte standards in FLJ-FF herb couple including flavones, organic acids, saponins, iridoids, phenylethanoid glycosides and lignans.

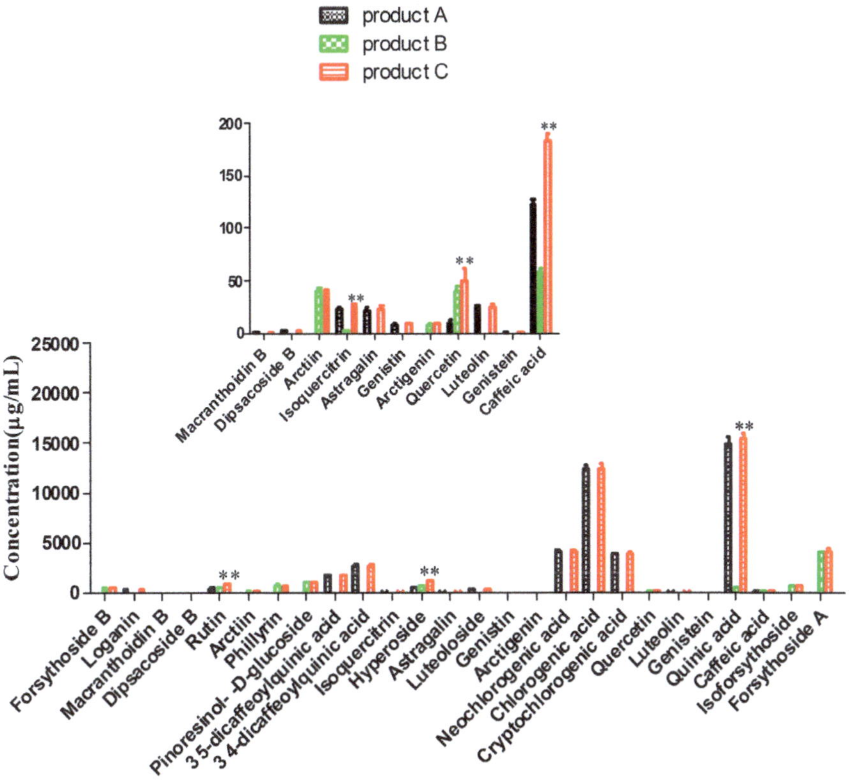

Figure 2. The contents of product A, B and C groups analyzed by UPLC-ESI-MS/MS. (*) $P<0.05$ and (**) $P<0.01$, compared with product C group.

a thick solution with the concentration of 2.5 g raw medicine per milliliter with 400 mL of extract used as follows, respectively [12], and the contents of caffeic acid, quinic acid, neochlorogenic acid, chlorogenic acid, cryptochlorogenic acid, 3, 5-dicaffeoylquinic acid, 3, 4-dicaffeoylquinic acid, genistin, luteoloside, astragalin, hyperoside, isoquercitrin, rutin, genistein, luteolin, quercetin, macranthoidin B, dipsacoside B and loganin (Fig. 1) in FLJ extract were 246.70, 29795, 8022.0, 24900, 7642.5, 3371.3, 5174.1, 17.313, 570.04, 43.595, 1044.0, 47.244, 789.64, 0.99522, 49.549, 20.007, 2.8651, 4.0725 and 542.44 μg/mL, respectively. And the contents of caffeic acid, quinic acid, rutin, hyperoside, isoquercitrin, quercetin, pinoresinol-β-D-glucoside, pillyrin, arctiin, arctigenin, isoforsythoside, forsythoside A and forsythoside B (Fig. 1) in FF extract were 118.16, 1092.2, 858.11, 1435.1, 4.2824, 79.045, 1958.9, 1380.1, 81.296, 17.313, 1356.1, 8036.0 and 826.97 μg/mL, respectively.

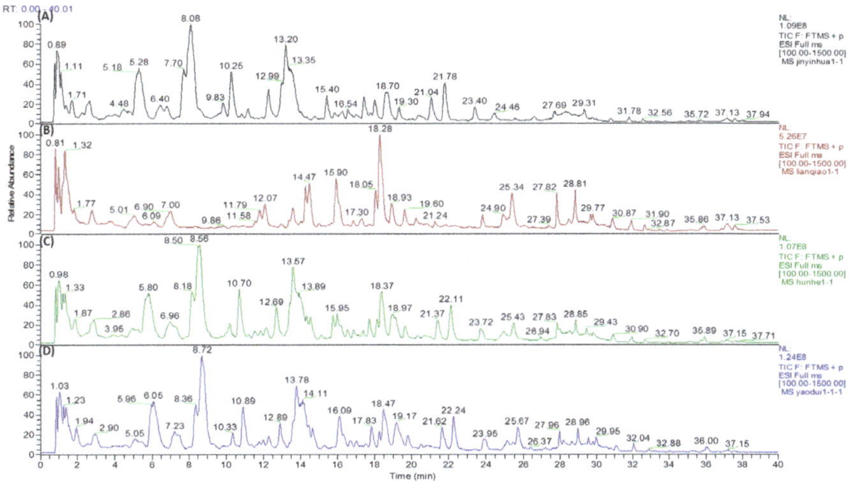

Figure 3. The TIC chromatographies of FLJ group (a), FF group (b), mixed decoction (c) and co-decoction (d) analyzed by UHPLC-ESI/LTQ-Orbitrap-MS.

Table 1. The chemical components identified from mixed decoction and co-decoction of *Flos Lonicera-Fructus Forsythiae* herb couple.

Peak no.	Components	Chemical formula	ESI^+, *m/z*	Ret. time	Source
			MS, MS^n		
1	Quinic acid	$C_7H_{12}O_6$	193.07066 $[M+H]^+$	1.16	FLJ, FF
2	Forsythoside D	$C_{20}H_{28}O_{13}$	499.14294 $[M+Na]^+$	2.32	FF
3	Neochlorogenic acid	$C_{16}H_{18}O_9$	355.10236 $[M+H]^+$, 162.97160	2.98	FLJ
4	Caffeic acid	$C_9H_8O_4$	181.04884 $[M+H]^+$	3.00	FLJ, FF
5	Forsythoside E	$C_{20}H_{30}O_{12}$	485.16295 $[M+Na]^+$, 185.12677	5.19	FF
6	Chlorogenic acid	$C_{16}H_{18}O_9$	355.10236 $[M+H]^+$, 162.97160	6.05	FLJ
7	Cryptochlorogenic acid	$C_{16}H_{18}O_9$	355.10236 $[M+H]^+$, 162.97160	7.23	FLJ
8	Sweroside	$C_{16}H_{22}O_9$	359.13366 $[M+H]^+$, 126.99121, 179.00241	10.89	FLJ
9	Loganin	$C_{17}H_{26}O_{10}$	391.15987 $[M+H]^+$	13.38	FLJ
10	Centauroside	$C_{34}H_{46}O_{19}$	759.27061 $[M+H]^+$	14.12	FLJ
11	Isoforsythoside	$C_{29}H_{36}O_{15}$	647.19324 $[M+Na]^+$, 321.08435, 347.21368	16.12	FF
12	Rutin	$C_{27}H_{30}O_{16}$	611.16066 $[M+H]^+$, 164.97000, 229.01273, 256.98975, 285.01004	16.23	FLJ, FF
13	Isoquercitin	$C_{21}H_{20}O_{12}$	465.10275 $[M+H]^+$, 57.06033, 164.96709, 229.02371, 285.05786	16.32	FLJ, FF
14	Hyperoside	$C_{21}H_{20}O_{12}$	465.10275 $[M+H]^+$, 257.06033, 164.96709, 229.02371, 285.05786	16.65	FLJ, FF
15	Luteoloside	$C_{21}H_{20}O_{11}$	449.10784 $[M+H]^+$, 152.88036	17.08	FLJ
16	Forsythoside B	$C_{34}H_{44}O_{19}$	779.23690 $[M+Na]^+$	18.21	FF
17	Forsythoside A	$C_{29}H_{36}O_{15}$	647.19464 $[M+Na]^+$, 321.08435, 347.21368	18.45	FF
18	3, 5-dicaffeoylquinic acid	$C_{25}H_{24}O_{12}$	517.13405 $[M+H]^+$, 162.96284, 319.11139	19.15	FLJ
19	Astragalin	$C_{21}H_{20}O_{11}$	449.10784 $[M+H]^+$, 152.88036	19.20	FLJ
20	Genistin	$C_{21}H_{20}O_{10}$	433.11292 $[M+H]^+$	19.99	FLJ
21	Pinoresinol-β-D-glucoside	$C_{26}H_{32}O_{11}$	543.18368 $[M+Na]^+$, 219.06879, 291.10626, 142.71555, 113.25488	20.46	FF
22	Epipinoresinol-β-D-glucoside	$C_{26}H_{32}O_{11}$	543.18231 $[M+Na]^+$, 142.98523, 219.06894, 231.05322, 266.29376, 281.40131, 291.15970	20.96	FF
23	3, 4-dicaffeoylquinic acid	$C_{25}H_{24}O_{12}$	517.13405 $[M+H]^+$, 162.96284, 319.11139	21.63	FLJ
24	Pinoresinol monomethyether-β-D-glucoside	$C_{25}H_{30}O_{11}$	529.16803 $[M+Na]^+$	23.31	FF
25	Arctiin	$C_{27}H_{34}O_{11}$	557.19933 $[M+Na]^+$	24.19	FF
26	Quercetin	$C_{15}H_{10}O_7$	303.04993 $[M+H]^+$	24.91	FLJ, FF
27	Luteolin	$C_{15}H_{10}O_6$	287.05501 $[M+H]^+$	25.20	FLJ
28	Genistein	$C_{15}H_{10}O_5$	271.06010 $[M+H]^+$	25.30	FLJ
29	Phillyrin	$C_{27}H_{34}O_{11}$	557.19933 $[M+Na]^+$, 291.15938, 249.07809, 218.97397, 143.08472	25.67	FF
30	Macranthoidin B	$C_{65}H_{106}O_{32}$	1421.65594 $[M+Na]^+$	28.82	FLJ
31	Dipsacoside B	$C_{53}H_{86}O_{22}$	1097.55030 $[M+Na]^+$	28.89	FLJ
32	Phillygenin	$C_{21}H_{24}O_6$	373.16456 $[M+H]^+$	28.90	FF
33	Pinoresinol	$C_{20}H_{22}O_6$	359.14891 $[M+H]^+$, 355.15335,	28.94	FF
34	Epipinoresinol	$C_{20}H_{22}O_6$	359.14847 $[M+H]^+$	29.29	FF
35	Arctigenin	$C_{21}H_{24}O_6$	373.16456 $[M+H]^+$	29.95	FF
36	Unknown	$C_{24}H_{30}O_6$	437.19244 $[M+Na]^+$, 168.99055, 259.07562, 243.24869, 285.09967, 200.95114	31.78	FLJ, FF
37	Unknown	$C_{24}H_{41}$	330.33511 $[M+H]^+$, 101.99937, 268.31992, 284.25348, 294.42615	32.64	FLJ, FF

Table 1. Cont.

Peak no.	Components	Chemical formula	ESI$^+$, *m/z* MS, MS^n	Ret. time	Source
38	Unknown	$C_{14}H_{22}O_2$	223.16858 [M+H]$^+$, 139.06036, 122.95891, 120.98438, 125.05688	33.24	FLJ, FF
39	Unknown	$C_{16}H_{22}O_4$	279.15869 [M+H]$^+$, 101.94276, 268.31708, 294.47253	33.91	FLJ, FF
40	Unknown	$C_{17}H_{37}O$	280.26303 [M+Na]$^+$, 263.10306, 245.16504	35.02	FLJ, FF
41	Unknown	$C_{17}H_{35}O$	256.26257 [M+H]$^+$, 70.93882	35.66	FLJ, FF
42	Unknown	$C_{27}H_{50}O_{15}$	637.30347 [M+Na]$^+$, 525.16754, 469.17981	35.80	FLJ, FF
43	Unknown	$C_{19}H_{37}O$	282.27856 [M+H]$^+$, 247.24356, 265.08508	35.86	FLJ, FF
44	Unknown	$C_{19}H_{39}O$	284.29425 [M+H]$^+$, 87.93765, 101.98130, 115.97544	36.79	FLJ, FF
45	Unknown	C_5O_9	226.95065 [M+Na]$^+$, 158.86320, 90.85480	37.13	FLJ, FF
46	Unknown	C_7H_4	111.01971 [M+Na]$^+$, 98.79458	37.51	FLJ, FF

Rat *in vivo* pharmacokinetics study

Product A (extract mixed with FLJ extract and water, (1:1, *v/v*)), product B (extract mixed with FF extract and water, (1:1, *v/v*)) and product C (extract mixed with FLJ and FF extracts, (1:1, *v/v*)) were given to oral administration to rats, respectively.

In order to study the pharmacokinetics *in vivo* based on drug-drug interaction of main ingredients between FLJ and FF, oral administration to rats at the same concentration was necessary, and we found that there was no significant difference of ingredients in product A or product B except caffeic acid, quinic acid, rutin, hyperoside, isoquercitrin and quercetin in quantity (Fig. 2), compared with that in product C group.

Male SD rats (~250 g) were kept in an environmentally controlled breeding room (temperature: 20±2°C, relative humidity: 60±5%) for 1 week. The animals were fasted for 12 h prior to drug administration. The rats were randomly divided into three groups with no less than six rats in each group to receive various administrations at a single oral dose (10 mL·kg^{-1}) by gastric gavage. After dosing for 0, 5, 10, 20, 30, 40, 55, 70, 100, 160, 250, 600 and 1440 min, blood was collected from the pre-intubated catheter and put into tubes with heparin sodium injection (10 μL) at predetermined time points. Subsequently, plasma was prepared by centrifugation at 1,816×g, 4°C for 7 min, and immediately analyzed or stored at −70°C for further analysis.

In vitro Caco-2 monolayer model

Caco-2 cells were cultured in high glucose DMEM with 10% fetal bovine serum, 1% nonessential amino acids. Cells were cultured in a humidified atmosphere of 5% CO_2 at 37°C. After reaching 80% confluens, Caco-2 cells were harvested with 0.05% trypsin-EDTA solution and seeded on top of CC inserts in 6-well plates, which has a surface area of 4.2 cm^2, at a density of 1.0×10^5 cells/cm^2. The protocols for cell culture in Transwell inserts were similar to those described previously [11].

Hank's balanced salt solution (HBSS) was used as the transport buffer for the transport study in Caco-2 cells monolayer model. It was prepared by dissolving 9.5 grams of commercial available HBSS powder in 1000 mL water. The pH value of the buffer was adjusted to pH 6.0 by 85% of phosphoric acid.

MTT test was used to estimate the potential cytotoxicities of the studied product A, product B and product C toward Caco-2 cells. The Caco-2 cells were seeded onto a 96-well plate at a seeding density of 5×10^4 cells/well in DMEM culture medium and cultured at 37°C for 24 h. Subsequently, the culture medium was replaced with 100 μL of product A, product B and product C dissolved in HBSS (pH 6.0) at different studied concentrations. Blank HBSS (pH 6.0) was employed as a negative control. Then the 96-well plate was incubated at 37°C for 24 h. Thereafter, 20 μL of 5 mg/mL MTT solution in HBSS was added to each well and the plate was incubated for another 4 h. The solutions in each well were then removed followed by dissolving the remained formazan crystals in the cells with 200 μL of DMSO. The absorbance of the mixture in the 96-well plate was then measured with a Kinetic microplate reader (Molecular Devices) at 570 nm. The cytotoxicity of each compound was calculated as the percentage of the absorbance relative to that of the negative control.

Cell culture experiments were described previously [11]. Briefly, after culture medium was aspirated, the cell monolayers were washed three times with blank HBSS. The transepithelial electrical resistance (TEER) values of cell monolayers were measured, which were more than 250 Ω×cm^2. The monolayers were incubated with the blank HBSS for 1 h with 37°C. Thereafter the incubation medium was aspirated. Afterwards, a solution containing the compound was loaded onto the apical side. The amounts of transported compound were measured as a function of time. Donor samples (400 μL) (Apical side) and receiver samples (400 μL) (Basolateral side) were taken at different times (typically 1 h), followed by the addition of 400 μL drug donor solution to the donor side (AP) and 400 μL of blank buffer to the receiver side (BL). The samples were taken at 0, 1, 2, 3 and 4 h after incubation. At the end of the transport experiment, integrity of the monolayer was monitored by TEER value.

Chemical sample (mixed decoction and co-decoction) analyzed by UHPLC-ESI/LTQ-Orbitrap-MS. Mixed decoction and co-decoction were diluted five times with methanol,

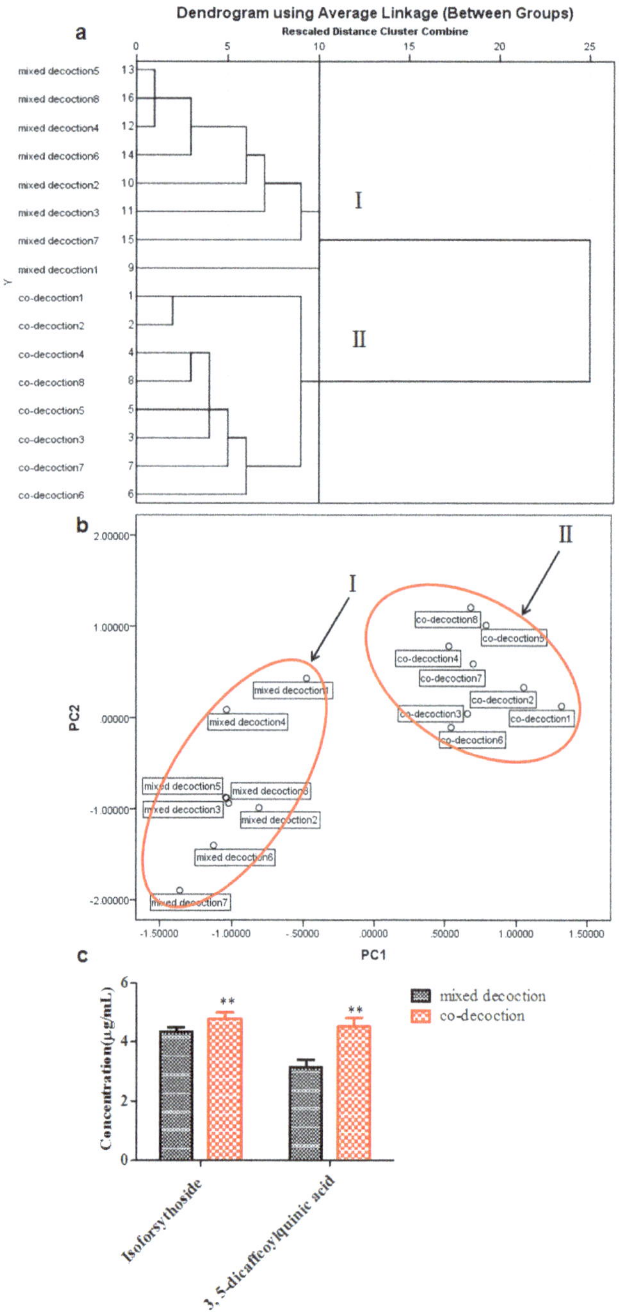

Figure 4. The chemical constitution differences between co-decoction and mixed decoction analyzed by both HCA and PCA. (A: HCA; B: PCA; C: the most important ingredients influencing the difference between co-decoction and mixed decoction).

respectively, and then filtered through 0.22 μm membrane before injection into the UHPLC-ESI/LTQ-Orbitrap-MS system for analysis.

The UHPLC analysis was performed on the Dionex UltiMate 3000 analytical system acquired from Fisher Scientific (Thermo Fisher scientific, Waltham, MA, USA) that consisted of an autosampler equipped with a column oven, a tray compartment cooler, and a quaternary pump with a built in solvent degasser, all piloted by Xcalibur software. The chromatographic separation was achieved using Syncronis C_{18} column (100×2.1 mm, 3 μm) (Thermo Scientific, Waltham, MA, USA). The injection volume used was 5 μL. The mobile phase was composed of A (acetonitrile) and solvent B (0.05% formic acid, *v*/*v*) with a linear gradient elution: 0–3 min, 5–5% A; 3–25 min, 5–22% A; 25–30 min, 22–60%; 30–35 min, 60–95% A; 35–36 min, 95–5% A, and hold for 4 min, at a flow rate of 400 μL/min, resulting chromatographic full-width-at-half-maximum (FWHM) of 3–5 s. The column oven and tray cooler temperatures were set to 30 and 4°C, respectively.

The Dionex UltiMate 3000 UHPLC system was hyphenated with a LTQ-Orbitrap XL mass spectrometer (Thermo Scientific, Waltham, MA, USA). The system was equipped with an ESI source, operated in positive ionization mode using the following parameters: capillary temperature 350°C, capillary voltage 47 V, sheath gas flow 30 arbitrary units, auxiliary gas 8 arbitrary units, source voltage 4.5 kV and tube lens voltage 130 V. Spectra was recorded in the range of *m/z* 50–1500 Da with a resolution of 30,000. For identification purposes, two scan events were applied for the MS experiments. The first was in a full scan MS mode and the second was a data dependent scan that selected the most intense ion or specified ions in another setting from the first scan event for the acquisition of MS/MS spectra. The collision energy for collision-induced dissociation or high-collision energy dissociation mode was adjusted to 35% of maximum, and the isolation width of precursor ions was *m/z* 2.0 Da. In the qualitative study, the compounds were identified by comparison with reference compounds when available and with literature data, from retention times, MS, MS/MS and MS^n analysis. In the quantitative study, full scan MS mode was applied, and then extracted ion chromatograms were generated from their theoretical exact masses using a mass tolerance of 5 ppm. After integration of the peaks, their respective areas were used for the quantifications.

Chemical sample (product A, product B and product C) quantified by UPLC-ESI-MS/MS. Product A, product B and product C were diluted five thousand times with 10% acetonitrile/methanol (4:1, *v*/*v*) containing 0.4% formic acid and 0.5 mM sodium formate, respectively, and then filtered through 0.22 μm membrane before injection into the UPLC-ESI-MS/MS system for analysis. The methodology validations have been studied and to be published elsewhere.

Biological samples (pharmacokinetics in vivo and Caco-2 cells in vitro) quantified by UPLC-ESI-MS/MS. The treatment and UPLC-ESI-MS/MS analysis for samples collected from *in vitro* and *in vivo* models, respectively have been studied and to be published elsewhere.

Calculation

For Caco-2 monolayer model, the apparent permeability coefficient (P_{app}) was calculated as $P_{app} = [(dQ/dt)]/[A\times C]$, dQ/dt (μg/S) was the flux rate, A was the effective surface area of the cell monolayer (4.2 cm^2), and C_0 (μg/mL) was the initial drug concentration in the donor chamber.

Pharmacokinetic analysis

The main pharmacokinetic parameters including the peak plasma concentration (C_{max}), the time to C_{max} (T_{max}), the *AUC* from 0 to infinity ($AUC_{0-\infty}$), the *AUC* form 0 to time (AUC_{0-t}), mean residence time (*MRT*), and terminal elimination half-life ($T_{1/2z}$) were calculated by the non-compartmental analysis of plasma concentration *vs.* time data using the "DAS 2.1.1" software (Mathematical Pharmacology Professional Committee of China, Shanghai, China). The comparison of pharmacokinetic

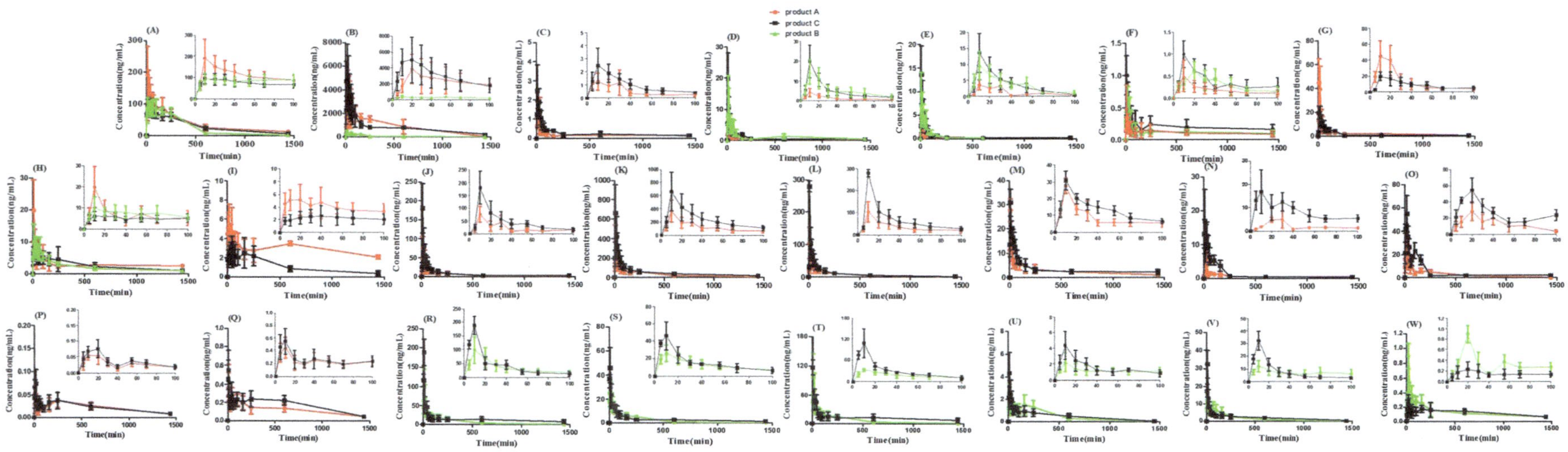

Figure 5. Mean pharmacokinetic profiles of caffeic acid (A), quinic acid (B), luteoloside (C), rutin (D), hyperoside (E), isoquercitrin (F), luteolin (G), quercetin (H), genistein (I), neochlorogenic acid (J), chlorogenic acid (K), cryptochlorogenic acid (L), 3, 5-dicaffeoylquinic acid (M), 3, 4-dicaffeoylquinic acid (N), loganin (O), genistin (P), astragalin (Q), forsythoside A (R), forsythoside B (S), isoforsythoside (T), pillyrin (U), pinoresinol-β-D-glucoside (V) and arctigenin (W) following oral administration of product A, B and C groups.

Table 2. Pharmacokinetic parameters of multi-compounds.

Parameters	C_{max} (ng·mL^{-1})			T_{max} (min)			MRT (min)			$AUC_{0\to\infty}$ (ng·min·mL^{-1})			$T_{1/2z}$ (min)		
Products	**A**	**B**	**C**	**A**	**B**	**C**	**A**	**B**	**C**	**A**	**B**	**C**	**A**	**B**	**C**
Caffeic acid	181±17.6**	91.1±6.74	98.1±16.2	10±0.0	10±0.0	10±0.0	399±27.5	334±45.1	377±51.5	71597±5695.4**	40993±10833	44196±2835.1	360±66.3	332±53.6	392±61.1
Quinic acid	383*10±182*10	358±157**	500*10±285*10	21±9.9	18±9.6	10±0.0	239±32.9**	270±18.2**	441±22.6	13808*10^2±19992*10	17980*10±34769**	14901*10^2±21646*10	229±16.8**	246±37.7**	330±76.3
Genistein	5.09±2.46*	–	2.30±1.00	14±5.3	–	15±5.8	650±18.6**	–	463±17.1	14425±1481.2	–	1715.2±417.45	600±76.4**	–	411±67.7
Luteolin	44.9±19.8**	–	19.5±5.43	10±0.0	–	10±0.0	347±28.4**	–	280±39.2	5296.2±737.73**	–	2816.7±543.87	423±56.6**	–	265±15.7
Quercetin	15.6±4.39**	12.6±2.23**	8.02±0.493	10±0.0	10±0.0	10±0.0	493±75.0	420±18.2	427±49.7	8667.6±1751.4**	3899.7±193.44	3143.6±592.07	277±52.6	316±55.8	280±62.9
Neochlorogenic acid	75.7±30.1**	–	181±65.0	10±0.0	–	10±0.0	322±33.8**	–	387±62.1	8298.0±1058.7**	–	24226±4891.0	458±38.2**	–	515±28.0
Chlorogenic acid	367±169	–	661±294*	10±0.0	–	10±0.0	347±28.3**	–	497±44.0	42426±5765.9**	–	10366*10±8547.5	322±44.0**	–	461±32.1
Cryptochlorogenic acid	352±29.4**	–	449±22.8	10±0.0	–	10±0.0	333±26.3**	–	453±27.2	11757±1572.1**	–	21078±1913.4	104±46.9**	–	279±17.2
Arctigenin	–	0.895±0.166**	0.231±0.144	–	20±0.0	20±0.0	–	560±32.1	564±26.6	–	266.53±5.8286**	239.53±9.7188	–	623±21.6	534±53.9
Genistin	0.0550±0.0154*	–	0.0753±0.0285	16±8.7	–	20±0.0	650±18.6**	–	463±17.1	37.8±1.94*	–	49.3±3.02	482±18.3*	–	552±27.3
Luteoloside	1.26±0.655	–	2.48±1.34	10±0.0	–	10±0.0	347±28.4**	–	280±39.2	177.91±30.147**	–	300.16±32.890	383±13.2**	–	579±85.7
Astragalin	0.441±0.166	–	0.551±0.207	10±0.0	–	10±0.0	489±29.3*	–	680±109	259.05±30.440**	–	375.45±42.516	460±15.8*	–	695±103
Hyperoside	5.25±0.859**	9.68±4.39**	22.1±1.90	10±0.0	–	10±0.0	436±24.4	409±60.9	387±41.8	593.59±19.662**	625.17±111.23**	1473.1±161.12	410±97.9	401±29.2	423±41.3
Isoquercitrin	0.504±0.351**	0.619±0.212**	1.00±0.300	10±0.0	20±0.0	16±8.7	557±46.9	498±66.7	555±46.9	158.09±27.790**	195.20±29.918**	330.89±56.587	436±26.3	471±30.9	455±52.1
3, 5-dicaffeoylquinic acid	27.6±4.73	–	30.8±5.66	10±0.0	–	10±0.0	438±25.9**	–	578±18.1	4291.1±243.43**	–	5384.9±198.59	292±77.6**	–	440±47.4
3, 4-dicaffeoylquinic acid	4.79±1.87**	–	12.5±4.07	15±4.6	–	12±4.1	422±13.5**	–	537±34.1	1376.6±251.42**	–	2327.6±152.15	295±37.0**	–	409±142.6
Rutin	4.08±1.99**	14.6±1.65	19.8±3.93	10±0.0	–	10±0.0	301±50.9	261±29.2	293±51.6	618.79±104.54**	1828.0±149.21	1366.6±329.59	476±50.2	490±92.9	453±36.8
Loganin	28.0±4.93**	–	54.7±8.63	21±3.8	–	16±8.1	349±36.4**	–	470±57.0	5571.8±490.50**	–	8381.5±1477.5	124±12.3**	–	440±16.4
Pinoresinol-β-D-glucoside	–	11.9±4.36**	32.3±7.57	–	10±0.0	10±0.0	–	246±33.4**	454±30.3	–	1917.7±480.53**	4067.3±345.77	–	202±12.6**	315±28.3
Phillyrin	–	2.24±0.978**	4.41±0.0769	–	10±0.0	10±0.0	–	316±11.8**	521±55.3	–	389.31±94.693**	1316.5±171.15	–	341±19.2**	450±52.4
Isoforsythoside	–	71.7±13.5**	188±33.7	–	10±0.0	10±0.0	–	240±15.5**	452±36.6	–	6736.9±861.30**	12347±1731.7	–	202±36.0**	455±38.5
Forsythoside A	–	102±6.19*	182±38.6	–	10±0.0	10±0.0	–	225±38.7**	452±27.0	–	13728±4154.2	46409±6015.3**	–	276±62.4**	359±21.4
Forsythoside B	–	25.5±9.37*	46.6±4.91	–	10±0.0	10±0.0	–	198±26.7**	380±43.3	–	3249.3±268.96*	5223.2±666.32	–	259±36.4**	425±50.7

(*) $p<0.05$ and (**) $p<0.01$ compared with product C.

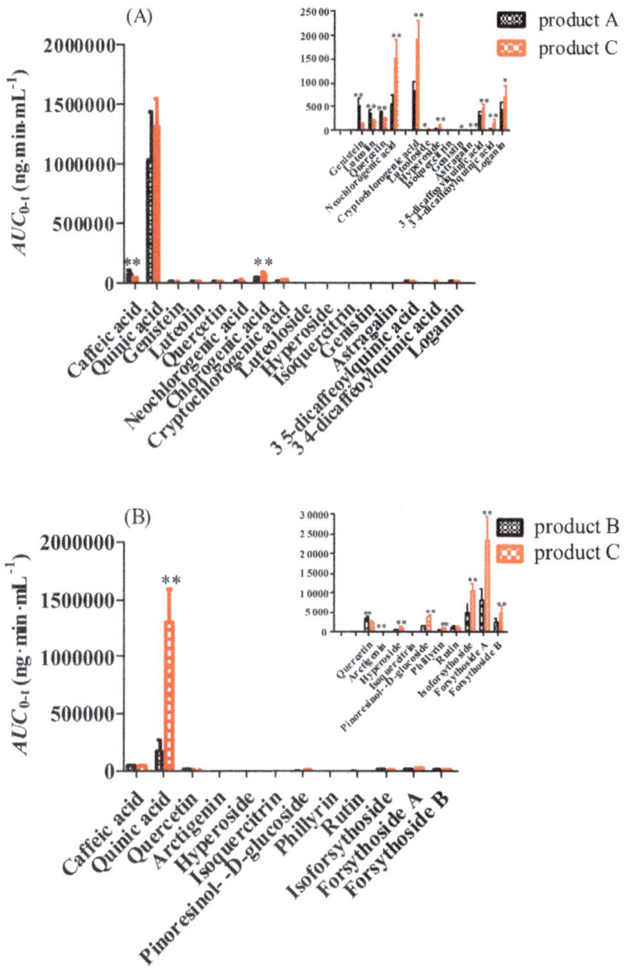

Figure 6. The Pharmacokinetic parameter (*AUC*) of main ingredients as variates analyzed by both HCA and PCA. (*) $P<0.05$ and (**) $P<0.01$, compared with product C group. (A: *AUC* between product A and product C group; B: *AUC* between product B and product C group).

parameters was possessed by SPSS 20.0 (Statistical Package for the Social Science).

Statistical analysis

Statistical significance in the P_{app} values and pharmacokinetic parameters were estimated by the analysis of variance (Student t-test) or one-way ANOVA. A p value of less than 0.05 was considered to be significantly different. All data were expressed as mean±SD.

Pattern recognition analysis

The data for chemical difference between co-decoction and mixed decoction, and intestinal absorption both *in vitro* and *in vivo* were all visualized by applying pattern recognition methods, such as HCA and PCA, which has been extensively applied to the biomolecules analysis [13–16]. Both HCA and PCA were done by SPSS 20.0 software. Between-group linkage method was applied, and squared Euclidean distance was selected as measurement.

Results

Chemical constitution difference between co-decoction and mixed decoction by pattern recognition analysis

As illustrated in Fig. 3A, B and Table 1, we found that 32 peaks and 31 peaks were detected in FLJ extract and FF extract in the positive ion model by UHPLC-ESI/LTQ-Orbitrap MS system, respectively and the influence of the co-decoction on the quality was little, compared with the mixed decoction (Fig. 3C, D). However, it was shown (Fig. 4a) that there was significant difference in quantity between mixed decoction and co-decoction analyzed by HCA, and we found (Fig. 4b, c) that the most possible ingredients resulted in the discrepancy between co-decoction and mixed decoction were isoforsythoside and 3, 5-dicaffeoylquinic acid analyzed by PCA combined with HCA. Besides, the contents of isoforsythoside and 3, 5-dicaffeoylquinic acid in co-decoction were significantly higher than that in mixed decoction, which indicated that isoforsythoside and 3, 5-dicaffeoylquinic acid might be the main chemical markers in herb couples.

The bioavailability interaction of main components from FLJ and FF using *in vivo* pharmacokinetics study

As shown in Fig. 5 and Table 2, $C_{\max}$, MRT, $T_{1/2z}$ and $AUC_{0\rightarrow\infty}$ of caffeic acid derivatives, flavonoids glucoside, lignins glucoside and iridoids glucoside were improved, but that of flavonoids aglycone and lignins aglycone were decreased in product C group compared with that in product A or B group (most of them had significant differences), which indicated that the intestinal absorption of caffeic acid derivatives, flavonoids glucoside, lignins glucoside and iridoids glucoside might be improved or the transformation from glucoside to aglycone by bacterial metabolism might be inhibited as FLJ combined with FF. In addition, the $AUC_{0\rightarrow t}$ (Fig. 6) as variates analyzed by both HCA and PCA of neochlorogenic acid, chlorogenic acid, cryptochlorogenic acid, 3, 5-dicaffeoylquinic acid, 3, 4-dicaffeoylquinic acid, luteoloside, genistin, astragalin, loganin, pillyrin, pinoresinol-β-D-glucoside, isoforsythoside, forsythoside A and forsythoside B in product C group were increased significantly to 286% (15542±3640.1) ng·min/mL, 215% (76148±14584) ng·min/mL, 235% (19248±4037.2) ng·min/mL, 162% (4944.7±595.54) ng·min/mL, 318% (1464.6±309.02) ng·min/mL, 137% (285.71±76.804) ng·min/mL, 131% (32.880±2.0100) ng·min/mL, 145% (250.30±28.344) ng·min/mL, 121% (6450.5±484.60) ng·min/mL, 213% (3374.0±265.32) ng·min/mL, 299% (1025.2±171.44) ng·min/mL, 203% (12320±1429.1) ng·min/mL, 230% (25229±426.79) ng·min/mL and 175% (5642.5±122.33) ng·min/mL, respectively, compared to that in product A or B groups, but the $AUC_{0\rightarrow t}$ of genistein, luteolin and arctigenin in product C group were lower significantly when the same dosages were administrated to rats. Besides, the bioavailability of caffeic acid in product C group had no significant difference, compared with that in product B group, and surprisingly significantly lower than that in product A group, and the bioavailability of quinic acid in product C group had no significant difference, compared with that in product A group, and higher significantly than that in product B group although the contents of caffeic acid and quinic acid (Fig. 3) in product C group were significantly higher than that in product A or B group. And the bioavailability of hyperoside in product C group was significantly higher than that in product A or B group, which corresponded to their administration dosages to rats, but that of quercetin was opposite. In addition, the bioavailability of rutin in product C group was significantly higher than that in product A group, but no significant difference compared to that in product B

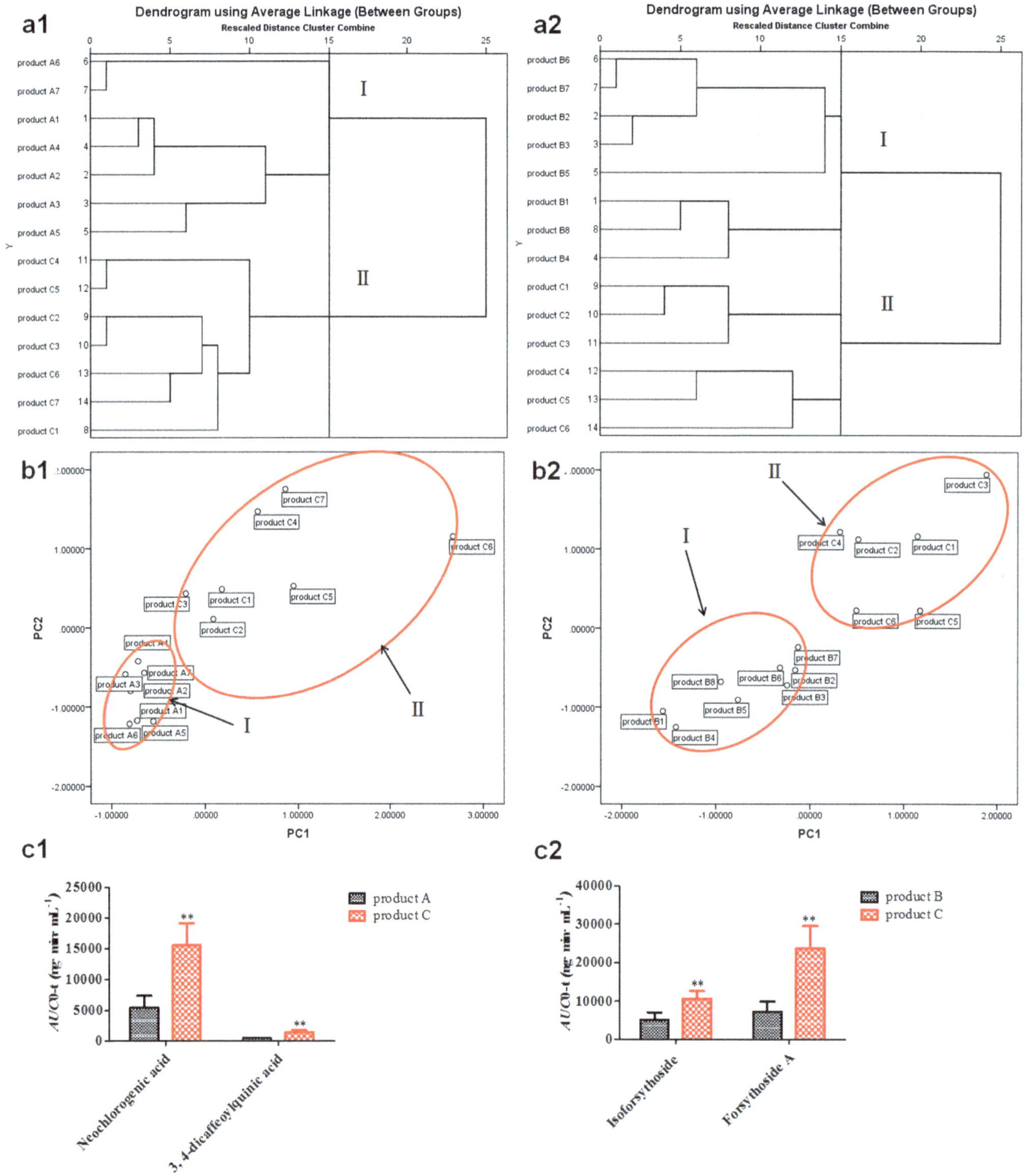

Figure 7. The pharmacokinetics differences among product A, B and C groups analyzed by both HCA and PCA. (a1, a2: HCA; b1, b2: PCA; The most important ingredients influencing the difference between product C and product A group (c1) or between product C and product B group (c2)).

group, and that of isoquercitrin was no significantly different among product A, B and C groups, though the dosage of product C group was higher than that of product A or B group. In short, it was found surprisingly that the bioavailability of some ingredients, such as caffeic acid and quercetin, *etc.* were significantly higher than that in product C, which was contrary to their administration dosages to rats. Therefore, it is necessary for us to consider caffeic

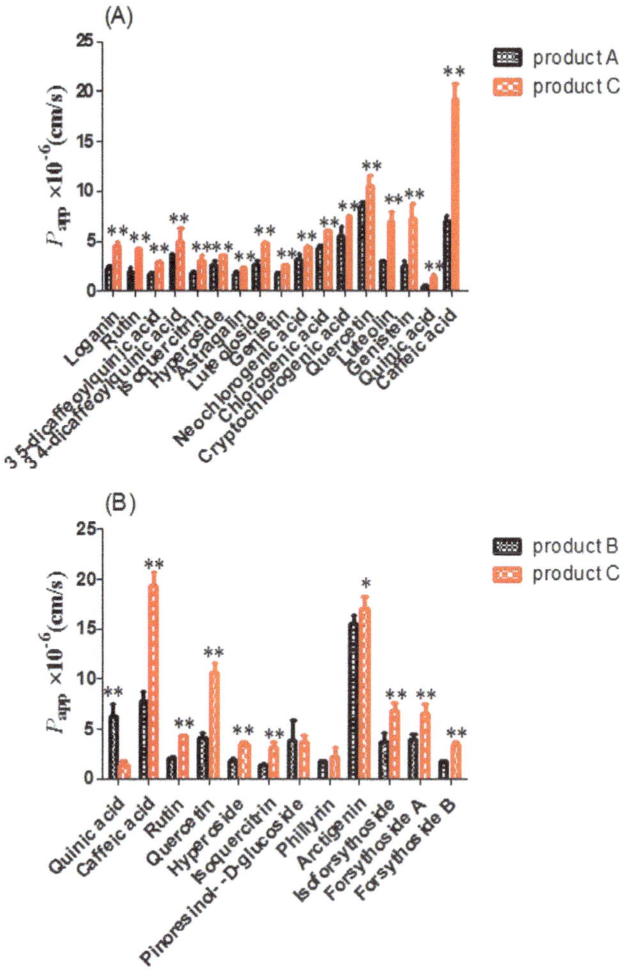

Figure 8. The intestinal absorption *in vitro* (P_{app}) of main ingredients as variates analyzed by both HCA and PCA. (*) $P<0.05$ and (**) $P<0.01$, compared with product C group. (A: P_{app} between product A and product C group; B: P_{app} between product B and product C group).

acid and quercetin, *etc.* as important variates in the process of PCA and HCA.

Pattern recognition analysis of pharmacokinetic profiling *in vivo*

Hierarchical clustering of the pharmacokinetics was presented in Fig. 7a1 and a2. The dendrogram showed the cluster relationships among product A, product B and product C groups *in vivo*. We found that the samples were divided into two main clusters, respectively. As shown in Fig. 7a1, cluster I represented product A1–A7, and cluster II grouped product C1–C7, which was illustrated by PCA (Fig. 7b1) by which samples were also clearly separated two domains, consistent with HCA analysis. Also in Fig. 7a2, product B1–B7 was marked in cluster I, and product C1–C6 was divided into cluster II, which was proved by PCA (Fig. 7b2) that samples were clearly grouped into two domains, correspondence to HCA analysis. In addition, it was displayed (Fig. 7c1) that the exposure level *in vivo* of one group of ingredients (neochlorogenic acid and 3, 4-dicaffeoylquinic acid) were the main influencing factor contributing to the difference between product C and product A group by both PCA and HCA. Similar results were obtained in the case of another group of ingredients (isoforsythoside and forsythoside A) between product C and product B group (Fig. 7c2).

The absorption interaction of main component from FLJ and FF using *in vitro* Caco-2 cells model

Caco-2 cells were exposed to various concentrations of product A, B and C (0.039, 0.078, 0.16, 0.31, 0.63, 1.3, 2.5, 5.0, 10 and 20 mg raw medicine per milliliter. It was shown that product A, B and C at different concentrations were all safe for the Caco-2 cells from MTT test.

As shown in Fig. 8A, the P_{app} for caffeic acid, genistein, luteolin, quercetin, neochlorogenic acid, chlorogenic acid, cryptochlorogenic acid, 3, 5-dicaffeoylquinic acid, 3, 4-dicaffeoylquinic acid, genistin, luteoloside, astragalin, hyperoside, isoquercitrin, rutin and loganin in product C group were increased significantly to 275%, 293%, 240%, 125%, 136%, 140%, 133%, 164%, 137%, 165%, 174%, 131%, 129%, 169%, 213% and 211% respectively compared to that in product A group, and the P_{app} (Fig. 8B) was increased to 247%, 256%, 195%, 234%, 210%, 110%, 187%, 165% and 210% for caffeic acid, quercetin, hyperoside, isoquercitrin, rutin, arctigenin, isoforsythoside, forsythoside A and forsythoside B, respectively compared with that in product B group, though some of them had different concentrations. Besides, the P_{app} for quinic acid in product C group was increased to 301% compared to that in product A group, but decreased to 24.0% compared to that in product B group. Meanwhile, there were no significant difference in P_{app} for pillyrin and pinoresinol-β-D-glucoside between product C group and B group. In addition, we found that dipsacoside B and macranthoidin B in product C or A group and arctiin in product C or B group might not be absorbed well into Caco-2 cells. The result above showed that the P_{app} for most of ingredients such as caffeic acid derivatives were improved significantly by FLJ combined with FF, which might be attributed to the influence of components in FLJ or FF on the efflux transporters.

Pattern recognition analysis of absorption profiling *in vitro*

Fig. 9a1 and a2 showed the hierarchical clustering of the absorption *in vitro*, and we found the samples were divided into two main clusters, respectively. As shown in Fig. 9a1, cluster I represented product A1–A4, and cluster II grouped product C1–C4, which was illustrated by PCA (Fig. 9b1) that samples were also clearly separated two domains, consistent with HCA analysis. Besides, it was shown (Fig. 9a2) that product B1–B4 was marked in cluster I, and product C1–C4 was divided into cluster II, which was also proved by PCA (Fig. 9b2) that samples were clearly grouped into two domains, correspondence to HCA analysis. Meanwhile, it was displayed (Fig. 9c1) that the intestinal absorption level *in vitro* for one group of ingredients (neochlorogenic acid and 3, 4-dicaffeoylquinic acid) were the main influencing factors leading to the difference between product C and product A group. Similar results were obtained in the case of another group of ingredients (isoforsythoside and forsythoside A) between product C and product B group (Fig. 9c2).

Discussion

In the present study, the systemic biopharmaceutics combined with HCA and PCA were firstly performed to rapidly elucidate the compatibility foundation of FLJ-FF herb couple, and it was found consistently (Fig. 4 & 7) that the caffeic acid derivatives including isoforsythoside, 3, 5-dicaffeoylquinic acid, neochlorogenic acid, 3, 4-dicaffeoylquinic acid and forsythoside A were the most

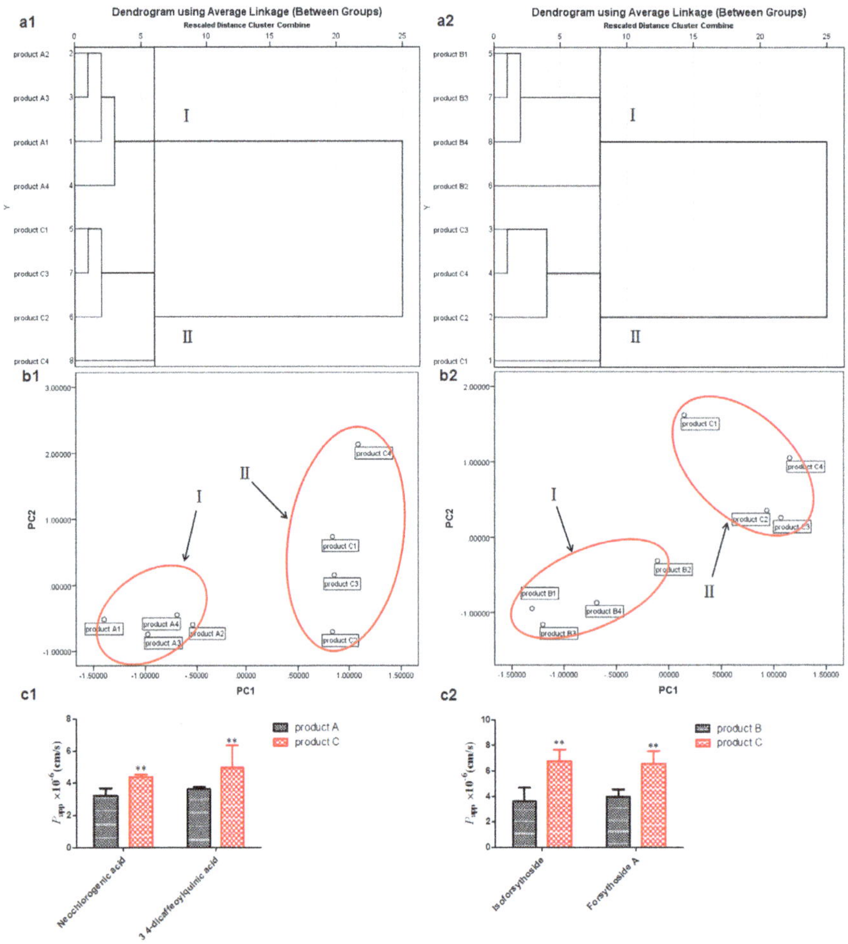

Figure 9. The absorption differences among product A, B and C groups analyzed by both HCA and PCA. (a1, a2: HCA; b1, b2: PCA; The most important ingredients influencing the difference between product C and product A group (c1) or between product C and product B group (c2)).

important ingredients resulting in difference between herb couple and single herbs, and interestingly, their exposure levels in the views of not only chemistry *in vitro* but also biology *in vivo* were all significantly higher than that in single herbs, highly consistent with the data that the pharmacological activities such as anti-inflammatory and antipyretic effects in FLJ-FF herb couple were significantly higher than that in FLJ or FF [17]. Besides, it was reported that caffeic acid derivatives such as isochlorogenic acids and forsythoside A had strong antioxidant, antibacterial and antiviral activities [18–20], and chito-oligosaccharide (COS) at dosage of 25 mg/kg could improve their pharmacological effects such as antiviral activity via enhancing the intestinal permeabilities and the *in vivo* bioavailabilities of caffeic acid derivatives significantly in FF-FLJ herb couple preparations [11]. The studies above indicated that the caffeic acid derivatives might be the most significant components contributing to the pharmacological effects.

It was shown (Fig. 9) from Caco-2 cells *in vitro* combined with HCA and PCA that neochlorogenic acid, 3, 4-dicaffeoylquinic acid, isoforsythoside and forsythoside A were the main ingredients resulting in the difference between single herbs and herb couple, and the values of intestinal absorption *in vitro* were significantly higher than that in single herbs, surprisingly consistent with the results obtained from pharmacokinetics *in vivo* (Fig. 7), which indicated that it was because of intestinal absorption improvement of neochlorogenic acid, 3, 4-dicaffeoylquinic acid, isoforsythoside and forsythoside A that the efficacies of herb couple were better than that of single herbs.

In the previous study, we found that the poor intestinal absorption of the caffeic acid derivatives was one of the most important factors resulting in the low oral bioavailability, and they permeated mainly via the paracellular pathways in the intestine, and the intestinal absorption of phenolic acid such as chlorogenic acid, neochlorogenic acid, cryptochlorogenic acid, 3, 4-dicaffeoylquinic acid and 3, 5-dicaffeoylquinic acid were influenced by P-gp, MRP2 and BCRP, but that of phenylethanoid glycosides such as forsythoside A, isoforsythoside and forsythoside B were affected by P-gp and MRP2, not BCRP [21–22]. Although the bioavailability of active ingredients (Fig. 6) (neochlorogenic acid, 3, 4-dicaffeoylquinic acid, isoforsythoside and forsythoside A) in herb couple were improved compared with that in single herbs, their intestinal absorptions (Fig. 8) were still unsatisfactory. Thus, the studies on how to improve the bioavailability of the caffeic acid derivatives in herb couple by pharmaceutical methods such as absorption enhancers based on tight junctions need to be further investigated.

Conclusion

Current findings from both the chemical and biological aspects consistently demonstrated that the biopharmaceutics characteristics (dissolution *in vitro* and intestinal absorptions both *in vivo* and *in vitro*) of caffeic acid derivatives in FLJ-FF herb couple, higher than that in FLJ or FF, contributed to the optimal efficacy of herb couples analyzed by both HCA and PCA, which indicated that caffeic acid derivatives should be considered as chemical markers to control the quality of its preparations.

Author Contributions

Conceived and designed the experiments: WZ BC LD. Performed the experiments: WZ XT AY. Analyzed the data: WZ JS SW. Contributed reagents/materials/analysis tools: LD. Wrote the paper: WZ.

References

1. Wang ZP. (2011) Studies on compatibility regulation and effective substance of Huangqi-Gegen herb pair. Guangzhou: Guangzhou University of Chinese Medicine (Doctoral dissertation (in Chinese)).
2. Li JB, Zhang L, Zhang J. (2013) Study on the compatibility regulation. J Tradit Chin Med 54: 1335–1340 (in Chinese).
3. Li YY. (2008) Studies on the extraction and separation of Gegen-Danshen herb pair and its capsule preparation. Beijing: Academy of Chinese Medical Sciences (Mater thesis (in Chinese)).
4. Shi XQ, Shang EX, Tang YP, Zhu HX, Guo JM, et al. (2012) Interaction of nourishing and tonifying blood effects of the combination of *Angelicae sinensis Radix* and *Astragali Radix* studied by response surface method. Yao Xue Xue Bao 47: 1375–1383.
5. Huang MY, Tang YP, Shang EX, Guo JM, Liu X, et al. (2013) Study on antioxidant interaction of different preparations and proportions of Danggui-Chuanxiong drug pair. Zhongguo Zhong Yao Za Zhi 38: 234–238.
6. Huang MY, Shang EX, Tang YP, Guo JM, Shi XQ, et al. (2013) Research on nourishing and tonifying blood effects of the herb pair consisting of Angelica sinensis and Ligusticum chuanxiong on the bisis of drug interaction. Zhongguo Zhong Xi Yi Jie He Za Zhi 33: 516–521.
7. Zhou W, Shan JJ, Wang SQ, Ju WZ, Meng MX, et al. (2014) Simultaneous determination of caffeic acid derivatives by UPLC-MS/MS in rat plasma and its application in pharmacokinetic study after oral administration of *Flos Lonicerae – Fructus Forsythiae* herb combination. J Chromatogr B 949–950: 7–15.
8. Wang XJ, Sun H, Fan YL, Li LJ, Makino T, et al. (2006) Analysis and bioactive evaluation of the compounds absorbed into blood after oral administration of the extracts of *Vaccinium vitis - idaea* in rat. Biol Pharm Bull 28: 1106–1108.
9. Shang XF, Pan H, Li MX, Miao XL, Ding H. (2011) *Lonicera japonica* Thunb.: Ethnopharmacology, phytochemistry and pharmacology of an important traditional Chinese medicine. J Ethnopharmacol 138: 1–21.
10. Zhou W, Qin KM, Shan JJ, Ju WZ, Liu SJ, et al. (2012) Improvement of intestinal absorption of forsythoside A in weeping forsythia extract by various absorption enhancers based on tight junctions. Phytomedicine 20: 47–58.
11. Zhou W, Wang HD, Zhu XX, Shan JJ, Yin AL, et al. (2013). Improvement of Intestinal Absorption of Forsythoside A and Chlorogenic Acid By Different Carboxymethyl Chitosan and Chito-oligosaccharide, Application to *Flos Lonicerae - Fructus Forsythiae* Herb Couple Preparations, Plos one 8(2013) e63348. doi:10.1371/journal.pone.0063348.
12. Lin LM. (2008) Study on an appropriate and quick method for illustrating the effective chemical substances of the complexity in Chinese herb medicine based on *Flos Lonicerae - Fructus Forsythiae* herb couples. China Academy of Chinese Medical Sciences (Doctoral dissertation (in Chinese)).
13. Wang L, Zhou GB, Liu P, Song SJ, Chen Z. (2008) Dissection of mechanisms of Chinese medicinal formula Realgar-Indigo naturalis as an effective treatment for promyelocytic leukemia. Proc Natl Acad Sci 105: 4826–4831.
14. Keith CT, Borisy AA, Stockwell BR. (2005) Multicomponent therapeutics for networked systems. Nat Rev Drug Discovery 4: 71–78.
15. Klayman DL. (1985) Qinghaosu (artemisinin): an antimalarial drug from China. Science 228: 1049–1055.
16. Pan SY, Chen SB, Dong HG, Yu ZL, Dong JC, et al. (2011) New perspectives on Chinese herbal medicine (zhong-yao) research and development. Evid Based Complement Alternat Med 403709.
17. Xia BH, Wang ZM, Lin LM, Guo Q, Chen SH. (2009) Pharmacological advances in the study of Lonicerae Flos, Forsythiae Fructus and their combination. Chin. J. Experi. Trad. Med. Formula. 15: 80–82.
18. Wang LM. (2008) Studies on antiviral effect and immunopotentiating activity of *Lonicera japonica* (Thunb). and *flos lonicerae in vitro*. Agri. Univ. Henan. (Master thesis (in Chinese)).
19. Wang L. (2010) Study of effective substances screening for *flos lonicerae* based on the "spectrum-effect" combination. Chengdu Univ. Trad. Chin. Med. (Master thesis (in Chinese)).
20. Zhang LW. (2002) Study on the extraction and separation of forsythoside A in *Forsythia suspense* (Thunb) Vahl and its pharmacological effects. Shanxi Univ. (Master thesis (in Chinese)).
21. Zhou W, Shan JJ, Tan XB, Zou JS, Yin AL, et al. (2014) Effect of chito-oligosaccharide on the oral absorptions of phenolic acids of *Flos Lonicerae* extract. Phytomedicine 21: 184–194.
22. Zhou W, Shan JJ, Tan XB, Zou JS, Yin AL, et al. (2014) Effect of chito-oligosaccharide on the intestinal absorptions of phenylethanoid glycosides in *Fructus Forsythiae* extract. Phytomedicine 21: 1549–1558.

19

A Network Pharmacology Study of Chinese Medicine QiShenYiQi to Reveal Its Underlying Multi-Compound, Multi-Target, Multi-Pathway Mode of Action

Xiang Li[1], Leihong Wu[1], Wei Liu[1], Yecheng Jin[1], Qian Chen[1], Linli Wang[1], Xiaohui Fan[1]*, Zheng Li[2]*, Yiyu Cheng[1]

1 Pharmaceutical Informatics Institute, College of Pharmaceutical Sciences, Zhejiang University, Hangzhou, China, **2** State Key Laboratory of Modern Chinese Medicine, Tianjin University of Traditional Chinese Medicine, Tianjin, China

Abstract

Chinese medicine is a complex system guided by traditional Chinese medicine (TCM) theories, which has proven to be especially effective in treating chronic and complex diseases. However, the underlying modes of action (MOA) are not always systematically investigated. Herein, a systematic study was designed to elucidate the multi-compound, multi-target and multi-pathway MOA of a Chinese medicine, QiShenYiQi (QSYQ), on myocardial infarction. QSYQ is composed of *Astragalus membranaceus* (Huangqi), *Salvia miltiorrhiza* (Danshen), *Panax notoginseng* (Sanqi), and *Dalbergia odorifera* (Jiangxiang). Male Sprague Dawley rat model of myocardial infarction were administered QSYQ intragastrically for 7 days while the control group was not treated. The differentially expressed genes (DEGs) were identified from myocardial infarction rat model treated with QSYQ, followed by constructing a cardiovascular disease (CVD)-related multilevel compound-target-pathway network connecting main compounds to those DEGs supported by literature evidences and the pathways that are functionally enriched in ArrayTrack. 55 potential targets of QSYQ were identified, of which 14 were confirmed in CVD-related literatures with experimental supporting evidences. Furthermore, three sesquiterpene components of QSYQ, Trans-nerolidol, (3S,6S,7R)-3,7,11-trimethyl-3,6-epoxy-1,10-dodecadien-7-ol and (3S,6R,7R)-3,7,11-trimethyl-3,6-epoxy-1,10-dodecadien-7-ol from *Dalbergia odorifera* T. Chen, were validated experimentally in this study. Their anti-inflammatory effects and potential targets including extracellular signal-regulated kinase-1/2, peroxisome proliferator-activated receptor-gamma and heme oxygenase-1 were identified. Finally, through a three-level compound-target-pathway network with experimental analysis, our study depicts a complex MOA of QSYQ on myocardial infarction.

Editor: Christina Chan, Michigan State University, United States of America

Funding: This work was financially supported by the National Basic Research Program of China (no. 2012CB518405) and the National Natural Science Foundation of China (no. 81373893). The funders had no role in study design, data collection and analysis, decision to publish, or preparation of the manuscript. The Microarray test was performed by National Engineering Center for Biochip at Shanghai by Dr. Huasheng Xiao's team.

Competing Interests: The authors have declared that no competing interests exist.

* E-mail: fanxh@zju.edu.cn (XF); lizheng1@gmail.com (ZL)

Introduction

Chinese medicine, an important branch of the healthcare system in China, has gradually gained popularity both at home and abroad [1]. Chinese medicine, a complex system with guidance from traditional Chinese medicine (TCM) theories, has proven to be especially effective to treat chronic and complex diseases. However, the underlying mechanisms of action (MOA) are rarely investigated systematically.

One of the consensus is that TCM produces its efficacy in a holistic way [2], taking the advantage of multi-target therapy being more effective in combating polygenic diseases than monotherapies [3]. With the advancements in understanding of pathobiology of human diseases, people find that most diseases are not simply caused by one single factor [4]. It is especially true for the complex multifactorial chronic diseases such as cardiovascular disease (CVD), cancer and diabetes [5,6]. The TCM treatments can be visualized as a complexity against complexity paradigm between multi-target therapy such as TCM and the complex biological networks of human diseases. The development of analytical tools such as systems biology [7], network biology [8] and network pharmacology [9,10] provide an opportunity to unravel the complex and holistic mechanisms of TCM in treating complex diseases. In today's post-genomic era, it has become much easier to obtain huge amounts of data related to the effect of drugs on transcriptome of target tissues. Data analysis becomes critical to identify the MOA of drugs. Recently, network models and network analysis of genomic data has been proven useful to translate the microarray information and identify potential targets [11,12] and enriched pathways involved in the MOA [13–15]. Tools such as Cytoscape have often been used to construct and analyze networks [16].

QiShenYiQi (QSYQ) dropping pills are a Chinese medicine prescription approved by the State Food and Drug Administration (SFDA) of China. QSYQ is widely and effectively used in China to treat CVD, including myocardial infarction, angina, myocarditis, myocardial fibrosis and heart failure [17–19]. QSYQ is composed of *Astragalus membranaceus* (Huangqi), *Salvia miltiorrhiza* (Danshen), *Panax notoginseng* (Sanqi), and *Dalbergia odorifera* (Jiangxiang). Twelve compounds including astragaloside IV (Ast), calycosin (Cal) and formononetin (For) from Huangqi; danshensu (DSS), protocatechuic aldehyde (PCA) and rosmarinic acid (RSA) from Danshen; ginsenoside Rg1 (Rg1), ginsenoside Rb1 (Rb1) and notoginsenoside R1 (R1) from Sanqi; trans-nerolidol (ENL), (3S,6S,7R)-3,7,11-trimethyl-3,6-epoxy-1,10-dodecadien-7-ol (SDL) and (3S,6R,7R)-3,7,11-trimethyl-3,6-epoxy-1,10-dodecadien-7-ol (RDL) from Jiangxiang are main components of QSYQ, and they were absorbed into blood and distributed into tissues after oral administration [20]. SDL and RDL were identified in Jiangxiang in our previous study [21]. However, the potential targets and the underlying molecular mechanisms of actions of these 12 compounds remain to be systematically elucidated.

In this study, the differentially expressed genes (DEGs) were identified from myocardial infarction (MI) rat model treated with QSYQ, followed by constructing a CVD related compound-target-pathway network linking main compounds to those DEGs supported with literature evidences and the pathways that are functionally enriched in ArrayTrack. The associations of DEGs with CVD were evaluated based on information in database CHD@ZJU of its version 1.0 (http://tcm.zju.edu.cn/chd/) developed by our group [22]. We also manually collected the information of targets reported for 9 compounds (i.e. Ast, Cal, For, DSS, PCA, RSA, Rg1, Rb1 and R1) from literatures in PubMed. The judging criteria of a gene being a target is that a CVD related DEG can be found directly influenced by a compound of QSYQ in literature. Furthermore, as there were no reports on the targets of ENL, SDL and RDL, the potential targets of these three sesquiterpenes were proposed based upon gene expression data and further experimentally validated in this study. Finally, we constructed the compound-target-pathway network on anti-MI of QSYQ to decipher the underlying multi-compound, multi-target and multi-pathway mechanism.

Materials and Methods

Cell Lines and Reagents

RAW264.7 cells were purchased from the cell bank of Chinese academy of sciences (Shanghai, China). Trans-nerolidol (ENL) was obtained from Sigma-Aldrich (Cat No. 18143, Sigma, Germany). (3S,6S,7R)-3,7,11-trimethyl-3,6-epoxy-1,10-dodecadien-7-ol (SDL) and (3S,6R,7R)-3,7,11-trimethyl-3,6-epoxy-1,10-dodecadien-7-ol (RDL) was extracted from volatile oil of *Dalbergia odorifera* T. Chen [21] (**Fig. 1A**). Lipopolysaccharide (LPS), U0126 monoethanolate (U0126), T0070907, DMSO, and Thiazolyl blue tetrazolium bromide (MTT) were obtained from Sigma. Pioglitazone hydrochloride (Pio) was purchased from National Institutes for Food and Drug Control (Beijing, China). Nitric oxide assay kit was purchased from Beyotime Institute of Biotechnology (Cat No. S0021, Haimen, Jiangsu, China). Primary antibodies, including anti-ERK1+ERK2 antibody (Cat No. ab17942) for ERK1/2, anti-ERK1+ERK2 (phospho T185+T202+Y204+Y187) antibody (Cat No. ab4819) for pERK1/2, anti-PPAR gamma antibody (Cat No. ab19481) for PPARγ, and anti-Heme Oxygenase 1 antibody [HO-1-1] (Cat No. ab13248) for HO-1, were purchased from Abcam (Hongkong, China).

Preparation of QiShenYiQi Extracts

QSYQ was prepared from four herbs, *Radix Astragalus membranaceus* (Chinse name Huangqi), *Radix Salvia miltiorrhiza* (Chinse name Danshen), *Panax notoginseng* (Chinse name Sanqi), and *Dalbergia odorifera* T. Chen (Chinse name Jiangxiang). Briefly, crude drug Huangqi were crushed, for Huangqi, we added water and extracted with refluxing twice, then the extract were filtrated on gauzes. Filtrate was concentrated on a rotary evaporator. In the alcohol sedimentation step, we slowly added 95% ethanol to the filtrate to make alcohol concentration to about 70%. Cooled the solution at room temperature and the supernatant was filtered through cotton gauzes. After recycling the alcohol, the residue was concentrated again to form Huangqi extract. As for crude drug Danshen and Sanqi, they were extracted together with the same procedure as that of Huangqi. For Jiangxiang, we boiled crushed crude drug Jiangxiang with refluxing, and essential oil was extracted in an extraction apparatus. Roots of Sanqi, the trunk and dry heartwood of root from Jiangxiang have been used.

Animal Study and Gene Expression Data Analysis

Male Sprague-Dawley rats (~250 g) were obtained from Zhejiang Experimental Animal Center. The Animal Ethic Review Committees of Zhejiang University approved all experimental procedures.

The rats were maintained in air-conditioned rooms (temperature, 22–26°C; humidity, 40%–70%) with a 12-h light-dark cycle, and were acclimatized to the setting. To provide comfortable conditions for rats, each cage contained 5 rats, and the bedding material sawdust was renewed every 2 days. Rats were free to get fresh foods and water, and the water was renewed everyday. All surgery was performed under 10% chloral hydrate anesthesia (300 mg/kg), and all efforts were made to minimize suffering. Rat myocardial infarction was made by occlusion of left anterior descending coronary artery (LAD) according to Yamaguchi [23,24]. Rats post-operation were laid flat on an electric blanket to help maintain the body temperature of rats. And for those rats which were really weak post-operation, we helped them to recover heart beating with chest cardiac massage and recover breath by connecting the animals with rodent ventilator. For the LAD ligation operation, the mortality was about 40%. Six surviving rats after LAD ligation were randomly divided into myocardial infarction group (MI) and QSYQ-treated group. Three sham-operated rats were treated in the same ways as the rats in MI group but without LAD ligation, which were served as control group (Control). In clinical, QSYQ pills are administered orally administrated to patients with unstable angina and heart failure to prevent acute coronary syndrome. In accordance with clinical recommendations, QSYQ was given intragastrically (i.g.) at a dose of 105.6 mg/kg once a day. Rats in control, and MI groups were administered with saline. Rats were sacrificed after 7 days of i.g. administration under 10% chloral hydrate anesthesia (300 mg/kg). Rats were fixed on a flat plate, and blood samples were collected by abdominal aortic method, then the chest was carefully dissected and the heart was cut quickly. Three tissue samples on the border between infarct and non-infarct area were dissected from left ventricles of each group. The tissue samples were stored at −80°C refrigerator.

Total RNA was extracted using TRIzol Reagent (Invitrogen) and purified using RNeasy Mini kit (QIAGEN), following manufacturers' protocols. RNA quality was evaluated using an Agilent 2100 Bioanalyzer and electrophoresis in 2% (w/v) agarose gels. Only RNA with RNA integrity number (RIN) greater than 7.0 and 28S/18S ratio greater than 0.7 was used for microarray analyses. Whole genome microarray analysis was performed using Affymetrix rat Genome 230 2.0 array. Briefly, total RNA were amplified, labeled, and purified using GeneChip 3′IVT Express Kit (Affymetrix) according to the manufacturer's instructions to obtain biotin labeled cRNA. Array hybridization and wash were performed using GeneChip Hybridization, Wash and Stain Kit in Hybridization Oven 645 (Affymetrix) and Fluidics Station 450 (Affymetrix) following the manufacturer's instructions. Slides were

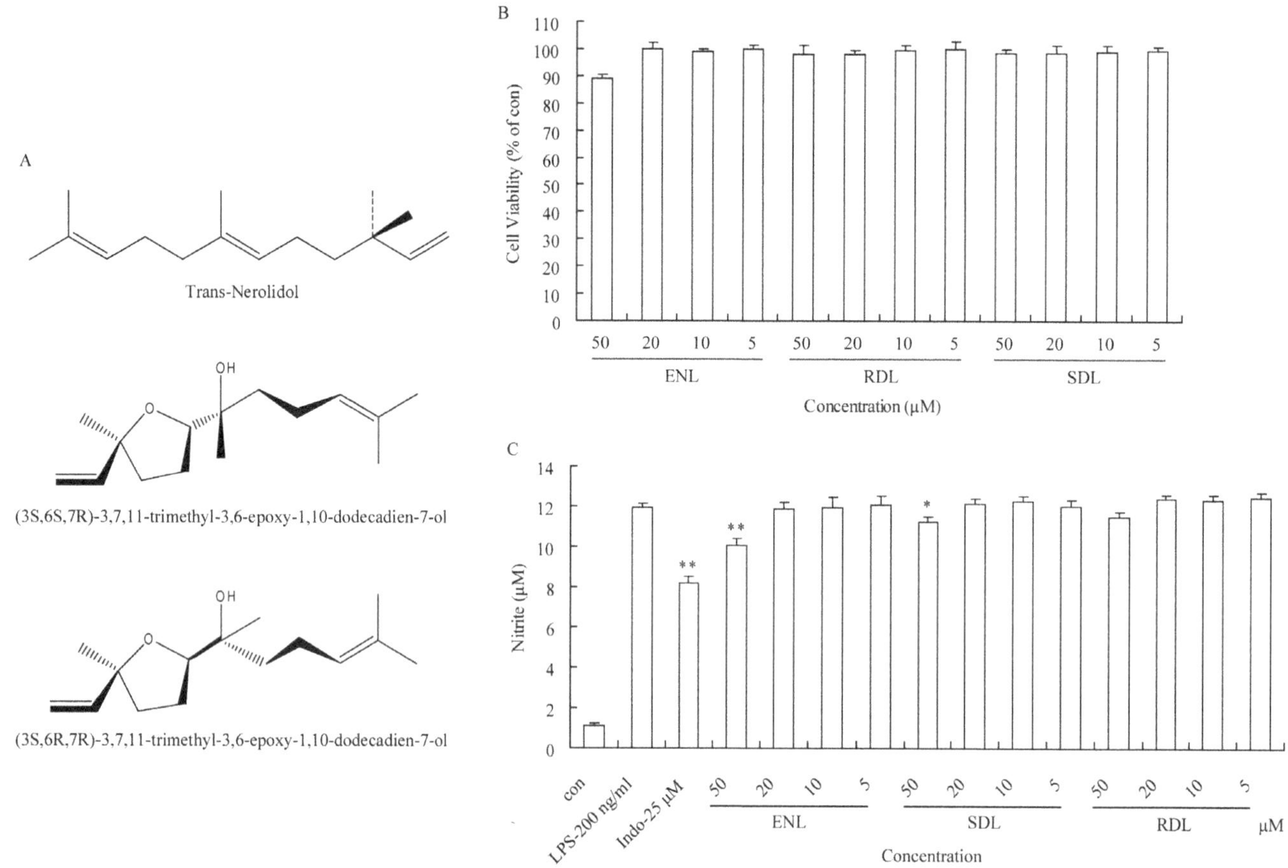

Figure 1. Effects of three sesquiterpene compounds from volatile oil of *Dalbergia odorifera* T. Chen on NO production in LPS-stimulated RAW264.7 macrophages. (A) Structure of ENL, SDL and RDL isolated from *Dalbergia odorifera* T. Chen. (B) Effects of ENL, SDL and RDL on RAW264.7 macrophages viability. (C) Effects of ENL, SDL and RDL on NO production in LPS-stimulated RAW264.7. Indo stands for indomethacin and was used as positive control. Each group was compared with model, and * stands for $p<0.05$, ** stands for $p<0.01$. Each assay was conducted in triplicate and repeated three times. ENL is trans-nerolidol; RDL is (3S,6R,7R)-3,7,11-trimethyl-3,6-epoxy-1,10-dodecadien-7-ol; SDL is (3S, 6S, 7R)-3,7,11-trimethyl-3,6-epoxy-1,10-dodecadien-7-ol.

scanned by GeneChip Scanner 3000 and Command Console Software 3.1 with default settings. Spike-in control transcripts were monitored to verify hybridization integrity. The dataset as CEL files was deposited to GEO and the access number is GSE54134. Significant genes were identified through an algorithm developed in-house[25].

As mentioned above, we validated the CVD-related DEGs by manually checking published literatures in PubMed (by April 10th, 2013). The keywords used to search papers in PubMed were: "Astragaloside IV", "Calycosin", "Formononetin", "Danshensu", "Salvianic Acid A", "Tanshinol", "Protocatechuic Aldehyde", "Protocatechualdehyde", "Rosmarinic Acid", "Ginsenoside Rg1", "Ginsenoside Rb1", "Notoginsenoside R1". The literatures related to pharmacology and activity of Ast, Cal, For, DSS, PCA, RSA, Rgl, Rb1 and R1 were manually read. A DEG was considered as a potential target of a compound if it was found to be affected directly by the compound in a paper. For each paper, the information of target, PubMed ID, and CVD relevancy were recorded. Detailed information on the references used in this study can be found in **Table S1**.

Experimental Target Validation

CVD-related DEGs were validated by manually checking published literature in PubMed (by April 10th, 2013). However, there were no previous studies reporting the targets of ENL, SDL and RDL. These three sesquiterpenes were isolated from volatile oils from Jiangxiang, which was reported to have anti-inflammatory activities, and was also used as a penetration enhancer [26]. Extracellular signal-regulated kinase-1/2 (ERK1/2), peroxisome proliferator-activated receptor-gamma (PPARγ) and heme oxygenase-1 (HO-1), which play important roles in inflammation, were identified as the potential targets of ENL and SDL. The anti-inflammatory activity of these targets was validated using LPS-stimulated RAW264.7 macrophage cells as models.

Cell Viability Analysis by MTT Assay

Murine macrophage cell line RAW264.7 was maintained in DMEM medium supplemented with 10% heat-inactivated fetal bovine serum at 37°C in 5% CO_2. To determine the effect of ENL and SDL on cell viability, RAW264.7 cells were seeded in 96-well plates at concentrations of 5000 cells/well. Following overnight incubation, cells were treated with several concentrations of ENL, RDL and SDL for 24 h. Cell viability was determined by the MTT assay. For MTT assay, the media were replaced with fresh DMEM medium that containing 10% FBS, penicillin/streptomycin, and MTT (0.5 mg/ml). After 4 h of incubation at 37°C, the media were removed, and replaced with 150 μL/well of DMSO. After mixing at 400 rpm in Thermomixer comfort (Eppendorf) at

37°C for 10 min, absorbance at 550 nm was measured on a Bio-Tek micro-plate reader. Each assay was conducted in triplicate and repeated three times.

Nitric Oxide Assay

RAW 264.7 cells (4×10^4 cells in 96-well microplate) were stimulated with 200 ng/ml LPS in 37°C CO_2 incubator for 24 h. Nitric oxide (NO) production was detected by measuring nitrite levels in the culture media using the Griess reagent according to the manufacturer's instructions (Beyotime Institute of Biotechnology, China). Absorbance was measured at 550 nm.

Effects of U0126, T0070907, and Pio on Nitric Oxide Secretion

U0126, a selective ERK1/2 phosphorylation inhibitor, was used to incubate with RAW264.7 macrophages together with LPS (200 ng/ml) or compounds with different concentrations plus LPS (200 ng/ml). PPARγ phosphorylation inhibitor T0070907 and PPARγ agonist Pio were also used in the same way as that of U0126. The concentration of U0126, T0070907 and Pio were used at 10 μM. NO production was determined using Griess Reagent. Each assay was conducted in triplicate and repeated three times, and outliers were excluded.

Western Blot Analysis

For western blot assay, RAW264.7 macrophages were seeded into 60-mm dishes, cells were cultured in the 37°C CO_2 incubator overnight. The second day, cells were treated with different compounds. The cells were collected after 24 h treatment. Cells were gently rinsed with ice-cold PBS. Then, 300 μL of cold RIPA buffer (RIPA lysis buffer, Cat No. P0013B, Beyotime Institute of Biotechnology, Haimen, Jiangsu, China) plus PMSF (Cat No. ST506, Beyotime Institute of Biotechnology, Haimen, Jiangsu, China), complete Mini (Cat No. 04693124001, Roche) and PhosSTOP (Cat No. 04906845001, Roche) were added to each dish. All steps of protein extraction were carried out on ice. Cells were lysed completely within 10 min, and the protein lysate was transferred to 1.5 ml centrifuge tubes, then the tubes were centrifuged at 12000 rpm for 10 min at 4°C. The supernatant in each tube was carefully collected without disturbing the sediments. Protein concentrations in the collected supernatants were determined using BCA protein assay kit (Cat No. P0012, Beyotime Institute of Biotechnology, Haimen, Jiangsu, China).

Protein samples containing LDS Sample Buffer (4×, NuPAGE, REF. NP0007) were heated at 70°C for 10 min and loaded onto a NuPAGE 10% Bis-Tris Gels, 1.5 mm, 15 well (Invitrogen, REF. NP0316BOX). PageRuler Prestained Protein Ladder (Fermentas, Cat No. SM0671) molecular weight marker used. The gels were run at 150 volts for 1 hour at room temperature (XCell SureLock Electrophoresis Cell). Proteins were transferred onto a PVDF membrane (iBlot, Gel Transfer Stacks, Mini, REF. IB401002) using an iBlot 7-minute Blotting System (Life technologies, Invitrogen). Primary antibodies for ERK1/2, pERK1/2, PPARγ and HO-1 were diluted in 5% BSA according to their manufacturer instructions respectively. GAPDH (Cat No. AG019, Beyotime) was used as the internal reference. Then the primary antibodies were incubated overnight at 4°C with 5% BSA. HRP-linked anti-rabbit IgG secondary antibody (Cat No. A0208, Beyotime) was used at 1:1000 for ERK1/2, pERK1/2 and PPARγ, while HRP-linked anti-mouse IgG secondary antibody (Cat No. A0216, Beyotime) was used at 1:1000 for HO-1. Detection was performed using SuperSignal West Femto Maximun Sensitivity Substrate (Cat No. 34095, Thermo Scientfic) on a BIO-RAD ChemiDoc XRS System.

Network Construction and Network Analysis

The DEGs related to CVD and the main compounds were used as input in ArrayTrack v.3.5.0 to carry out pathway enrichment analysis, in which the MI or CVD associated pathways were selected for further analysis. Then, we constructed compound-target-pathway network and compound-pathway network in Cytoscape [16]. A compound and a target were connected with a solid line if the link was reported in at least one paper (≥1 literature) when they were; and the edge between target and pathway was constructed using the relationship found in ArrayTrack v.3.5.0 pathway enrichment analysis [27].

Statistical Analysis

All experiments were performed three times in triplicate. Results are expressed as mean ± SD. Two-tailed unpaired Student's t tests were used to compare two distinct groups. When more than three groups were compared, One-Way ANOVA was performed between different treatment groups using PASW Statistics 18 (SPSS Inc., USA). A p value <0.05 was considered to be statistically significant.

Results

DEGs Analysis

312 genes (442 probe sets) in CHD@ZJU V1.0 database were found to be differentially expressed, out of which 83 genes with reverse rate (RR)>0.5 and fold change (FC)>1.1 after the QSYQ treatment were selected for further analysis (**Table S2**). Combined with the targets information about the compounds collected manually from published papers, 52 genes were included in this study, with additional information about compound, target, pathway, category and Fisher P-value (**Table S3**). The number of targets and the pathways of the compounds are listed in **Table 1**.

Effect of ENL, RDL and SDL on RAW264.7 Macrophages Viability

After 24 h co-incubation with different concentrations (50, 20, 10, 5 μM) of ENL, RDL and SDL, MTT assay results showed that there was no obvious cytotoxicity of the three compounds (**Fig. 1B**) at these concentrations. Concentrations ≤50 μM were used for subsequent experiments.

Effects of ENL and SDL on NO Production in LPS-stimulated RAW264.7 Macrophages

Two sesquiterpene compounds (ENL and SDL) from the volatile oil of *Dalbergia odorifera* T. Chen were able to suppress NO secretion from LPS-induced RAW264.7 macrophages. Both ENL and SDL significantly inhibited the NO secretion by LPS-stimulated RAW264.7 cells at 50 μM ($p<0.01$ for ENL, $p<0.05$ for SDL compared to model) (**Fig. 1C**). However, RDL at all concentrations had no obvious inhibition effect on NO secretion by LPS-stimulated RAW264.7 cells. Indomethacin at 25 μM was used as the positive control. More details of indomethacin, NEL and SDL on NO production can be found in **Fig. 1C**.

Effects of ENL, RDL and SDL on ERK1/2, pERK1/2, PPARγ and HO-1 Expression

Western blot results (**Fig. 2**) showed that LPS treatment significantly increased pERK1/2 to ERK1/2 ratio (*$p<0.05$ vs.

Table 1. The number of targets and pathways of 9 main compounds from QSYQ.

	Potential targets			
	Total	Confirmed in CVD-related references	Confirmed in non-CVD-related references	Pathways
Astragaloside IV	16	7	9	16
Calycosin	10	8	2	14
Formononetin	13	1	12	14
Danshensu	7	0	7	13
Protocatechuic Aldehyde	5	1	4	12
Rosmarinic Acid	21	0	21	15
Ginsenoside Rg1	26	7	19	16
Ginsenoside Rb1	21	4	17	16
Notoginsenoside R1	5	3	2	9

The numbers listed in the column of Pathway stands for CVD related pathways enriched in ArrayTrack v.3.5.0 pathway enrichment analysis of the targets of certain compound.

control) and HO-1 levels (** $p<0.01$ vs. control), but decreased PPARγ expression in RAW 264.7 macrophages (** $p<0.01$ vs. control). Both ENL and SDL attenuated the increased ratio of pERK1/2 to ERK1/2 at 50 μM compared to LPS treated alone (# $p<0.05$ for SDL), but RDL had no effect on the increased ratio (**Fig. 2A**). While ENL, RDL, SDL all partially increased PPARγ expression, ENL showed the strongest effect (# $p<0.05$ vs. model) (**Fig. 2B**). ENL, RDL, SDL further promoted HO-1 expression (for ENL $p<0.05$, and for RDL, SDL $p<0.01$, comparing with model) (**Fig. 2C**).

Effects of U0126, T0070907, and Pio on Nitric Oxide Secretion

U0126, an antagonist of ERK1/2 phosphorylation, Pio, a PPARγ agonist, and T0070907, a PPARγ phosphorylation inhibitor, were able to inhibit NO secretion by LPS-induced RAW264.7 macrophages. So these three tool drugs were used to validate the effects of ENL and SDL. 200 ng/ml LPS significantly induced NO secretion ($^{§§}p<0.01$, vs control by student's t test) (**Fig. 3**). Combined-treatment with either of the three drugs, U0126, T0070907, and Pio, significantly strengthened the effect of ENL on suppressing NO secretion except 20 μM ENL plus Pio (**Fig. 3A, B, C**). U0126 also significantly enhanced the effect of SDL on inhibition of NO production (## $p<0.01$, vs. the group with SDL treated alone) (**Fig. 3D**).

Network Construction and Pathway Analysis

Combining the relationships in **Table S3** and the relationships from the experimental validation part, that is the potential targets such as PPARG (targets of ENL and SDL), HMOX1 (targets of ENL, RDL and SDL), MAPK3 and MAPK1 (targets of ENL and SDL) were also used to construct the network (**Fig. 4**). Then the paired relationships information (link between compound and target genes, link between target gene and pathways) was imported to Cytoscape software, and a compound-target-pathway network was constructed (**Fig. 4**). The three-level network consisted of 84 nodes (12 compounds, 55 genes and 17 pathways) and 230 edges. The detailed information of the compound names, gene names, pathway names and their category, and Fisher P-values can be found in **Table S3**. Through the visualization and network analysis of the relationships among compound, target gene and pathway in the constructed network, 52 DEGs were affected by at least one compound, in which 14 genes (*DUSP1, EPO, FGF1, FLT1, FN1, HIF1A, LDHA, LDHB, PLAT, PRKCB, RELA, VEGFA* and *VWF*) were the potential targets of the compounds based on the CVD-related literatures in PubMed. Among the 52 genes, RELA was influenced by 9 compounds. RELA is associated with cell growth and death, immune system, and endocrine system. IL6, PTGS2 and VEGFA were affected by 6 compounds, which maybe related with inflammation and angiogenesis. GPX1, HIF1A, IL1B, LDHA, LDHB and PPARG were affected by 5 compounds. FN1 and PLAT were influenced by 4 compounds. While five targets were influenced by 3 compounds, nine targets were influenced by 2 compounds, and the rest twenty six were affected by only one compound.

Using the 52 DEGs, 16 KEGG pathways were enriched in the ArrayTrack v.3.5.0 pathway enrichment analysis (**Table 2**), in which apoptosis signaling pathway is a critical pathway in regulating cell death. Most of the pathways, such as Cytokine-cytokine receptor interaction, NOD-like receptor signaling pathway, PPAR signaling pathway, Toll-like receptor signaling pathway, MAPK signaling pathway, Hematopoietic cell lineage, Cytosolic DNA-sensing pathway, Complement and coagulation cascades and Arachidonic acid metabolism, are either directly involved in immune and inflammation or play important roles there. In addition, there are several energy metabolism associated pathways including PPAR signaling pathway, Adipocytokine signaling pathway, Pyruvate metabolism. The Glutathione metabolism is antioxidant related, Focal adhesion plays role in cell motility and structure, VEGF signaling pathway has function in vasodilation, Complement and coagulation cascades is related with coagulation, and mTOR signaling pathway plays a role in hypoxia induced angiogenesis.

Discussion

Based on the results of microarray data and published literature information available in PubMed, a compound-target-pathway network (**Fig 4**) was constructed for the multi-compound-multi-target-multi-pathway mode of action (MOA) of the Chinese medicine QSYQ. The cardioprotective or anti-MI function of QSYQ is complex, involving modulation of groups of targets and a number of associated pathways. Cardiomyocytes apoptosis occurs promptly following acute myocardial infarction (AMI), and

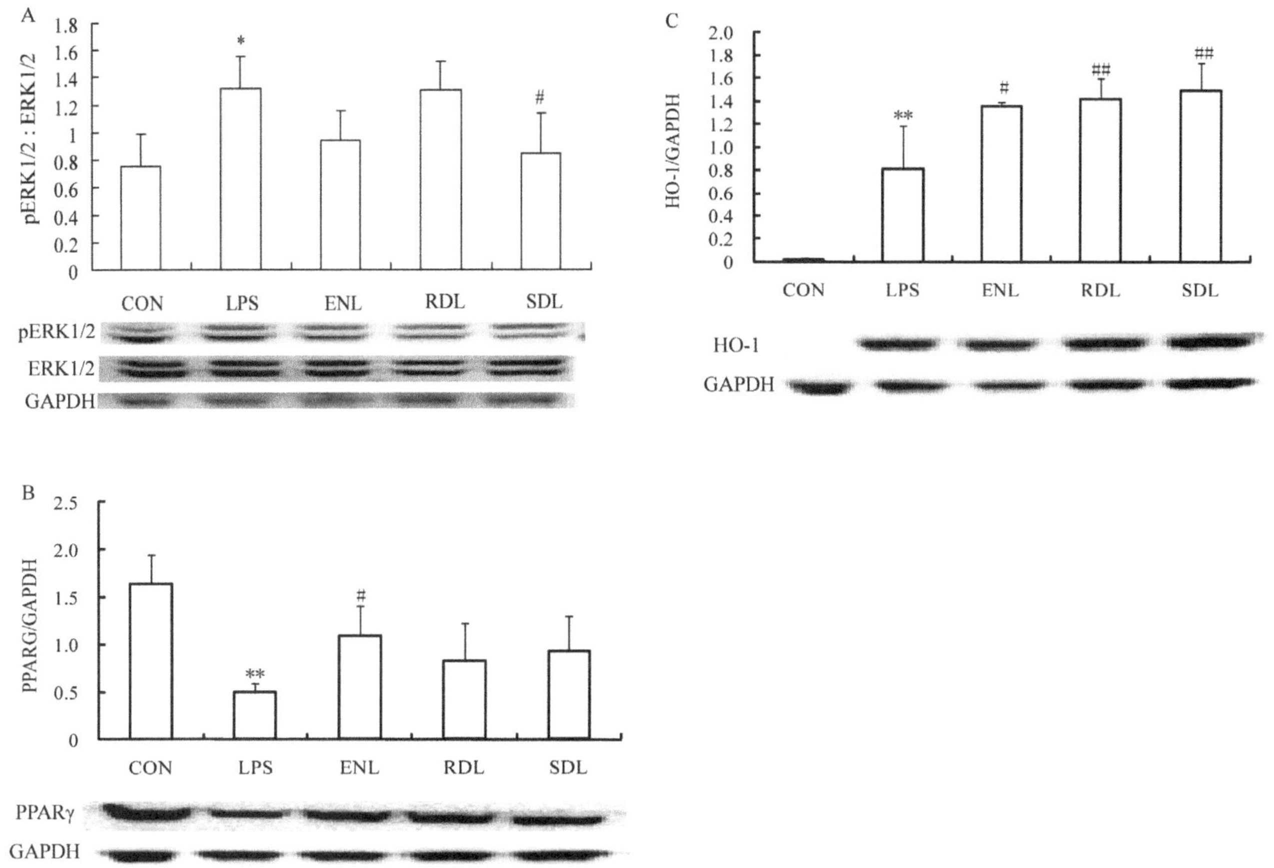

Figure 2. Effects of three sesquiterpene compounds from volatile oil of *Dalbergia odorifera* T. Chen on pERK1/2, ERK1/2, PPARγ and HO-1 expression in LPS-stimulated RAW264.7 macrophages. (A). LPS co-incubation induced significant increase of pERK1/2 expression, the ratio of pERK1/2 to ERK1/2 was higher than that in the control group (*$p<0.05$). 50 μM ENL attenuated the increased ratio of pERK1/2 to ERK1/2, while 50 μM SDL suppressed this ratio compared to LPS treated alone (#$p<0.05$), and RDL had no effect on the increased ratio. (B). LPS decreased PPARγ expression (**$p<0.01$ vs. control), and ENL, RDL, SDL all partially increased PPARγ expression, ENL showed the most strong effect (#$p<0.05$ vs. model). (C). The expression of HO-1 was induced to increase with 200 ng/ml LPS stimulation (**$p<0.01$ vs. control), and ENL, RDL, SDL further promoted HO-1 expression (for ENL $p<0.05$, and for RDL, SDL $p<0.01$, comparing with model). The RAW264.7 was stimulated with 200 ng/ml LPS for 24 h, and the concentration of ENL, RDL and SDL were all at 50 μM. Each assay was conducted in triplicate and repeated three times. ENL is trans-nerolidol; RDL is (3S,6R,7R)-3,7,11-trimethyl-3,6-epoxy-1,10-dodecadien-7-ol. SDL is (3S, 6S, 7R)-3,7,11-trimethyl-3,6-epoxy-1,10-dodecadien-7-ol.

apoptosis pathway (including the mitochondrial death pathway) plays a pivotal role in this pathological process [28–30]. Inflammation accompanies from the initial stage of AMI and participates in the development of ischemia injury, one of the mechanisms is post-AMI hypoxia elicited inflammatory response [31].

Among the 16 pathways, nine are immune and inflammation related, including Cytokine-cytokine receptor interaction, NOD-like receptor signaling pathway [32,33], PPAR signaling pathway [34–36], Toll-like receptor signaling pathway [37,38], MAPK signaling pathway [39], Hematopoietic cell lineage, Cytosolic DNA-sensing pathway [40], Complement and coagulation cascades [41,42] and Arachidonic acid metabolism [43]. Compounds from *Dalbergia odorifera* suppressed NO production in our in vitro target validation experiments. Anti-inflammation effect of QSYQ has been reported. QSYQ can reduce high sensitivity C reactive protein level in atherosclerotic rabbit to prevent the progress of atherosclerosis by inhibiting inflammatory reaction[44]. Also, it was reported that QSYQ can inhibit inflammatory effect through reducing TNF-α and IL-6 levels in rat after acute myocardial infarction[45,46]. In clinical settings, QSYQ can improve cardiac function through anti-inflammatory effects by reducing TNF-α and IL-6 levels both in AMI and chronic heart failure patients[47,48]. QSYQ could decrease the levels of high sensitivity C reactive protein, plasminogen activator inhibitor-1 and endothelin-1 in acute coronary syndrome patients[49].

Myocardial energy metabolism is another important event during and post-AMI, including fatty acid and glucose utilization. Acetyl-CoA is common end product of fatty acid, glucose and pyruvate to supply ATP. PPAR signaling pathway may prevent ischemic insult involving anti-inflammatory effect and promoting glucose utilization [36]. Adiponectin is a key adipocytokine having beneficial effect to facilitate fatty acid beta-oxidation and increase glucose utilization [50].

As for Glutathione metabolism pathway, glutathione has antioxidant activity [51] which is beneficial to prevent further myocardial injury elicited by reactive oxygen species (ROS) post-AMI. Focal adhesion plays a role in cell motility, cell proliferation, cell differentiation, and tissue remodeling after injury [52,53]. VEGF signaling pathway has a function in vasculature vasodilatation through modulation of PKC, cPLA2, COX-2 and PGI2 [54–56]. Complement and coagulation cascades are activated early after injury. The modulation of coagulation may prevent secondary injury post AMI [41,57]. mTOR signaling pathway

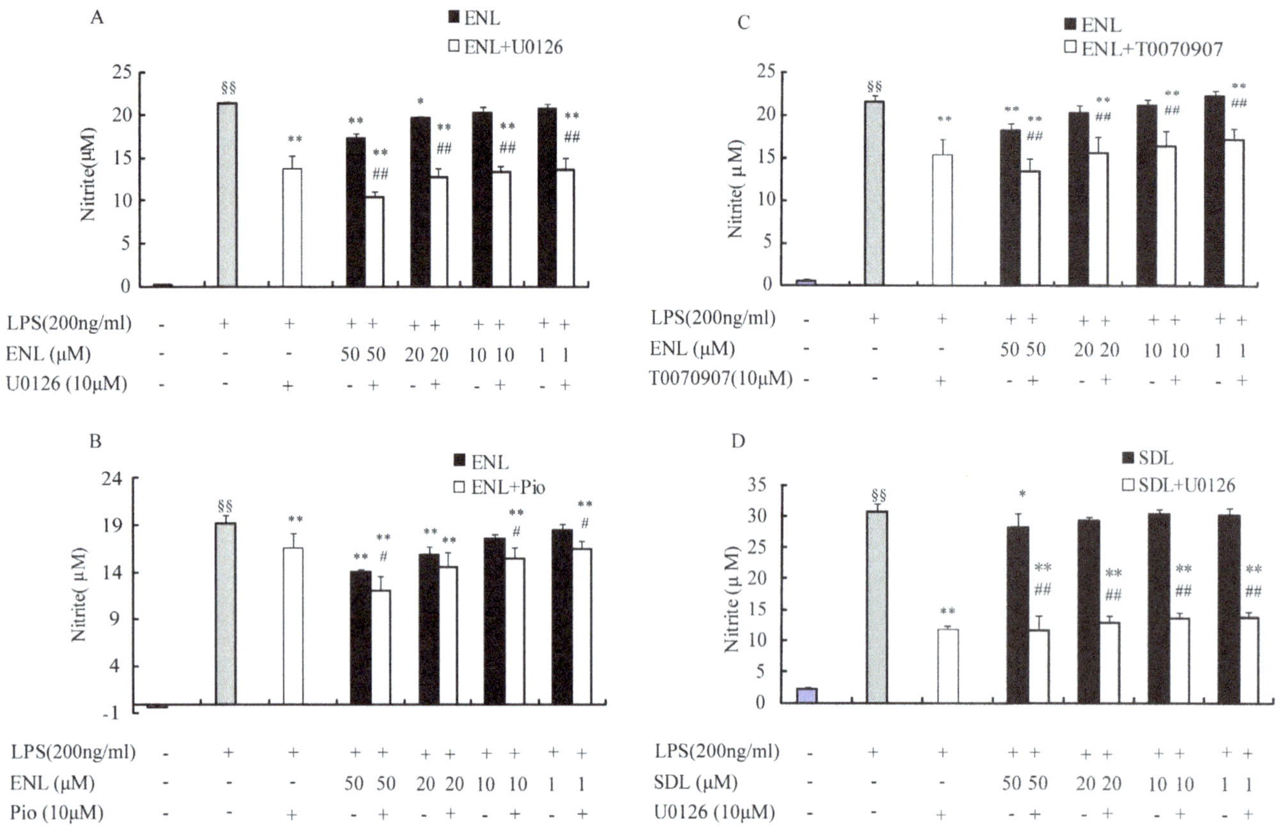

Figure 3. Effects of U0126, T0070907, and Pioglitazone hydrochloride (Pio) on NO production in LPS-stimulated RAW264.7 macrophages. LPS significantly induced NO secretion (§§p<0.01 vs control). ERK1/2 phosphorylation antagonist U0126 significantly inhibited NO production (**p<0.01 vs. LPS treated alone) (A and D). PPARγ phosphorylation inhibitor T0070907 strongly suppressed NO release (**p<0.01 vs. model) (C), while PPARγ agonist Pio decreased NO secretion (**p<0.01 vs. model) (B). ENL does-dependently attenuated NO secretion, U0126, T0070907, and Pio further strengthened ENL's effect. 50 μM SDL also showed NO inhibition activity, while U0126 enhanced SDL's effect. * Means compared with model group (200 ng/ml LPS treated alone), and # stands for statistic significance analysis between two groups with and without small molecular tool drugs (*i.e.* U0126, T0070907, and Pio). ENL is trans-nerolidol; RDL is (3S,6R,7R)-3,7,11-trimethyl-3,6-epoxy-1,10-dodecadien-7-ol.

plays a role in hypoxia-induced angiogenesis, which can help to recover blood supply to the ischemic myocardium post-MI [58,59]. In addition, Hypoxia-Inducible Factor-1 signaling is also an important pathway which can be triggered by both hypoxia and inflammation conditions. The activation of Hypoxia-Inducible Factor-1 signaling could minimize the ischemic tissue damage and plays a protective role in inflammatory diseases[60].

The potential targets of those 9 main compounds from Huangqi, Danshen, Sanqi were validated using CVD-ralated literatures, and there was no reference reporting the targets of two main sesquiterpenes from Jiangxiang. In our experimental study, we investigated the anti-inflammatory effects of two main sesquiterpenes in volatile oils of Jiangxiang, i.e. ENL and SDL. SDL was newly identified from Jiangxiang in our previous study [21]. To the best of our knowledge, the pharmacological activities of ENL and SDL, and their potential protein targets have not been previously reported. We used nitric oxide assay, Western blot technology and small molecular compounds specific to the proteins of interest to validate the identified targets. As discussed above, ENL and SDL could suppress NO production in LPS-stimulated RAW264.7 macrophages.

Extracellular signal-regulated kinase-1/2 (ERK1/2) phosphorylation participates in stimuli induced inflammation. ERK1/2 phosphorylation was increased in lipopolysaccharide (LPS)-induced RAW264.7 macrophages. U0126 can suppress NO production in LPS-stimulated RAW264.7 macrophages by selectively inhibiting ERK1/2 phosphorylation, followed by inhibition of NF-κB transactivation and iNOS expression [61]. Inhibition of MAPKs (ERK1/2, p38MAPK, JNK) phosphorylation and NF-κB activation could decrease production of pro-inflammatory mediators (TNF-α, IL6, NO, *etc.*) [62–64]. In our study, U0126 suppressed NO production significantly (p<0.01 vs LPS treated alone) (**Fig. 3A, D**), and U0126 further reinforced NO inhibition induced by ENL (p<0.01 vs. ENL treated alone) and SDL (p<0.01 vs. SDL treated alone) (**Fig. 3A, D**). Therefore, ENL and SDL may attenuate LPS-induced NO release from RAW264.7 macrophages via inhibiting ERK1/2 phosphorylation; and NF-κB and iNOS may be involved in this process [65]. Furthermore, PPARγ plays an important role in inflammation [66,67]. Activation of PPARγ leads to anti-inflammatory effects of PPARγ ligands (such as thiazolidinediones (TZDs), GW1929, indomethacin, ibuprofen and fenoprofen) [34,35,68]. LPS treatment has been shown to decrease PPARγ expression both in vivo and in vitro [69], the latter was repeated in our study (**Fig. 2B**). PPARγ ligand Pioglitazone inhibited LPS-stimulated microglia inflammation by inhibiting inflammatory mediators, including NO [70]. The effect of pioglitazone on NO synthase inhibition is potentially mediated through blocking of p38 MAPK activity [71]. Here in our study, 10 μM pioglitazone hydrochloride significantly inhibited NO production (p<0.01, **Fig. 3B**). ENL at 50 μM and 20 μM

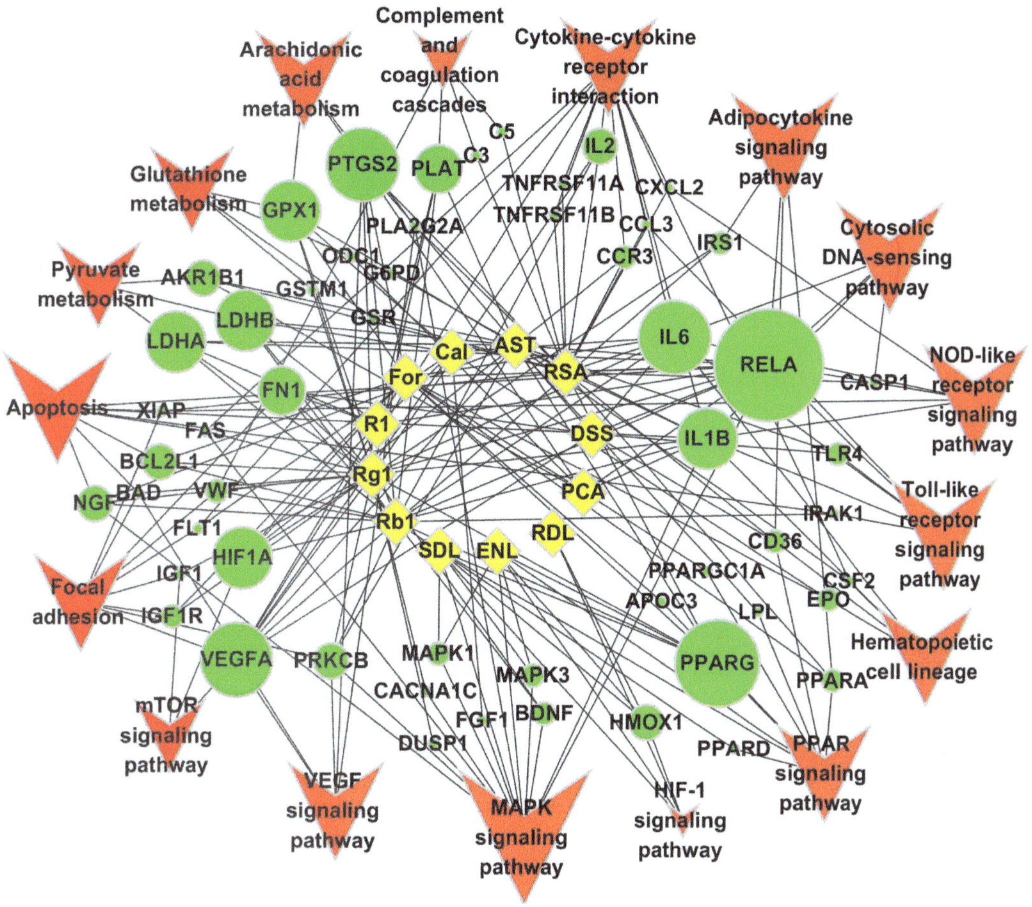

Figure 4. Multi-compound-multi-target-multi-pathway network of TCM QSYQ on treating myocardial infarction. There were 52 differentially expressed genes which were validated in published literatures. Node size of targets and pathways are proportional to the number of compounds associated with the node. This network depicted a clear three-level structure of the mode of action of main compounds of QSYQ, that is multi-compound regulated multi-pathways through modulating of groups of genes to show their pharmacological and clinical effects. Compound was linked to targets, while target were linked to pathways, a certain compound linked indirect link to pathways through certain targets. Diamond represents compounds; Circle represents target genes; Vee represents CVD related pathways. The edge went through compound to target, and target to pathway.

significantly suppressed NO secretion ($p<0.01$) (**Fig. 3B**). Combined use of Pio further enhanced the anti-NO production effect of ENL (**Fig. 3B**). Interestingly, phosphorylation of PPARγ decreases its transcriptional activity [72,73]. T0070907 is the antagonist of PPARγ phosphorylation, it also inhibits ERK1/2 phosphorylation dose-dependently [74]. The results obtained in this study are consistent with those previously reported, as 10 µM T0070907 significantly inhibited NO release from LPS-stimulated RAW264.7 macrophages ($p<0.01$, **Fig. 3C**). 50 µM ENL attenuated NO secretion significantly ($p<0.01$, **Fig. 3C**), while 10 µM T0070907 further strengthened the effect of ENL ($p<0.01$, **Fig. 3C**). Therefore, ENL may inhibit NO production partially via inhibiting PPARγ phosphorylation and inducing PPARγ activity.

In cardiovascular disease, heme oxygenase-1 (HO-1) is another beneficial factor, it also plays an important role in anti-inflammation process [75]. LPS could enhance NO production through ROS generation, and induced HO-1 expression in RAW264.7 macrophages was able to inhibit iNOS expression [76]. Flavonoids could promote HO-1 expression, which suppresses LPS-induced NO production [77]. HO-1 was transcriptionally regulated by PPARγ [78], and PPARγ was able to stabilize HO-1 mRNA in monocytes/macrophages [79]. Carbon monoxide (CO) was proposed to be involved in the protective effects of HO-1, including its anti-inflammatory actions [80,81]. LPS induced an increase in HO-1 expression in RAW264.7 macrophages, while ENL, RDL and SDL further enhanced HO-1 expression ($p<0.05$, $p<0.01$, and $p<0.01$, respectively, comparing with LPS treated alone, **Fig. 2C**).

We propose herein that the three sesquiterpene compounds (especially ENL and SDL) from volatile oil of Jiangxiang may suppress LPS-stimulated NO production from RAW264.7 macrophages at least partially via inhibition of ERK1/2 and PPARγ phosphorylation, and increasing expression of PPARγ and HO-1, in which NF-κB, ROS and iNOS maybe involved (**Fig. S1.**).

Chinese medicine treats diseases in a holistic way to make body recovery from imbalanced state by modulating a complex MOA including multiple pathways. Therefore, rodent animal models mimicking human disease are more suitable to evaluate the therapeutic effects of TCM and discover its MOA than cell culture. In our study, the underlying MOA of a clinical effective Chinese medicine QSYQ is systematically investigated combining mRNA expression profiles at molecular level on a rat myocardial infarction model. Using rat model is more convenient and easy to

Table 2. 16 KEGG pathways enriched in ArrayTrack v.3.5.0 pathway enrichment analysis using the 52 differentially expressed genes (DEGs) affected by nine compounds from the TCM QSYQ.

Pathway	Category	Fisher P-value
Apoptosis	Cell Growth and Death/Cellular Processes	0.00001765
Cytokine-cytokine receptor interaction	Signaling Molecules and Interaction/Environmental Information Processing	0.0000376
NOD-like receptor signaling pathway	Immune System/Cellular Processes	0.00015053
PPAR signaling pathway	Endocrine System/Cellular Processes	0.00027289
Glutathione metabolism	Metabolism of Other Amino Acids/Metabolism	0.00047522
Focal adhesion	Cell Communication/Cellular Processes	0.00122324
Adipocytokine signaling pathway	Endocrine System/Cellular Processes	0.00182003
Toll-like receptor signaling pathway	Immune System/Cellular Processes	0.0020686
MAPK signaling pathway	Signal Transduction/Environmental Information Processing	0.00263886
VEGF signaling pathway	Signal Transduction/Environmental Information Processing	0.00317584
Hematopoietic cell lineage	Immune System/Cellular Processes	0.0059589
Cytosolic DNA-sensing pathway	Immune System/Cellular Processes	0.00622074
Complement and coagulation cascades	Immune System/Cellular Processes	0.01287548
Pyruvate metabolism	Carbohydrate Metabolism/Metabolism	0.01558565
mTOR signaling pathway	Signal Transduction/Environmental Information Processing	0.03115849
Arachidonic acid metabolism	Lipid Metabolism/Metabolism	0.04113971

perform research to get rich information about the drug investigated both at phenotype and molecular base. On the other hand, cell culture model can be used to mimic a certain biological step of the drug investigated. Cell culture experiment has its merit as it is much easier to manipulate and to set investigation conditions. The results from animal experiments can be confirmed and studied in depth within cell culture experiments. However the results from animal studies should be carefully interpreted and concluded to explain the potential MOA of drug in treating human disease.

For the additional predicted targets as shown in **Fig. 4**, it is also important to validate them for a better understanding of the underlying MOA of QSYQ. Cell culture models play an important role in target validation. For example, inflammation related targets validation can be done with LPS-stimulated macrophage RAW264.7 cell culture model. TNF-α injured endothelial cell models are also used for anti-inflammatory related targets validation. The other two important processes mentioned in our study, apoptosis and energy metabolism can be studied with H9C2 cell line and primary neonatal rat heart cells to investigate cardioprotective effects and mechanisms of active compounds and drugs. Hypoxia or hypoxia-reoxygenation conditions are used to mimic in vivo ischemia or ischemia-reperfusion conditions. In addition, siRNA technology and target specific small molecular tool drugs could help to further confirm the validation results. Secondly, the targets validated at the in vitro experiments need further in vivo experiments confirmation. Rat MI model can be used to investigate the contributions of several targets to the anti-MI effects of compounds. The mRNA and protein expression profiles of specific targets after the intervention of single compounds or compounds combinations are tested using RT-PCR and western blot technologies. Finally, transgenetic mice models (both knock out and knock in) if available would provide more conclusive information for validating predicted targets with regard to cardioprotective effects.

The approach described in this paper provided an example on discovering the multi-compound, multi-target, multi-pathway MOA of a clinically effective Chinese medicine. A few steps have to be followed to ensure successful results. First, it is important to choose a clinically effective Chinese medicine with appropriate animal model available. Second, there should be reasonable understanding of the chemical compositions of the Chinese medicine. Third, in vitro experiments using cell culture models should be applied to test the pharmacological protective effects of potential compounds. Animal models (usually rodents) mimicking human disease are also used to confirm the effectiveness of potential compounds. Through these investigations, we understand the efficacious material basis of the Chinese medicine. Finally, network pharmacology analysis can be applied to integrate all these information to gain a full understanding of the MOA of the Chinese medicine.

In conclusion, the potential targets of 12 major compounds of QSYQ were identified by integrating gene expression data analysis and literature mining. These compounds may regulate multiple pathways through modulation of groups of genes to exert their anti-MI effects, involving biological processes of anti-apoptosis, anti-inflammation, antioxidant, anti-coagulation, energy utilization facilitation and angiogenesis promotion. Potential targets of 9 main compounds were validated by CVD-related references, while potential targets of three sesquiterpene compounds were further experimentally validated for their roles in mediation of inflammation.

Supporting Information

Figure S1 Proposed molecular mechanisms of the anti-inflammatory effects of two sesquiterpene compounds from volatile oil of *Dalbergia odorifera* T. Chen. ENL is proposed as an inhibitor of ERK1/2 phosphorylation and PPARγ phosphorylation, an agonist of PPARγ, via which ENL could suppress NO production from LPS-stimulated RAW264.7 macrophages. SDL is also an antagonist of ERK1/2 phosphorylation, through which SDL may attenuate NO secretion. HO-1 may also participated in the regulation process of these two naturally occurring products in anti-inflammation. ENL is trans-nerolidol; SDL is (3S, 6S, 7R)-3,7,11-trimethyl-3,6-epoxy-1,10-dodecadien-7-ol.
(TIF)

Table S1 The target, PubMed ID, and CVD relevancy about the 9 main compounds of QSYQ.
(XLS)

Table S2 Differentially expressed genes(DEGs) slected from CHD@ZJU V1.0 database with fold change (FC) and reverse rate (RR) information after the QSYQ treatment.
(XLS)

Table S3 52 Differentially expressed genes(DEGs) with corresponding compounds,together with the information of pathways, categories and Fisher P-value.
(XLS)

Acknowledgments

The Microarray test was performed by National Engineering Center for Biochip at Shanghai by Dr. Huasheng Xiao's team. We sincerely thank Shireesh Srivastava (DBT-ICGEB Centre For Advanced Bioenergy Research, International Centre For Genetic Engineering and Biotechnology (ICGEB), Aruna Asaf Ali Marg, New Delhi), for his great help with language editing.

Author Contributions

Conceived and designed the experiments: XL L. Wang WL YJ QC L. Wu. Contributed reagents/materials/analysis tools: XL L. Wu WL. Wrote the paper: XL L. Wu ZL XF.

References

1. Cheung F (2011) TCM: made in China. Nature 480: S82–S83.
2. Jiang W-Y (2005) Therapeutic wisdom in traditional Chinese medicine: a perspective from modern science. Trends in pharmacological sciences 26: 558–563.
3. Zimmermann GR, Lehar J, Keith CT (2007) Multi-target therapeutics: when the whole is greater than the sum of the parts. Drug Discov Today 12: 34–42.
4. Goh K-I, Cusick ME, Valle D, Childs B, Vidal M, et al. (2007) The human disease network. Proceedings of the National Academy of Sciences 104: 8685–8690.
5. Terzic A, Waldman S (2011) Chronic diseases: the emerging pandemic. Clin Transl Sci 4: 225–226.
6. Waldman SA, Terzic A (2011) Cardiovascular health: the global challenge. Clin Pharmacol Ther 90: 483–485.
7. Kitano H (2002) Systems biology: a brief overview. Science 295: 1662–1664.
8. Barabási A-L, Oltvai ZN (2004) Network biology: understanding the cell's functional organization. Nature Reviews Genetics 5: 101–113.
9. Hopkins AL (2007) Network pharmacology. Nature biotechnology 25: 1110–1110.
10. Hopkins AL (2008) Network pharmacology: the next paradigm in drug discovery. Nature chemical biology 4: 682–690.
11. Gardner TS, Di Bernardo D, Lorenz D, Collins JJ (2003) Inferring genetic networks and identifying compound mode of action via expression profiling. Science 301: 102–105.
12. di Bernardo D, Thompson MJ, Gardner TS, Chobot SE, Eastwood EL, et al. (2005) Chemogenomic profiling on a genome-wide scale using reverse-engineered gene networks. Nature biotechnology 23: 377–383.
13. Zhao S, Iyengar R (2012) Systems pharmacology: network analysis to identify multiscale mechanisms of drug action. Annual review of pharmacology and toxicology 52: 505–521.
14. Diez D, Wheelock ÅM, Goto S, Haeggström JZ, Paulsson-Berne G, et al. (2010) The use of network analyses for elucidating mechanisms in cardiovascular disease. Molecular BioSystems 6: 289–304.
15. Berger SI, Iyengar R (2009) Network analyses in systems pharmacology. Bioinformatics 25: 2466–2472.
16. Cline MS, Smoot M, Cerami E, Kuchinsky A, Landys N, et al. (2007) Integration of biological networks and gene expression data using Cytoscape. Nature protocols 2: 2366–2382.
17. Zhang L, Wang Y, Yu L, Liu L, Qu H, et al. (2010) QI-SHEN-YI-QI accelerates angiogenesis after myocardial infarction in rats. International journal of cardiology 143: 105–109.
18. Yunfei L, Haibin Q, Yiyu C (2008) Identification of major constituents in the traditional Chinese medicine QI-SHEN-YI-QI dropping pill by high-performance liquid chromatography coupled with diode array detection-electrospray ionization tandem mass spectrometry. Journal of pharmaceutical and biomedical analysis 47: 407–412.
19. Li Y, Wang Y, Qu H, Cheng Y (2008) Simultaneous determination of seven bioactive compounds in Chinese medicine "QI-SHEN-YI-QI" dropping pill by LC-UV and LC-ELSD. Chromatographia 67: 293–297.
20. Zhang Y, Shi P, Yao H, Shao Q, Fan X (2012) Metabolite Profiling and Pharmacokinetics of Herbal Compounds Following Oral Administration of a Cardiovascular Multi-herb Medicine (Qishen Yiqi Pills) in Rats. Current Drug Metabolism 13: 510–523.
21. Tao Y, Wang Y (2010) Bioactive sesquiterpenes isolated from the essential oil of *Dalbergia odorifera* T. Chen. Fitoterapia 81: 393–396.
22. Wu L, Li X, Yang J, Liu Y, Fan X, et al. (2013) CHD@ ZJU: a knowledgebase providing network-based research platform on coronary heart disease.Database: The Journal of Biological Databases and Curation 2013.
23. Pfeffer MA, Pfeffer JM, Fishbein MC, Fletcher PJ, Spadaro J, et al. (1979) Myocardial infarct size and ventricular function in rats. Circulation Research 44: 503–512.
24. Yamaguchi F, Sanbe A, Takeo S (1997) Cardiac sarcoplasmic reticular function in rats with chronic heart failure following myocardial infarction. Journal of molecular and cellular cardiology 29: 753–763.
25. Wang L, Li Z, Zhao X, Liu W, Liu Y, et al. (2013) A network study of Chinese medicine Xuesaitong Injection to elucidate a complex mode-of-action with multi-compound, multi-target and multi-pathway. Evidence-Based Complementary and Alternative Medicine 2013: Article ID 652373.
26. Zheng X, Zhao X, Wang S, Luo K, Wei Y, et al. (2007) Co-administration of Dalbergia odorifera Increased Bioavailability of Salvia miltiorrhizae in Rabbits. The American Journal of Chinese Medicine 35: 831–840.
27. Tong W, Cao X, Harris S, Sun H, Fang H, et al. (2003) ArrayTrack—supporting toxicogenomic research at the US Food and Drug Administration National Center for Toxicological Research. Environmental health perspectives 111: 1819.
28. Yaoita H, Ogawa K, Maehara K, Maruyama Y (2000) Apoptosis in relevant clinical situations contribution of apoptosis in myocardial infarction. Cardiovascular research 45: 630–641.
29. Palojoki E, Saraste A, Eriksson A, Pulkki K, Kallajoki M, et al. (2001) Cardiomyocyte apoptosis and ventricular remodeling after myocardial infarction in rats. American Journal of Physiology-Heart and Circulatory Physiology 280: H2726–H2731.
30. Crow MT, Mani K, Nam Y-J, Kitsis RN (2004) The mitochondrial death pathway and cardiac myocyte apoptosis. Circulation Research 95: 957–970.
31. Schwartz RS, Eltzschig HK, Carmeliet P (2011) Hypoxia and inflammation. New England Journal of Medicine 364: 656–665.
32. Chen G, Shaw MH, Kim Y-G, Nuñez G (2009) NOD-like receptors: role in innate immunity and inflammatory disease. Annual Review of Pathological Mechanical Disease 4: 365–398.
33. Fritz JH, Ferrero RL, Philpott DJ, Girardin SE (2006) Nod-like proteins in immunity, inflammation and disease. Nature immunology 7: 1250–1257.
34. Murphy GJ, Holder JC (2000) PPAR-gamma agonists: therapeutic role in diabetes, inflammation and cancer. Trends in pharmacological sciences 21: 469.
35. Wahli W, Michalik L (2012) PPARs at the crossroads of lipid signaling and inflammation. Trends in Endocrinology & Metabolism.
36. Finck BN (2007) The PPAR regulatory system in cardiac physiology and disease. Cardiovascular research 73: 269–277.
37. Chao W (2009) Toll-like receptor signaling: a critical modulator of cell survival and ischemic injury in the heart. American Journal of Physiology-Heart and Circulatory Physiology 296: H1–H12.
38. Timmers L, Sluijter JP, van Keulen JK, Hoefer IE, Nederhoff MG, et al. (2008) Toll-like receptor 4 mediates maladaptive left ventricular remodeling and impairs cardiac function after myocardial infarction. Circulation Research 102: 257–264.
39. Kaminska B (2005) MAPK signalling pathways as molecular targets for anti-inflammatory therapy–from molecular mechanisms to therapeutic benefits. Biochimica et biophysica acta 1754: 253.
40. Barber GN (2011) Innate immune DNA sensing pathways: STING, AIMII and the regulation of interferon production and inflammatory responses. Current opinion in immunology 23: 10–20.
41. Amara U, Rittirsch D, Flierl M, Bruckner U, Klos A, et al. (2008) Interaction between the coagulation and complement system. Current topics in complement II: Springer. pp. 68–76.
42. Markiewski MM, Nilsson B, Nilsson Ekdahl K, Mollnes TE, Lambris JD (2007) Complement and coagulation: strangers or partners in crime? Trends in immunology 28: 184–192.
43. Needleman P, Jakschik B, Morrison A, Lefkowith J (1986) Arachidonic acid metabolism. Annual review of biochemistry 55: 69–102.
44. Yan F, Liu Y, Liu Y, Zhao Y (2007) Effects of "Qishen Yiqi Droplet" on High Sensitivity C Reactive Protein in Experimenytal Atherosclerosis Rabbits. Shanghai Journal of Traditional Chinese Medicine 41: 59–60.
45. Liu M, Du W, Zhu M, Song Q, Wei Y, et al. (2009) Effect of QiShenYiQi dropping pills on TNF-alpha of AMI Rat. Li Shi Zhen Medicine and Materia Medica Research 20: 829–830.
46. Zhu M, Du W, Liu C, Zhang J, Feng L, et al. (2013) A dymatic mornitoring of effects of QiShenYiQi dripping pills on cardiac inflammation factors in AMI rat. Li Shi Zhen Medicine and Materia Medica Research 24: 22–25.
47. Chen T, Ma Z, Zhong Z, Sun G, Zhou Y, et al. (2011) Affect on heart function and serum cytokines in the patients after acute myocardial infarct treated with compound Qishenyiqi dripping pills. Jiangxi Medical Journal 46: 3.

48. Guan X, Deng B, Zhou X, Bao Y (2013) Effect of QiShenYiQi dripping pills on cardiac remodelling and inflammatory factors of chronic heart failure patients. 24: 2.
49. Wei W, Zhang W, Zhang T, Tian G, Meng Q, et al. (2009) Effect of "Qishen Yiqi Droplet" on Inflammatory Factors in Patients With Acute Coronary Syndrome After Percutaneous Coronary Intervention. Chinese Circulation Journal 24: 182–184.
50. Yamauchi T, Kamon J, Minokoshi Ya, Ito Y, Waki H, et al. (2002) Adiponectin stimulates glucose utilization and fatty-acid oxidation by activating AMP-activated protein kinase. Nature medicine 8: 1288–1295.
51. Wu G, Fang Y-Z, Yang S, Lupton JR, Turner ND (2004) Glutathione metabolism and its implications for health. The Journal of nutrition 134: 489–492.
52. Wozniak MA, Modzelewska K, Kwong L, Keely PJ (2004) Focal adhesion regulation of cell behavior. Biochimica et Biophysica Acta (BBA)-Molecular Cell Research 1692: 103–119.
53. Petit V, Thiery JP (2000) Focal adhesions: structure and dynamics. Biology of the Cell 92: 477–494.
54. Robinson ES, Khankin EV, Karumanchi SA, Humphreys BD, Hypertension induced by vascular endothelial growth factor signaling pathway inhibition: mechanisms and potential use as a biomarker. 2010. Elsevier. pp. 591–601.
55. Aramoto H, Breslin JW, Pappas PJ, Hobson RW, Durán WN (2004) Vascular endothelial growth factor stimulates differential signaling pathways in in vivo microcirculation. American Journal of Physiology-Heart and Circulatory Physiology 287: H1590–H1598.
56. Olsson A-K, Dimberg A, Kreuger J, Claesson-Welsh L (2006) VEGF receptor signalling? In control of vascular function. Nature Reviews Molecular Cell Biology 7: 359–371.
57. Suefuji H, Ogawa H, Yasue H, Kaikita K, Soejima H, et al. (1997) Increased plasma tissue factor levels in acute myocardial infarction. American heart journal 134: 253–259.
58. KIEFER FN, BERNS H, RESINK TJ, BATTEGAY EJ (2002) Hypoxia enhances vascular cell proliferation and angiogenesis in vitro via rapamycin (mTOR)-dependent signaling. The FASEB Journal 16: 771–780.
59. Laplante M, Sabatini DM (2009) mTOR signaling at a glance. Journal of cell science 122: 3589–3594.
60. Hirota SA, Beck PL, MacDonald JA (2009) Targeting hypoxia-inducible factor-1 (HIF-1) signaling in therapeutics: implications for the treatment of inflammatory bowel disease. Recent patents on inflammation & allergy drug discovery 3: 1–16.
61. Suh S-J, Chung T-W, Son M-J, Kim S-H, Moon TC, et al. (2006) The naturally occurring biflavonoid, ochnaflavone, inhibits LPS-induced iNOS expression, which is mediated by ERK1/2 via NF-κB regulation, in RAW264.7 cells. Archives of Biochemistry and Biophysics 447: 136–146.
62. Tang S, Shen X-Y, Huang H-Q, Xu S-W, Yu Y, et al. (2011) Cryptotanshinone suppressed inflammatory cytokines secretion in RAW264. 7 macrophages through inhibition of the NF-κB and MAPK signaling pathways. Inflammation 34: 111–118.
63. Hong SC, Jeong JB, Koo JS (2012) Inhibitory effect of essential oil from Agastache rugosa against nitric oxide (NO) production induced by inducible nitric oxide synthase (iNOS) over-expression through NF-κB and mitogen-activated protein kinase (MAPK) activation in lipopolysaccharide (LPS)-stimulated RAW264.7 cells. Journal of Medicinal Plants Research 6: 4494–4500.
64. Lee M-Y, Yuk J-E, Kwon O-K, Oh S-R, Lee H-K, et al. (2012) Zuonin B inhibits lipopolysaccharide-induced inflammation via downregulation of the ERK1/2 and JNK pathways in RAW264. 7 macrophages. Evidence-Based Complementary and Alternative Medicine 2012.
65. Jeong JB, Shin YK, Lee S-H (2013) Anti-inflammatory activity of patchouli alcohol in RAW264. 7 and HT-29 cells. Food and Chemical Toxicology 55: 229–233.
66. Martin H (2009) Role of PPAR-gamma in inflammation. Prospects for therapeutic intervention by food components. Mutation Research/Fundamental and Molecular Mechanisms of Mutagenesis 669: 1–7.
67. Campbell I (2005) The clinical significance of PPAR gamma agonism. Current molecular medicine 5: 349–363.
68. Jiang C, Ting AT, Seed B (1998) PPAR-γ agonists inhibit production of monocyte inflammatory cytokines. Nature 391: 82–86.
69. Miksa M, Wu R, Cui X, Dong W, Das P, et al. (2007) Vasoactive hormone adrenomedullin and its binding protein: anti-inflammatory effects by up-regulating peroxisome proliferator-activated receptor-γ. The Journal of Immunology 179: 6263–6272.
70. Ji H, Wang H, Zhang F, Li X, Xiang L, et al. (2010) PPARγ agonist pioglitazone inhibits microglia inflammation by blocking p38 mitogen-activated protein kinase signaling pathways. Inflammation Research 59: 921–929.
71. Xing B, Xin T, Hunter RL, Bing G (2008) Pioglitazone inhibition of lipopolysaccharide-induced nitric oxide synthase is associated with altered activity of p38 MAP kinase and PI3K/Akt. J Neuroinflammation 5: 1–11.
72. Burns KA, Vanden Heuvel JP (2007) Modulation of PPAR activity via phosphorylation. Biochimica et Biophysica Acta (BBA)-Molecular and Cell Biology of Lipids 1771: 952–960.
73. Adams M, Reginato MJ, Shao D, Lazar MA, Chatterjee VK (1997) Transcriptional activation by peroxisome proliferator-activated receptor γ is inhibited by phosphorylation at a consensus mitogen-activated protein kinase site. Journal of Biological Chemistry 272: 5128–5132.
74. ZAYTSEVA YY, WALLIS NK, SOUTHARD RC, KILGORE MW (2011) The PPARγ antagonist T0070907 suppresses breast cancer cell proliferation and motility via both PPARγ-dependent and-independent mechanisms. Anticancer research 31: 813–823.
75. Abraham NG, Kappas A (2008) Pharmacological and clinical aspects of heme oxygenase. Pharmacological Reviews 60: 79–127.
76. Kim B-C, Choi J-W, Hong H-Y, Lee S, Hong S, et al. (2006) Heme oxygenase-1 mediates the anti-inflammatory effect of mushroom *Phellinus linteus* in LPS-stimulated RAW264. 7 macrophages. Journal of ethnopharmacology 106: 364–371.
77. Lin H-Y, Juan S-H, Shen S-C, Hsu F-L, Chen Y-C (2003) Inhibition of lipopolysaccharide-induced nitric oxide production by flavonoids in RAW264. 7 macrophages involves heme oxygenase-1. Biochemical pharmacology 66: 1821–1832.
78. Krönke G, Kadl A, Ikonomu E, Blüml S, Fürnkranz A, et al. (2007) Expression of heme oxygenase-1 in human vascular cells is regulated by peroxisome proliferator-activated receptors. Arteriosclerosis, thrombosis, and vascular biology 27: 1276–1282.
79. von Knethen A, Neb H, Morbitzer V, Schmidt MV, Kuhn A-M, et al. (2011) PPARγ stabilizes HO-1 mRNA in monocytes/macrophages which affects IFN-β expression. Free Radical Biology and Medicine 51: 396–405.
80. Otterbein LE, Soares MP, Yamashita K, Bach FH (2003) Heme oxygenase-1: unleashing the protective properties of heme. Trends in immunology 24: 449–455.
81. Sawle P, Foresti R, Mann BE, Johnson TR, Green CJ, et al. (2005) Carbon monoxide-releasing molecules (CO-RMs) attenuate the inflammatory response elicited by lipopolysaccharide in RAW264. 7 murine macrophages. British journal of pharmacology 145: 800–810.

A Systems Biology-Based Approach to Uncovering the Molecular Mechanisms Underlying the Effects of Dragon's Blood Tablet in Colitis, Involving the Integration of Chemical Analysis, ADME Prediction, and Network Pharmacology

Haiyu Xu[1,2⁋], Yanqiong Zhang[1⁋], Yun Lei[1,3⁋], Xiumei Gao[1,4], Huaqiang Zhai[3], Na Lin[1], Shihuan Tang[1], Rixin Liang[1], Yan Ma[1], Defeng Li[1], Yi Zhang[1], Guangrong Zhu[5], Hongjun Yang[1]*, Luqi Huang[2]*

1 Institute of Chinese Materia Medica, China Academy of Chinese Medical Sciences, Beijing, P.R. China, **2** National resource center for Chinese Materia Medica, China Academy of Chinese Medical Sciences, Beijing, P.R. China, **3** Beijing University of Chinese Medicine, Beijing, P.R. China, **4** Tianjin University of Traditional Chinese Medicine, Tianjin, P.R. China, **5** Yunnan Datang Hanfang Pharmacy co.ltd, Yunnan, P.R. China

Abstract

Traditional Chinese medicine (TCM) is one of the oldest East Asian medical systems. The present study adopted a systems biology-based approach to provide new insights relating to the active constituents and molecular mechanisms underlying the effects of dragon's blood (DB) tablets for the treatment of colitis. This study integrated chemical analysis, prediction of absorption, distribution, metabolism, and excretion (ADME), and network pharmacology. Firstly, a rapid, reliable, and accurate ultra-performance liquid chromatography-electrospray ionization-tandem mass spectrometry method was employed to identify 48 components of DB tablets. *In silico* prediction of the passive absorption of these compounds, based on Caco-2 cell permeability, and their P450 metabolism enabled the identification of 22 potentially absorbed components and 8 metabolites. Finally, networks were constructed to analyze interactions between these DB components/metabolites absorbed and their putative targets, and between the putative DB targets and known therapeutic targets for colitis. This study provided a great opportunity to deepen the understanding of the complex pharmacological mechanisms underlying the effects of DB in colitis treatment.

Editor: Jan P. A. Baak, Stavanger University Hospital, Norway

Funding: Financial support was provided by Key Projects in the National Science & Technology Pillar Program during the 11th Five-Year Plan Period (No. 2008BAI51B03), the National Natural Science Foundation of China (No. 81202793), Beijing Joint Project Specific Funds and independent topics supported by Operational expenses for basic research of China Academy of Chinese Medical Sciences (No. Z02063), Beijing Joint Project Specific Funds and the Fundamental Research Funds for the Central public welfare research institutes (Nos. ZZ070819, ZZ070831 and ZZ070830). Support was also provided in the form of salary for Guangrong Zhu as an employee at Datang Hanfang Pharmacy co.ltd. The funders had no role in study design, data collection and analysis, decision to publish, or preparation of the manuscript.

Competing Interests: Guangrong Zhu is an employee of Datang Hanfang Pharmacy co.ltd, and received funding in the form of salary. This does not alter the authors' adherence to all the PLoS ONE policies on sharing data and materials.

* Email: hongjun0420@vip.sina.com (HY); huangluqi@263.net (LH)

⁋ These authors contributed equally to this work.

Introduction

Traditional Chinese medicine (TCM) is one of the oldest medical systems of health care, and it has been used in East Asian countries such as China, Japan, and Korea for thousands of years [1,2]. However, acceptance of traditional Chinese medicines within Western biomedical practice has been restricted by a lack of knowledge of the active compounds involved, and their therapeutic mechanisms of action [3]. TCM is characterized by the usage of multi-component, multi-target agents that collectively modulate molecular networks. Recently, network pharmacology has provided a means to improve understanding of the molecular mechanisms underlying the therapeutic effects of traditional Chinese medicines [3–5]. TCM chemical databases such as TCM Database@Taiwan [6] and HerbBioMap database [7] and some literature generally provide the main sources of information on the chemical profiles of traditional Chinese medicines. However, these are not always accurate because the chemical profiles of traditional Chinese medicines can vary significantly, depending on the geographical origin of the materials used, the harvest time, pretreatments, and manufacturing processes employed. In addition, most TCM formulations are taken orally, estimation of intestinal absorption and cytochrome P450 metabolism provide more in-depth insights into their therapeutic

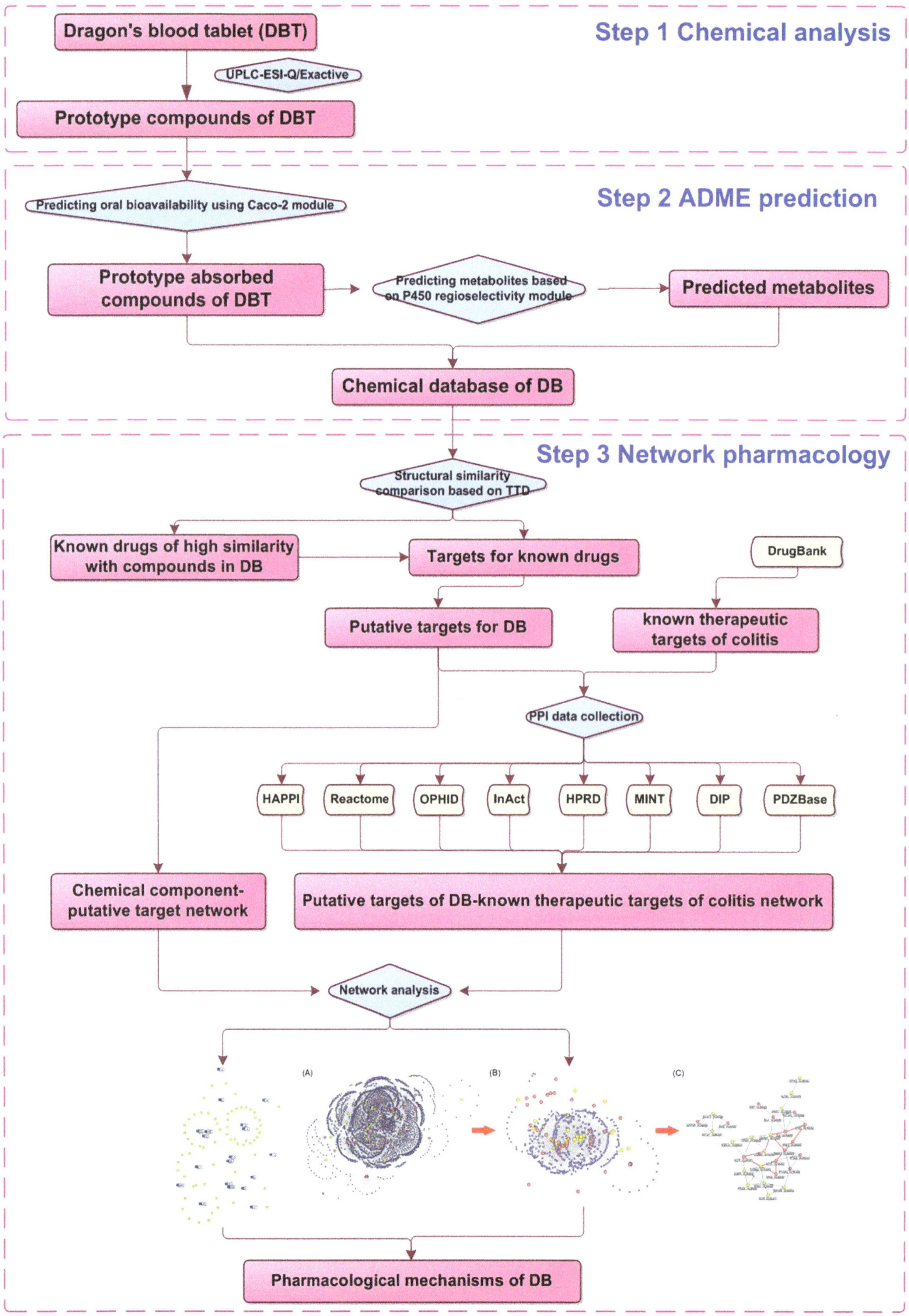
Step 1 Chemical analysis
Dragon's blood tablet (DBT)
UPLC-ESI-Q/Exactive
Prototype compounds of DBT
Step 2 ADME prediction
Predicting oral bioavailability using Caco-2 module
Prototype absorbed compounds of DBT
Predicting metabolites based on P450 regioselectivity module
Predicted metabolites
Chemical database of DB
Step 3 Network pharmacology
Structural similarity comparison based on TTD
Known drugs of high similarity with compounds in DB
Targets for known drugs
DrugBank
Putative targets for DB
known therapeutic targets of colitis
PPI data collection
HAPPI
Reactome
OPHID
InAct
HPRD
MINT
DIP
PDZBase
Chemical component-putative target network
Putative targets of DB-known therapeutic targets of colitis network
Network analysis
(A)
(B)
(C)
Pharmacological mechanisms of DB

Figure 1. A schematic diagram of this systems biology-based investigation into the molecular mechanisms of DB tablet for colitis by integrating chemical analysis, ADME prediction and network pharmacology.

mechanisms [8,9]. However, experimental determination using these systems can be costly and time-consuming. To obtain a rapid estimation of human absorption and metabolism, high throughput screening methods using Caco-2 cell monolayers and P450 enzymes provide the most advanced *in vitro* approaches to assessing new chemical entities [10–12]. Thus, the development of rapid high-throughput approaches to studying TCM compositions and mechanisms, combining chemical analysis, prediction of absorption, distribution, metabolism, and excretion (ADME), and network pharmacology is required.

According to the Pharmacopoeia of the People's Republic of China, commercially available longxuejie or dragon's blood (DB) includes plant resins from four species; *Dracaena* spp., *Daemonorops* spp., *Croton* spp., and *Pterocarpus* spp., and has long been used as an ethnomedicine in China to invigorate blood circulation in the treatment of traumatic injuries, blood stasis, and pain [13,14]. DB has also been used to treat chronic colitis in recent decades and many clinical studies have reported good therapeutic effects [15–17]. Chemically, flavonoids, phenols, steroides, and terpenoids have been identified as the main constituents of DB [18–22]. Some analytical methods have been developed to identify and characterize DB composition and assess its quality [23–25]. Pharmacologic studies of these components have identified a wide variety of actions, including anti-inflammatory, antiulcer, antimicrobial, hemostatic, and analgesic activities, which could contribute to their efficacy in the treatment of chronic colitis [26–28]. However, the precise active constituents of DB that have benefits in chronic colitis, and their molecular mechanisms of action, are still unclear. In particular, the lack of elucidation of the ingredient-target network has hindered understanding of the molecular mechanisms of DB in chronic colitis treatment.

The present study employed high-throughput analysis, *in silico* ADME models, and a network pharmacology technique to investigate the active constituents of DB and their actions on molecular networks in chronic colitis, as shown in **Figure 1**.

Materials and Methods

1. Reagents and chemicals

High performance liquid chromatography (HPLC)-grade acetonitrile, formic acid, and methanol were obtained from Merck (Darmstadt, Germany). Water was purified using a Milli-Q system (Millipore, Billerica, MA, USA). 7,4′-Dihydroxyflavan, loureirin A, loureirin B, dracaenin A and pterostilbene standards were purchased from the National Institute for the Control of Pharmaceutical and Biological Products (Beijing, China). The purities of all standards were no less than 98% and suitable for liquid chromatography-tandem mass spectrometry (LC-MS/MS) analysis. DB enteric-coated tablets were supplied from Yunnan Datang Hanfang Pharmaceutical Co. Ltd. (Yunnan, China).

2. Preparation of samples and standard solution

Six different batches of DB enteric-coated tablets were pulverized with a 60 mesh, respectively. Each sample of this powder (0.1 g) was weighed precisely and ultrasonically extracted in 10 ml methanol for 20 min at room temperature. The solution was centrifuged at 12000 rpm for 10 min, and then filtered through 0.22 μm nylon membrane filters. The filtrate was analyzed directly by UPLC-ESI-MS/MS, as described in section 2.3. At the same time, a stock solution containing five standards (7,4′-dihydroxyflavan, loureirin A, loureirin B, pterostilbene, and dracaenin A) was prepared in methanol. All solutions were stored at 4°C prior to analysis.

3. Instrument and UPLC-ESI-MS/MS conditions

UPLC was performed on a Dionex UltiMate 3000 system (Dionex Corporation, Sunnyvale, USA) equipped with a quaternary pump, an online vacuum degasser, an autosampler, and an automatic thermostatic column oven. A Thermo Hyper Gold C18 column was used (100×2.1 mm, 1.9 μm) at 30°C with a flow rate of 0.4 ml/min and an injection volume of 5 μl. The mobile phase was a mixture of 0.1% formic acid in water (A) and acetonitrile (B). The mobile phase gradient program was 5% B, 0–3 min; 5–95% B, 3–20 min; 95% B, 20–25 min. High-resolution accurate-mass full scan LC-MS and LC-MS/MS analyses were performed using Thermo Q-Exactive (Thermo Fisher Scientific, Bremen, Germany). Full scans were acquired in the mass analyzer at 100–1500 m/z with a resolution of 70000 in both positive and negative ion modes, and MS/MS scans were obtained with a resolution of 17500 using a normalized collision energy of 30% for high-energy collisional dissociation fragmentation. Based on the best response for most compounds, the final parameters were set as follows: spray voltage, 3.2 kV in the positive mode and 3.0 kV in the negative mode; capillary temperature, 350°C; sheath gas pressure, 35 arbitrary units; auxiliary gas pressure, 10 arbitrary units; and heater temperature, 300°C. Xcalibur 2.2 software (Thermo Fisher Scientific) was used for data acquisition.

4. Prediction of absorbed constituents and their metabolites using in silico ADME models

Structural information (*.mol or *.sdf files) relating to the DB components(identified by UPLC-ESI-MS/MS) were downloaded from ChemSpider (http://www.chemspider.com/). ADME evaluation of these constituents was carried out using ACD/Percepta software 5.07 (ACD/Labs, Toronto, Canada), including the passive intestinal permeability of Caco-2 module and the P450 regioselectivity module to predict their oral bioavailability. The apparent permeability coefficient (Papp) of one constituent was greater than 9.0×10^{6} cm/s, which indicated good absorption characteristics. The score and the reliability of metabolic reaction were set at greater than 0.6 and 0.5, respectively, in order to increase prediction credibility.

5. Known therapeutic targets for colitis treatment

Known therapeutic targets were obtained from the DrugBank database [29] (http://www.drugbank.ca/, version: 3.0). We only included drug-target interactions where the drugs were approved by the Food and Drug Administration, USA (FDA) for the treatment of colitis, with human gene/protein targets. To facilitate data analysis, all protein identification codes were converted to a common UniProtKB-Swiss-Prot code, and detailed target information is provided in the supplementary **Table S1.**

6. PPI data collection

PPI data were imported from eight existing PPI databases, including the Human Annotated and Predicted Protein Interaction Database (HAPPI) [30], Reactome [31], Online Predicted Human Interaction Database (OPHID) [32], InAct [33], Human Protein Reference Database (HPRD) [34], Molecular Interaction

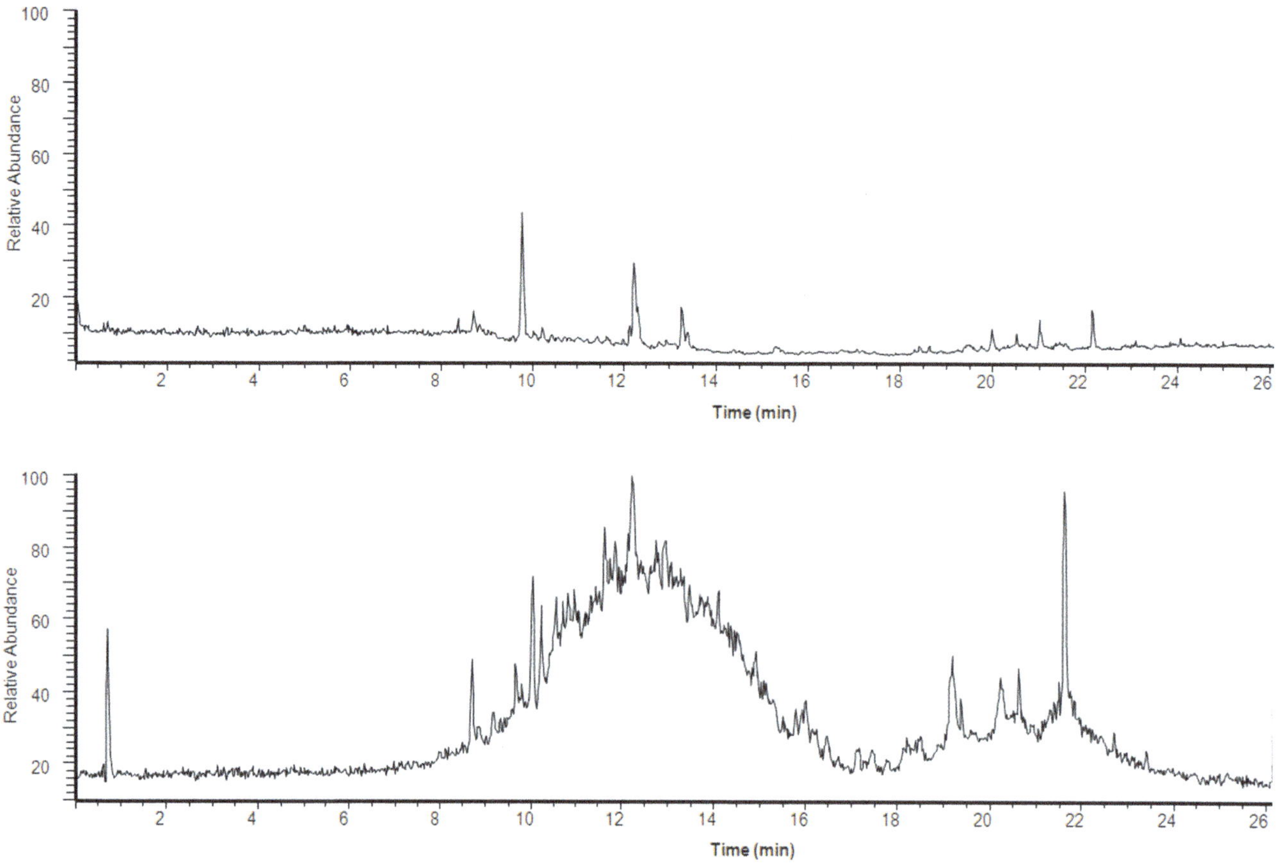

Figure 2. UPLC-ESI-MS/MS of DB in positive ion mode (A) and negative ion mode (B).

Database (MINT) [35], Database of Interacting Proteins (DIP) [36], and PDZBase [37]. Detailed information on these PPI databases is provided in the supplementary **Table S2**.

7. Pharmacological mechanism analysis

7.1. Prediction of putative DB targets. As described in our previous study [38], we used the Drug Similarity Search tool in the Therapeutic Targets Database [39] (TTD, http://xin.cz3.nus.edu.sg/group/cjttd/ttd.asp, Version 4.3.02, released on Aug 25th 2011) to screen drugs similar to DB via structural similarity comparisons. We only selected drugs with a high structural similarity score (>0.85, similar to very similar) with the potentially absorbed DB constituents and their metabolites. The therapeutic targets of these similar drugs were also included as putative DB targets.

7.2. Network construction and analysis. The absorbed DB components and their metabolites, their putative targets, and known therapeutic targets for colitis treatment were used to construct a chemical component-putative target network, and a putative DB targets-known colitis therapeutic targets PPI network, respectively. PPI data were obtained from eight existing PPI databases, as described in section 2.6. Navigator software (Version 2.2.1) and Cytoscape (Version 2.8.1) were utilized to visualize the networks.

For each node "i" in these two networks, we defined four measures of topology: (1) "degree," defined as the number of links to node i; (2) "betweenness," defined as the capacity of node i to be located in the shortest communication paths between different pairs of nodes in the network [40]. The betweenness centrality of node i is computed as following formula:

$$B(i)=\frac{(\sum_{s\neq i\neq t}(\sigma_{st}(i)/\sigma_{st}))}{((N-1)(N-2)/2)}$$

where σ_{st} denotes the number of the shortest paths between node s and node t in the PPI network, $\sigma_{st}(i)$ denotes the number of the shortest paths across node i between node s and node t, and N is the total number of nodes in the PPI network. This property correlates more closely with essentiality than connectivity, exposing critical nodes that usually belong to the group of scaffold proteins or proteins involved in crosstalk between signal pathways (called bottlenecks) [41]. (3) "closeness," defined as the inverse of the sum of node i distances to all other nodes. Closeness can be regarded as a measure of how long it would take to spread information from node i to all other nodes sequentially. Degree, betweenness and closeness centralities correlate with a protein's topological importance in the PPI network [40]. (4) K-core analysis is an iterative process in which nodes were removed from the network in order of the least-connected [42]. The core of maximum order is defined as the main (highest) k-core in the network. A k-core sub-network of the original network can be generated by recursively deleting vertices from the network whose degree is less than k. This results in a series of sub-networks that gradually reveal the globally central region of the original network. On this basis, "k value" is used to measure the centrality of node i.

Table 1. MS data of ESI-MS spectra and identification of the Longxuejie enteric-coated tablet.

No.	RT (Measured)	m/z (Measured)	m/z (Expected)	m/z (Delta, ppm)	polarity	Formula	Compound Name	Papp (10^{-6} cm/s)
1	8.11	311.11395	311.11363	1.046	negative	$C_{15}H_{20}O_7$	3,4-dihydroxyallylbenzene 4-O—D-Glucopyranoside	3.8494
2	8.38	285.07592	285.07575	0.594	positive	$C_{16}H_{12}O_5$	unknown	—
		283.06137	283.0612	0.606	negative			
3	8.68	229.08608	229.08592	0.702	positive	$C_{14}H_{12}O_3$	3,5,4′-trihydroxystilbene	148.9186
		227.07154	227.07137	0.752	negative			
4	8.68	273.07713	273.07685	1.054	negative	$C_{15}H_{14}O_5$	4′-methoxy-3′7-dihydroxyflavan	115.6472
5	8.72	255.06525	255.06519	0.241	positive	$C_{15}H_{10}O_4$	7,4′-dihydroxyflavan	137.4393
		253.05074	253.05063	0.408	negative			
6	8.74	259.09663	259.09649	0.563	positive	$C_{15}H_{14}O_4$	2,4,4′-Trihydroxydihydrochalcone	94.5322
		257.08211	257.08193	0.707	negative			
7	8.83	314.13891	314.13868	0.703	positive	$C_{18}H_{19}NO_4$	norisoboldine	30.448
		312.12448	312.12413	1.11	negative			
8	9.27	149.06084	149.0608	0.219	negative	$C_9H_{10}O_2$	unknown	—
9	9.66	269.08209	269.08193	0.594	negative	$C_{16}H_{14}O_4$	unknown	—
10	9.78	525.19107	525.19078	0.558	positive	$C_{32}H_{28}O_7$	dracaenin A	134.7937
		523.1766	523.17623	0.709	negative			
11	10.02	273.11223	273.11214	0.359	positive	$C_{16}H_{16}O_4$	unknown	—
		271.09769	271.09758	0.385	negative			
12	10.21	303.1228	303.1227	0.339	positive	$C_{17}H_{18}O_5$	unknown	—
		301.10831	301.10815	0.531	negative			
13	10.21	392.20704	392.20676	0.696	positive	$C_{21}H_{26}O_6$	3,4-O-dimethylcedrusin	149.4172
14	10.21	167.0704	167.07027	0.788	positive	$C_9H_{10}O_3$	Ethyl 4-hydroxybenzoate	216.6625
15	10.57	287.09152	287.0914	0.414	positive	$C_{16}H_{14}O_5$	unknown	—
		285.07703	285.07685	0.638	negative			
16	10.73	532.23343	532.23298	0.849	positive	$C_{31}H_{30}O_7$	cochinchinenin	21.059
		513.19218	513.19188	0.587	negative			
17	10.95	301.10837	301.10815	0.733	negative	$C_{17}H_{18}O_5$	unknown	—
18	11.2	241.08608	241.08592	0.665	positive	$C_{15}H_{12}O_3$	(2S)-7-hydroxyflavanone	227.3156
		239.07151	239.07137	0.616	negative			
19	11.45	199.07646	199.07645	0.057	negative	$C_{13}H_{12}O_2$	4,4′-Dihydroxydiphenylmethane	201.7499
20	11.64	529.22251	529.22208	0.817	positive	$C_{32}H_{32}O_7$	unknown	—
		527.20758	527.20753	0.102	negative			
21	11.65	511.21352	511.21261	1.776	negative	$C_{32}H_{32}O_6$	homoisosocotrin-4-ol	17.1673
22	11.86	283.09773	283.09758	0.507	negative	$C_{17}H_{16}O_4$	unknown	—
23	12	516.23823	516.23806	0.321	positive	$C_{31}H_{30}O_6$	socotrin 4-ol	7.5670
24	12.13	287.12781	287.12779	0.077	positive	$C_{17}H_{18}O_4$	Loureirin A	228.3831

Table 1. Cont.

No.	RT (Measured)	m/z (Measured)	m/z (Expected)	m/z (Delta, ppm)	polarity	Formula	Compound Name	Papp (10^{-6} cm/s)
		285.11337	285.11323	0.492	negative			
25	12.13	151.07542	151.07536	0.442	positive	$C_9H_{10}O_2$	3,4-Dihydroxy-allylbenzene	140.4007
26	12.23	227.10674	227.10666	0.351	positive	$C_{15}H_{14}O_2$	7-hydroxyflavanone	227.3156
27	12.23	317.13839	317.13835	0.136	positive	$C_{18}H_{20}O_5$	Loureirin B	227.8266
		315.12406	315.1238	0.833	negative			
28	12.93	257.11728	257.11722	0.227	positive	$C_{16}H_{16}O_3$	pterostilbene	236.2931
		255.10277	255.10267	0.396	negative			
29	13	885.45033	885.44894	1.572	negative	$C_{44}H_{70}O_{18}$	26-O—D-Glucopynanosyl-furostan-5,25(27)-diene-1,3,22,26-tetrol-1-O-[-L-rhamnopyranosyl(12)]—L-Arabinopyranoside	0.0073
30	13.25	167.0704	167.07027	0.799	positive	$C_9H_{10}O_3$	unknown	—
31	14.08	265.14798			negative		unknown	—
32	14.39	462.32139	462.3214	−0.029	positive	$C_{27}H_{40}O_5$	dracaenol B	141.9713
33	14.90	571.23383			negative		unknown	—
34	14.91	527.24323	527.24282	0.786	positive	$C_{33}H_{34}O_6$	cochinchinenin E	8.2809
35	15.77	532.92554			negative		unknown	—
36	15.92	325.18451	325.18569	−3.642	negative	$C_{14}H_{29}O_8$	unknown	—
37	16.27	415.32104	415.32067	0.894	positive	$C_{27}H_{42}O_3$	Diosgenin	112.3202
38	16.44	325.18448	325.18569	−3.734	negative	$C_{14}H_{29}O_8$	unknown	—
39	17.44	339.20010	339.20134	−3.668	negative	$C_{15}H_{31}O_8$	unknown	—
40	19.18	698.91071			negative		unknown	—
41	19.95	323.25817	323.25807	0.292	positive	$C_{20}H_{34}O_3$	bincatriol	172.7858
42	20.25	445.29987			negative		unknown	—
43	20.49	628.19489			positive		unknown	—
44	20.63	383.18988	383.19117	−4.807	negative	$C_{16}H_{31}O_{10}$	unknown	—
45	21	461.32938			positive		unknown	—
46	21.6	116.92857			negative		unknown	—
47	22.14	394.3465	394.34415	4.577	Positive	$C_{25}H_{46}O_3$	unknown	—
48	24.99	427.3939	427.39344	1.082	positive	$C_{30}H_{50}O$	lupeol	0.0386

Papp: apparent permeability coefficient at the indicated concentrations in the basolateral-to-apical (B-A) direction across a Caco-2 cell monolayer.

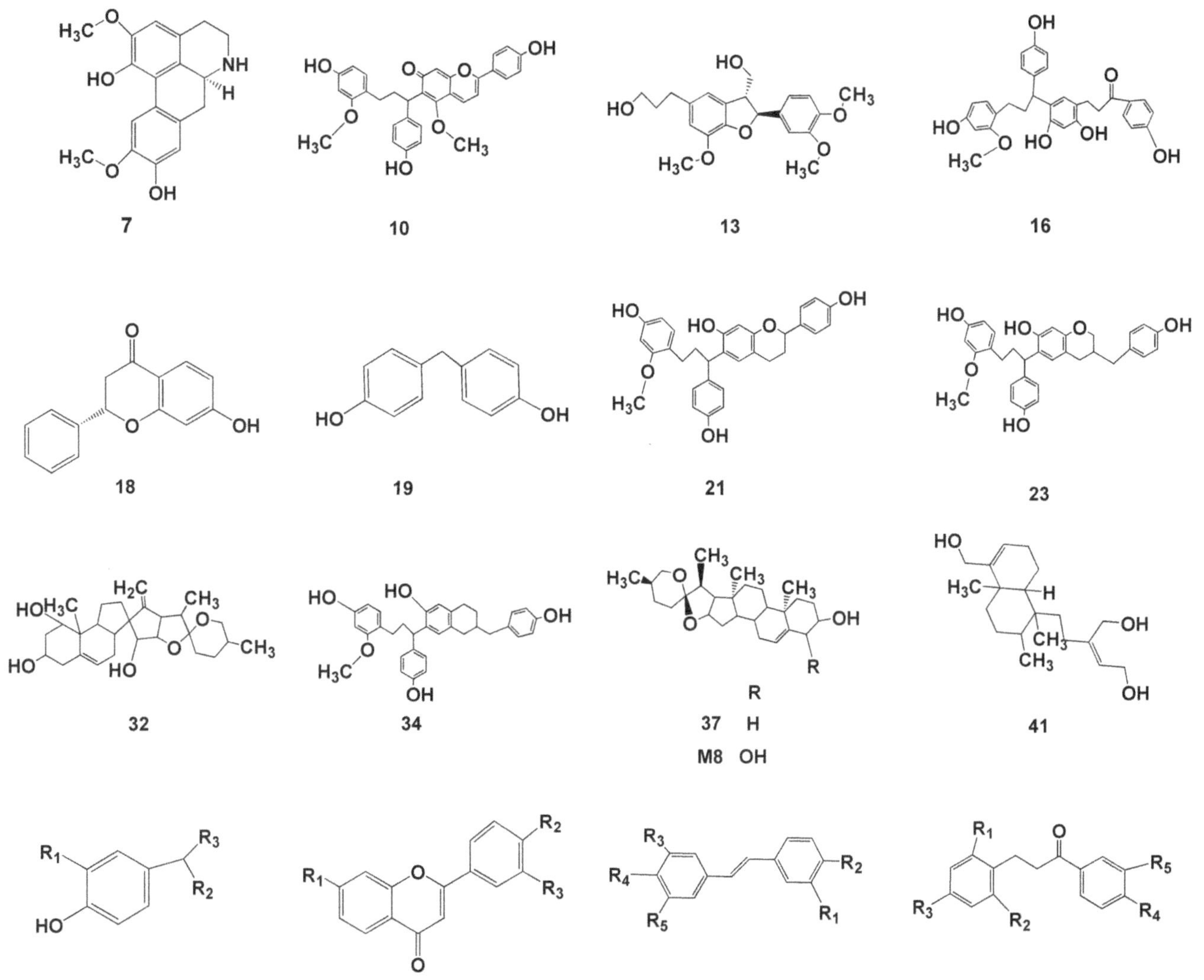

	R_1	R_2	R_3
25	OH	H	CH=CH2
M5	OH	OH	CH=CH2
14	H	H	O-C2H5

	R1	R2	R3
4	OH	OCH3	OH
5	OH	OH	H
26	OH	H	H
M3	H	OH	OH
M4	OH	OH	OH

	R1	R2	R3	R4	R5
3	H	OH	OH	H	OH
28	H	OH	OCH3	H	OCH3
M1	OH	OH	OH	H	OH
M2	H	OH	OH	OH	OH
M7	OH	OH	OCH3	H	OCH3

	R1	R2	R3	R4	R5
6	OH	H	OH	OH	H
24	OCH3	H	OCH3	OH	H
M6	OCH3	OCH3	OCH3	OH	OH
27	OCH3	OCH3	OCH3	OH	H

Figure 3. The structures of the 20 potentially absorbed DB constituents and 8 metabolites. **3.** 3,5,4′-trihydroxystilbene; **4.** 4′-methoxy-3′7-dihydroxyflavan; **5.** 7,4′-dihydroxyflavan; **6.** 2,4,4′-trihydroxydihydrochalcone; **7.** norisoboldine; **10.** dracaenin A; **13.** 3,4-*o*-dimethylcedrusin; **14.** ethyl 4-hydroxybenzoate; **16.** cochinchinenin; **18.** (2*S*)-7-hydroxyflavanone; **19.** 4,4′-dihydroxydiphenylmethane; **21.** homoisosocotrin-4-ol; **24.** loureirin A; **25.** 3,4-dihydroxy-allylbenzene; **26.** 7-hydroxyflavanone; **27.** loureirin B; **28.** pterostilbene; **32.** dracaenol B; **34.** cochinchinenin E; **37.** diosgenin; **41.** bincatriol. M1 and M2 were metabolites of compound **3**; M3, M4, M5, M6, M7, and M8 were metabolites of compounds **4**, **5**, **25**, **27**, **28**, and **37**, respectively.

7.3 Pathway enrichment analysis for the major putative DB targets and the major known therapeutic targets for colitis. We performed pathway enrichment analysis using pathway data obtained from the FTP service of KEGG [43] (Kyoto Encyclopedia of Genes and Genomes, http://www.genome.jp/kegg/, Last updated: Oct 16, 2012).

Results and Discussion

1. Optimization of UPLC-ESI-MS/MS conditions

To obtain reliable chromatographic results and appropriate ionization, four mobile phase systems of acetonitrile-water, methanol-water, acetonitrile-acid aqueous solution, and methanol-acid aqueous solution were tested and compared. The results suggested that acetonitrile-formic acid aqueous solution was superior to the others. Different concentration of formic acid aqueous solution (0.05%, 0.1%, and 0.5%) were investigated,

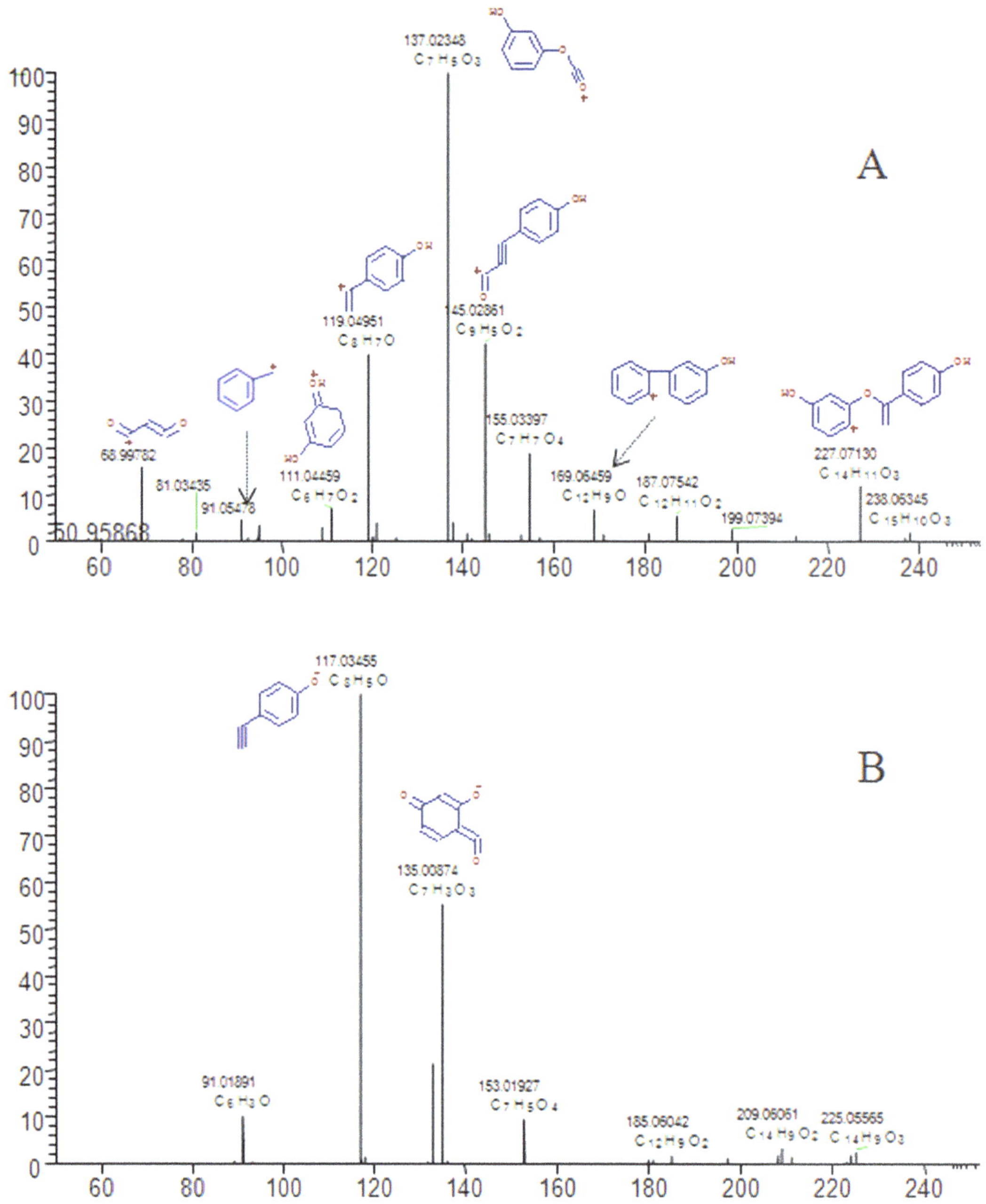

Figure 4. The MS/MS spectrum and possible fragmentation pathways of 7,4′-dihydroxyflavan.

indicating that use of 0.1% formic acid aqueous solution produced the optimal peak shape and reduced peak tailing, as well as increasing ion response for most compounds. Meanwhile, the process of gradient elution was optimized to obtain better separation over shorter time periods. The MS parameters were optimized to improve ion intensity. These optimized parameters were described in section 2.3. Base peak chromatograms of DB in positive and negative ion modes are shown in **Figure 2**.

2. Screening and identification of DB using UPLC-ESI-MS/MS

Recently, the UPLC-Q-Exactive system was reported to provide a rapid, reliable and accurate technique for identification of herbal constitutions, because of its separation efficiency, high resolution and high mass accuracy [44–46]. In the present study, a total of 48 components of DB were identified. These were mainly flavonoids, such as flavones, flavonols, flavanones, chalcones, and isoflavones, as listed in **Table 1**. For some compounds (7,4′-dihydroxyflavan, loureirin A, loureirin B, pterostilbene, and dracaenin A), purified standards were available and these were identified by comparing sample retention time and accurate mass with that of the standard. For compounds where standards were unavailable, identification was based on accurate mass and tandem mass spectra. The molecular formula was established by high-accuracy quasi-molecular ion such as $[M-H]^-$, $[M+CH_3COO]^-$, $[M+H]^+$, and $[M+Na]^+$ within a mass error of 5.0 ppm and fractional isotope abundance. The most rational molecular formula was identified using chemical or herbal databases, such as Chemspider (www.

Table 2. Prediction of the score, reliability, reaction site and reaction type of excellent oral absorbed constituents of LXJ by the P450 regioselectivity module in ACD/Percepta, respectively.

No.	Compound No	Compound name	Score	Reliability	Reaction site	Reaction type	Metabolizing enzymes
M1	3	3,5,4'-trihydroxyStilbene	0.94	0.86	3	Aromatic Hydroxylation	CYP1A2
			0.94	0.86	7	Aromatic Hydroxylation	CYP1A2
M2	3	3,5,4'-trihydroxyStilbene	0.65	0.87	14	Aromatic Hydroxylation	CYP1A2
M3	4	4'-methoxy-3'7-dihydroxyflavan	0.92	0.78	21	O-dealkylation	CYP1A2
M4	5	7,4'-Dihydroxyflavan	0.92	0.79	13	Aromatic Hydroxylation	CYP1A2
			0.92	0.79	15	Aromatic Hydroxylation	CYP1A2
M5	25	3,4-Dihydroxy-allylbenzene	0.85	0.74	4	Aliphatic Hydroxylation	CYP2C19
			0.91	0.86	4	Aliphatic Hydroxylation	CYP2C9
M6	27	Loureirin B	0.74	0.5	18	Aromatic Hydroxylation	CYP1A2
			0.74	0.5	19	Aromatic Hydroxylation	CYP1A2
M7	28	pterostilbene	0.90	0.74	10	Aromatic Hydroxylation	CYP1A2
			0.90	0.74	13	Aromatic Hydroxylation	CYP1A2
M8	37	Diosgenin	0.64	0.52	24	Aliphatic Hydroxylation	CYP3A4

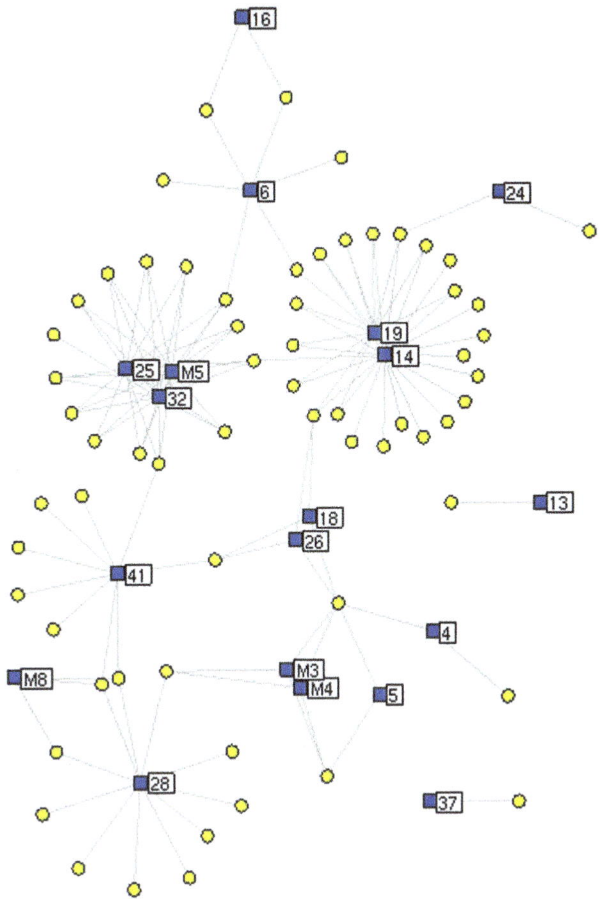

Figure 5. DB chemical component-putative target network. Blue squares refer to the DB compounds and metabolites; yellow spherical nodes refer to the predicted targets.

chemspider.com) and TCM Database@Taiwan (http://tcm.cmu.edu.tw). When several isomers were matched, a compound that had previously been identified in DB was considered more likely to be correct. Finally, ion fragments were used to provide further confirmation of the chemical structure. The structures of the main constitutions of DB are shown in **Figure 3**. For example, 7,4′-dihydroxyflavan (compound **5**) was firstly identified by comparing its retention time and accurate mass with that of the appropriate standard. Then, the MS/MS spectrum and possible fragmentation pathways of 7,4′-dihydroxyflavan were depicted in **Figure 4**. Only $[M+H]^+$ and $[M-H]^-$ were observed in positive and negative ion modes, respectively. The loss of 128 Da and 136 Da were the characteristic neutral loss of 7,4′-dihydroxyflavan in positive and negative ion modes.

3. Prediction of absorbed DB constituents and their metabolites by in silico ADME models

Quantitative structure-permeability relationships (QSPerR) have been established for permeability across Caco-2 monolayers (Papp) by the application of new molecular descriptors [47]. Among them, the passive Caco-2 absorption model provides a useful drug discovery tool by predicting human oral absorption of new chemical entities [48–49]. Yazdanian *et al.* [50] reported that compounds with Papp values less than 0.4×10^{-6} cm/s exhibited very poor oral absorption, whereas compounds with Papp values

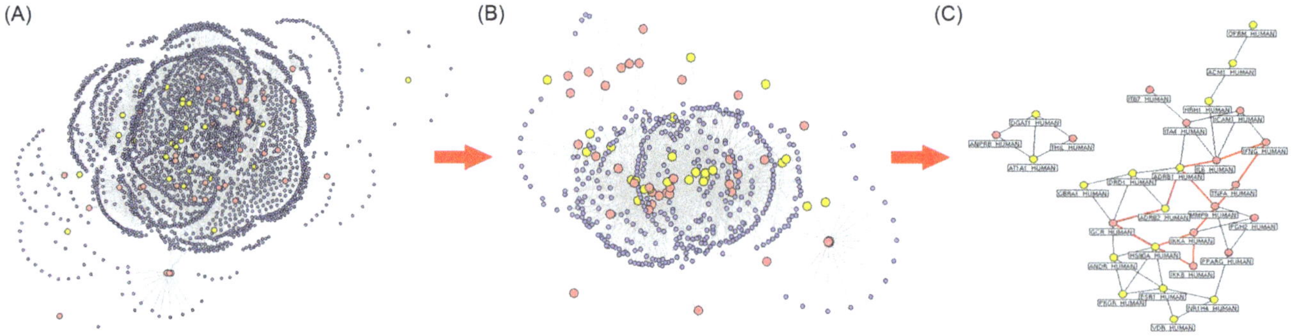

Figure 6. Putative DB targets-known colitis therapeutic targets protein-protein interaction (PPI) network. (A) The network between all targets and other human proteins. (B) The network of hub proteins in network (A). (C) The network of the major putative DB targets and the major known colitis therapeutic targets in network (B). Yellow spherical nodes indicate the putative targets; pink spherical nodes indicate the known therapeutic targets; purple spherical nodes indicate other human proteins that interact with putative targets or known therapeutic targets. Red edges in (C) indicate the PPIs of targets involved in the NOD-like receptor signaling pathway.

greater than 7×10^{-6} cm/s had excellent oral absorption. The present study employed an *in silico* passive Caco-2 absorption model within the ACD/Percepta software to identify DB constituents with excellent oral absorption values (greater than 7×10^{-6} cm/s) and the results were shown in **Table 1**. Subsequently, the ACD/Percepta software P450 regioselectivity module was applied to predict the metabolites of these well-absorbed DB constituents. These results were listed in **Table 2** and the structures of the metabolites were shown in **Figure 3**.

4. Analysis of DB pharmacological mechanisms in colitis

In order to analyze the synergistic effects and pharmacological mechanisms of DB in colitis, we constructed a chemical component-putative target network, and a putative DB targets-known colitis therapeutic targets PPI network. Detailed information relating to these similar drugs and putative targets is provided in supplementary **Table S3**. The performance of this prediction method was evaluated in our previous study [34].

4.1. DB chemical component-putative target network. As shown in **Figure 5**, this network consisted of 67 nodes (15 absorbed components, 4 metabolites and 48 putative targets) and 120 edges. The mean number of putative targets per chemical component/metabolite was 2.53. The absorbed DB component 14 and the metabolite M5 of compound **25** (3,4-dihydroxy-allylbenzene) both had the highest degree distributions, and hit 23 and 14 putative targets, respectively. Since chemical components or metabolites with a higher degree in the network have been demonstrated to be more pharmacologically important, and our data indicated that components 25, 32, and the M5 metabolite had the shortest paths between each other, they may play major roles in this pharmacological network, with synergistic effects.

4.2. Putative DB targets-known colitis therapeutic targets PPI network. Putative DB targets-known colitis therapeutic targets PPI network was constructed using PPIs between putative DB targets and known colitis therapeutic targets. As shown in **Figure 6A**, this network consisted of 2397 nodes and 4005 edges. According to the previous study of Li et al. [51], if the degree of a node is more than 2 fold of the median degree of all nodes in a network, such node is believed to play a critical role in the network structure, and can be treated as a hub node. Thus, we identified 463 hub proteins. Then, the PPI network of these hub proteins was constructed using the direct PPIs between them. As a result, this network consisted of 463 nodes and 1574 edges (**Figure 6B**). In addition, we calculated four topological feature values of all 463 nodes in the PPI network of hub proteins according to the definition described in section 2.7.2. We defined a hub protein, the four topological feature values of which were all larger than the corresponding median values, as a major hub protein. After the calculation, the median values of the four topological features were 3, 0.06, 31.30, and 3 for "degree," "betweenness," "closeness," and "k value," respectively. Therefore, we determined that hub proteins with "degree" >3, "betweenness" >0.06, "closeness" > 31.30, and "k value" >3 were major hubs. As a result, 106 proteins were identified as major hubs, including 18 putative DB targets and 16 known therapeutic targets for colitis. Detailed information on the topological features of these major hubs is provided in supplementary **Table S4**.

To investigate the pharmacological mechanisms of DB in colitis further, we analyzed the direct PPIs between the major putative DB targets and the major known therapeutic targets for colitis. As shown in **Figure 6C**, this network contained 34 nodes and 42 edges. According to the results of enrichment analysis based on the KEGG pathway [43], these major target proteins were frequently involved in the NOD-like receptor signaling pathway (KEGG ID: map04621). The intracellular NOD-like receptor (NLR) family contains more than 20 members in mammals and plays a pivotal role in the recognition of intracellular ligands. NOD1 and NOD2, two prototypic NLRs, sense the cytosolic presence of bacterial peptidoglycan fragments that have escaped from endosomal compartments, driving the activation of NF-kappa-B and MAPK, cytokine production, and apoptosis [52]. Accumulating studies have demonstrated that several members of the NOD-like receptor signaling pathway, such as heat shock protein 90 (Hsp90) [53], interleukin-6 (IL-6) [54], tumor necrosis factor alpha (TNF-α) [55], NF-kappa-B inhibitor kinase alpha (IKKA) [56], IKKB [56], and adrenergic receptors [57], may be associated with the pathogenesis of colitis. Of these proteins, Hsp90, ADRB1, and ADRB2 were identified as putative DB targets. Moreover, a number of putative DB targets also interacted with members of the NOD-like receptor signaling pathway, as shown in **Fig. 6C**. These findings suggested that the therapeutic effects of DB on colitis may involve this pathway.

Conclusion

High-throughput analysis, *in silico* ADME prediction, and network pharmacology techniques have recently emerged as powerful tools to provide new insights into the active compounds and the molecular mechanisms involved in the therapeutic actions of traditional Chinese medicines. In this study, a rapid, sensitive, and high-throughput analytical method using UPLC-ESI-MS/MS was firstly developed to characterize 48 constituents and accurately identify 24 constituents of DB tablet. Then, 22 components of DB tablet were predicted to be absorbed by an *in silico* passive absorption model, based on the Caco-2 cell monolayer. Eight metabolites were predicted using a computational module of P450 regioselectivity. Finally, these compounds were predicted to interact with 26 putative targets. Using this information, pharmacological networks were built to visualize the synergistic interactions between DB components and their targets. Furthermore, a PPI network of putative DB targets and known therapeutic targets for colitis was constructed to pinpoint the key targets and pathways. This approach offered a valuable opportunity to deepen understanding of the pharmacological mechanisms of DB in colitis.

In summary, this research provided a more accurate analysis of DB constituents, compared to using TCM databases. Consideration of ADME using the passive absorption and P450 metabolism modules *in silico* predicted the *in vivo* situation more closely. Finally, network pharmacology analysis was applied effectively and helped to interpret the essence of "synergy" in Chinese medicine. This provided a new way to identify the key candidate targets and possible molecular pathways utilized by DB in the treatment of colitis.

Supporting Information

Table S1 The detailed target information for colitis.
(XLSX)

Table S2 The detailed PPI information of colitis based on eight existing PPI databases.
(XLSX)

Table S3 Detailed information relating to these similar drugs and putative targets for DB curing colitis.
(XLSX)

Table S4 Detailed information on the topological features of these major hubs including 18 putative DB targets and 16 known therapeutic targets for colitis.
(XLSX)

Author Contributions

Conceived and designed the experiments: XG GZ HY LH. Performed the experiments: HX Yanqiong Z. YL HZ RL DL Yi Z. Analyzed the data: NL ST. Contributed to the writing of the manuscript: YM.

References

1. Barnes PM, Powell-Griner E, McFann K, Nahin RL (2004) Complementary and alternative medicine use among adults: United States, 2002. Adv Data 27:1–19.
2. US Food and Drug Administration (2006) Guidance for industry on complementary and alternative medicine products and their regulation by the Food and Drug Administration.
3. Xu H, Tao Y, Lu P, Wang P, Zhang F, et al. (2013) A computational drug-target network for yuanhu zhitong prescription. Evid Based Complement Alternat Med e658531: 1–15.
4. Zhang B, Wang X, Li S (2013) An integrative platform of TCM network pharmacology and its application on a herbal formula, Qing-Luo-Yin. Evid Based Complement Alternat Med e456747: 1–12.
5. Zhang GB, Li QY, Chen QL, Su SB (2013) Network Pharmacology: A New Approach for Chinese Herbal Medicine Research. Evid Based Complement Alternat Med e621423: 1–9.
6. Chen CY (2011) TCM database Taiwan: the world's largest traditional Chinese medicine database for drug screening In Silico. PLoS ONE 6(1): e15939.
7. Li S, Zhang B, Yuan J (2011) A HerbBioMap database. China Copyright of Computer Software. 2011SR076502.
8. Tao Y, Xu H, Wang S, Wang B, Zhang Y, et al. (2013) Identification of the absorbed constituents after oral administration of Yuanhu Zhitong prescription extract and its pharmacokinetic study by rapid resolution liquid chromatography/quadrupole time-of-flight. J Chromatogr B Analyt Technol Biomed Life Sci 935:1–9.
9. Xu H, Li K, Chen Y, Zhang Y, Tang S, et al. (2013) Study on the absorbed fingerprint-efficacy of Yuanhu Zhitong tablet based on chemical analysis, vasorelaxation evaluation and data mining. PLoS One 8(12): e81135.
10. Artursson P, Karlsson J (1991) Correlation between oral drug absorption in humans and apparent drug permeability coefficient in human intestinal epithelial (Caco-2) cells. Biochem Biophys Res Commun 175: 880–885.
11. U.S. Department of Health and Human Services, FDA (2000) Center for Drug Evaluation and Research (CDER) Waiver of In Vivo Bioavailability and Bioequivalence Studies for Immediate-Release Solid Oral Dosage Forms Based on a Biopharmaceutics Classification System. US FDA Guidance for Industry 1–16.
12. Marrero Ponce Y, Cabrera Pérez MA, Romero Zaldivar V, González Díaz H, Torrens F (2004) A new topological descriptors based model for predicting intestinal epithelial transport of drugs in Caco-2 cell culture. J Pharm Pharm Sci 7(2):186–99.
13. State Pharmacopoeia Committee (2010) Pharmacopoeia of the People's republic of china. Beijing: China Medical Science and Technology Press 133.
14. The Editorial Committee (1999) Materia medica of china (volume 8). Shanghai: Shanghai Science and Technology Publishing House 455.
15. Zhu ZY (2012) Nursing experience of longxuejie combined with levofloxacin retention enema in treating ulcerative colitis. J Clin Med Prac 16: 47–49.
16. Hu WB, Gao SH, Gao YL (2011) Treating 40 Cases of Chronic Colitis by Longxuejie plus Western Medicine. J Prac Trad Chin Med 25: 56–57.
17. Feng SH, Liu B, Du R, Sun J (2011) Clinical Observation of Choroidal Neovasularization Treated with Herbal Medicine Longxuejie Tablets. World - J Integra Trad Med 6: 496–498.
18. Arnone A, Nasini G, Merlini L (1990) Constituents of dragon's blood. Part 4. Dracoflavan a, a novel secotri flavanoid. J Chem Soc Perkin 10: 2637–2640.
19. Shen CC, Tsai SY, Wei SL, Wang ST, Shieh BJ, et al. (2007) Flavonoids isolated from draconis resina. Nat Prod Res 21: 377–380.
20. Piozzi F, Passannanti S, Paternostro MP, Nasini G (1974) Diterpenoid resin acids of daemonorops Draco. Phytochemistry 13: 2231–2233.
21. Nasini G, Piozzi F (1981) Pterocarpol and triterpenes from daemonorops. Draco. Phytochemistry 20: 514–516.
22. Shi J, Hu R, Lu Y, Sun C, Wu T (2009) Single-step purification of dracorhodin from dragon's blood resin of Daemonorops draco using high-speed counter-current chromatography combined with pH modulation. J Sep Sci 32: 4040–4047.
23. De Marino S, Gala F, Zollo F, Vitalini S, Fico G, et al. (2008) Identification of minor secondary metabolites from the latex of Croton lechleri (Muell-Arg) and evaluation of their antioxidant activity. Molecules 13:1219–1229.
24. Baumer U, Dietemann P (2010) Identification and differentiation of dragon's blood in works of art using gas chromatography/mass spectrometry. Anal Bioanal Chem 397:1363–76.
25. Yi T, Tang Y, Zhang J, Zhao Z, Yang Z, et al. (2012) Characterization and determination of six flavonoids in the ethnomedicine "Dragon's Blood" by UPLC-PAD-MS. Chem Cent J 6: 116.
26. Milburn M (1984) Dragon's Blood in East & West Africa, Arabia and the Canary Islands. Africa 39: 486–493.
27. Badib AS (1991) Medicinal plants of the Yemen Maktabah Alirsaid: Sanaa 15.
28. Wangensteen H, Klarpås L, Alamgir M, Samuelsen ABC, Malterud KE (2013) Can Scientific Evidence Support Using Bangladeshi Traditional Medicinal Plants in the Treatment of Diarrhoea? A Review on Seven Plants. Nutrients 5: 1757–1800.
29. Wishart DS, Knox C, Guo AC, Cheng D, Shrivastava S, et al. (2008) DrugBank: a knowledgebase for drugs, drug actions and drug targets. Nucleic Acids Res 36: D901–D906.
30. Chen JY, Mamidipalli SR, Huan TX (2009) HAPPI: an online database of comprehensive human annotated and predicted protein interactions. BMC Genomics (Suppl 1): S16.
31. Matthews L, Gopinath G, Gillespie M, Caudy M, Croft D, et al. (2009) Reactome knowledgebase of human biological pathways and processes. Nucleic Acids Res 37: D619–D622.
32. Brown KR, Jurisica I (2005) Online predicted human interaction database. Bioinformatics 21: 2076–2082.
33. Aranda B, Achuthan P, Alam-Faruque Y, Armean I, Bridge A, et al. (2010) The IntAct molecular interaction database in 2010. Nucleic Acids Res 38: D525–D531.
34. Keshava Prasad TS, Goel R, Kandasamy K, Keerthikumar S, Kumar S, et al. (2009) Human Protein Reference Database-2009 update. Nucleic Acids Res 37: D767–D772.

35. Ceol A, Chatr Aryamontri A, Licata L, Peluso D, Briganti L, et al. (2010) MINT, the molecular interaction database: 2009 update. Nucleic Acids Res 38: D532–D539.
36. Lehne B, Schlitt T (2009) Protein-protein interaction databases: keeping up with growing interactomes. Hum. Genomics 3: 291–297.
37. Beuming T, Skrabanek L, Niv MY, Mukherjee P, Weinstein H (2005) PDZBase: a protein-protein interaction database for PDZ-domains. Bioinformatics 21: 827–828.
38. Zhang Y, Wang D, Tan S, Xu H, Liu C, et al. (2013) A systems biology-based investigation into the pharmacological mechanisms of Wu Tou Tang acting on rheumatoid arthritis by integrating network analysis. Evid Based Complement Alternat Med e548498: 1–12.
39. Zhu F, Shi Z, Qin C, Tao L, Liu X, et al. (2012) Therapeutic target database update 2012: a resource for facilitating target-oriented drug discovery. Nucleic Acids Res 40: D1128–D1136.
40. Wang Y1, Liu Z, Li C, Li D, Ouyang Y, et al (2012) Drug target prediction based on the herbs components: the study on the multitargets pharmacological mechanism of qishenkeli acting on the coronary heart disease. Evid. Based Complement Alternat. Med. 2012: 698531.
41. Azuaje FJ, Zhang L, Devaux Y, Wagner DR (2011) Drug-target network in myocardial infarction reveals multiple side effects of unrelated drugs. Scientific Reports 1: 1–10.
42. Wuchty S, Almaas E (2005) Evolutionary cores of domain co-occurrence networks. BMC Evol Biol 5: 24.
43. Wixon J, Kell D (2000) The Kyoto encyclopedia of genes and genomes—KEGG. Yeast 17: 48–55.
44. Guillarme D, Schappler J, Rudaz S, Veuthey JL (2010) Coupling ultra-high-pressure liquid chromatography with mass spectrometry. TrAC Trends Anal Chem 29:15–27.
45. Theodoridis GA, Gika HG, Want EJ, Wilson ID (2012) Liquid chromatography-mass spectrometry based global metabolite profiling: a review. Anal Chim Acta 711: 7–16.
46. Michalski A, Damoc E, Hauschild JP, Lange O, Wieghaus A, et al. (2011) Mass spectrometry-based proteomics using Q Exactive, a high-performance benchtop quadrupole Orbitrap mass spectrometer. Mol Cell Proteomics 10: M111.011015.
47. Yovani Marrero P, Miguel Angel C, Vicente Romero Z, Ernest O, Luis AM (2003) Total and local quadratic indices of the "molecular pseudograph's atom adjacency matrix". Application to prediction of Caco-2 permeability of drugs. Int. J Mol Sci 4: 512–536.
48. Zhang J, Zhang Y, Zhang S, Wang S, He L (2010) Discovery of novel taspine derivatives as antiangiogenic agents. Bioorg Med Chem Lett 20: 718–721.
49. Zhou L, Chow MS, Zuo Z (2009) Effect of sodium caprate on the oral absorptions of danshensu and salvianolic acid B. Int J Pharm 379:109–118.
50. Yazdanian M, Glynn SL, Wright JL, Hawi A (1998) Correlating Partitioning and Caco-2 Cell Permeability of Structurally Diverse Small Molecular Weight Compounds. Pharm Res 15: 1490–1494.
51. Li S, Zhang ZQ, Wu LJ, Zhang XG, Li YD, et al. (2007) Understanding ZHENG in traditional Chinese medicine in the context of neuro-endocrine-immune network. IET Syst Biol 1: 51–60.
52. Rubino SJ, Selvanantham T, Girardin SE, Philpott DJ (2012) Nod-like receptors in the control of intestinal inflammation. Curr Opin Immunol 24: 398–404.
53. Tomasello G, Sciumé C, Rappa F, Rodolico V, Zerilli M, et al. (2011) Hsp10, Hsp70, and Hsp90 immunohistochemical levels change in ulcerative colitis after therapy. Eur J Histochem 55: e38.
54. Wine E, Mack DR, Hyams J, Otley AR, Markowitz J, et al. (2013) Interleukin-6 is associated with steroid resistance and reflects disease activity in severe pediatric ulcerative colitis. J Crohns Colitis 7: 916–922.
55. Lv R, Qiao W, Wu Z, Wang Y, Dai S, et al. (2014) Tumor necrosis factor alpha blocking agents as treatment for ulcerative colitis intolerant or refractory to conventional medical therapy: a meta-analysis. PLoS One 9: e86692.
56. Horwitz B (2005) NF-kappa B, an inhibitor of microflora-induced colitis. J Pediatr Gastroenterol Nutr 40 (Suppl 1): S22–3.
57. Sikander A, Rana SV, Sharma SK, Sinha SK, Arora SK, et al. (2010) Association of alpha 2A adrenergic receptor gene (ADRAlpha2A) polymorphism with irritable bowel syndrome, microscopic and ulcerative colitis. Clin Chim Acta 411: 59–63.

Screening Active Components from Yu-Ping-Feng-San for Regulating Initiative Key Factors in Allergic Sensitization

Dandan Shen[1,6], Xuejian Xie[2], Zhijie Zhu[1], Xi Yu[1], Hailiang Liu[1], Huizhu Wang[1], Hongwei Fan[3]*, Dawei Wang[5], Guorong Jiang[4], Min Hong[1]*

1 National Standard Laboratory of Pharmacology for Chinese Materia Medica, Jiangsu Key Laboratory for Pharmacology and Safety Evaluation of Chinese Materia Medica, Nanjing University of Chinese Medicine, Nanjing, China, **2** Nanjing General Hospital of Nanjing Military Command, Nanjing, China, **3** Department of Clinical Pharmacology Lab, Nanjing First Hospital, Nanjing Medical University, JiangSu Nanjing, China, **4** Suzhou Hospital of Tradional Chinese Medicine, Suzhou, China, **5** Jiangsu Academy of Traditional Chinese Medicine, Nanjing, China, **6** Pharmacy Department, The First People's Hospital of Taicang, Taicang, China

Abstract

Yu-ping-feng-san (YPFS) is a Chinese medical formula that is used clinically for allergic diseases and characterized by reducing allergy relapse. Our previous studies demonstrated that YPFS efficiently inhibited T helper 2 cytokines in allergic inflammation. The underlying mechanisms of action of YPFS and its effective components remain unclear. In this study, it was shown that YPFS significantly inhibited production of thymic stromal lymphopoietin (TSLP), an epithelial cell-derived initiative factor in allergic inflammation, *in vitro* and *in vivo*. A method of human bronchial epithelial cell (16HBE) binding combined with HPLC-MS (named 16HBE-HPLC-MS) was established to explore potential active components of YPFS. The following five components bound to 16HBE cells: calycosin-7-glucoside, ononin, claycosin, sec-o-glucosylhamaudol and formononetin. Serum from YPFS-treated mice was analyzed and three major components were detected claycosin, formononetin and cimifugin. Among these, claycosin and formononetin were detected by 16HBE-HPLC-MS and in the serum of YPFS-treated mice. Claycosin and formononetin decreased the level of TSLP markedly at the initial stage of allergic inflammation *in vivo*. Nuclear factor (NF)-κB, a key transcription factor in TSLP production, was also inhibited by claycosin and formononetin, either in terms of transcriptional activation or its nuclear translocation *in vitro*. Allergic inflammation was reduced by claycosin and formononetin when they are administered only at the initial stage in a murine model of atopic contact dermatitis. Thus, epithelial cell binding combined with HPLC-MS is a valid method for screening active components from complex mixtures of Chinese medicine. It was demonstrated that the compounds screened from YPFS significantly attenuated allergic inflammation probably by reducing TSLP production via regulating NF-κB activation.

Editor: Patricia T. Bozza, Fundação Oswaldo Cruz, Brazil

Funding: This research was funded by Project 81073121, 81373549 and 81102885 supported by National Natural Science Foundation of China, Project Funded by the Priority Academic Program Development of Jiangsu Higher Education Institutions and Qing Lan Project. The funders had no role in study design, data collection and analysis, decision to publish, or preparation of the manuscript.

Competing Interests: The authors have declared that no competing interests exist.

* Email: hongmin72@hotmail.com (MH); fanhongwei178@sina.com (HF)

These authors contributed equally to this work.

Introduction

Yu-ping-feng-san (YPFS) is a well-known Chinese prescription that consists of *Radix Astragali* (RA, Huangqi), *Rhizoma Atractylodis Macrocephalae* (RAM, Baizhu), and *Radix Saposhnikoviae* (RS, Fangfeng). Clinically, YPFS is mainly used in allergic diseases, such as allergic rhinitis [1], urticaria [2,3] and asthma [4,5], especially in reducing the relapse rate and disease severity. Recent studies have indicated that YPFS affects expression of T cell receptor (TCR) and major histocompatibility complex (MHC) class II expression on $CD4^+$ T cells in a mouse model of asthma, regulates the balance of T helper(Th)1/Th2 cells in murine allergic airway disease [6], and decreases interleukin(IL)-17 level [7]. Our previous studies have demonstrated that YPFS significantly inhibits Th2-cell-mediated atopic contact dermatitis (ACD) [8] and ovalbumin (OVA)-induced allergic asthma. YPFS markedly decreased the IL-4 level and consequently increased the ratio of interferon-γ/IL-4 [9]. However, these studies were focused on the inflammatory phase of allergy, which does not explain the mechanisms underlying the effect of YPFS on relapse.

The pharmacological effects of some components of YPFS have been reported. For example, flavonoids show antioxidant [10] and antiviral [11] activity. Total saponin in RA promotes antibody production and immune responses [12,13]. Chromone glucosides in RS and atractylenolide I and III are anti-inflammatory components [14]. Polysaccharide in these herbs has an effect on the immune system [15–17]. However, these components have no direct activity against relapse of allergic diseases.

Most allergic diseases are mediated by Th2 lymphocytes. Researchers have come to realize that epithelial cells (ECs) play a critical role in stimulating and regulating local immune responses [18]. Studies of thymic stromal lymphopoietin (TSLP) derived from ECs have provided important evidence that ECs can regulate the immune response to initiate the allergic response. TSLP mRNA is highly expressed in human primary skin keratinocytes and bronchial ECs [18,19]. TSLP contributes directly to the activation of dendritic cells (DCs), which then migrate into the lymph nodes and prime allergen-specific Th2 responses [20]. Therefore, TSLP might be a master switch for allergic inflammation at the EC–DC interface [21]. It was presumed that the key mechanism involved in the reduction of allergy recurrence by YPFS might be related to regulation of TSLP derived from ECs. Therefore, we examined the effect of YPFS on TSLP production in the present study. ECs were utilized to screen for potential active components in YPFS, and their effects on TSLP production and allergic inflammation were determined.

We selected human bronchial epithelial cells (16HBE cells) to screen for potential active components in YPFS effective on ECs. This method combined 16HBE cell binding with HPLC-MS, therefore it was called 16HBE-HPLC-MS. Previously, our group has successfully established some cell-binding methods to screen for potential active components in Chinese medicine, including hepatocyte [22,23], erythrocyte [24], macrophage [25] and splenocyte [26] binding. By utilizing these methods, some components from Chinese medicine were identified and demonstrated to be active. The components in serum of mice treated with YPFS were analyzed to determine whether they were absorbed into the blood. The effects of these detected components on allergic inflammation and TSLP production were evaluated *in vitro* and *in vivo*.

Methods

Materials

Radix Astragali (RA; Inner Mongolia, China), Rhizoma Atractylodis Macrocephalae (RAM; Zhejiang, China), and Radix Saposhnikoviae (RS; Heilongjiang, China) were purchased from the Herbal Decoction Slices division of Nanjing Pharmaceutical Company (Nanjing, China). Botanic identification was confirmed by Professor Chungen Wang (Nanjing University of Chinese Medicine, China). Calycosin-7-glucoside, ononin, claycosin, sec-o-glucosylhamaudol and formononetin were purchased from Tianjin Marker Bio-Tech Co. Ltd (Tianjin, China). Cimifugin was purchased from National Institutes For Food And Drug Control (Beijing, China).

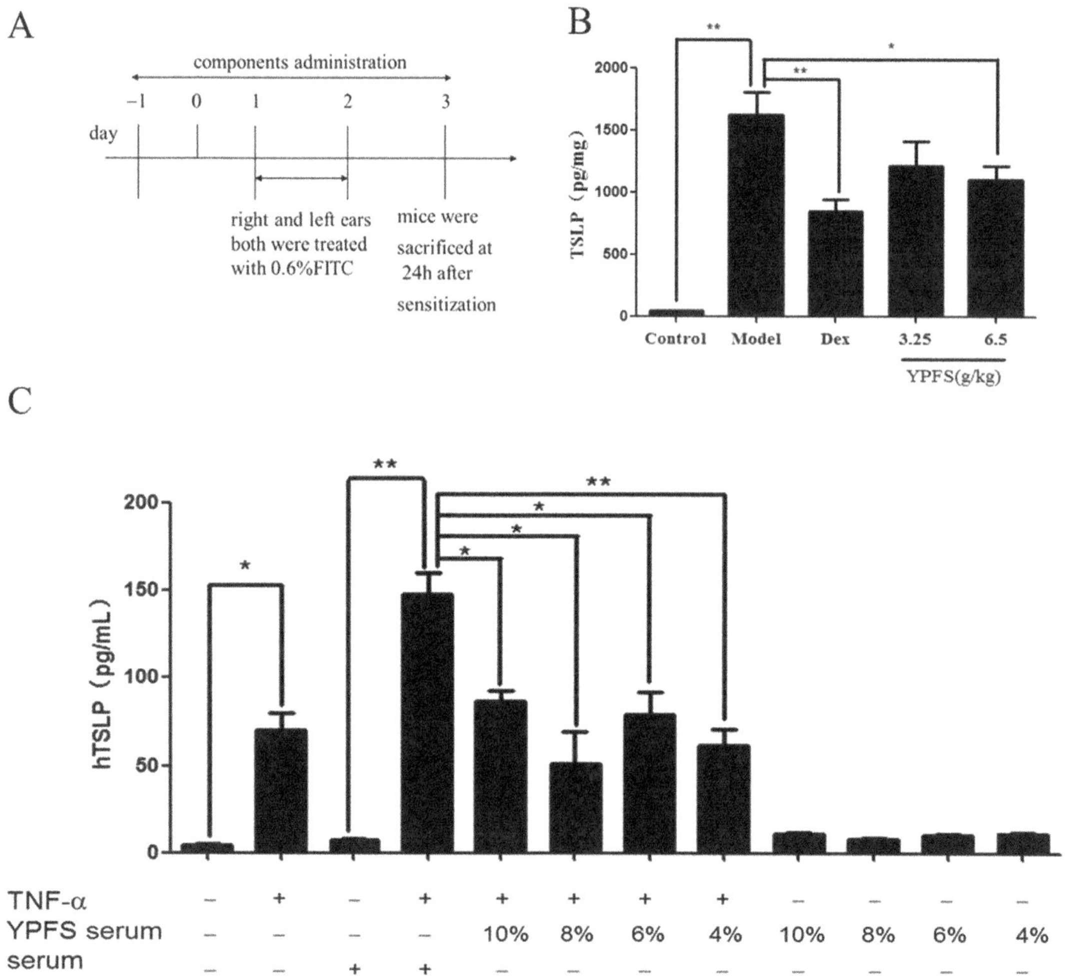

Figure 1. Effect of YPFS on TSLP *in vivo* and *in vitro*. (A) Flow charts of the TSLP production model. (B) Effect of YPFS on the production of TSLP in ear tissue at the initial stage in a murine model of ACD. TSLP in ear homogenates was analyzed by ELISA and total protein were examined by BCA kit. TSLP level was assessed with the formula: concentration of TSLP in the homogenate/total protein (pg/mg). (mean±SD, n = 8, *p<0.05, **p<0.01). (C) Effect of YPFS on TSLP production induced by TNF-α in 16HBE cells. 16HBE cells were treated with 1.25 µg/mL TNF-α and YPFS serum (4%, 6%, 8% or 10%) or control serum for 12 h. TSLP protein level was analyzed by ELISA. (mean±SD, n = 3, *p<0.05, **p<0.01) All the experiments were performed in triplicates.

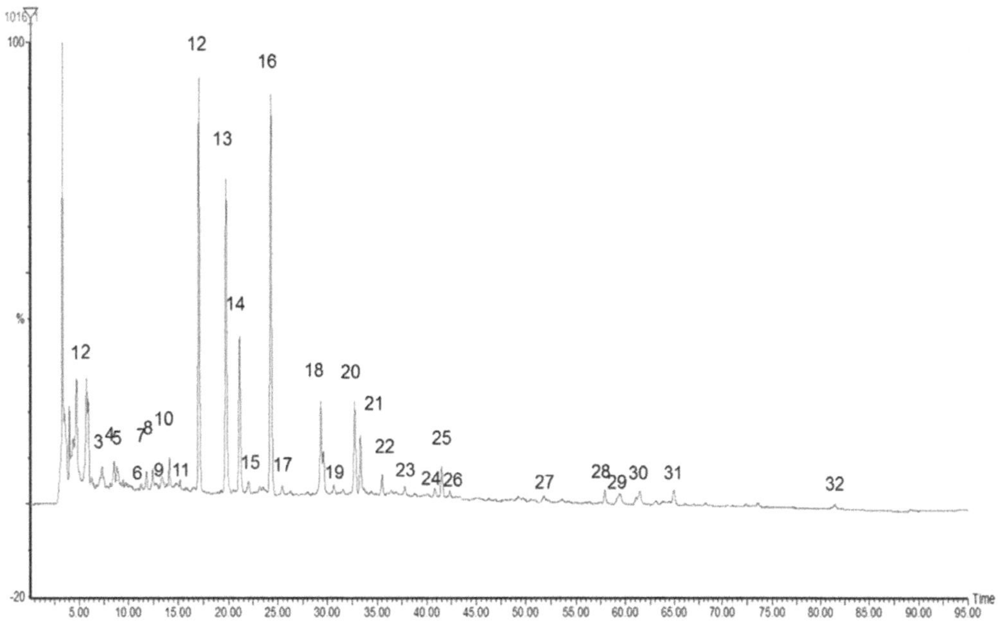

Figure 2. HPLC fingerprint of YPFS extract at 254 nm. YPFS was detected by HPLC-MS with an optimal condition for obtaining maximum peaks. There were 32 main peaks in YPFS extract. All the experiments were performed in triplicates.

Animals and cells

All procedures involving animals were approved by the Animal Care and Use Committee of Nanjing University of Chinese Medicine and strictly performed according to the Guide for the Care and Use of Laboratory Animals. BALB/c mice were purchased from Beijing Military Medical Academy and Shanghai Slac Laboratory Animal Company. All animals were maintained at Nanjing University of Chinese Medicine under specific pathogen-free conditions at 18°C–25°C and 50%–60% humidity, and were used at 6–10 weeks of age. 16HBE cells were purchased from the Cell Bank of the Chinese Academy of Medical Sciences (Beijing, China) and cultured in RPMI 1640 medium (Wisent, Saint-Jean-Baptiste, QC, Canada) supplemented with 10% fetal bovine serum (Wisent) at 37°C and 5% CO_2.

Preparation of YPFS extracts

Five hundred grams of YPFS (3:1:1) were immersed in 3.25 L ethanol:water (95:5, v/v) for 1 h and then refluxed for 2 h. The extraction process was repeated twice and the extracts were combined, filtered, and evaporated to dryness using a vacuum concentrator system (CH-9230; BUCHI Labortechnik, Flawil, Switzerland) at 60°C. The extract was then subjected to analysis at a concentration of 1.5 g crude drug/g extract.

TSLP production model *in vivo*

BALB/c mice were treated with 0.6% fluorescein isothiocyanate (FITC; Sigma, St. Louis, MO, USA) in 20 μL acetone and dibutyl phthalate (1:1, vehicle) on both ears on day 1 and 2, and sacrificed on day 3. Mice were treated once daily with YPFS or formononetin and claycosin 2 days before treatment with FITC until day 3 of the model. Both ears were removed and ground into homogenates with ice–phosphate–buffered saline (PBS), and the homogenates were centrifuged at 4000 g at 4°C for 15 min. The supernatant was stored at −80°C before analysis. The concentration of TSLP in ear homogenate was analyzed by mouse TSLP ELISA kits (eBioscience, San Diego, CA) according to the manufacturer's instructions. Total protein level in the homogenates was examined by BCA kit (Jiancheng, Nanjing, China). TSLP level was assessed with the formula: concentration of TSLP in the homogenate/total protein (pg/mg).

Measurement of TSLP production induced by tumor necrosis factor-alpha (TNF-α) in 16HBE cells *in vitro*

16HBE cells were seeded into 96-well plates at a density of 8×10^5cells/mL and incubated at 37°C under 5% CO_2. At 80%–90% confluency, cells were stimulated with TNF-α (1.25 μg/mL; PeproTech, Rocky Hill, NJ, USA) and 4%–10% serum from YPFS-treated mice simultaneously for 12 h. The concentration of TSLP in culture supernatant was detected by Human TSLP ELISA kit (eBioscience) according to the manufacturer's instructions.

16HBE cell binding assay

16HBE cell suspensions (8×10^6cells/mL) were incubated with YPFS extract at a concentration of 0.1 g/mL with gentle shaking at 37°C for 1 h and then centrifuged at 1100 g for 5 min. Cell pellets were washed three times with D-Hank's Solution to remove unbound components, followed by centrifugation at 200 g for 5 min. The final washing eluate was collected as one of the controls. Cells were incubated with 8 mL hydrochloride acid D-Hanks' (pH 4.0) for 1 h at 37°C, followed by centrifugation at 400 g for 5 min to liberate the components bound to the cells. The supernatant was collected by centrifugation and was referred to as the desorption eluate. The blank desorption eluate, in which YPFS extract was replaced by RPMI 1640, was generated using the method described above.

The desorption solution or the final washing eluate (2 mL) was separately mixed with ethyl acetate (4 mL), vortexed for 3 min, and centrifuged at 1600 g for 5 min. Supernatants were collected and dried under nitrogen at 45°C. Residues were dissolved with 300 μL methanol and centrifuged at 10000 g for 5 min and

Table 1. RRT and RPA of each peak in fingerprint of YPFS extract.

No.	RRT	RPA	Identified compound
1	0.195039	0.409416	
2	0.237648	0.4078	
3	0.301521	0.077928	
4	0.35163	0.056677	
5	0.363823	0.0987593	
6	0.463535	0.0121612	
7	0.486958	0.039583	
8	0.511683	0.041818	
9	0.54162	0.037255	
10	0.581036	0.047355	
11	0.625051	0.031994	
12	0.7019	0.843082	Prim-O-glucosylcimifugin
13	0.813162	0.766692	Calycosin-7-glucoside copyranoside
14	0.869494	0.394774	Cimifugin
15	0.906581	0.035079	
16	1	1	4′-O-glucopyranosyl-5-O-methylvisamminol
17	1.048749	0.02977	
18	1.208102	0.367158	Ononin
19	1.263032	0.025007	
20	1.348869	0.247059	Claycosin
21	1.372934	0.129639	Sec-o-glucosylhamaudol
22	1.462892	0.047043	
23	1.55697	0.021852	
24	1.681296	0.020301	
25	1.710141	0.082697	Formononetin
26	1.743808	0.018922	
27	2.134322	0.017997	
28	2.386657	0.038159	
29	2.448469	0.067835	
30	2.531545	0.056232	
31	2.675114	0.04355	
32	3.351017	0.02101	

filtered by 0.45 μm nylon membrane filter before HPLC-MS analysis.

Preparation of serum from YPFS-treated mice

Serum from YPFS-treated mice was prepared as described previously [27]. BALB/c mice were administered 34.1 g crude drug/kg YPFS intragastrically twice daily for 3 days, and normal saline was administered as a control (control serum). One hour after the final administration, blood was collected and centrifuged at 2200 g for 15 min after standing for 1 h. The serum was filtered through a 0.22 μm nylon filter membrane and stored at −80°C. Serum from YPFS-treated mice was used to evaluate the effect of YPFS on TNF-α induced TSLP production in 16HBE cells.

Part of the serum from YPFS-treated mice (200 μL) was mixed with ethyl acetate (400 μL), vortexed for 3 min, and centrifuged at 1600 g for 5 min. Supernatants were collected and dried under nitrogen at 45°C. Residues were dissolved in 200 μL methanol and centrifuged at 10000 g for 5 min and filtered through a 0.45 μm nylon membrane filter before HPLC-MS analysis.

HPLC-MS analysis

Analysis were performed on an Waters ZQ2000 LC-MS system equipped with a quaternary gradient pump, an autosampler, and a column incubator, a diode-array detector (DAD) and an electrospray ionization (ESI) ion source, connect to Masslynx 4.0 workstation. A chromatographic column (4.6×250 mm, 5μm; Chrom-Matrix) was used. The liquid phase conditions were (A) acetonitrile (Tedia, USA); (B) water:formic acid (100:0.05, v/v). The flow rate was 1 mL/min and elution conditions were: 0–10 min, linear gradient 3%–15% (v/v) A in B; 10–20 min, linear gradient 15%–20% A; 20–30 min, linear gradient 20%–28% A; 30–40 min, linear gradient 28%–40% A; 40–60 min, linear gradient 40%–60% A; 60–85 min, 60%–95% A isocratic; 85–95 min, linear gradient 95%–3% A. The system operated at 30°C

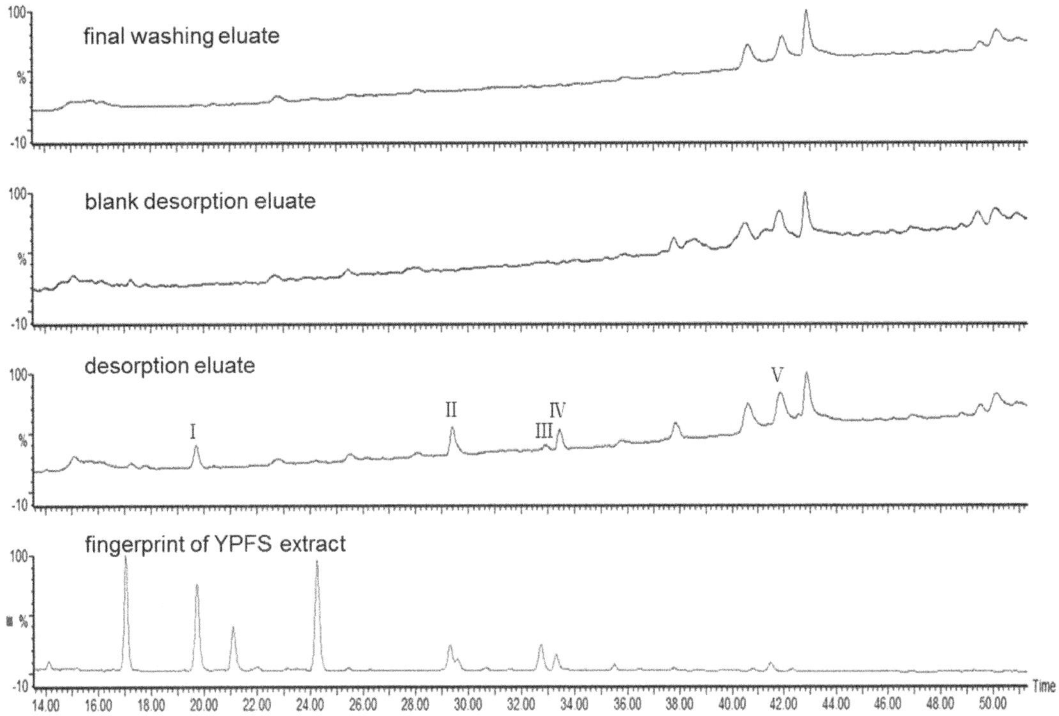

Figure 3. Comparative chromatograms of fingerprint of YPFS extract, final wash eluate, blank desorption eluate (in which YPFS extract was replaced by RPMI 1640) and 16HBE-binding desorption eluate. Detection was at 254 nm. All the experiments were performed in triplicates.

and the injection volume was 10 μL. The DAD was set to scan from 200 to 400 nm.

The mass spectrometry conditions were: capillary voltage 3 kV, cone voltage 40 V, source temperature 120°C, desolvation temperature 400°C, desolvation gas flow 400 L/h, cone gas flow 50 L/h. The ESI was performed in the positive and negative ionization modes in the scan range 100–1000 nm.

Luciferase reporter assay *in virto*

Functional nuclear factor (NF) -κB activation was determined by luciferase reporter assay. 16HBE cells were seeded at a density of 1×10^5cells/mL in 24-well plates and transfected with pNFκB-TA-luc plasmid (Beyotime Biotechnology, Haimen, China) containing the response element that drives transcription of the luciferase reporter gene, along with Renilla using Lipofectamine TM 2000 (Invitrogen Carlsbad, CA) according to the manufacturer's instructions for 6 h. Cells were further incubated with fresh medium for 24 h. Cells were pretreated with different concentrations of claycosin or formononetin for 2 h or with culture medium as a control before stimulated with TNF-α (100 ng/mL) for 1 h. The luciferase activity was measured in the cellular extracts using a dual luciferase reporter assay system (Promega, Madison, WI, USA) with GloMax 20/20 n Luminometer (Promega).

Immunofluorescence assay *in virto*

NF-κB nuclear translocation was evaluated by immunofluorescence assay. 16HBE cells were starved with serum-free medium overnight and were pretreated with claycosin or formononetin for 2 h or with culture medium as a control before stimulated with TNF-α (100 ng/mL) for 1 h. The cells were fixed in ice-cold paraformaldehyde (PFA) for 1 h. The coverslips were washed with PBS before permeabilizing the cells with Triton X-100 (Genview, Scientific Inc, USA) and blocked with 5% bovine serum albumin (BSA) for 1 h at 37°C. The cells were probed with 4 μg/mL rabbit monoclonal antibody to NF-κB (Santa Cruz Biotechnology, Santa Cruz, CA, USA) at 4°C overnight. After repeated washes with PBS, the cells were probed with 1 μg/mL goat anti-rabbit IgG conjugated to FITC (Santa Cruz Biotechnology) and 4′,6-diamidino-2-phenylindole (DAPI, Santa Cruz Biotechnology) at a concentration of 5 μg/mL for 1 h. The labeled sections were viewed with fluorescence confocal microscopy (Olympus, Tokyo, Japan).

Cytotoxicity assay *in vitro*

Cytotoxicity was determined with the methyl tetrazolium (MTT) assay. Cells were seeded in 96-well plates (1×10^4 cells/well) and were incubated for 12 or 24 h in the presence of indicated doses of calycosin and formononetin. 20 μL MTT (5 mg/mL; Sigma) stock solution was added to each well, and plates were incubated at 37°C. After 4 h incubation, cells were lysed with dimethyl sulfoxide (DMSO, Sigma). Absorbance was measured at 490 nm using Synergy HT Multi-Mode Microplate Reader (Bio-Tek, Winooski, VT, USA). All experiments were performed in triplicate.

Experimental ACD model *in vivo*

To establish the ACD model, BALB/c mice were topically sensitized with 1.5% FITC solution on the abdominal skin on days 1 and 2 and elicited on the right ear with 0.5% FITC solution on day 6. Mice were treated once daily with calycosin (0.5, 5 or 10 mg/kg, intraperitoneally), formononetin (0.5, 5 or 10 mg/kg, intraperitoneally) or normal saline 2 days before sensitization until day 3 of the model (only administrated at initiation stage of sensitization phase). Ear thickness was measured 24 h after

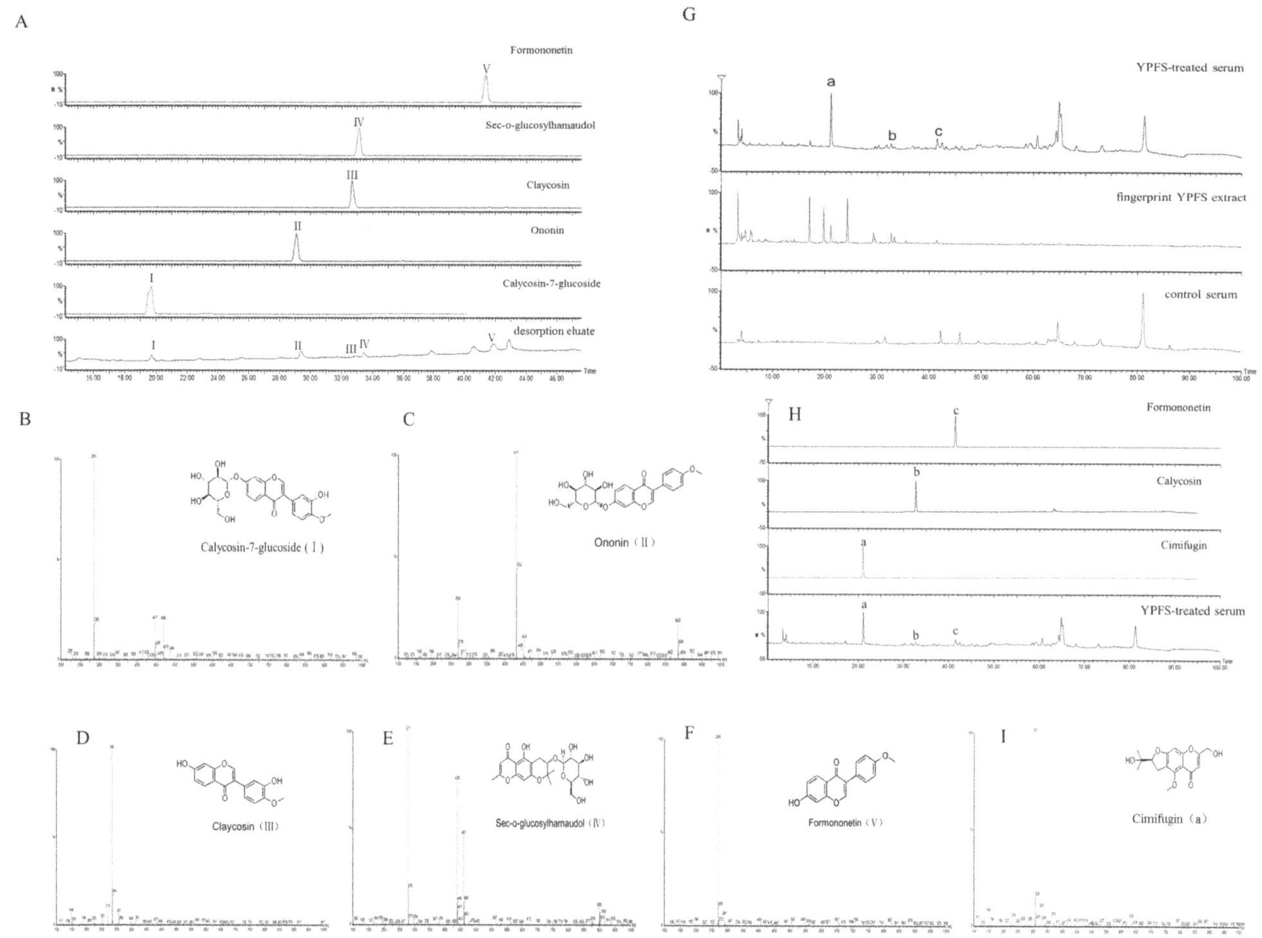

Figure 4. Determination of components in serum from YPFS-treated mice and identification of YPFS extract chemicals binding to 16HBE cells by HPLC-MS. (A) UV visible spectrum of YPFS components I–V in the 16HBE-binding desorption eluate corresponding to the standard materials at 254 nm. (B) ESI-MS negative ionization spectrum of compound I and its structural formula (inset). Calycosin-7-glucoside, (+)ESI-MS m/z was 447[M+H]$^+$(m/z). (C) ESI-MS negative ionization spectrum of compound II and its structural formula (inset). Ononin, (+)ESI-MS m/z was 431[M+H]$^+$(m/z). (D) ESI-MS negative ionization spectrum of compound III and its structural formula (inset). Claycosin, (+)ESI-MS m/z was 285[M+H]$^+$(m/z). (E) ESI-MS negative ionization spectrum of compound IV and its structural formula (inset). Sec-o-glucosylhamaudol, (+)ESI-MS m/z was 439[M+H]$^+$(m/z). (F) ESI-MS negative ionization spectrum of compound V and its structural formula (inset). Formononetin, (+)ESI-MS m/z was 269[M+H]$^+$(m/z). (G) UV spectrum of serum from YPFS-treated mice, compared with fingerprint of YPFS extract and control serum at 254 nm. (H) UV spectrum of components a–c detected in serum of YPFS-treated mice corresponding to the standard materials at 254 nm. (I) ESI-MS negative ionization spectrum of compound "a" and its structural formula (inset). Cimifugin, (+)ESI-MS m/z was 307[M+H]$^+$(m/z). All the experiments were performed in triplicates.

elicitation (Harbin Measuring & Cutting Tool Group Co. Ltd. Harbin, China) and changes in ear thickness were calculated. Histopathological changes in the ears were examined by hematoxylin and eosin (H&E) staining.

Statistical analysis

The data were expressed as means ± SD. Multiple groups' comparisons were analyzed by one-way analysis of variance, and Dunnett's test was used for comparison between two groups, with

Table 2. Peak assignment for the components from desorption eluate.

Peak no.	Compound name	t_R(min)	(+)ESI-MS m/z	Other ions	UV λ_{max}(nm)
I	Calycosin-7-glucoside	19.73	447[M+H]$^+$(m/z)	285	260,290
II	Ononin	29.40	431[M+H]$^+$(m/z)	269	255,301
III(b)	Claycosin	32.90	285[M+H]$^+$(m/z)	-	250,290
IV	Sec-o-glucosylhamaudol	33.45	439[M+H]$^+$(m/z)	277	250,298
V(c)	Formononetin	41.87	269[M+H]$^+$(m/z)	-	250,303
a	Cimifugin	20.99	307[M+H]$^+$(m/z)	-	216,229

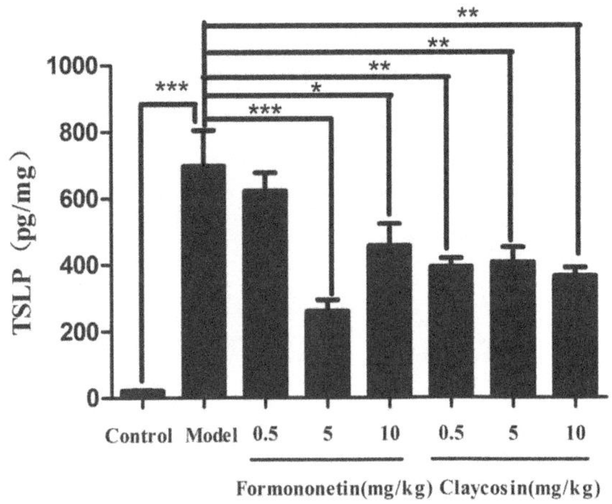

Figure 5. Effect of claycosin and formononetin on the production of TSLP at the initial stage in a murine model of ACD *in vivo*. TSLP in ear homogenates was analyzed by ELISA and total protein was determined by BCA kit. TSLP level was assessed with the formula: concentration of TSLP in homogenate/total protein (pg/mg). (mean±SD, n = 8, *p<0.05, **p<0.01, ***p<0.001). All the experiments were performed in triplicates.

GraphPad Prism 5 (GraphPad Software, San Diego, CA, USA). Statistical significance was set at p<0.05.

Results

1 Effect of YPFS on TSLP production *in vivo* and *in vitro*

1.1 YPFS inhibited TSLP production at the initial stage of sensitization *in vivo*. A murine model of TSLP production at the initial stage of ACD was established to observe the effect of YPFS on TSLP production *in vivo*. Mice were treated once daily with 3.25 or 6.5 g/kg YPFS, intragastrically, or 0.67 mg/kg dexamethasone, intraperitoneally, 2 days before treatment with FITC until day 3 of the model (Fig. 1A). The level of TSLP was significantly higher in the model compared with the control group. YPFS (6.5 g/kg) decreased the level of TSLP in this model (Fig. 1B). The result implies that YPFS might affect allergic sensitization process by regulating TSLP.

1.2 TSLP production in 16HBE cells was reduced by serum from YPFS-treated mice *in vitro*. We studied the effect of serum from YPFS-treated mice on TNF-α-induced TSLP production in 16HBE cells. Serum pharmacology is a widely used method to evaluate effects of Chinese medicine *in vitro* to exclude the disturbance of irrelevant factors, such as pH, osmolality, ion and so on [28]. Cells were treated with 4%–10% serum from YPFS-treated mice and 1.25 μg/mL TNF-α simultaneously for 12 h. Serum from YPFS-treated mice did not alter the TSLP basal levels when there was no stimulation. A substantial amount of TSLP was detected in the supernatant following stimulation of 16HBE cells with 1.25 μg/mL TNF-α. Serum from YPFS-treated mice significantly decreased TSLP level in the presence of TNF-α (Fig. 1C). These results were consistent with previous observations *in vivo* and implied that regulation of TSLP might be an important mechanism of YPFS.

2 Probing potential active components of YPFS by 16HBE cell binding combined with HPLS-MS (16HBE-HPLC-MS)

2.1 HPLC fingerprint of YPFS extract. We performed 16HBE-HPLC-MS to screen for active components of YPFS that interacted with ECs. We established the fingerprint of YPFS as the background information for 16HBE-HPLC-MS. There were 32 main peaks in the fingerprint of YPFS extract at 254 nm (Fig. 2). Among these, eight components were identified after comparison with the standard materials (Table 1). All of the main peaks were well separated.

The injection precision was determined by five replicate injections of the same sample in one day. The relative standard deviations (RSDs) of relative retention time (RRT) and relative peak area (RPA) were 0.01%–0.32% and 0.28%–2.83%, respectively, and there were no significant changes. The repeatability was assessed by analyzing five independently prepared samples of YPFS extract. The RSDs of RRT and RPA were 0.01%–0.28% and 0.15%–2.88%, respectively, and there were no significant changes. The sample stability was assessed by successive injections

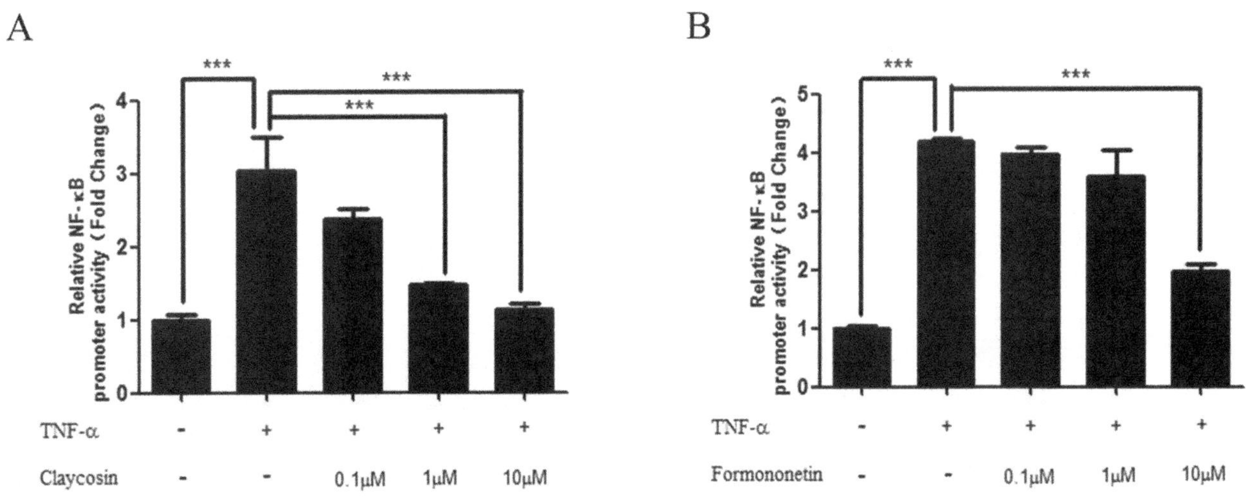

Figure 6. Effect of claycosin and formononetin on the transcriptional activation of NF-κB induced by TNF-α. 16HBE cells transfected with pNFκB-TA-luc were pretreated with claycosin or formononetin for 2 h or treated with medium only as a control, then stimulated with TNF-α(100 ng/mL) for 1 h. Transcriptional activation of NF-κB was measured in the cellular extracts using a dual luciferase reported gene assay kit. (A) Effect of claycosin on the transcriptional activation of NF-κB. (B) Effect of formononetin on the transcriptional activation of NF-κB. (mean±SD, n = 3, ***p<0.001). All the experiments were performed in triplicates.

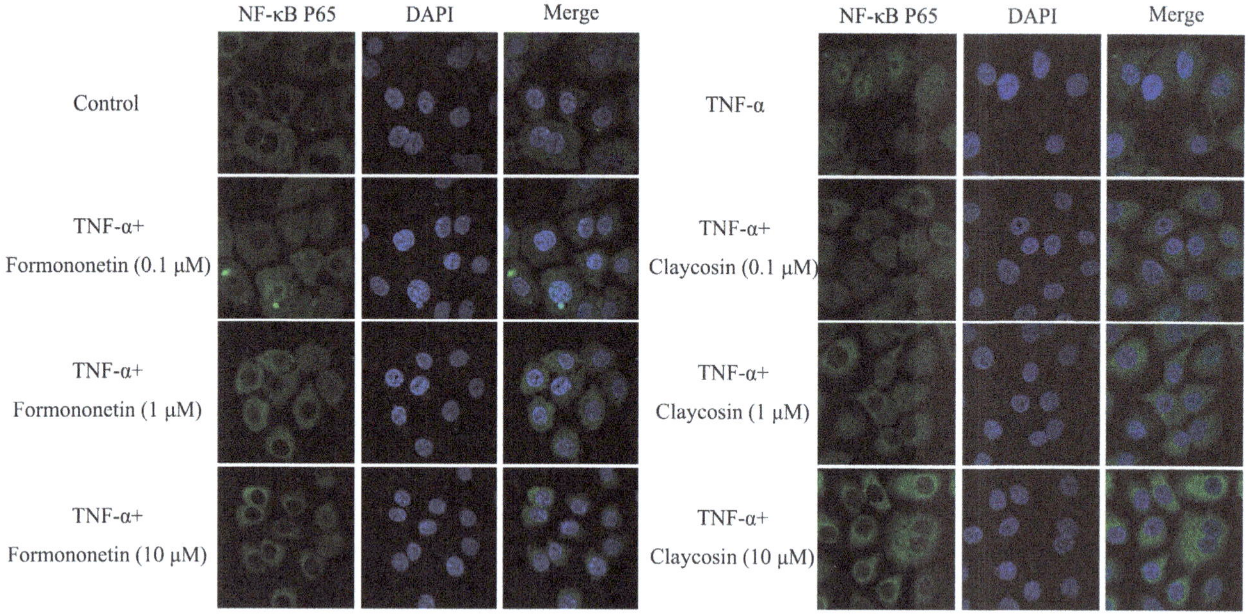

Figure 7. Effect of claycosin and formononetin on NF-κB translocation. NF-κB translocation in 16HBE cells was examined by immunofluorescence assay. n = 3. All the experiments were performed in triplicates.

of the same sample at 0, 3, 6, 9, 12 and 24 h. During this period, the solution was stored at room temperature. The RSDs of RRT and RPA were 0.04%–0.71% and 0.42%–2.81%, respectively, and there were no significant changes. The results of injection precision, repeatability and stability indicated that this method was adequate, valid and applicable. The RRT and RPA of the 32 peaks are shown in Table 1.

2.2 Probing 16HBE-binding components of YPFS. We selected 16HBE cells to explore the potential active components of YPFS. Five principal peaks (I–V) were detected at 254 nm in the YPFS 16HBE-binding desorption eluate, and no comparable peaks were detected in the chromatograms of the two control samples (final wash and blank desorption eluates) (Fig. 3). All the captured peaks were also found in the fingerprint of YPFS, which indicated that these components were from YPFS.

2.3 Identification of chemicals binding to 16HBE cells by HPLC-MS. To identify the above chemicals, we analyzed the molecular weight by MS and compared it with reference values [29]. Retention time and UV spectrum of the five peaks in HPLC were corresponded with the standard materials (Fig. 4A). In

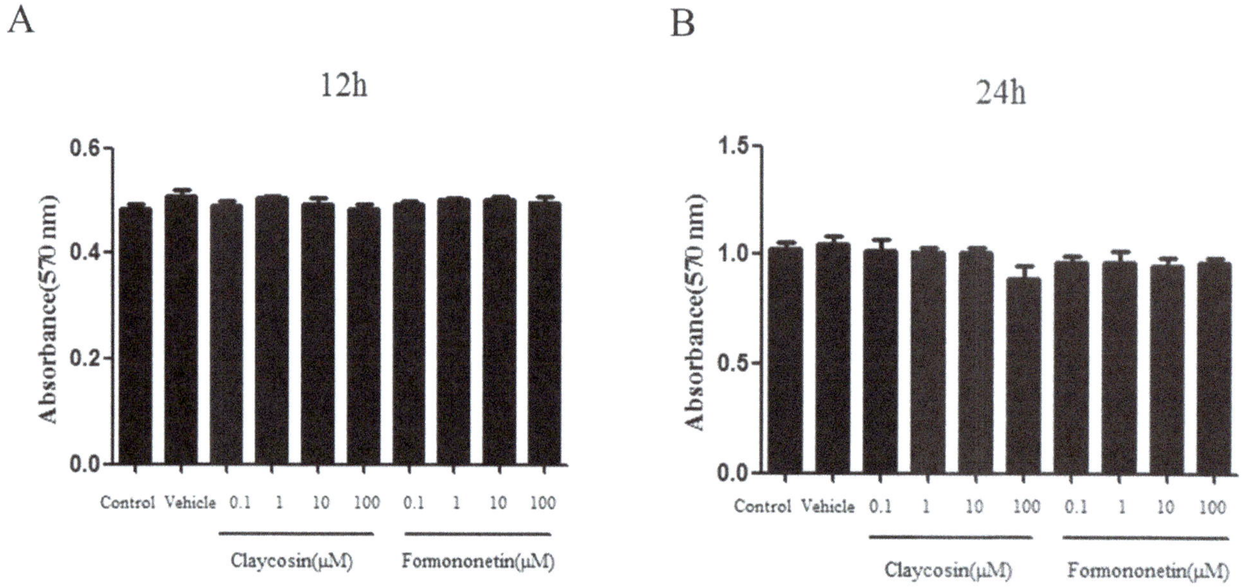

Figure 8. Effect of claycosin and formononetin on 16HBE cell proliferation. (A) Effect of claycosin and formononetin on 16HBE cell proliferation for 12 h. (B) Effect of claycosin and formononetin on 16HBE cell proliferation for 24 h. (mean±SD, n = 3). All the experiments were performed in triplicates.

negative ion mode, the product ion $[M+H]^+$ at m/z 447 was calycosin-7-glucoside; the transition m/z 447→285 was chosen. The subtraction of the two ions was m/z 162 (neutral loss glucose). The product ion $[M+H]^+$at m/z 431was ononin; the transition m/z 431→269 was chosen. The subtraction of the two ions was m/z 162 (neutral loss glucose). The product ion $[M+H]^+$at m/z 285 was claycosin. The product ion $[M+H]^+$ at m/z 439 was sec-o-glucosylhamaudol; the transition m/z 439→277 was chosen. The product ion $[M+H]^+$ at m/z 269 was formononetin (Fig. 4B–F). In conclusion, the five peaks were identified as calycosin-7-glucoside (I), ononin (II), claycosin (III), sec-o-glucosylhamaudol (IV) and formononetin (V) (Table 2).

2.4 Analysis of components in serum from YPFS-treated mice. Generally, the components of Chinese medicine need to be absorbed into the blood to exert their effects. Therefore, serum from YPFS-treated mice was analyzed to establish which components were present in blood. Three main peaks (a–c) were detectable in serum from YPFS-treated mice, as opposed to none in control serum (Fig. 4G). These peaks were also found in the fingerprint of YPFS. Retention time and UV spectrum of the three peaks in HPLC corresponded with the standard materials (Fig. 4H). In negative ion mode, the product ion $[M+H]^+$ at m/z 285 was claycosin (Fig. 4D). The product ion $[M+H]^+$ at m/z 285 was formononetin (Fig. 4F). The product ion $[M+H]^+$ at m/z 307 was cimifugin (Fig. 4I). Consequently, the major components in serum from YPFS-treated mice were claycosin, formononetin and cimifugin.

Among these components, claycosin and formononetin were both detected by 16HBE-HPLC-MS and analysis of serum from YPFS-treated mice. It is reasonable to speculate that these two compounds are the most likely to be active components in YPFS. Claycosin and formononetin were studied to explore further their effect on regulating TSLP and allergic inflammation.

3 Claycosin and formononetin are effective in regulating TSLP and attenuating allergic inflammation

3.1 Claycosin and formononetin reduced TSLP production at the initial stage of allergic inflammation *in vivo*. To verify the effects of these two compounds *in vivo*, a TSLP production model at the initial stage of allergic inflammation was utilized. Mice were treated once daily with formononetin and claycosin (0.5, 5 or 10 mg/kg, intraperitoneally) or vehicle 2 days before treatment with FITC, until day 3 of the model. After FITC treatment, mice exhibited increased TSLP production in the ears. TSLP levels in the ear homogenates were reduced markedly by formononetin (5 mg/kg) and claycosin (0.5, 5 and 10 mg/kg) (Fig. 5), which indicated that these two compounds could inhibit TSLP production in the initial stage of allergic inflammation.

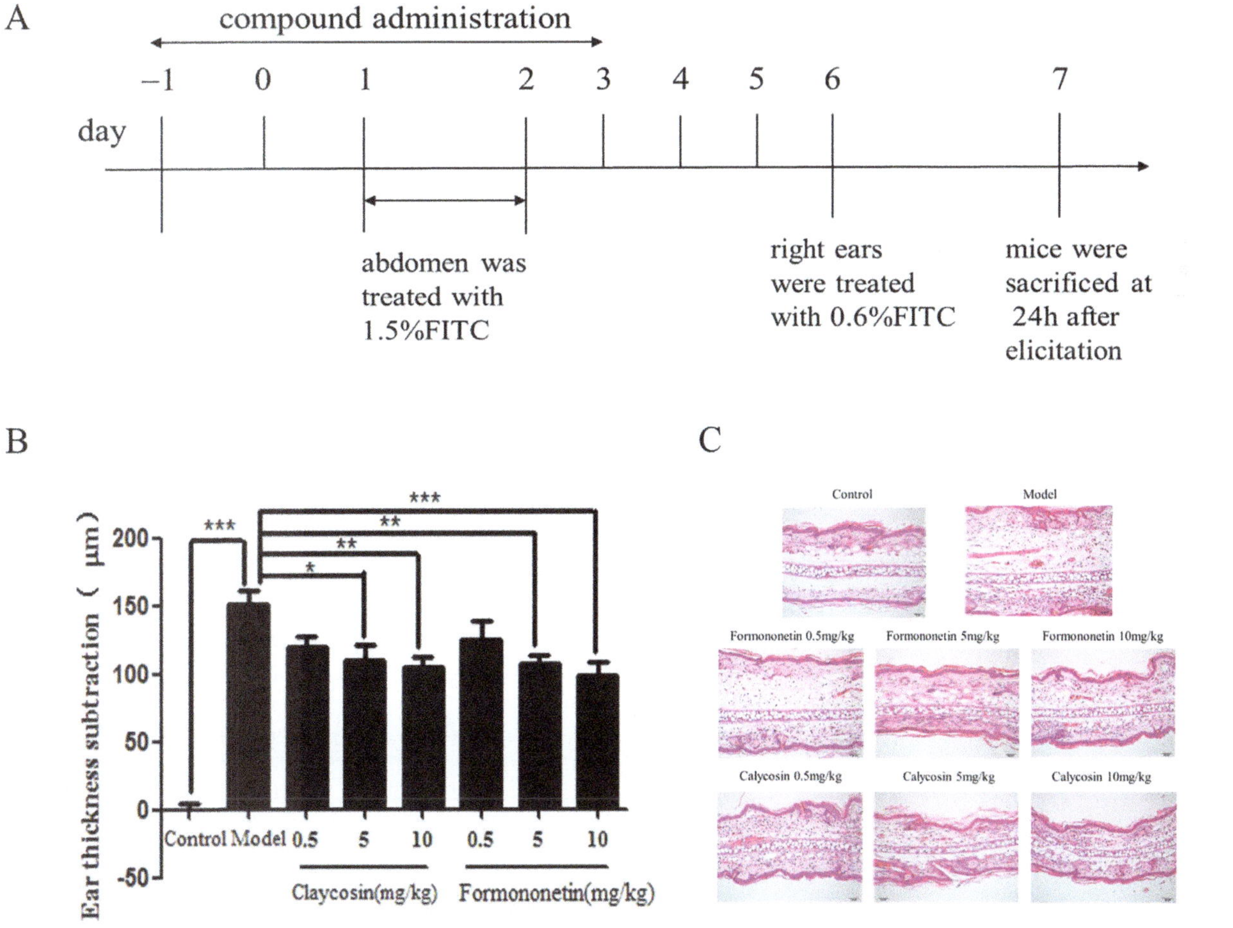

Figure 9. Effect of calycosin and formononetin administered at the initial stage of sensitization on ear thickness and histopathological changes in ACD mice. (A) Flow charts of compound administration in ACD murine model. (B) Effect of calycosin and formononetin on ear thickness. (mean±SD, n = 8, *p<0.05, **p<0.01, ***p<0.001). (B) Histopathological changes of dermatitis examined by H&E staining. All the experiments were performed in triplicates.

3.2 Claycosin and formononetin suppressed transcriptional activation of NF-κB induced by TNF-α *in vitro*. We explored whether claycosin and formononetin affected NF-κB signaling in 16HBE cells. After transfection with pNFκB-TA-luc plasmid, 16HBE cells were pretreated with different concentrations of claycosin or formononetin for 2 h or with culture medium as a control before TNF-α stimulation. NF-κB transcriptional activity was strongly induced after stimulation of transfected cells with TNF-α (100 ng/mL) for 1 h. The transcriptional activity of NF-κB was significantly reduced in cells treated with calycosin (1 and 10 μM) (Fig. 6A) and formononetin (10 μM) (Fig. 6B). The results indicated that calycosin and formononetin were able to inhibit NF-κB transcriptional activity, which might subsequently suppress the production of TSLP.

3.3 Claycosin and formononetin restricted NF-κB translocation *in vitro*. The above studies showed that claycosin and formononetin downregulated transcriptional activation of NF-κB *in vitro* and reduced TSLP production *in vivo*. However, it was unclear whether these two compounds affected nuclear translocation of NF-κB. Translocation of NF-κB was analyzed in 16HBE cells, which were pretreated with claycosin or formononetin for 2 h or with culture medium as a control before stimulation. After 1 h stimulation of the 16HBE cells with 100 ng/mL TNF-α, immunofluorescence revealed that NF-κB (p65) was predominantly present in the nucleus, compared to the control cells. Formononetin and claycosin at 0.1 μM partially inhibited translocation of NF-κB to the nucleus. More obviously, formononetin and claycosin at 1 and 10 μM significantly suppressed NF-κB nuclear translocation, wherein NF-κB (p65) was predominantly present in the cytosol (Fig. 7). Hence, formononetin and claycosin downregulation of TSLP expression might be due to blocking nuclear translocation of NF-κB.

3.4 Evaluation of claycosin and formononetin cytotoxicity in 16HBE cells. We studied the effect of claycosin and formononetin on cytotoxicity of 16HBE cells by modified MTT assay. 16HBE cells were incubated with different concentrations (0.1–100 μM) of these compounds for 12 and 24 h. Vehicle control groups were treated with DMSO (0.01%, v/v; Sigma) and control groups were treated with RPMI 1640. Claycosin and formononetin had no significant effect on 16HBE proliferation at 12 h (Fig. 8A) or 24 h (Fig. 8B). Thus, their effect on TSLP and NF-κB should not be attributed to cytotoxicity.

3.5 Allergic inflammation was attenuated by calycosin and formononetin administered only at the initial stage of sensitization. Calycosin and formononetin had a significant effect on TSLP at the initial stage of allergic inflammation in this study, and affected transcriptional activation and translocation of NF-κB. Nevertheless, are these effects sufficient to interfere with allergic inflammation? If yes, administering the compounds at the initial stage of the sensitization phase in the ACD model would suppress eventual inflammation.

Mice were treated once daily with calycosin (0.5, 5 or 10 mg/kg, intraperitoneally), formononetin (0.5, 5 or 10 mg/kg, intraperitoneally) or normal saline 2 days before sensitization until day 3 of the model (only administrated at initiation stage of sensitization phase, Fig. 9A). Ear thickness of ACD mice was significantly decreased by treatment with the two compounds (Fig. 9B). In terms of pathological changes, thickening of the epidermis and infiltration of inflammatory cells were evident compared with the normal ear in control mice. After treatment with calycosin and formononetin, the thickening of epidermis and infiltration of inflammatory cells were alleviated (Fig. 9C). These results indicated that the effects of calycosin and formononetin at the initial stage of sensitization are sufficient to suppress the eventual allergic inflammation in the ACD model.

Discussion

YPFS affected TCR and MHC class II expression on CD4$^+$ T cells in a mouse model of asthma, and regulated the balance of Th1/Th2 cells in murine allergic airway disease [6]. However, the relevant mechanism underlying these functions has not yet been identified. TSLP derived from ECs is a key allergic inflammation master switch [20,21,30], suggesting that it is the most important target interfering with the initial phase of allergic diseases [31–33]. Most studies have shown that epithelial cells are the main source of TSLP production [34–36]. These results directly confirm the link between TSLP and allergic inflammation. In this study, we reported that YPFS significantly inhibited TSLP production *in vivo* and serum from YPFS-treated mice decreased TSLP production *in vitro*, which indicated that regulating TSLP is the underlying mechanism of YPFS in reducing allergy relapse.

Although both clinical and experimental studies attest to the prophylactic and/or therapeutic efficacy of YPFS, the bioactive molecules have not yet been identified. Previous studies have suggested that purified YPFS polysaccharides have immunostimulatory activity and represent the active components of YPFS [37]. However, the molecules responsible for the immunosuppressive effect of YPFS have not been identified. The active molecules are inferred to interact with target cells, therefore, cell-based affinity purification and assay techniques have been used as a screener to capture the bioactive components in Chinese medicines. Our group has established the cell-binding methods to screen for the potential active components in Chinese medicine including hepatocyte [22,23] and erythrocyte [24] binding. Here, we used ECs to establish a method called 16HBE-HPLC-MS to capture the potential bioactive components. Five components were found to bind to 16HBE cells. They were identified as calycosin-7-glucoside, ononin, claycosin, sec-o-glucosylhamaudol and formononetin. We analyzed serum from YPFS-treated mice and three main components were detected. Claycosin and formononetin were both detected by 16HBE-HPLC-MS and in serum from YPFS-treated mice. This indicated that these two compounds were most likely to be the potential active components in YPFS.

There are some reports about the bioactivities of these compounds. Calycosin at low concentrations promotes the proliferation of MCF-7 cells and inhibits apoptosis [38]. Formononetin has estrogen-like effects in the body that improve dyslipidemia in high-fat diet rats [39], and inhibits migration and proliferation of vascular smooth muscle cells induced by platelet-derived growth factor BB [40]. However, these results had no direct relationship with inhibition of relapse of allergic diseases. Our data suggested that TSLP level in the ears was significantly reduced by claycosin and formononetin at the initial stage in a murine model of TSLP production. NF-κB signaling is essential for epithelial production of TSLP, thus, we assessed the transcriptional activity and translocation of NF-κB to explore the effect of these compounds. Calycosin and formononetin reduced the transcriptional activity of NF-κB and blocked its nuclear translocation. The results implied that these compounds might be active in inhibiting TSLP through regulating NF-κB, consequently contributing to the antiallergic effect of YPFS.

We found that claycosin and formononetin administered only at the initial stage of sensitization attenuated thickening of the epidermis and decreased infiltration of inflammatory cells in the ear of the ACD model. These results indicate that effects of calycosin and formononetin at the initial stage of sensitization are sufficient for suppression of allergic inflammation. Therefore, regulation of TSLP might be the mechanism for this effect on allergic inflammation. We will explore further the signaling pathway and the mechanisms of these detected components for regulating TSLP.

In summary, EC binding combined with HPLC-MS is a valid method for screening active components from complex mixtures of Chinese medicine. The compounds screened from YPFS alleviated allergic inflammation by inhibiting TSLP through regulating NF-κB activation and translocation. These components might have important implications for screening promising drugs in allergic diseases.

Acknowledgments

We thank Mengying Wu for assistance with HPLC-MS experiments and Xiaoyan Jiang for assistance with field experiments. We also thank reviewers for valuable input that improved the manuscript.

Author Contributions

Conceived and designed the experiments: MH DDS. Performed the experiments: DDS ZJZ HZW HLL XJX. Analyzed the data: DDS ZJZ XY HLL. Contributed reagents/materials/analysis tools: XJX ZJZ HWF GRJ DWW. Wrote the paper: DDS MH.

References

1. Zhang ZL, Yao BQ, Zhong L, Zang ZH (2009) Clincical effect observation of YPFS to cure 123 patients of allergic rhinitis. Liaoning Journal of Traditional Chinese Medicine 36: 937–938.
2. Sun ZL, Yang ZB (2009) Yuping Feng San plus and minus in treatment of chronic urticaria measles in 33 cases. Guiding Journal of Traditional Chinese Medicine and Pharmacy 15: 39–40.
3. Zeng WJ, Wang LJ (2008) Yupingfeng Powder Prescription in Treatment of Chronic Urticaria and Effects on Serum Levels of Interleukin- 4, Interferon-γand IgE. Chin J Dermato Venerol Integ Trad W Med 7: 16–18.
4. Sheng LX (2009) Discuss preventive and treatment thought of children asthma from theory "Treat Pre-disease". Zhejiang Chinese Medical University 33: 701–702.
5. Yuan XJ (2009) Professor Wang teachs the experience of treating children asthma in remission from asthenia of pulmonosplenic qi. Guiding Journal of Traditional Chinese Medicine and Pharmacy 15: 8–9.
6. Gu J, Jiang JJ, Shen CB, Lu L, Dai Q, et al. (2005) Effects of"Jude-Screen Powder"on Th1/Th2 Balance in Mice Model of Systemic Allergic Airway Disease. ShangHai Journal of Traditional Chinese Medicine 39: 50–52.
7. Shen CB, Gu J, Xia YJ, Cai H, Wang QE, et al. (2009) Effects of "Jade Screen Powder" on IL-17 and IL-6 in mice model of systemic allergic airway disease. ShangHai Journal of Traditional Chinese Medicine 43: 58–61.
8. Shao JH, Hong M, Niu Y, Yu LY, Liao XJ, et al. (2011) Yupingfeng San Inhibits Th2 Cell-mediated Allergic Contact Dermatitis in Mice. China Journal of Experimental Traditional Medical Formulae 17: 173–175.
9. Wang HZ, Hong M, Gui L, Hua YQ, Xu HQ (2013) Effect of Yupingfeng San against OVA-induced allergic asthma in mice. China Journal of Chinese Materia Medica 38: 1052–1055.
10. Brigadeau F, Gele P, Marquie C, Soudan B, Lacroix D (2005) Ventricular arrhythmias following exposure of failing hearts to oxidative stress in vitro. J Cardiovasc Electrophysiol 16: 629–636.
11. Wang ZJ, Huang TN (2003) The therapeutic effects on human simplex virus cutaneous infection of guniea pigs of various components in the root ofAstragalus membranaceus. Chin JMAP 20: 452–455.
12. Yesilada E, Bedir E, Calis I, Takaishi Y, Ohmoto Y (2005) Effects of triterpene saponins from Astragalus species on in vitro cytokine release. J Ethnopharmacol 96: 71–77.
13. Kong XF, Hu YL, Rong R, Wang DY, Li XR (2004) Effect of Chinese herbal medicinal ingredients on peripheral lymphocyte proliferation and serum antibody titer after vaccination in chicken. International Immunopharmacology 4: 975–982.
14. Tang DF, Hao YY, Liu ZY (1984) Constituents and antitumor effect of the Pingjiang Atractylodes rhizome volatile oil. Chinese Pharmaceutical Journal 19: 43–46.
15. Zhang Y, Liang HP (1995) The effect of astragalus Polysaccharides(APS) on cell mediated immunity(CMI) in burned mice. Chinese Pharmacological Bulletin 11: 136–138.
16. Zhang YZ, Qi J, Huang QF (1997) Effects of Xinmailing Solution on Amino Aeids and Caleium Tissue of the Endotoxic shock rat. Joumal of Beijing University of TCM 20: 39–40.
17. Tang XH (1998) Effects of Rhizoma Atractylodis Macrocephalae polysaccharide on immune function in mice Traditional Chinese Medicinal Research 11: 7–9.
18. Saenz SA, Taylor BC, Artis D (2008) Welcome to the neighborhood: epithelial cell-derived cytokines license innate and adaptive immune responses at mucosal sites. Immunological Reviews 226: 172–190.
19. Soumelis V, Liu YJ (2004) Human thymic stromal lymphopoietin: a novel epithelial cell-derived cytokine and a potential key player in the induction of allergic inflammation. Springer Semin Immunopathol 25: 325–333.
20. Soumelis V, Reche PA, Kanzler H, Yuan W, Edward G, et al. (2002) Human epithelial cells trigger dendritic cell mediated allergic inflammation by producing TSLP. Nat Immunol 3: 673–680.
21. Liu YJ (2006) Thymic stromal lymphopoietin: master switch for allergic infl ammation. The Journal of Experimental Medicine 203: 269–273.
22. Hong M, Ma HY, Wu XR, Hua YQ, Zhu Q, et al. (2008) Establishment of hepatocyte extraction combined with HPLC(HE-HPLC) and application in analysis of active components in the fruits of Gardenia jasminoides extract. China Journal of Chinese Materia Medic 34: 450–453.
23. Hong M, Ma HY, Wu XR, Hua YQ, Zhu Q, et al. (2012) A Method of Hepatocyte Extraction Conjugated with HPLC is Established for Screening Potential Active Components in Chinese Medicines – Probing Herba Artemisiae Scopariae as an Exemplifying Approach. Molecules: 1468–1482.
24. Dong ZB, Li SP, Hong M, Zhu Q (2005) Hypothesis of potential active components in Angelica sinensis by using biomembrane extraction and high performance liquid chromatography. Journal of Pharmaceutical and Biomedical Analysis 38: 664–669.
25. Li Y, Zhao J, Zhu Q (2007) Macrophage biospecific extraction and high performance liquid chromatography for hypothTSIs of immunological active components in Cordyceps sinensis. J Pharm and Biomed Anal 44: 439–443.
26. Fan HW, Zhu Q, Hong M, Yu L (2004) Analysis of Active Components in Mailuoning Injection by Platelet Membrane Immobilized Chromatography. Chinese Pharmaceutical Journal 41: 63–65.
27. Li YK (1999) Some problems of the experimental method for the China medicine serum pharmacology. Traditional Chinese Drug Research Clinical Pharmacology 10: 95–98.
28. Huang CH, Lu Y, Gao XJ, Sun ZG (2011) Advances of Serum Pharmacology of Chinese Medicine. Chinese Journal of Experimental Traditional Medical Formulae 17: 266–271.
29. Xiao WH, Han LJ (2008) Analysis ofHydrolysis Products of F lavone G lycosides ofRadix Astragali Using High Performance Liquid Chromatography-E lectrospray Ionization-Mass Spectrometry. Chinese Journal of Analytical Chemistry 36: 1399–1402.
30. Zhou B, Comeau MR, De ST (2005) Thymic stromal lymphopoietin as a key initiator of allergic airway inflammation in mice. Nat Immunol 6: 1047–1053.
31. Wang YH, Ito T, Homey B, Watanabe N, Martin R, et al. (2006) Maintenance and polarization of human TH2 central memory T cells by thymic stromal lymphopoietin-activated dendritic cells. Immunity 24: 827–838.
32. Hulse KE, Reefer AJ, Engelhard VH, Patrie JT, Ziegler SF, et al. (2010) Targeting allergen to FcgammaRI reveals a novel T(H)2 regulatory pathway linked to thymic stromal lymphopoietin receptor. J Allergy Clin Immunol 125: 247–256 e241–248.
33. Wang YH, Liu YJ (2007) OX40-OX40L interactions: a promising therapeutic target for allergic diseases? J Clin Invest 117: 3655–3657.
34. Zhang D, Cai SX, Zhao HJ, Liu LY (2010) Dimethylsulfoxide-induced expression of thymic stromal lymphopoietin in human bronchial epithelial cells. J South Med Univ 30: 963–965.
35. Comeau MR, Ziegler SF (2010) The influence of TSLP on the allergic response. Mucosal Immunol 3: 138–147.
36. Allakhverdi Z, Comeau MR, Jessup HK, Yoon BR, Brewer A, et al. (2007) Thymic stromal lymphopoietin is released by human epithelial cells in response to microbes, trauma, or inflammation and potently activates mast cells. J Exp Med 204: 253–258.
37. Chen XT, Li J, Wang HL, Cheng WM, Zhang L, et al. (2006) Immunomodulating effects of fractioned polysaccharides isolated from Yu-Ping-Feng-Powder in cyclophosphamide-treated mice. Am J Chin Med 34: 631–641.
38. Kuang WJ, Liu LT, Tan XS, Duan Y, Zhou LM (2011) Effect of calycosin on human breast cancer cell line MCF-7 in vitro. TUMOR 31: 789–793.
39. Xia DX, Gao ZL, Kuan CX (2009) Formononetin estrogen-like effect and lipid-related research. Chinese Journal of Gerontology 29: 2340–2342.
40. Sun L, Zhao R, Xin WY (2012) Formononetin inhibits Vascular Smooth Muscle Cells migration and proliferation induced by PDGF-BB Molecular Cardiology of China 3: 186–189.

Full Toxicity Assessment of Genkwa Flos and the Underlying Mechanism in Nematode *Caenorhabditis elegans*

Yan Qiao[1,2], Yunli Zhao[2], Qiuli Wu[2], Lingmei Sun[2], Qinli Ruan[1], Yanyan Chen[1], Meng Wang[1]*, Jinao Duan[1]*, Dayong Wang[2]*

1 Jiangsu Key Laboratory for High Technology Research of TCM Formulae, Nanjing University of Chinese Medicine, Nanjing, China, **2** Key Laboratory of Developmental Genes and Human Disease in Ministry of Education, Medical School of Southeast University, Nanjing, China

Abstract

Genkwa Flos (GF), the dried flower bud from *Daphne genkwa* Sieb. et Zucc. (Thymelaeaceae), is a well-known and widely used traditional Chinese medicine. However, we know little about the *in vivo* mechanism of GF toxicity. Nematode *Caenorhabditis elegans* has been considered as a useful toxicity assay system by offering a system best suited for asking the *in vivo* questions. In the present study, we employed the prolonged exposure assay system of *C. elegans* to perform the full *in vivo* toxicity assessment of raw-processed GF. Our data show that GF exposure could induce the toxicity on lifespan, development, reproduction, and locomotion behavior. GF exposure not only decreased body length but also induced the formation of abnormal vulva. The decrease in brood size in GF exposed nematodes appeared mainly at day-1 during the development of adult nematodes. The decrease of locomotion behavior in GF exposed nematodes might be due to the damage on development of D-type GABAergic motor neurons. Moreover, we observed the induction of intestinal reactive oxygen species (ROS) production and alteration of expression patterns of genes required for development of apical domain, microvilli, and apical junction of intestine in GF exposed nematodes, implying the possible dysfunction of the primary targeted organ. In addition, GF exposure induced increase in defecation cycle length and deficits in development of AVL and DVB neurons controlling the defecation behavior. Therefore, our study implies the usefulness of *C. elegans* assay system for toxicity assessment from a certain Chinese medicine or plant extract. The observed toxicity of GF might be the combinational effects of oxidative stress, dysfunction of intestine, and altered defecation behavior in nematodes.

Editor: Aamir Nazir, CSIR-Central Drug Research Institute, India

Funding: This work was supported by grants from National Basic Research Program of China (973 Program) (No. 2011CB505303), and National Natural Science Foundation of China (No. 81172698, 81202233, 81302814). The funders had no role in study design, data collection and analysis, decision to publish, or preparation of the manuscript.

Competing Interests: The authors have declared that no competing interests exist.

* E-mail: mengwang.drug@hotmail.com (MW); dja@njutcm.edu.cn (JD); dayongw@seu.edu.cn (DW)

These authors contributed equally to this work.

Introduction

Genkwa Flos (GF), the dried flower bud from *Daphne genkwa* Sieb. et Zucc. (Thymelaeaceae), is widely distributed in the regions of Yangtze River and Yellow River in China. GF is a well-known traditional Chinese medicine (TCM). GF has been used for the purposes of diuretic, antitussive, expectorant, abortifacient, and antitumor for centuries [1]. In GF, a series of compounds including flavonoids and daohne diterpene esters have been identified and isolated [2–3]. GF or compounds from GF can be potentially used for anti-inflammation, anti-complement, anti-melanogenesis, anti-virus, and anti-leukemia [4–8]. Moreover, because *Daphne genkwa* plants can be used as the effective remedy to treat various tumors [9], some compounds have also been isolated from *Daphne genkwa* plants because of their antitumor activity [10–15].

It has been commonly recognized that *Daphne genkwa* is a toxic shrub [15]. Previous study has investigated the cytotoxicity of compounds from *Daphne genkwa* with the aid of cancer cell lines [16]. The excessive or chronic application of GF also resulted in the hepatotoxicity on animals [17–18]. Recently, the toxicity of daphnane-type diterpenoids extracted from GF was further examined in rat with the aid of mortality and time to death as the toxicity assessment endpoints [19]. However, so far the toxicity information on GF is still very limited. Especially, we still know little about the *in vivo* mechanism for GF toxicity.

Free-living nematode *Caenorhabditis elegans*, a thoroughly studied model animal, has been considered as a useful alternative toxicity assay system for mammalians [20–22]. The experimental potential of *C. elegans* can offer a system best suited for asking the *in vivo* questions [20–22]. *C. elegans* has been used in both toxicity assessment and toxicological study for many toxicants including metals [23–36], organic pollutants [37–42], and engineered nanomaterials (ENMs) [43–53]. It has been proven that *C. elegans* can be further used for toxicological study of drugs [54–58]. Especially, several studies have been performed on the investigations on beneficial or adverse effects of components isolated from specific plants and beneficial effects of specific Chinese medicines with the aid of *C. elegans* as the assay system [59–66].

In the present study, we employed the *C. elegans* assay system to perform the full *in vivo* toxicity assessment of raw-processed GF. Moreover, we tried to examine the possible underlying mechanism for the GF toxicity in nematodes. Our data here will be helpful for our understanding the possible underlying *in vivo* mechanism of GF toxicity. In addition, our study further implies the usefulness of *C. elegans* assay system for the assessment of adverse effects from a certain Chinese medicine or plant extract.

Results

GF Exposure at the Examined Concentrations did not Induce Lethality of Nematodes

Considering the property of long-term application for Chinese medicines, we performed the prolonged exposure for toxicity assessment of GF in nematodes. Prolonged exposure was performed from L1-larvae to young adult (Fig. S1A). Concentrations selected for GF exposure were 0.12, 0.14, 0.16, 0.18, 0.2, 0.22, and 0.24 g/mL (Fig. S1B). After prolonged exposure to the examined concentrations of GF, we did not observe the lethality of nematodes (Fig. S1B), implying that GF at the examined concentrations may be not lethal to the exposed organisms.

Effects of GF Exposure on Lifespan of Nematodes

We further investigated the effects of GF exposure on lifespan of nematodes. Lifespan is an important endpoint to reflect the long-term effects of a specific toxicant. Prolonged exposure to 0.12–0.18 g/mL of GF did not significantly alter lifespan of nematodes (Fig. 1). In contrast, prolonged exposure to 0.24 g/mL of GF significantly reduced the lifespan of nematodes (Fig. 1).

Effects of GF Exposure on Development of Nematodes

To examine the effects of prolonged exposure to GF on development, we first investigated the body length in control and GF-exposed nematodes. Although prolonged exposure to 0.12 g/mL of GF did not noticeably influence the body length of nematodes, prolonged exposure to 0.18–0.24 g/mL of GF significantly reduced the body length of nematodes (Fig. 2A). Moreover, we observed that prolonged exposure to 0.18–0.24 g/mL of GF significantly induced the formation of abnormal vulva (Fig. 2B). Prolonged exposure to 0.12 g/mL of GF did not obviously affect the morphology of exposed nematodes (Fig. 2B). Compared with the control vulva having a slightly smooth surface, the abnormal vulva induced by GF exposure had a large protuberance (Fig. 2C).

Effects of GF Exposure on Reproduction of Nematodes

In nematodes, reproductive organ is one of the important secondary targeted organs for toxicants [22,67–69]. We further investigated the effects of prolonged exposure to GF on reproduction with the aid of brood size as the endpoint. Prolonged exposure to 0.12 g/mL of GF did not obviously influence the brood size of nematodes (Fig. 3A). In contrast, prolonged exposure to 0.18–0.24 g/mL of GF significantly reduced the brood size of nematodes (Fig. 3A). More interestingly, the decrease in brood size in GF exposed nematodes appeared mainly at day-1 during the development of adult nematodes (Fig. 3B). We did not observe the significant differences of brood size at day-2 or day-3 during the development of adult nematodes between control and GF exposure (Fig. 3B).

Effects of GF Exposure on Locomotion Behavior of Nematodes

In nematodes, neuron may be another secondary targeted organ for toxicants [22,42,51,70]. Previous studies have demonstrated that locomotion behavior is a relatively sensitive endpoint for toxicity assessment in nematodes [36,48,53]. We next investigated the effects of prolonged exposure to GF on locomotion behavior in nematodes. Prolonged exposure to all the examined concentrations of GF significantly decreased both head thrash and body bend of nematodes (Figs. 4A and 4B). Our data here further suggest the sensitivity of locomotion behavior for toxicity assessment in nematodes.

GF Exposure Affects the Development of D-type GABAergic Motor Neurons in Nematodes

In *C. elegans*, locomotion behavior is under the control of D-type GABAergic motor neurons [71]. Prolonged exposure to 0.24 g/mL of GF obviously influenced the development of D-type GABAergic motor neurons (Fig. 4C). The severe deficits in axon development were observed in 0.24 g/mL of GF exposed nematodes (Fig. 4C). Prolonged exposure to 0.24 g/mL of GF significantly decreased the fluorescent intensity of cell bodies for ventral cord D-type GABAergic motor neurons (Fig. 4D). Moreover, prolonged exposure to 0.24 g/mL of GF noticeably induced the neuronal loss and the gap formation on both ventral and dorsal cords of D-type GABAergic motor neurons (Figs. 4E and 4F). Thus, GF exposure can potentially cause damage on development of D-type GABAergic motor neurons in nematodes.

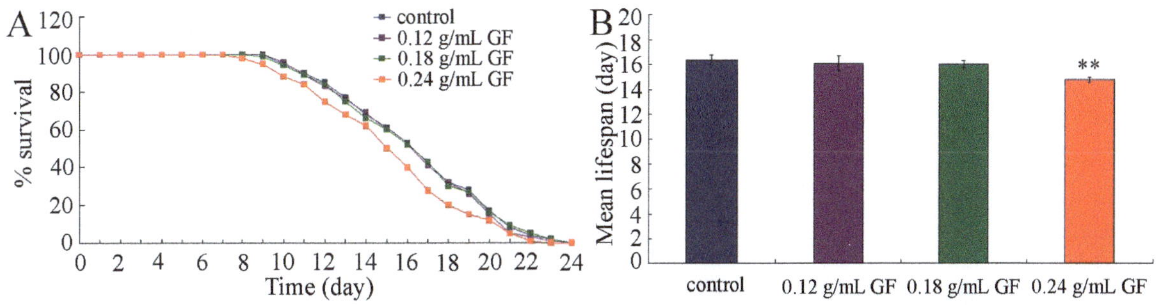

Figure 1. Comparison of lifespan in nematodes exposed to GF. (A) Lifespan curves of nematodes exposed to GF. (B) Comparison of mean lifespans in nematodes exposed to GF. Exposures were performed from L1-larvae to young adult. GF, Genkwa Flos. Bars represent means ± S.E.M. $^{**}p<0.01$.

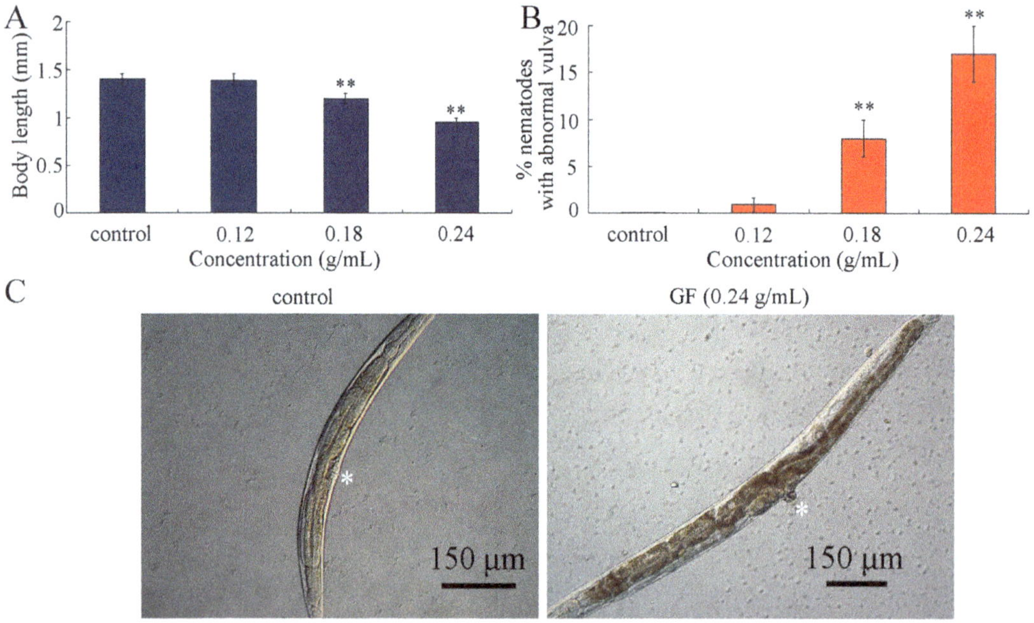

Figure 2. Effects of prolonged exposure to GF on development of nematodes. (A) Effects of GF exposure on body length. (B) Effects of GF exposure on percentage of nematodes with abnormal vulva. (C) Pictures showing the nematodes with abnormal vulva induced by GF. Asterisks show the positions of vulva. GF, Genkwa Flos. Exposures were performed from L1-larvae to young adult. Bars represent means ± S.E.M. ***p*<0.01.

Effects of GF Exposure on Intestinal Reactive Oxygen Species (ROS) Production in Nematodes

In nematodes, intestine is the primary targeted organ for toxicants [22,46,67–69,72]. Previous studies have implied that the functional state of intestinal barrier is required for nematodes to protect themselves from the damage of toxicants [67–69]. To examine the possible mechanism explaining the GF toxicity, we investigated the effects of prolonged exposure to GF on intestinal ROS production. After prolonged exposure, GF at concentrations of 0.12–0.24 g/mL significantly induced the intestinal ROS production (Figs. 5A and 5B), implying the damage from GF exposure on intestinal development in nematodes.

Alteration of Expression Patterns of Genes Required for Intestinal Development in Nematodes

Moreover, we found that prolonged exposure to 0.24 g/mL of GF significantly altered the expression patterns of some genes required for intestinal development in nematodes [73]. Although GF exposure did not influence the expression patterns of *vha-6*, *let-413*, *inx-3*, *abts-4*, *gem-4*, *egl-8*, *nhx-2*, *par-6*, *act-5*, *par-3*, *ifb-2*, and *nfm-1* genes, GF exposure significantly increased expression levels of *pkc-3*, *eps-8*, *pgp-3*, and *erm-1* genes and decreased expression levels of *ajm-1*, *lin-7*, *dlg-1*, *gtl-1*, *pgp-1*, *mtm-6*, and *opt-2* genes (Fig. 5C, Fig. S2). In *C. elegans*, *pkc-3* gene encodes an atypical protein kinase, *eps-8* gene encodes a homolog of mouse epidermal growth factor receptor kinase substrate, *pgp-1* and *pgp-3* genes encode transmembrane protein, *erm-1* gene encodes an ortholog of the ERM family of cytoskeletal linker, *ajm-1* gene encodes a member of the apical junction molecule class, *lin-7* gene encodes a protein containing a PDZ domain and an L27 domain, *dlg-1* gene encodes a MAGUK protein, *gtl-1* gene encodes a TRPM subfamily member of the TRP channel family, *mtm-6* gene encodes a myotubularin lipid phosphatase orthologous, and *opt-2* gene encodes a high-affinity, proton-coupled oligopeptide transporter (Table S1).

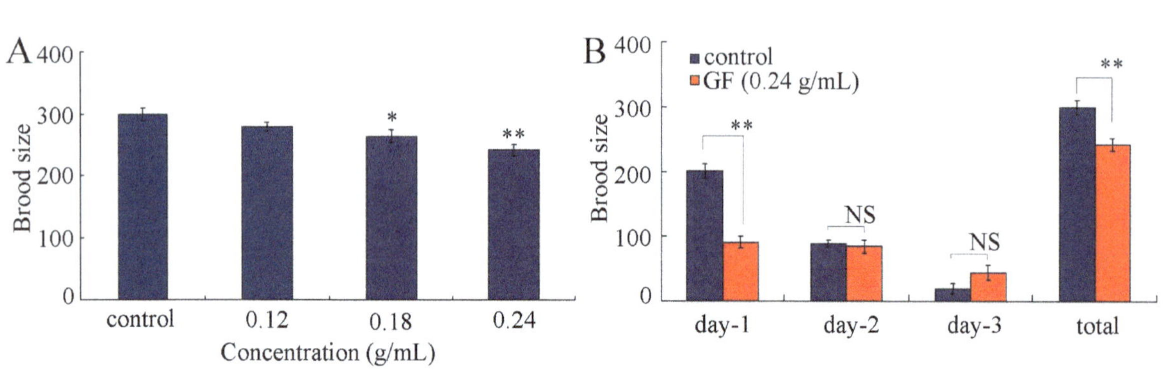

Figure 3. Effects of prolonged exposure to GF on reproduction of nematodes. (A) Effects of GF exposure on brood size of nematodes. (B) Effects of GF exposure on brood size of day-1, day-2 and day-3 adult nematodes. GF, Genkwa Flos. Exposures were performed from L1-larvae to young adult. Bars represent means ± S.E.M. NS, no significance. **p*<0.05, ***p*<0.01.

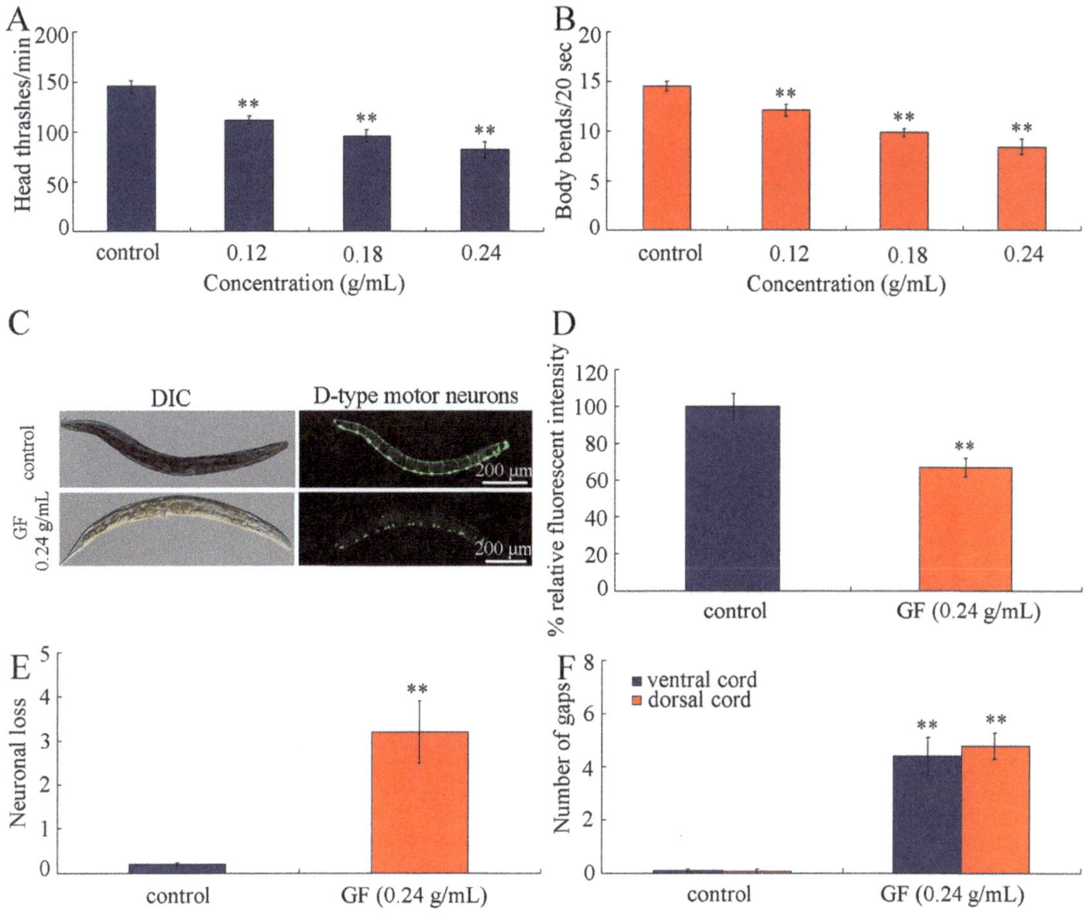

Figure 4. Effects of prolonged exposure to GF on locomotion behavior and development of D-type GABAergic motor neurons in nematodes. (A) Effects of GF exposure on head thrash. (B) Effects of GF exposure on body bend. (C) Effects of GF exposure on development of D-type GABAergic motor neurons. (D) Effects of GF exposure on relative fluorescent intensity of cell bodies at ventral cord of D-type GABAergic motor neurons. (E) Effects of GF exposure on neuronal loss of D-type GABAergic motor neurons. (F) Effects of GF exposure on gap formation on ventral or dorsal cord of D-type GABAergic motor neurons in nematodes. GF, Genkwa Flos. Exposures were performed from L1-larvae to young adult. Bars represent means ± S.E.M. $^{**}p<0.01$.

Effects of GF Exposure on Defecation Behavior in Nematodes

Besides the intestinal development, defecation behavior may also be an important regulator for toxicity formation of toxicants in nematodes [68]. We further investigated the effects of prolonged exposure to GF on defecation behavior with the aid of mean defecation cycle length as the assay endpoint. After prolonged exposure, GF at concentrations of 0.12–0.24 g/mL significantly increased the mean defecation cycle length (Fig. 6A), which implies the possible damage of GF on structures controlling defecation behavior or the difficulty of toxic components of GF to be excreted out of the body.

Damage of GF Exposure on Development of Neurons Controlling Defecation Behavior in Nematodes

In nematodes, the defecation behavior is controlled by both AVL neuron in head and DVB neuron in tail [52]. To determine whether GF exposure would cause damage on structures controlling defecation behavior, we examined the effects of prolonged exposure to GF on development of AVL and DVB neurons. After prolonged exposure, GF at the concentration of 0.24 g/mL significantly decreased the relative size of fluorescent puncta for both AVL neurons and DVB neurons in nematodes (Figs. 6B–6D). These results suggest that prolonged exposure to GF can result in the damage on neurons controlling the defecation behavior.

Molecular Basis for GF to Reduce the Lifespan in Nematodes

To determine whether certain genes playing key roles in detoxification are required for the control of GF toxicity, we examined the effects of mutations of *daf-16* [74], *skn-1* [75], or *mdt-15* [76] gene on GF toxicity formation in nematodes. With the aid of lifespan as the endpoint, interestingly, we found that the *daf-16(mu86)*, *skn-1(zu67)*, and *mdt-15(tm2182)* mutants had the susceptible property to the GF toxicity (Fig. 7). These data confirm the possible involvement of *daf-16*, *skn-1* and *mdt-15* mediated signaling pathways in regulating the GF toxicity formation.

Identification of Chemical Components in Raw-processed GF

Using the reverse phase high-performance liquid chromatography (RP-HPLC) method, we finally identified the possible

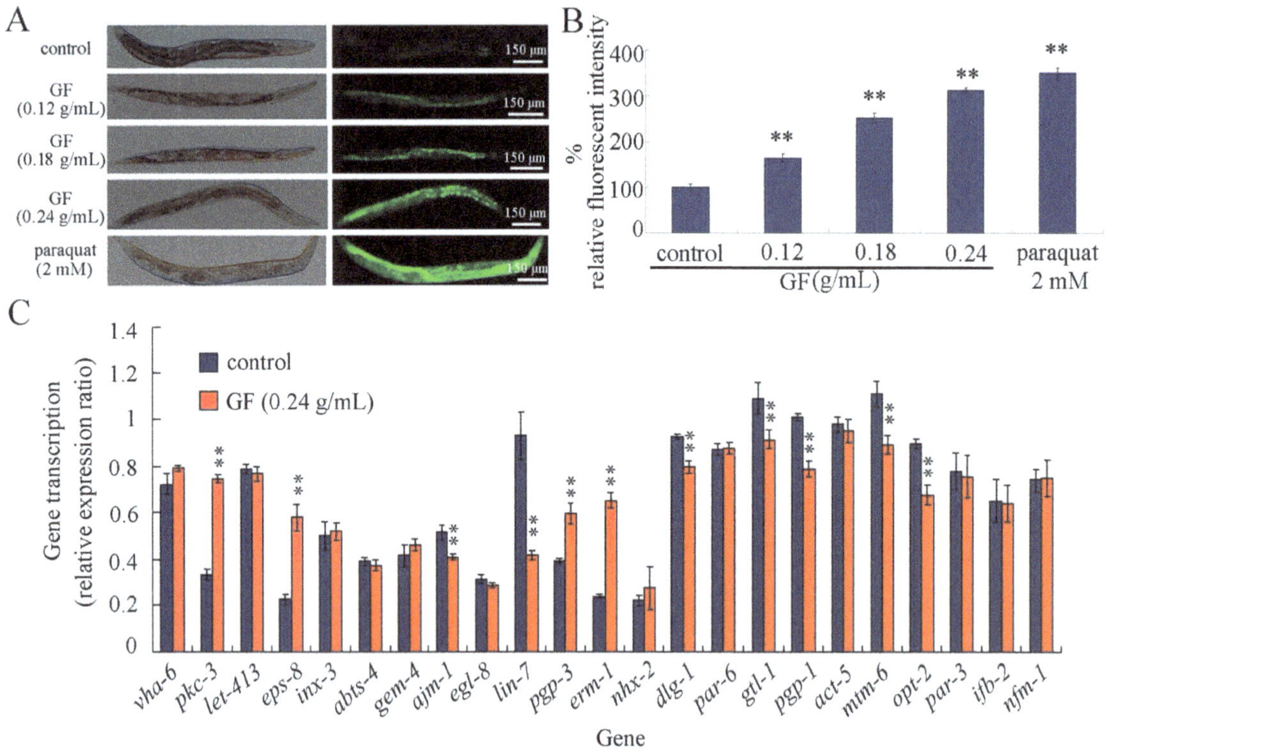

Figure 5. Effects of prolonged exposure to GF on intestinal development in nematodes. (A) Pictures showing the effects of GF exposure on intestinal ROS production. Paraquat (2 mM) treatment for 12-hr from L4-larvae was used as a positive control. Paraquat is a commonly used ROS-generator. (B) Comparison of intestinal ROS production between control and GF exposed nematodes. (C) Expression patterns of genes required for intestinal development in control and GF exposed nematodes. The results were expressed as the relative expression ratio between the targeted gene and the reference *tba-1* gene. GF, Genkwa Flos. Exposures were performed from L1-larvae to young adult. Bars represent means ± S.E.M. **$p<0.01$.

chemical components in our prepared GF solution. Based on the chromatographic fingerprint, the prepared GF solution contained the chemical components of luteolin-5-O-β-D-glucoside, apigenin-5-O-β-D-glucoside, genkwanin-5-O-β-D-primeveroside, genkwa-

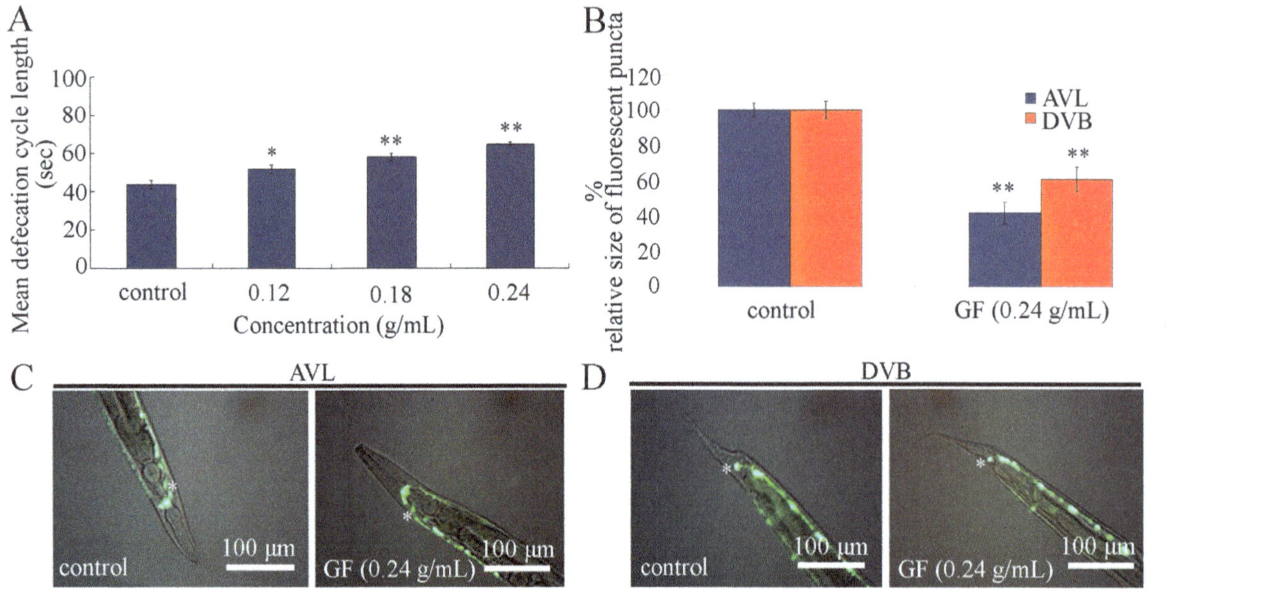

Figure 6. Effects of prolonged exposure to GF on defecation behavior and development of neurons controlling defecation behavior in nematodes. (A) Effects of GF exposure on mean defecation cycle length. (B) Effects of GF exposure on relative size of fluorescent puncta of AVL or DVB neurons. (C) Effects of GF exposure on development of AVL neurons. (D) Effects of GF exposure on development of DVB neurons. GF, Genkwa Flos. Exposures were performed from L1-larvae to young adult. Bars represent means ± S.E.M. *$p<0.05$, **$p<0.01$.

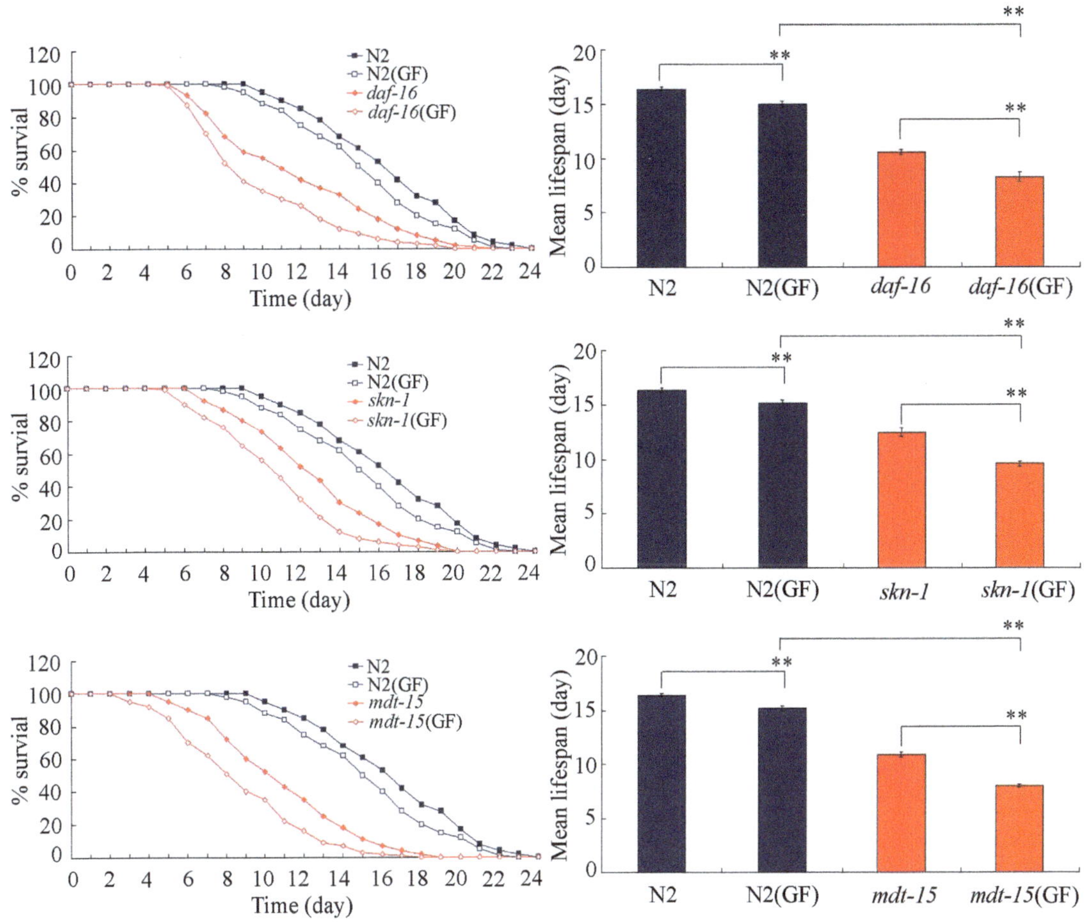

Figure 7. Comparison of lifespan in wild-type and mutant nematodes exposed to GF. GF, Genkwa Flos. Exposures were performed from L1-larvae to young adult. Bars represent means ± S.E.M. ** $p<0.01$.

nin-5-O-β-D-glucoside, genkwanin-4′-O-β-D- lutinoside, apigenin, 3′-hydroxygenkwanin, and genkwanin, and some other still unknown compounds (Fig. 8).

Discussion

Previous studies have demonstrated that *C. elegans* can be used for toxicity assessment of metals [23–36], organic pollutants [37–42], ENMs [43–53], or specific components extracted from plants [62]. In this study, our data further imply that *C. elegans* can be used for toxicity assessment of specific Chinese medicines or plant

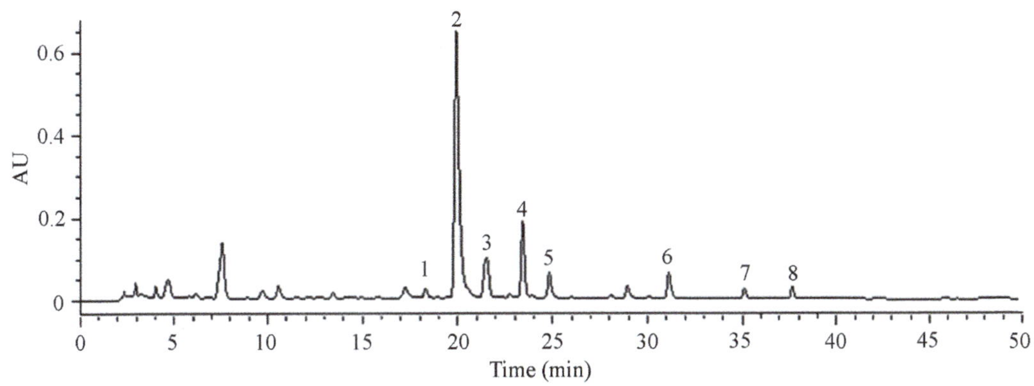

Figure 8. Chemical components in GF analyzed by HPLC. 1, luteolin-5-O-β-D-glucoside; 2, apigenin-5-O-β-D-glucoside, 3, genkwanin-5-O-β-D-primeveroside; 4, genkwanin-5-O-β-D-glucoside; 5, genkwanin-4′-O-β-D- lutinoside; 6, apigenin; 7, 3′-hydroxygenkwanin; 8, genkwanin. GF, Genkwa Flos.

extracts. Thus, *C. elegans* can be used for evaluation of both the beneficial effects [59–61,63–66] and the adverse effects of specific Chinese medicines or plant extracts. Because most of the Chinese medicines or plant extracts still lack the detailed toxicity data, *C. elegans* will serve as a rapid and systematic assay system for toxicity assessment of specific Chinese medicines or plant extracts.

In the present study, we performed the full assessment of GF toxicity utilizing the *in vivo C. elegans* assay system. Considering the property of long-term application for GF in clinical, we performed the prolonged exposure from L1-larvae to young adult for toxicity assessment of GF. L1-larvae may be more sensitive than adults for toxicity evaluation in nematodes [25,77]. Our data demonstrate that prolonged exposure to GF could induce the toxicity on lifespan, development, reproduction and locomotion behavior (Figs. 1–4). Especially, GF exposure induced the formation of abnormal vulva (Fig. 2C). Such a deficit was also observed in heavy metal exposed nematodes [33,78], which suggests that the induction of abnormal vulva may be a common phenotype for adverse effects of toxicants on nematodes.

For the mechanism explaining the GF toxicity, we raised several possibilities. One of the possibilities is the induction of structural deficits caused by GF exposure. For the decrease in locomotion behavior in GF exposed nematodes, we found that prolonged exposure to GF caused the damage on development of D-type GABAergic motor neurons (Figs. 4C–4F), which specially function in the control of locomotion behavior. The second possibility is that prolonged exposure to GF may result in the damage on intestinal development. We observed the severe induction of intestinal ROS production (Figs. 5A–5B) and alteration of expression patterns of some genes required for the intestinal development (Fig. 5C). In *C. elegans*, *mtm-6*, *pkc-3*, *pgp-1*, *opt-2*, *pgp-3*, and *gtl-1* genes are required for the development of apical domain of intestine, *erm-1* and *eps-8* are required for the microvilli development, and *ajm-1*, *dlg-1*, and *lin-7* genes are required for the development of apical junction of intestine [73]. These data suggest that GF exposure may at least result in the damage on development of apical domain, microvilli, and apical junction of intestine in nematodes. In addition, these data may also imply that the response of intestinal development and function may serve as an important physiological basis for the possible adaptation of nematodes to GF. The third possibility is that GF exposure induced the increase in mean defecation cycle length, which may in turn cause the deficits in AVL and DVB neurons controlling defecation behavior and the difficulty of excretion of GF out of the body in nematodes. Moreover, the phenotypic analysis of *daf-16*, *skn-1*, and *mdt-15* mutants suggests that at least *daf-16*, *skn-1*, and *mdt-15* mediated signaling pathways may function as the important molecular basis for the control of GF toxicity in nematodes. Therefore, the toxicity of GF is possibly the combinational effects of oxidative stress, dysfunction of intestine, and altered defecation behavior.

Our data here suggest the potential adverse effects of GF on nematodes after prolonged exposure. These results will be helpful for our understanding and attention of the careful use of this drug in clinical. At least based on our data, the duration, dose, and developmental stage of patients should be carefully considered before use of this drug. Meanwhile, some strategies, such as modulation of the processing procedure, can be also designed and considered to reduce the possible adverse effects from GF.

In the present study, the raw-processed GF was extracted after boiling treatment. During this extraction process, some possible thermolabile molecules having the bioactivity may be broken down. Therefore, the data provided here may be not able to reflect the possible biological effects of those possible thermolabile molecules in GF. Moreover, the GF can be extracted with different strategies. Besides the water boiling, the ethanolic extraction can also be used for GF preparation. The chemical components in raw-processed GF solutions prepared with different extraction strategies may be somewhat different, which implies that the obtained data here may be not able to completely reflect the biological effects of raw-processed GF solutions prepared with the other extraction strategies on nematodes.

In conclusion, with the Chinese medicine of GF as a sample, our data here provide the evidence to indicate the value of *C. elegans* assay system for the *in vivo* toxicity assessment of specific Chinese medicines or plant extracts. After prolonged exposure, GF induced multiple toxicities on nematodes, which may be due to the combinational effects of several mechanisms including oxidative stress, intestinal dysfunction, and abnormal defecation behavior. In the prepared GF solution, many chemical components may exist. In the future, examination of the beneficial or adverse effects of specific chemical components in GF will be further helpful for our understanding and controlling the toxicity formation and the clinical use of this drug.

Materials and Methods

Plant Materials and Chemicals

The dried flower buds of *Daphne* genkwa Sieb et Zucc. were collected from Liuan city, Anhui province, China. No specific permissions were required for the location/activity to collect the plants, because the location does not belong to any national park or protected area of land or sea. We also confirm that the field did not involve endangered behavior to the protected species. The flower buds were authenticated, and the voucher specimen (No. 110326) has been deposited at the Herbarium in Jiangsu Key Laboratory for High Technology Research of Traditional Chinese Medicine Formulae, Nanjing University of Chinese Medicine. The raw-processed GF (24 g) was decocted 2 times with 240 mL of boiling distilled water for 2-hr. The decocted suspensions were filtered, collected, and concentrated by decompressive rotary evaporation. The prepared solutions were stored at $-20°C$ before use. The prepared raw-processed GF can be directly used in the clinical. All the other chemicals were obtained from Sigma-Aldrich (St. Louis, MO, USA).

Strain Preparation

Nematodes used in the present study were wild-type N2, mutants of *daf-16(mu86)*, *skn-1(zu67)*, and *mdt-15(tm2182)*, and transgenic strain of *oxIs12*[Ex(P*unc-47::GFP*)], originally obtained from *Caenorhabditis* Genetics Center. They were maintained on nematode growth medium (NGM) plates seeded with *Escherichia coli* OP50 at 20°C as described [79]. Age synchronous populations of L1- or L4-larvae were obtained as described previously [80]. Exposures were performed from L1-larvae to young adult in 12-well sterile tissue culture plates at 20°C in the presence of food. Exposed nematodes were used for toxicity assessment of GF with lethality, lifespan, growth, brood size, locomotion behavior, defecation, and intestinal ROS production as the endpoints.

Lethality and Growth

For lethality assay, a 1.0 mL aliquot of test solution was added to each well of tissue culture plate, which was subsequently loaded with 50 nematodes for each treatment. Following exposure, wells were observed under a dissecting microscopy, where inactive ones were scored. Nematodes were judged to be dead if they did not respond to stimulus using a small, metal wire.

Growth was assessed by the body length, which was determined by measuring flat surface area of nematodes using Image-Pro® Express software. Twenty nematodes were examined per treatment.

Lifespan Assay

In the test, the hermaphrodites were transferred daily for the first 4 days of adulthood. Nematodes were checked every day and would be scored as dead when they did not move even after repeated taps with a pick. Thirty nematodes were examined per treatment. For lifespan, graphs are representative of three trials.

Reproduction and Locomotion Behavior

Reproduction was assessed by the brood size. To assay brood size, the number of offspring at all stages beyond the egg was counted. Twenty nematodes were examined per treatment.

Locomotion behavior was evaluated by both the head thrash and the body bend. To assay head thrash, the examined nematodes were washed with K medium, and transferred into a microtiter well containing 60 μL of K medium on the top of agar. After a 1-min recovery period, head thrash, defined as a change in the direction of bending at the mid body, was counted for 1-min. To assay body bend, the examined nematodes were picked onto a second plate and scored for the number of body bends in an interval of 20-sec. A body bend was counted as a change in the direction of the part of nematodes corresponding to the posterior bulb of the pharynx along the *y*-axis, assuming that nematode was traveling along the *x*-axis. Thirty nematodes were examined per treatment.

Defecation

To assay mean defecation cycle length, individual animal was examined for a fixed number of cycles, and a cycle period was defined as the interval between initiations of two successive posterior body-wall muscle contraction steps. Thirty nematodes were examined per treatment.

Intestinal ROS Production

The examined nematodes were transferred to 1 mL of M9 buffer containing 1 μM 5′,6′-chloromethyl-2′,7′dichlorodihydro-fluorescein diacetate (CM-H_2DCFDA; Molecular Probes) in 12-well sterile tissue culture plates to pre-incubate for 3-hr at 20°C in the dark. CM-H_2DCFDA can specially detect the presence of various intracellular produced ROS species. The intracellular ROS can oxidate the H_2DCF without fluorescence to generate the DCF with green fluorescence. The nematodes were then mounted on 2% agar pads for examination with a laser scanning confocal microscope (Leica, TCS SP2, Bensheim, Germany) at 488 nm of excitation wavelength and 510 nm of emission filter. The relative fluorescent intensities of intestines were semi-quantified, and the semiquantified ROS was expressed as relative fluorescent units (RFU). Twenty nematodes were examined per treatment.

Quantitative Real-time Polymerase Chain Reaction (PCR)

Total RNA was extracted using RNeasy Mini Kit (Qiagen). Total nematode RNA (~1 μg) was reverse-transcribed using cDNA synthesis kit (Bio-Rad Laboratories). Quantitative reverse transcription PCR was run at the optimized annealing temperature of 58°C. The relative quantification of targeted genes in comparison to the reference *tba-1* gene encoding the tubulin protein or *act-1* gene encoding the actin protein was determined. The final results were expressed as the relative expression ratio (between targeted gene and reference gene). The designed primers for targeted genes and reference *tba-1* or *act-1* gene were shown in Table S2.

Analysis of the Axonal Degeneration and Neuronal Loss of D-type GABAergic Motor Neurons

The method was performed as described [81]. D-type GABAergic motor neurons were visualized using a transgenic strain of *oxIs12* [82]. Gap numbers of ventral or dorsal cord were quantified to reflect the axonal degeneration. Neuronal loss was examined by counting the number of cell bodies in D-type GABAergic nervous system. Images were photographed and examined on the same day to avoid effects of light source variance on fluorescent intensity. Thirty nematodes were examined per treatment.

Fluorescent Images of Neurons Controlling Defecation Behavior

The fluorescent images of AVL and DVB neurons controlling defecation behavior were captured with a Zeiss Axiocam MRm camera on a Zeiss Axioplan 2 Imaging System using SlideBook software (Intelligent Imaging Innovations). Images were acquired with a Quantix cooled charge-coupled device (CCD) camera, and illumination was provided by a 175 W xenon arc lamp and GFP filter sets. The relative sizes of fluorescent puncta for cell bodies of AVL and DVB neurons were measured as the maximum radius for assayed fluorescent puncta. Twenty nematodes were examined per treatment.

Analysis of Chemical Components of Raw-processed GF

Before analysis of chemical components of GF, we added 600 μL methanol to 200 μL prepared GF, and then the suspensions were centrifugated for 10-min at 13000 rpm. The RP-HPLC method was applied to establish the chromatographic fingerprint. The separation was performed on a Elite C18 column with a mobile phase composed of methanol (A) and 0.25% acetic acid (B). Gradient elution condition was 0-min, 20% (A); 30-min, 60% (A); 45-min, 100% (A); and 50-min, 20% (A). The column temperature was set at 30°C and the flow rate was 1.0 mL/min. The detective wavelength was set at 260 nm. The injection volume was 10 μL. According to the HPLC data, the main components of prepared GF were determined.

Statistical Analysis

All data in this article were expressed as means ± standard error of the mean (S.E.M.). Graphs were generated using Microsoft Excel (Microsoft Corp., Redmond, WA). Statistical analysis was performed using SPSS 12.0 (SPSS Inc., Chicago, USA). Differences between groups were determined using analysis of variance (ANOVA). Probability levels of 0.05 and 0.01 were considered statistically significant.

Supporting Information

Figure S1 Prolonged exposure to GF did not induce lethality in nematodes. (A) Schematic drawing showing the prolonged exposure to GF. (B) Effects of GF exposure on lethality. GF, Genkwa Flos. Exposures were performed from L1-larvae to young adult. Bars represent means ± S.E.M.
(DOC)

Figure S2 Expression patterns of genes required for intestinal development in control and GF exposed nematodes. The results were expressed as the relative expression ratio between the targeted gene and the reference *act-1* gene. GF,

Genkwa Flos. Exposures were performed from L1-larvae to young adult. Bars represent means ± S.E.M. **$p<0.01$.
(DOC)

Table S1 Information on genes required for intestinal development in *C. elegans*.
(DOC)

Table S2 Primers used for quantitative real-time polymerase chain reaction (PCR).
(DOC)

Author Contributions

Conceived and designed the experiments: MW JD DW. Performed the experiments: YQ YZ QW LS QR YC. Analyzed the data: QR YC. Contributed reagents/materials/analysis tools: MW JD. Wrote the paper: DW.

References

1. Jiangsu New Medical College (1985) The encyclopedia of traditional Chinese medicine. 2nd ed., Shanghai Science and Technology Press, Shanghai.
2. Wang R, Li J, Qi H, Shi Y (2013) Two new tigliane diterpene esters from the flower buds of *Daphne genkwa*. J Asian Nat Produt Res 15: 502–506.
3. Xie H, Liang Y, Ito Y, Wang X, Chen R, et al. (2011) Preperative isolation and purification of four flavonoids from *Daphne genkwa* Sieb. et Zucc. by high-speed countercurrent chromatography. J Liq Chromatogr Relat Technol 34: 2360–2372.
4. Lee M, Yuk J, Kwon O, Oh S, Lee H, et al. (2012) Zuonin B inhibits lipopolysaccharide-induced inflammation via downregulation of the ERK1/2 and JNK pathways in RAW264.7 macrophages. Evid-Based Compl Alt Med 2012: 728196.
5. Park B, Min B, Oh S, Kim J, Bae K, et al. (2006) Isolation of flavonoids, a biscoumarin and an amide from the flower buds of *Daphne genkwa* and the evaluation of their anti-complement activity. Phytother Res 20: 610–613.
6. Bang KK, Yun C, Lee C, Jin Q, Lee JW, et al. (2013) Melanogenesis inhibitory daphnane diterpenoids from the flower buds of *Daphne genkwa*. Bioorg Med Chem Lett 23: 3334–3337.
7. Chang C, Leu Y, Horng J (2012) *Daphne genkwa* Sieb. et Zucc. water-soluble extracts act on enterovirus 71 by inhibiting viral entry. Viruses 4: 539–556.
8. Park B, Oh S, Ahn K, Kwon O, Lee H (2008) (-)-syringaresinol inhibits proliferation of human promyelocytic HL-60 leukemia cells via G1 arrest and apoptosis. Int Immunopharmacol 8: 967–973.
9. Yang CL (1993) Toxic herbal medicine. Traditional Chinese Medicine Press, Beijing.
10. Zhang S, Li X, Zhang F, Yang P, Gao X, et al. (2006) Preparation of yuanhuacine and relative diterpene esters from *Daphne genkwa* and structure-activity relationship of potent inhibitory activity against DNA topoisomerase I. Bioorg Med Chem 14: 3888–3895.
11. Zheng W, Gao X, Chen C, Tan R (2007) Total flavonoids of *Daphne genkwa* root significantly inhibit the growth and metastasis of Lewis lung carcinoma in C57BL6 mice. Int Immunopharmacol 7: 117–127.
12. Zheng W, Gao X, Gu Q, Chen C, Wei Z, et al. (2007) Antitumor activity of daphnodorins from *Daphne genkwa* roots. Int Immunopharmacol 7: 128–134.
13. Hong J, Nam J, Seo E, Lee S (2010) Daphnane diterpene esters with anti-proliferative activities against human lung cancer cells from *Daphne genkwa*. Chem Pharm Bull 58: 234–237.
14. Hong J, Chung H, Lee H, Park H, Lee S (2011) Growth inhibition of human lung cancer cells via down-regulation of epidermal growth factor receptor signaling by Yuanhuadine, a daphnane diterpene from *Daphne genkwa*. J Nat Prod 74: 2102–2108.
15. Li F, Sun Q, Hong L, Li L, Wu Y, et al. (2013) Daphnane-type diterpenes with inhibitory activities against human cancer cell lines from *Daphne genkwa*. Bioorg Med Chem Lett 23: 2500–2504.
16. Zhan Z, Fan C, Ding J, Yue J (2005) Novel diterpenoids with potent inhibitory activity against endothelium cell HMEC and cytotoxic activities from a well-known TCM plant *Daphne genkwa*. Biorag Med Chem 13: 645–655.
17. Geng L, Ma C, Zhang L, Yang G, Cui Y, et al. (2013) Metabonomic study of Genkwa Flos-induced hepatotoxicity and effect of herb-processing procedure on toxicity. Phytother Res 27: 521–529.
18. Li Z, Li Q, Geng L, Chen X, Bi K (2013) Use of the local false discovery rate for identififcation of metabolic biomarkers in rat urine following Genkwa Flos-induced hepatotoxicity. PLoS ONE 8: e67451.
19. Chen Y, Guo J, Qian Y, Guo S, Ma C, et al. (2013) Toxicity of daphnane-type diterpenoids from Genkwa Flos and their pharmacokinetic profile in rat. Phytomedicine 21: 82–89.
20. Leung MCK, Williams PL, Benedetto A, Au C, Helmcke KJ, et al. (2008) *Caenorhabditis elegans*: an emerging model in biomedical and environmental toxicology. Toxicol Sci 106: 5–28.
21. Zhao Y-L, Wang D-Y (2012) Formation and regulation of adaptive response in nematode *Caenorhabditis elegans*. Oxid Med Cell Longev 2012: 564093.
22. ZhaoY-L, Wu Q-L, Li Y-P, Wang D-Y (2013) Translocation, transfer, and *in vivo* safety evaluation of engineered nanomaterials in the non-mammalian alternative toxicity assay model of nematode *Caenorhabditis elegans*. RSC Adv 3: 5741–5757.
23. Hu Y-O, Wang Y, Ye B-P, Wang D-Y (2008) Phenotypic and behavioral defects induced by iron exposure can be transferred to progeny in *Caenorhabditis elegans*. Biomed Environ Sci 21: 467–473.
24. Xing X-J, Du M, Zhang Y-F, Wang D-Y (2009) Adverse effects of metal exposure on chemotaxis towards water-soluble attractants regulated mainly by ASE sensory neuron in nematode *Caenorhabditis elegans*. J Environ Sci 21: 1684–1694.
25. Xing X-J, Wang D-Y (2009) The lethality toxicities induced by metal exposure during development in nematode *Caenorhabditis elegans*. Bull Environ Contam Toxicol 83: 530–536.
26. Wang D-Y, Xing X-J (2009) Pre-treatment with mild metal exposure suppresses the neurotoxicity on locomotion behavior induced by the subsequent severe metal exposure in *Caenorhabditis elegans*. Environ Toxicol Pharmacol 28: 459–464.
27. Helmcke KJ, Syversen T, Miller III DM, Aschner M (2009) Characterization of the effects of methylmercury on *Caenorhabditis elegans*. Toxicol Appl Pharmacol 240: 265–272.
28. Wang S, Wu L, Wang Y, Luo X, Lu Y (2009) Copper-induced germline apoptosis in *Caenorhabditis elegans*: the independent roles of DNA damage response signaling and the dependent roles of MAPK cascades. Chemico-Biol Interactions 180: 151–157.
29. Wang D-Y, Xing X-J (2010) Pre-treatment with mild UV irradiation suppresses reproductive toxicity induced by subsequent cadmium exposure in nematodes. Ecotoxicol Environ Safety 73: 423–429.
30. Wang D-Y, Liu P-D, Yang Y-C, Shen L-L (2010) Formation of combined Ca/Cd toxicity on lifespan of nematode *Caenorhabditis elegans*. Ecotoxicol Environ Safety 73: 1221–1230.
31. Zeitoun-Ghandour S, Charnock JM, Hodson ME, Leszczyszyn OI, Blindauer CA, et al. (2010) The two *Caenorhabditis elegans* metallothioneins (CeMT-1 and CeMT-2) discriminate between essential zinc and toxic cadmium. FEBS J 277: 2531–2542.
32. Zhang H, He X, Bai W, Guo X, Zhang Z, et al. (2010) Ecotoxicological assessment of lanthanum with *Caenorhabditis elegans* in liquid medium. Metallomics 2: 806–810.
33. Wu Q-L, He K-W, Liu P-D, Li Y-X, Wang D-Y (2011) Association of oxidative stress with the formation of reproductive toxicity from mercury exposure on hermaphrodite nematode *Caenorhabditis elegans*. Environ Toxicol Pharmacol 32: 175–184.
34. Jiang B, Ren C, Li Y, Lu Y, Li W, et al. (2011) Sodium sulfite is a potential hypoxia inducer that mimics hypoxic stress in *Caenorhabditis elegans*. J Biol Inorg Chem 16: 267–274.
35. Liu P-D, He K-W, Li Y-X, Wu Q-L, Yang P, et al. (2012) Exposure to mercury causes formation of male-specific structural deficits by inducing oxidative damage in nematodes. Ecotoxicol Environ Safety 79: 90–100.
36. Wu Q-L, Qu Y-Y, Li X, Wang D-Y (2012) Chromium exhibits adverse effects at environmental relevant concentrations in chronic toxicity assay system of nematode *Caenorhabditis elegans*. Chemosphere 87: 1281–1287.
37. Li Y-H, Ye H-Y, Du M, Zhang Y-F, Ye B-P, et al. (2009) Induction of chemotaxis to sodium chloride and diacetyl and thermotaxis defects by microcystin-LR exposure in nematode *Caenorhabditis elegans*. J Environ Sci 21: 971–979.
38. Ruan Q-L, Ju J-J, Li Y-H, Liu R, Pu Y-P, et al. (2009) Evaluation of pesticide toxicities with differing mechanisms using *Caenorhabditis elegans*. J Toxicol Environ Health A 72: 746–751.
39. Boyd WA, Smith MV, Kissling GE, Rice JR, Snyder DW, et al. (2009) Application of mathematical model to describe the effects of chlorpyrifos on *Caenorhabditis elegans* development. PLoS ONE 4: e7024.
40. Allard P, Colaiacovo MP (2010) Bisphenol A impairs the double-strand break repair machinery in the germline and causes chromosome abnormalities. Proc Natl Acad Sci USA 107: 20405–20410.
41. Ruan Q-L, Ju J-J, Li Y-H, Li X-B, Liu R, et al. (2012) Chlorpyrifos exposure reduces reproductive capacity owing to a damaging effect on gametogenesis in the nematode *Caenorhabditis elegans*. J Appl Toxicol 32: 527–535.
42. Ju J-J, Ruan Q-L, Li X-B, Liu R, Li Y-H, et al. (2013) Neurotoxicological evaluation of microcystin-LR exposure at environmental relevant concentrations on nematode *Caenorhabditis elegans*. Environ Sci Pollut Res 20: 1823–1830.
43. Ma H, Bertsch PM, Glenn TC, Kabengi NJ, Williams PL (2009) Toxicity of manufactured zinc oxide nanoparticles in the nematode *Caenorhabditis elegans*. Environ Toxicol Chem 28: 1324–1330.
44. Mohan N, Chen C, Hsieh H, Wu Y, Chang H (2010) In vivo imaging and toxicity assessments of fluorescent nanodiamonds in *Caenorhabditis elegans*. Nano Lett 10: 3692–3699.

45. Qu Y, Li W, Zhou Y, Liu X, Zhang L, et al. (2011) Full assessment of fate and physiological behavior of quantum dots utilizing *Caenorhabditis elegans* as a model organism. Nano Lett 11: 3174–3183.
46. Yu S-H, Rui Q, Cai T, Wu Q-L, Li Y-X, et al. (2011) Close association of intestinal autofluorescence with the formation of severe oxidative damage in intestine of nematodes chronically exposed to Al_2O_3-nanoparticle. Environ Toxicol Pharmacol 32: 233–241.
47. Yang X, Gondikas AP, Marinakos SM, Auffan M, Liu J, et al. (2012) Mechanism of silver nanoparticle toxicity is dependent in dissolved silver and surface coating in *Caenorhabditis elegans*. Environ Sci Technol 46: 1119–1127.
48. Wu Q-L, Li Y-P, Tang M, Wang D-Y (2012) Evaluation of environmental safety concentrations of DMSA coated Fe_2O_3-NPs using different assay systems in nematode *Caenorhabditis elegans*. PLoS ONE 7: e43729.
49. Li Y-X, Wang W, Wu Q-L, Li Y-P, Tang M, et al. (2012) Molecular control of TiO_2-NPs toxicity formation at predicted environmental relevant concentrations by Mn-SODs proteins. PLoS ONE 7: e44688.
50. Wu Q-L, Wang W, Li Y-X, Ye B-P, Tang M, et al. (2012) Small sizes of TiO_2-NPs exhibit adverse effects at predicted environmental relevant concentrations on nematodes in a modified chronic toxicity assay system. J Hazard Mater 243: 161–168.
51. Li Y-X, Yu S-H, Wu Q-L, Tang M, Wang D-Y (2013) Transmissions of serotonin, dopamine and glutamate are required for the formation of neurotoxicity from Al_2O_3-NPs in nematode *Caenorhabditis elegans*. Nanotoxicology 7: 1004–1013.
52. Zhao Y-L, Wu Q-L, Tang M, Wang D-Y (2014) The *in vivo* underlying mechanism for recovery response formation in nano-titanium dioxide exposed *Caenorhabditis elegans* after transfer to the normal condition. Nanomedicine: Nanotechnol Biol Med 10: 89–98.
53. Rui Q, Zhao Y-L, Wu Q-L, Tang M, Wang D-Y (2013) Biosafety assessment of titanium dioxide nanoparticles in acutely exposed nematode *Caenorhabditis elegans* with mutations of genes required for oxidative stress or stress response. Chemosphere 93: 2289–2296.
54. Ye H-Y, Ye B-P, Wang D-Y (2008) Trace administration of vitamin E can retrieve and prevent UV-irradiation- and metal exposure-induced memory deficits in nematode *Caenorhabditis elegans*. Neurobiol Learn Mem 90: 10–18.
55. Onken B, Driscoll M (2010) Metformin induces a dietary restriction-like state and the oxidative stress response to extend *C. elegans* healthspan via AMPK, LKB1, and SKN-1. PLoS ONE 5: e8758.
56. Kumar S, Aninat C, Michaux G, Morel F (2010) Anticancer drug 5-fluorouracil induces reproductive and developmental defects in *Caenorhabditis elegans*. Reprod Toxicol 29: 415–420.
57. Lublin A, Isoda F, Patel H, Yen K, Ngugen L, et al. (2011) FDA-approved drugs that protect mammalian neurons from glucose toxicity slow aging dependent on cbp and protect against proteotoxicity. PLoS ONE 6: e27762.
58. Li Y-P, Li Y-X, Wu Q-L, Ye H-Y, Sun L-M, et al. (2013) High concentration of vitamin E decreases thermosensation and thermotaxis learning and the underlying mechanisms in nematode *Caenorhabditis elegans*. PLoS ONE 8: e71180.
59. Rui Q, Lu Q, Wang DY (2009) Administration of *Bushenkangshuai Tang* alleviates the UV irradiation- and oxidative stress-induced lifespan defects in nematode *Caenorhabditis elegans*. Front Med China 3: 76–90.
60. Dostal V, Roberts CM, Link CD (2010) Genetic mechanisms of coffee extract protection in a *Caenorhabditis elegans* model of β-amyloid peptide toxicity. Genetics 186: 857–866.
61. Zhang W-M, Lv T, Li M, Wu Q-L, Yang L-S, et al. (2013) Beneficial effects of wheat gluten hydrolysate to extend lifespan and induce stress resistance in nematode *Caenorhabditis elegans*. PLoS ONE 8: e74553.
62. Mukai D, Matsuda N, Yoshioka Y, Sato M, Yamasaki T (2008) Potential anthelmintics : polyphenols from the tea plant *Camellia sinensis* L. are lethally toxic to *Caenorhabditis elegans*. J Nat Med 62: 155–159.
63. Fan D, Hodges DM, Zhang J, Kirby CW, Ji X, et al. (2011) Commercial extract of the brown seaweed *Ascophyllum nodosum* enhances phenolic antioxidant contents of spinach (*Spinacia oleracea* L.) which protects *Caenorhabditis elegans* against oxidative and thermal stress. Food Chem 124: 195–202.
64. Sangha JS, Sun X, Wally OSD, Zhang K, Ji X, et al. (2012) Liuwei Dihuang (LWDH), a traditional Chinese medicinal formula, protects against β-amyloid toxicity in transgenic *Caenorhabditis elegans*. PLoS ONE 7: e43990.
65. Dharmalingam K, Yan B, Mahmud MZ, Sedek SAM, Majid MIA, et al. (2012) *Swietenia macrophylla* extract promotes the ability of *Caenorhabditis elegans* to survive *Pseudomonas aeruginosa* infection. J Ethnopharmacol 139: 657–663.
66. Kandasamy S, Khan W, Evans F, Critchley AT, Prithiviraj B (2012) Tasco®: a product of *Ascophyllum nodosum* enhances immune response of *Caenorhabditis elegans* against *Pseudomonas aeruginosa* infection. Mar Drugs 10: 84–105.
67. Wu Q-L, Li Y-X, Li Y-P, Zhao Y-L, Ge L, et al. (2013) Crucial role of biological barrier at the primary targeted organs in controlling translocation and toxicity of multi-walled carbon nanotubes in nematode *Caenorhabditis elegans*. Nanoscale 5: 11166–11178.
68. Wu Q-L, Yin L, Li X, Tang M, Zhang T, et al. (2013) Contributions of altered permeability of intestinal barrier and defecation behavior to toxicity formation from graphene oxide in nematode *Caenorhabditis elegans*. Nanoscale 5: 9934–9943.
69. Nouara A, Wu Q-L, Li Y-X, Tang M, Wang H-F, et al. (2013) Carboxylic acid functionalization prevents the translocation of multi-walled carbon nanotubes at predicted environmental relevant concentrations into targeted organs of nematode *Caenorhabditis elegans*. Nanoscale 5: 6088–6096.
70. Li Y-X, Yu S-H, Wu Q-L, Tang M, Pu Y-P, et al. (2012) Chronic Al_2O_3-nanoparticle exposure causes neurotoxic effects on locomotion behaviors by inducing severe ROS production and disruption of ROS defense mechanisms in nematode *Caenorhabditis elegans*. J Hazard Mater 219–220: 221–230.
71. McIntire SL, Jorgensen E, Kaplan J, Horvitz HR (1993) The GABAergic nervous system of *Caenorhabditis elegans*. Nature 364: 337–341.
72. Pluskota A, Horzowski E, Bossinger O, von Mikecz A (2009) In *Caenorhabditis elegans* nanoparticle-bio-interactions become transparent: silica-nanoparticles induce reproductive senescence. PLoS ONE 4: e6622.
73. McGhee JD (2007) The *C. elegans* intestine. WormBook, ed. The *C. elegans* Research Community, WormBook, doi: 10.1895/wormbook.1.133.1.
74. Lapierre LR, Hansen M (2012) Lessons from *C. elegans* : signaling pathways for longevity. Trend Endocrinol Metab 23: 637–644.
75. Tullet JM, Hertweck M, An JH, Baker J, Hwang JY, et al. (2008) Direct inhibition of the longevity-promoting factor SKN-1 by insulin-like signaling in *C. elegans*. Cell 132: 025–1038.
76. Goh GY, Martelli KL, Parhar KS, Kwong AW, Wong MA, et al. (2013) The conserved mediator subunit MDT-15 is required for oxidative stress responses in *Caenorhabditis elegans*. Aging Cell doi: 10.1111/acel.12.
77. Wu S, Lu J-H, Rui Q, Yu S-H, Cai T, et al. (2011) Aluminum nanoparticle exposure in L1 larvae results in more severe lethality toxicity than in L4 larvae or young adults by strengthening the formation of stress response and intestinal lipofuscin accumulation in nematodes. Environ Toxicol Pharmacol 31: 179–188.
78. Wang D-Y, Wang Y (2008) Phenotypic and behavioral defects caused by barium exposure in nematode *Caenorhabditis elegans*. Arch Environ Contam Toxicol 54: 447–453.
79. Brenner S (1974) The genetics of *Caenorhabditis elegans*. Genetics 77: 71–94.
80. Donkin S, Williams PL (1995) Influence of developmental stage, salts and food presence on various end points using *Caenorhabditis elegans* for aquatic toxicity testing. Environ Toxicol Chem 14: 2139–2147.
81. Williams PL, Dusenbery DB (1990) Aquatic toxicity testing using the nematode *Caenorhabditis elegans*. Environ Toxicol Chem 9: 1285–1290.
82. Du M, Wang D-Y (2009) The neurotoxic effects of heavy metal exposure on GABAergic system in nematode *Caenorhabditis elegans*. Environ Toxicol Pharmacol 27: 314–320.

23

Methodological Reporting of Randomized Trials in Five Leading Chinese Nursing Journals

Chunhu Shi[1,2,3], Jinhui Tian[1,2,3], Dan Ren[4], Hongli Wei[5], Lihuan Zhang[5], Quan Wang[1,2,4], Kehu Yang[1,2,3]*

1 Evidence-Based Medicine Center, Lanzhou University, Lanzhou, China, **2** Key Laboratory of Evidence Based Medicine and Knowledge Translation of Gansu Province, Lanzhou University, Lanzhou, China, **3** School of Basic Medical Sciences, Lanzhou University, Lanzhou, China, **4** The First Clinical Medicine School, Lanzhou University, Lanzhou, China, **5** The Second Clinical Medical School, Lanzhou University, Lanzhou, China

Abstract

Background: Randomized controlled trials (RCTs) are not always well reported, especially in terms of their methodological descriptions. This study aimed to investigate the adherence of methodological reporting complying with CONSORT and explore associated trial level variables in the Chinese nursing care field.

Methods: In June 2012, we identified RCTs published in five leading Chinese nursing journals and included trials with details of randomized methods. The quality of methodological reporting was measured through the methods section of the CONSORT checklist and the overall CONSORT methodological items score was calculated and expressed as a percentage. Meanwhile, we hypothesized that some general and methodological characteristics were associated with reporting quality and conducted a regression with these data to explore the correlation. The descriptive and regression statistics were calculated via SPSS 13.0.

Results: In total, 680 RCTs were included. The overall CONSORT methodological items score was 6.34±0.97 (Mean ± SD). No RCT reported descriptions and changes in "trial design," changes in "outcomes" and "implementation," or descriptions of the similarity of interventions for "blinding." Poor reporting was found in detailing the "settings of participants" (13.1%), "type of randomization sequence generation" (1.8%), calculation methods of "sample size" (0.4%), explanation of any interim analyses and stopping guidelines for "sample size" (0.3%), "allocation concealment mechanism" (0.3%), additional analyses in "statistical methods" (2.1%), and targeted subjects and methods of "blinding" (5.9%). More than 50% of trials described randomization sequence generation, the eligibility criteria of "participants," "interventions," and definitions of the "outcomes" and "statistical methods." The regression analysis found that publication year and ITT analysis were weakly associated with CONSORT score.

Conclusions: The completeness of methodological reporting of RCTs in the Chinese nursing care field is poor, especially with regard to the reporting of trial design, changes in outcomes, sample size calculation, allocation concealment, blinding, and statistical methods.

Editor: Robert K. Hills, Cardiff University, United Kingdom

Funding: The authors have no support or funding to report.

Competing Interests: The authors have declared that no competing interests exist.

* Email: kehuyangebm2006@126.com

Introduction

The randomized controlled trial (RCT) is the most appropriate design for evaluating the effectiveness of a nursing intervention among eligible primary study designs for evidence-based practice [1]. Evidence-based nursing practitioners believe that randomization and unbiased allocation of interventions assure methodological quality and the subsequent findings of RCTs [2,3]. However, well-conducted trials may be reported poorly [4], and failing to report all of the study's methods, details, and findings, especially for RCTs, seriously distorts the evidence base for clinical decision-making [5].

As a set of evidence-based reporting guidelines for RCTs, the Consolidated Standards of Reporting Trials (CONSORT) [6] was developed to improve the transparency of reporting and interpreting RCTs, minimize biased conclusions, ultimately facilitate clinical decision making, and indirectly drive better design of trials. The CONSORT guidelines have been associated with improving the quality of RCT reporting [7]. To date, CONSORT has been accepted by 600 medical journals, including 20 nursing care journals in English [8], and it has been revised twice, in 2001 and 2010 [9].

For RCTs in various disciplines (e.g., diagnostic procedures, interventions, cancer trials, and alternative medicine), the reporting quality has been assessed via CONSORT [5] to ensure their transparency, and found widespread inadequate reporting of methodological issues. However, evidence is still deficient on the reporting quality of RCTs in nursing care, especially in China. Existing reviews have focused on only a specific discipline [10,11], were not conducted systematically [12,13], used a modified CONSORT checklist according to the purposes of the study [14], or focused on only a specific methodological issue [15,16].

This study was thus conducted to investigate (1) the adherence to methodological reporting complying with CONSORT on Chinese nursing RCTs, and (2) the correlation between CONSORT adherence and key indicators regarding characteristics and methodological factors.

Methods

Information Source

According to their total number of citations and impact factors (IFs) in the "Chinese S&T Journal Citation Reports 2012" [17], we selected the following five leading Chinese nursing journals(see Appendix S1): Chinese Journal of Nursing (CJN, 1954–), Chinese Journal of Modern Nursing (CJMN, 1995–), International Journal of Nursing (IJN, 1980–), Chinese Journal of Practical Nursing (CJPN, 1985–) and Journal of Nurses Training (JNT, 1986–). In June 2012, a comprehensive electronic search strategy for the Chinese Bio-Medicine disc (CBM; see Appendix S2) was performed using "randomized controlled trial" or "clinical trial" as keywords, limited to these five targeted journals.

Eligibility Criteria

Inclusion criteria.

1) Citations claiming to be RCTs in the titles and/or abstracts, according to the "Cochrane definitions and criteria for randomized controlled trials and controlled clinical trials" [18].
2) Controlled trials with two comparators.
3) Trials of both nursing interventions (e.g., drug interventions, social and psychological interventions, traditional Chinese medicine interventions, complex interventions) and non-nursing interventions (e.g., nursing education program interventions).

Exclusion criteria.

1) "Quasi-random" trials: when "random" was mentioned with a high-risk randomization method, such as alternation, assignment based on date of birth, case record number, or date of presentation.
2) Irrelevant study reports: reports that are published in a summary form, reviews of randomized trials, and randomized trials on animals, even though they may be reported as "random."
3) Other study designs, such as cohort study and case series report.

Study Selection and Data Extraction

All citations from the CBM were allocated evenly to three units. By first screening titles and abstracts and then screening fulltexts, three groups consisting of two authors each selected eligible studies from these units of citations independently. When a disagreement arose in any of groups, another group would participate to arrive at an agreement. Then, two authors extracted relevant information and data from the included studies. A well-designed extraction form (Appendix S3) was formulated to assess the reporting quality of RCTs according to CONSORT [6]. The extraction form included (1) general characteristics [5] (i.e., journal name, IF, publication date, number of authors, multicenter trials, types of interventions, sample size, and funding source) and a description of the interventions [19], including length of descriptions of interventions and controls in words and the reproducibility of the interventions, which authors evaluated by assessing whether the intervention was described in enough detail to be reproducible; (2) CONSORT methodological items; and (3) methodological quality measurements [20], including allocation concealment and intention-to-treat (ITT) analysis. The overall CONSORT methodological items score was the total score of 17 items with response options of "yes" (scored as 1) or "no" (scored as 0) on whether the component had been reported as recommended. Items were scored as "no" (i.e., 0) if the item was only partly met by the research report. Disagreements during data extraction were resolved by discussion.

Quality Control

We implemented rigorous quality control throughout the study. Before selecting the eligible studies, investigators were trained to distinguish RCTs from irrelevant study designs using the definitions from the Centre for Evidence-Based Medicine, Oxford, UK (University of Oxford) [21]. Before data extraction, the extraction form (Appendix S3) following CONSORT guidelines was established via three rounds of pre-survey and team discussion.

Data Analysis

Using SPSS 13.0, we performed a descriptive analysis, obtaining frequencies and percentages for categorical variables, and means, medians, standard deviations, and inter-quartile ranges (IQR) for continuous variables. Then, exploratory regression was conducted to examine whether general and methodological characteristics are associated with reporting quality, as measured by the CONSORT methodological items score. Univariate regression was performed for each potentially associated variable, and variables with P values lower than 0.25 were then included in a stepwise backward linear regression. Any P value lower than 0.05 was regarded as statistically significant. In this study, the sample sizes of the trials were included to power the exploratory linear regression.

Results

Study Inclusion

In total, 58,823 citations published in the five leading nursing journals from 1954 to June 2012 were retrieved via the "Journal Search Engine" function of the CBM disc. After screening abstracts and fulltexts, 5519 fulltexts that mentioned "random" were initially identified. Among them, 5502 trials described "randomization" in both abstracts and fulltexts, and 17 described "randomization" in only the fulltexts. Six hundred and eighty trials met the criteria for "details of randomization" and were included in the final analysis. Figure 1 depicts a flow diagram of the inclusion decisions.

Characteristics of Included Studies

Most of the included trials (99.9%) were published after the 2001 CONSORT (Appendix S4). Furthermore, 27.6% (188/680) of trials were published in CJN and JNT, which had higher IFs than the average (mean $\pm$ SD $=1.20\pm1.05$); 61% (415/680) of trials were reported by no more than three authors (i.e., the median number of authors). Two point five percent (17/680) of trials reported a collaboration between multicenter studies. However, 21.6% of these trials did not specify the number of clinical trial centers. Most trials (83.4%) studied the implementation of non-pharmacological interventions. The median sample size of the included studies was 90 (IQR $=62.75$). Most trials (75.6%) did not mention financial support. By our judgment,

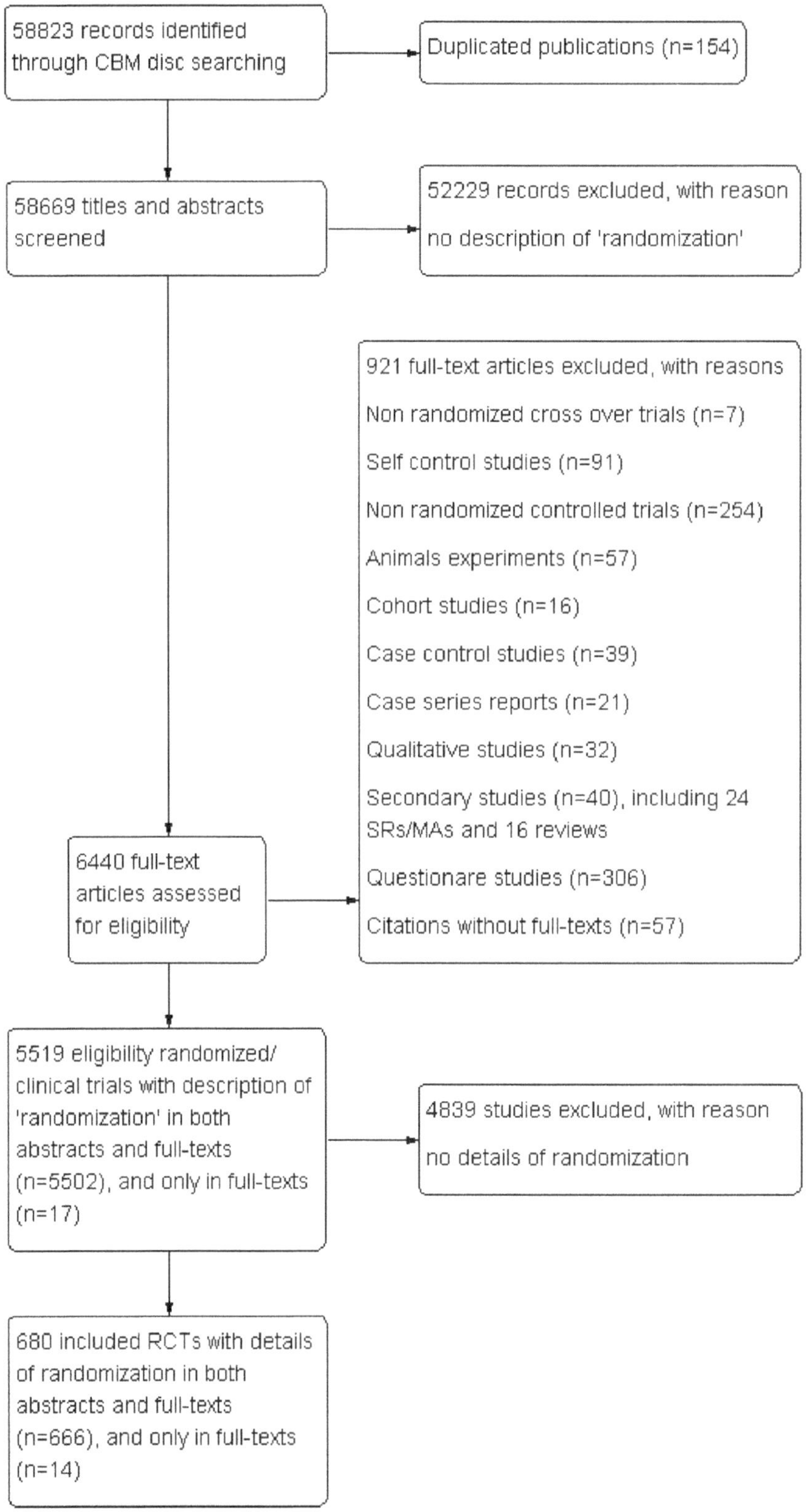

Figure 1. Flow diagram of included studies.

85.4% of trials provided enough details in the description of interventions to facilitate replication; however, only 48.2% of control group protocols were sufficiently described. Nisnety percent of trials from CJPN described the control group protocol as "the control group used standard nursing inventions for this disease." There were significant differences in the number of words used to describe the interventions and controls (median = 215.0 and IQR = 422.75 for interventions, and median = 32.0

Table 1. Characteristics of Included Studies.

Predictors		n* (Total N = 680)	Percent (%)
Journal	CJMN	255	37.5
	JNT	73	10.7
	CJN	115	16.9
	IJN	106	15.6
	CJPN	131	19.3
Publication year§	-1996	1	0.1
	1996–2000	0	0
	2001–2005	44	6.5
	2006–2010	373	54.9
	2010–	262	38.5
No. of authors		Median = 3	IQR = 3
	≤3 authors	415	61
	>3 authors	265	39
Multicenter trials	Yes	17	2.5
	No	516	75.9
	Unclear	147	21.6
Type of interventions	Non-pharmacological interventions	567	83.4
	Pharmacological interventions	113	16.6
Sample size		Median = 90	IQR = 62.75
Funding support	Industry support	3	0.4
	Public support	163	24
	Unclear	514	75.6
Length of descriptions of interventions in words		Median = 215.0	IQR = 422.75
Reproducibility of interventions	Yes	581	85.4
	No	99	14.6
Length of descriptions of controls in words¶		Median = 32.0	IQR = 47.0
Reproducibility of control	Yes	328	48.2
	No	352	51.8
Allocation concealment	Yes	2	0.3
	No/unclear	678	99.7
ITT analysis	Yes/no drop outs	580	85.3
	Per protocol analysis	39	5.7
	Unclear	61	9

*Items are reported as frequency and proportion for categorical variables and are otherwise specified for continuous variables.
§CONSORT was published in 1996 and revised twice in 2001 and 2010, respectively; the number of RCTs in each publication year is depicted in Appendix S4.
¶There is a significant difference between the number of words used to describe interventions and controls,as indicated by two related-samples tests ($Z = -21.192$, $P < 0.001$);
IQR indicates interquartile range.

and IQR = 47.0 for controls, $Z = -21.192$, $P < 0.001$). For methodological quality measurements, only two trials (0.3%) reported the details of the allocation concealment mechanism; 85.3% of trials had no dropouts, and 5.7% conducted per protocol analysis. Table 1 depicts the characteristics of the included studies.

Reporting of CONSORT Methodological Items

When screening abstracts rather than fulltexts, 97.9% of RCTs could be identified. Only two trials (0.3%) reported "randomized control trial" in the title. Overall, the mean CONSORT methodological score was 6.34±0.97 out of 17 sub-items. Additionally, in order to explore the influence of the score of "blinding (11a, 11b)", an analysis excluding data on blinding showed that the mean and SD of the CONSORT score were 6.28 and 0.94 respectively, which were similar to the mean score obtained while including data on blinding. No RCT reported descriptions and changes in "trial design," changes in "outcomes" and "implementation," or descriptions of the similarity of interventions for "blinding." For the description of trial design, 99.7% of the studies used a parallel design while 0.3% used a crossover design. Sub-standard reporting was also found regarding the details of "settings of participants" (13.1%), "type of randomization sequence generation" (1.8%), calculation methods of "sample size" (0.4%), explanation of any interim analyses and stopping guidelines of "sample size" (0.3%), additional analyses of "statistical methods" (2.1%), and targeted subjects and methods of "blinding" (5.9%). In addition, no central randomization that implied allocation concealment was reported. Only two studies conducted allocation concealment through sequentiallynumbered opaque sealed envelopes. More than 50% of trials described randomization sequence generation, the eligibility criteria of participants, "interventions," and definitions of "outcomes" and "statistical methods." Table 2 depicts the reporting of individual CONSORT methodological items.

Predictors Associated with CONSORT Methodological Score

We explored the association of predictors, including general characteristics and methodological quality measurements, with CONSORT methodological score with a linear regression and found that publication year and ITT analysis were weakly associated with CONSORT score. Each predictor was associated with a small increase of 0.047 and 0.601 points to the overall CONSORT methodological score. The two predictors associated with CONSORT score (i.e. publication year and ITT analysis) remained after the data on "blinding" were excluded, and their P values were 0.005 and <0.001 respectively. Table 3 depicts the results of our linear regression.

Discussion

In this review, we investigated 680 RCT fulltexts using CONSORT methodological items and found that RCTs of nursing interventions in Chinese nursing care journals reported

Table 2. Reporting of individual CONSORT methodological items.

Methodological items		**n (Total N = 680)**	**Percent (%)**
RCT*		666	97.9
Title		2	0.3
Trial design	Description (3a)	0	0
	Parallel design¶	678	99.7
	Crossover design¶	2	0.3
	Changes and reasons (3b)	0	0
Participants	Eligibility criteria (Item 4a)	370	54.4
	Settings (4b)	89	13.1
Interventions	Item 5	643	94.6
Outcomes	Definition (6a)	484	71.2
	Changes(6b)	0	0
Sample size	Calculation (7a)	3	0.4
	Interim analyses (7b)	2	0.3
Randomization sequence generation	Methods of randomization (8a)		
	Coin toss	47	6.9
	Computerized random number generator	28	4.1
	Drawing lots	61	9
	Random number table	543	79.9
	Minimization	1	0.1
	Type of randomization (8b)		
	Blocked randomization	10	1.5
	Simple randomization	668	98.2
	Stratified randomization	2	0.3
Allocation concealment mechanism	Item 9	2	0.3
Implementation	Item 10	0	0
Blinding	Targeted subjects and methods (11a)		
	Double blinding	4	0.6
	Single blinding	36	5.3
	Unclear	640	94.1
	Similarity of interventions (11b)	0	0
Statistical methods	Statistical methods (12a)	627	92.2
	Additional analyses (12b)	14	2.1
Overall score**		Mean = 6.34	SD = 0.97

*RCTs according to abstracts.
¶Parallel and crossover design are judged by authors.
**In order to explore the influence of the score of "blinding (11a, 11b)," we excluded data on blinding and found the mean and SD to be 6.28 and 0.94, respectively, which are similar to the mean and SD obtained when including data on blinding.

Table 3. Results of linear regression for predictors associated with CONSORT methodological score.

Predictor	Univariate		Multivariate	
	beta (95%CI)	P	beta (95%CI)	P
Journal	−0.027 (−0.074, 0.020)	0.257	-	-
Impact factor	−0.104 (−0.174, −0.034)	0.004	−0.054 (−0.123, 0.015)	0.232
Publication year	0.059 (0.026, 0.091)	<0.001	0.047 (0.016, 0.078)	0.004[¶]
No. of authors	0.003 (−0.036, 0.042)	0.881	-	-
Multicenter trials	−0.047 (−0.517, 0.423)	0.845	-	-
Type of interventions	−0.025 (−0.223, 0.172)	0.801	-	-
Sample size	0.000 (−0.001, 0.000)	0.155	−0.067 (−0.001, 0.000)	0.080
Funding support	0.039 (−0.047, 0.125)	0.376	-	-
Allocation concealment	−0.341 (−1.696, 1.015)	0.622	-	-
ITT analysis	0.586 (0.383, 0.788)	<0.001	0.601 (0.404, 0.799)	<0.001[¶]
Length of descriptions of interventions in words	0.000 (0.000, 0.000)	0.091	0.065 (−0.132, 0.263)	0.157
Reproducibility of interventions	0.055 (−0.153, 0.263)	0.606	-	-
Length of descriptions of controls in words	0.000 (−0.002, 0.001)	0.871	-	-
Reproducibility of control	−0.056 (−0.202, 0.091)	0.458	-	-

Note: [¶]When data on "blinding" were deleted, two predictors associated with CONSORT score (i.e., publication year and ITT analysis) remained, and their P values were 0.005 and <0.001 respectively.

"trial design," "participant settings," changes in "outcome," "sample size," "allocation concealment mechanism," "implementation," "blinding," and additional analyses of "statistical methods" poorly. The overall CONSORT score was low. Weak correlations between CONSORT score and two variables (i.e., publication year and ITT analysis) were found.

Concordant with our findings, Zhang et al. [11] showed that the reporting of methodological items in cancer nursing care literature was also poor in terms of outcomes, sample size, randomization sequence generation, allocation concealment mechanism, implementation, and blinding. Zhu et al. [15] demonstrated that only 3.8% of RCTs of nursing interventions described randomization sequence generation methods; furthermore, in traditional Chinese medicine nursing studies [10], 7.8% of RCTs described randomization sequence generation, 1.4% described the allocation concealment mechanism, and 3.1% described blinding. Evidence from RCTs of nursing interventions in English [13,14,16] also supported our findings. Samaan et al. [5] reviewed systematic reviews of adherence to reporting guidelines across different clinical areas and found a prevailing lack of reporting quality in most disciplines. Additionally, Samaan et al. [5] showed that 80% of the studies that did not adhere to CONSORT guidelines had negative conclusions, such as "some improvements are needed, reporting inadequate/poor/medium/suboptimal, etc." Our findings are consistent with other systematic reviews in other specializations [19,22]. Given these findings, we have provided important evidence to alert Chinese nursing researchers of the urgent need for improving the reporting of RCTs on nursing interventions. This is especially true for randomization, as we found that 87.7% (4839/5519) of RCTs that mentioned "random" in abstracts and/or fulltexts did not actually include details of the randomization or used incorrect randomized methods, such as alternate allocation and allocation by record number. Similar results were reported by Wu et al. [24].

We found poorer reporting of blinding in 83.4% of non-pharmacological interventions, but no correlation was established via the regression analysis. Due to some methodological challenges, such as the complexity of the intervention [23], expertise of the care provider [23], and difficulties with blinding [16], it is believed that non-pharmacological interventions always limit the blinding of participants and caregivers; however, the blinding of data collectors is often achievable. Regardless of whether blinding is possible, authors can and should state who was blinded. Therefore, although it seemed unnecessary in some included studies, blinding was judged as impracticable because the authors did not report its details. Our regression analysis indicated that publication year had a weak correlation with reporting quality. This demonstrates that reporting quality is improving yearly. We also examined the relationship between reporting quality and methodological quality of RCTs by regression of allocation concealment and ITT analysis. The regression indicated only weak correlations with ITT analysis, and no correlations with the other variable. In order to explore the influence of the score of "blinding (11a, 11b)" on regression analysis, data on "blinding" were deleted, and the results showed that the two same predictors (i.e. publication year and ITT analysis) were associated with CONSORT score analysis.

The main strengths of this study were the comprehensive search strategy, determination of associations of CONSORT score with various predictors, and the well-conducted quality control assessment. However, this review had some limitations. First, nursing interventions are often far more complicated than drug interventions are. We did not investigate the reporting of items related to external validity. Second, as our eligible criteria was not restricted to any specific nursing intervention such as drug interventions, social and psychological interventions, traditional Chinese medicine interventions, or complex interventions, we did not use CONSORT extensions for social and psychological interventions, non-pharmacological interventions, herbal interventions, and CReDECI criteria [25–28]. In addition, we did not find a pragmatic trial among the included studies, so the CONSORT extension for pragmatic trials [29] was also not used. Third, according to our eligibility criteria, no dissertation in nursing care was included. A search on the Internet in the Doctoral Dissertations and Masters' Theses sub-set of the China Knowledge Resource Integrated Database yielded 2312 citations dating up to June 2013 that mentioned "random." Finally, because none of the studied nursing journals endorsed CONSORT as a requirement for a manuscript submission in China, we did not investigate differences in the reporting between each item by comparing CONSORT-endorsing journals with CONSORT non-endorsing journals.

Conclusions

In conclusion, the completeness of methodological reporting of RCTs in Chinese nursing care journals was very poor, especially in terms of trial design, outcome changes, sample size calculation, allocation concealment, blinding, and statistical methods. Authors are highly recommended to use the CONSORT criteria when submitting reports of RCTs. Editors should also present their peer-reviewed manuscripts under the guidance of CONSORT to ensure that journal articles contain the key clinical and methodological details that readers need. Initiatives recommended by Altman [30] should be accepted; these suggest that authors should sign a publication transparency declaration as part of every journal submission and journals should update their instructions to authors.

Supporting Information

Appendix S1 The total cites and impact factors in five Chinese nursing journals.
(DOC)

Appendix S2 Comprehensive electronic search strategy for CBM disc.
(DOC)

Appendix S3 Data extraction form.
(DOC)

Appendix S4 Number of RCTs in each publication year.
(TIF)

Checklist S1 PRISMA Checklist.
(DOC)

Acknowledgments

Thanks to Daniel James Green and Editage for providing important comments and English editing. We paid for the services of Editage and there were no conflicts of interest.

Author Contributions

Conceived and designed the experiments: CS JT LZ. Performed the experiments: CS JT LZ HW DR QW KY. Analyzed the data: CS LZ KY. Contributed reagents/materials/analysis tools: KY HW. Wrote the paper: CS DR QW KY. Addressed disagreements: KY.

References

1. DiCenso A, Cullum N, Ciliska D (1998) Implementing evidence-based nursing: some misconceptions. Evidence-Based Nursing 1: 38–40.
2. Cullum N (2000) Evaluation of studies of treatment or prevention interventions. Evidence Based Nursing 3: 100–102.
3. Borglin G, Richards DA (2010) Bias in experimental nursing research: Strategies to improve the quality and explanatory power of nursing science. Int J Nurs Stud 47: 123–128.
4. Huwiler-Müntener K, Jüni P, Junker C, Egger M (2002) Quality of reporting of randomized trials as a measure of methodologic quality. JAMA 287: 2801–2804.
5. Samaan Z, Mbuagbaw L, Kosa D, Borg Debono V, Dillenburg R, et al. (2013) A systematic scoping review of adherence to reporting guidelines in health care literature. J Multidiscip Healthc 6: 169–188.
6. Schulz KF, Altman DG, Moher D; CONSORT Group (2010) CONSORT 2010 statement: updated guidelines for reporting parallel group randomized trials. Ann Intern Med 152: 726–732.
7. Turner L, Shamseer L, Altman DG, Weeks L, Peters J, et al. (2012) Consolidated standards of reporting trials (CONSORT) and the completeness of reporting of randomised controlled trials (RCTs) published in medical journals. Cochrane Database Syst Rev 11:MR000030.
8. CONSORT Group. CONSORT Endorsers - Journals. Available: http://www.consort-statement.org/about-consort/consort-endorsement/consort-endorsers-journals/. Accessed: 2013 Dec 26.
9. Altman DG, Moher D, Schulz KF (2012) Improving the reporting of randomised trials: the CONSORT Statement and beyond. Stat Med 31: 2985–2997.
10. Mei LJ, Zheng GH, Chen QY, Lin R, Yan Y, et al. (2012) Methodological Evaluation on Domestic Clinical Trials on Traditional Chinese Medicine Nursing from 2006 to 2011. Chin J Evid-based Med 12: 735–739.
11. Zhang XX, Yin WR, Liu YQ (2009) Reporting quality assessment on randomized controlled trials of cancer nursing care: based on CONSORT statement. Chinese Journal of Practical Nursing 25: 72–73.
12. Li XL, Tian YM, Zen JH, Liu L (2002) Evaluation on the randomized controlled trials papers published in Journal of Nurses Training. Journal of Nurses Training 17: 16–18.
13. Parent N, Hanley JA (2009) Assessing quality of reports on randomized clinical trials in nursing journals. Can J Cardiovasc Nurs 19: 25–39.
14. Smith BA, Lee HJ, Lee JH, Choi M, Jones DE, et al. (2008) Quality of reporting randomized controlled trials (RCTs) in the nursing literature: application of the consolidated standards of reporting trials (CONSORT). Nurs Outlook 56: 31–37.
15. Zhu D, Huang WX, Li XL, Jiang XL, Wang SP (2003) Investigation on randomized controlled trials of nursing care field in China. Journal of Practical Nursing 19: 60–61.
16. Polit DF, Gillespie BM, Griffin R (2011) Deliberate ignorance: a systematic review of blinding in nursing clinical trials. Nurs Res 60:9–16.
17. Institute of Scientific and Technical Information of China (2012) Chinese S&T journal citation reports. Beijing: Scientific and Technical Documents Publishing House 350 p.
18. Higgins JPT, Green S (2011) Cochrane Handbook for Systematic Reviews of Interventions Version 5.1.0 [updated March 2011]. The Cochrane Collaboration, 2011. Available: www.cochrane-handbook.org. Accessed: 2013 Dec 26.
19. Adie S, Harris IA, Naylor JM, Mittal R (2013) CONSORT compliance in surgical randomized trials: are we there yet? A systematic review. Ann Surg. 258: 872–878.
20. Boutron I, Tubach F, Giraudeau B, Ravaud P (2003) Methodological differences in clinical trials evaluating nonpharmacological and pharmacological treatments of hip and knee osteoarthritis. JAMA 290: 1062–1070.
21. University of Oxford (2010) Study Designs. The Centre for Evidence Based Medicine, University of Oxford, Available: http://www.cebm.net/index.aspx?o=1039. Accessed: 2012 Jul 1.
22. Xu L, Li J, Zhang M, Ai C, Wang L (2008) Chinese authors do need CONSORT: reporting quality assessment for five leading Chinese medical journals. Contemp Clin Trials 29: 727–731.
23. Stephenson J, Imrie J (1998) Why do we need randomised controlled trials to assess behavioural interventions? BMJ 316: 611–613.
24. Wu T, Li Y, Bian Z, Liu G, Moher D (2009) Randomized trials published in some Chinese journals: how many are randomized? Trials 10: 46.
25. Mayo-Wilson E, Montgomery P, Hopewell S, Macdonald G, Moher D, et al. (2013) Developing a reporting guideline for social and psychological intervention trials. Br J Psychiatry 203: 250–254.
26. Möhler R, Bartoszek G, Köpke S, Meyer G (2012) Proposed criteria for reporting the development and evaluation of complex interventions in healthcare (CReDECI): guideline development. Int J Nurs Stud 49: 40–46.
27. Gagnier JJ, Boon H, Rochon P, Moher D, Barnes J, et al. (2006) Reporting randomized, controlled trials of herbal interventions: an elaborated CONSORT statement. Ann Intern Med 144: 364–367.
28. Boutron I, Moher D, Altman DG, Schulz K, Ravaud P, for the CONSORT group. (2008) Methods and Processes of the CONSORT Group: Example of an Extension for Trials Assessing Nonpharmacologic Treatments. Ann Intern Med 2008: W60–W67.
29. Zwarenstein M, Treweek S, Gagnier JJ, Altman DG, Tunis S, et al. (2008) Improving the reporting of pragmatic trials: an extension of the CONSORT statement. BMJ 337: a2390.
30. Altman DG, Moher D (2013) Declaration of transparency for each research article. BMJ 347: f4796.

Practitioner Perspectives on Strategies to Promote Longer-Term Benefits of Acupuncture or Counselling for Depression

Hugh MacPherson[1]*, Liz Newbronner[1,2], Ruth Chamberlain[2], Stewart J. Richmond[1], Harriet Lansdown[1], Sara Perren[1], Ann Hopton[1], Karen Spilsbury[1]

1 Department of Health Sciences, University of York, York, United Kingdom, 2 Firefly Research & Evaluation, North Yorkshire, United Kingdom

Abstract

Background: Non-pharmacological interventions for depression may help patients manage their condition. Evidence from a recent large-scale trial (ACUDep) suggests that acupuncture and counselling can provide longer-term benefits for many patients with depression. This paper describes the strategies practitioners reported using to promote longer-term benefits for their patients.

Methods: A qualitative sub-study of practitioners (acupuncturists and counsellors) embedded in a randomised controlled trial. Using topic guides, data was collected from telephone interviews and a focus group, altogether involving 19 counsellors and 17 acupuncturists. Data were audio recorded, transcribed verbatim and analysed using thematic content analysis.

Results: For longer-term impact, both acupuncturists and counsellors encouraged insight into root causes of depression on an individual basis and saw small incremental changes as precursors to sustained benefit. Acupuncturists stressed the importance of addressing concurrent physical symptoms, for example helping patients relax or sleep better in order to be more receptive to change, and highlighted the importance of Chinese medicine theory-based lifestyle change for lasting benefit. Counsellors more often highlighted the importance of the therapeutic relationship, emphasising the need for careful "pacing" such that the process and tools employed were tailored and timed for each individual, depending on the "readiness" to change. Our data is limited to acupuncture practitioners using the principles of traditional Chinese medicine, and counsellors using a humanistic, non-directive and person-centred approach.

Conclusions: Long-term change appears to be an important focus within the practices of both acupuncturists and counsellors. To achieve this, practitioners stressed the need for an individualised approach with a focus on root causes.

Editor: Fan Qu, Women's Hospital, School of Medicine, Zhejiang University, China

Funding: This research is supported by the National Institute for Health Research (NIHR) under Programme Grants for Applied Research (Grant No. RP-PG-0707-10186). The views expressed in this presentation are those of the author(s) and not necessarily those of the NHS, the NIHR or the Department of Health. The funders had no role in study design, data collection and analysis, decision to publish, or preparation of the manuscript.

Competing Interests: Liz Newbronner and Ruth Chamberlain worked for Firefly Research & Evaluation and were commissioned by the Department of Health Sciences, University of York, to conduct the interviews and work with the authors to analyse the data and prepare this manuscript. This does not alter the authors' adherence to PLOS ONE policies on sharing data and materials.

* Email: hugh.macpherson@york.ac.uk

Background

Depression is a common illness in primary care. Some of the optimism regarding the potential of selective serotonin re-uptake inhibitors (SSRIs) as a treatment for depression has faded in the light of concerns about effectiveness and safety. [1] A recent meta-analysis has concluded that antidepressants have only a modest advantage over placebo, with the magnitude of benefit increasing with severity of depression. [2] There is an ongoing interest, especially among patients, in the potential of non-pharmacological treatments for depression, with the hope that they might avoid some of the concerns about antidepressants regarding safety and dependency. [3] Furthermore, for many patients, depression is a chronic and recurring illness, and non-pharmacological treatments that seek to improve longer-term outcomes are potentially of interest.

Evidence from a recent large-scale trial (ACUDep) [4] has suggested that acupuncture and counselling can provide longer-term benefits for many patients with on-going depression in primary care. The ACUDep trial recruited 755 patients with depression via 27 participating primary care practices; 302 were randomised to up to 12 acupuncture sessions; 302 to up to 12 counselling sessions; and 151 to usual care alone. The counselling was delivered within a recognised, manualised competency framework developed by Roth et al. at the University College of London's Centre for Outcomes Research and Effectiveness. [5] The acupuncture diagnosis and treatment, including selection of points, was based on the principles of traditional Chinese medicine, the details of which are reported elsewhere. [6]

Both acupuncture and counselling were found to be effective in reducing the symptoms of depression when compared to usual care, and these differences were significant at the 3 and 6 month time points, as well as when averaged over the 12 month period. [4][7] The trial focused on the effectiveness and cost effectiveness of the interventions. However, we were keen to understand the experiences of those providing treatments (acupuncture or counselling) within the trial, and in particular the aspects of these interventions that practitioners perceived to be associated with their longer-term benefit. In doing so, these insights will help understanding of the interventions and help inform both clinical practice and any future research design.

Underreported within randomised controlled trials are qualitative analyses of strategies employed by acupuncturists and counsellors within treatment for depression that are intended to promote longer-term change. In one qualitative study, interviews with patients receiving counselling in routine practice were used to identify the key characteristics of the intervention that were experienced as beneficial in the longer term. [8] In the authors' interpretation, a key component was the client's active engagement during and between counselling sessions. In turn this enabled a change to take place in the way they conducted their lives and relationships. We are unaware of any published qualitative studies of the processes of care associated with long-term change in the case of acupuncture for depression.

This qualitative study, embedded within a clinical trial, was designed to explore the perceptions and experiences of counsellors and acupuncturists who provided the treatment interventions within the trial. The aim was to understand better the key aspects of their work and their perceptions of the 'active ingredients' of counselling or acupuncture that were intended to promote longer-term benefits for the patients and may help in our understanding of the trial results. The study also provided an opportunity to identify important issues relating to professional practice and future policy, which are not reported here, including support needs and working arrangements; the acceptability and feasibility of different treatment options; the implications for the provision of acupuncture or humanistic counselling for treating depression within primary care settings; and related commissioning issues.

Methods

Recruitment of participants

To provide treatments for trial participants, 41 counsellors and 23 acupuncturists were recruited from across the regions of Yorkshire and the North East of England. Altogether these practitioners treated 497 (out of 604) patients participating in the intervention arms of the ACUDep trial. After the end of the trial's treatment phase, acupuncturists and counsellors who had consulted with at least two patients in the trial were invited to take part in the qualitative sub-study. They were sent an information sheet and consent form and asked to indicate whether they would prefer to be involved in a one-to-one telephone interview or a focus group. The aim was to recruit up to 30 counsellors and acupuncturists (approximately 15 in each group). Ethical approval was obtained from the York NHS Research Ethics Committee (REC ref: 09/H1311/75), which included approval for procedures that required written consent from all participants.

Interview and focus group data collection

The topic guides for the interviews and focus group were developed by the ACUDep research team to address the main research question of practitioner strategies intended to promote longer-term benefits for patients – a key finding of the trial results. The initial ideas were developed into topic guides for the interviews, one for each of the practitioner groups, and one for the focus group discussion which comprised both acupuncturists and counsellors. Along with questions, the topic guides also included prompts.These were then refined further at face-to-face meetings, such that the guides covered the practitioner's professional background and experience of working with depression, their approach to treating depression, their perceptions of working within the trial, and their thoughts on the implications for policy and professional practice. These issues were considered important for interpretation of the qualitative data.

All participants provided written consent. Those who agreed to take part in a telephone interview were contacted (either by telephone or email) to arrange a convenient time for the one-to-one interview. Arrangements were confirmed by email and the topic guide to be used in the interview was attached. Only small numbers of practitioners expressed a preference for a focus group discussion and so only one group discussion was held. Many issues covered in the group discussion were similar to those expressed in the individual interviews. However, the group discussion provided an opportunity for therapists to explore together any differences and similarities in their perceptions and experiences. This added to the richness of the data. The interviews and focus group were conducted by two experienced health services researchers from the research team who were not involved in the conduct of the trial itself (LN and RC). The interviews commonly lasted around 45 minutes (range 40 to 90) and the focus group 90 minutes. They were all audio-recorded (with participants' permission) and transcribed verbatim.

Data analysis

The transcripts were analysed thematically. [9] The main areas of inquiry covered in the topic guides were used for a framework approach to thematic content analysis, which involved analysing the data across the two groups of practitioners contributing to the study. [10] The framework was created in an Excel spreadsheet and coded and populated with data from the transcripts by the two researchers who had conducted the interviews (LN and RC). An inductive process was used to identify themes, drawing on shared experiences or points of difference identified from the data. As this study was intended to broaden our understanding of practice in relation to the treatment of patients with depression, the analysis also sought to draw out findings which might inform the practice of acupuncturists and counsellors.

Results

Practitioner characteristics

Forty-one therapists consented to be involved in the study but five therapists later withdrew or didn't respond when the fieldwork was being set up. The sub-study included individual telephone interviews with15 counsellors and13 acupuncturists (n = 28) and one focus group with 4 counsellors and 4 acupuncturists (n = 8) (Table 1). The sample for the qualitative sub-study included over half (56%) of the total number of therapists involved in the main trial.

The 17 participating acupuncturists were registered members of the British Acupuncture Council with at least three years' post-qualification experience and practising with the theoretical

Table 1. Breakdown of study participants.

	Number involved in main trial	Number involved in one-to-one interviews	Number involved in the focus group	Total number participating
Counsellors	41	15	4	19
Acupuncturists	23	13	4	17
Total	64	28	8	36

approach of traditional Chinese medicine. [6] The acupuncturists were predominantly male (39% were female), with an average duration of practice of 12 years. In the trial they treated on average 9 patients, who attended on average for 10 sessions. The 19 counsellors were members of the British Association for Counselling and Psychotherapy, who were accredited or were eligible for accreditation having completed 400 supervised hours post-qualification, and provided clients a humanistic style of counselling based on competences developed for Skills for Health. [11] They were predominantly female practitioners (79%), with an average duration of practice of 7 years. In the trial they treated on average 7 patients, who attended on average for 9 sessions.

Trial patient characteristics

Practitioners were treating patients in the trial who had ongoing depression for at least 3 months and a score of 20 or more on the Beck Depression Inventory (BDI-II), with 38% having depression categorised as "moderate" and 62% "severe". [4] The mean age was 44 years and 73% were female. They were (on average) 25 years old when they experienced their first episode of depression. In terms of prescribed medication, 69% were on anti-depressants and 48% were on analgesics.

Overview of the findings from thematic analysis

A cluster of eight themes emerged from the framework analysis. Almost all of the acupuncturists and counsellors stressed the importance they attached to promoting longer-term benefits. To achieve this, practitioners commonly reported on the need to focus on the root causes, to address treatment for each individual patient, and to value small incremental changes from one session to the next as precursors to sustained benefit over the longer term. Acupuncturists more commonly reported on the need to address concurrent physical symptoms, for example helping patients relax or sleep better in order to be more receptive to change. Most also highlighted the importance of Chinese medicine theory-based lifestyle change as an approach to promoting more lasting benefit. Counsellors more often highlighted the importance of the therapeutic relationship, emphasising the need for careful "pacing" such that the process and tools employed were tailored and timed for each individual, depending on the "readiness" to change. These findings are presented in more detail below.

Importance of a long-term focus

Long-term change appears to be an important focus within the practices of both acupuncturists and counsellors. Almost all of the practitioners mentioned the long-term perspective as inherent to the way they worked.

> *with something like depression, longer term for me, longer term approach is very fundamental.*(acupuncturist1)

For acupuncturists, this perspective was drawn from the theoretical approach of traditional Chinese medicine, in which long-term change needed to be facilitated by lifestyle changes related to acupuncture theory. For counsellors it was drawn from the humanistic approach, which many contrasted with what was perceived as the "quick fix" of cognitive behavioural therapy (CBT).

> *I would like to think that the whole approach is based on longer term change, in terms of the client learning ways of coping. Not just with the present crisis, whatever it might be, but hopefully that they would take something from it that they could apply in the future.*(counsellor1)

When comparing acupuncturists and counsellors, the reported long-term focus involved some differences in approach, as described above, as well as some similarities, especially with regard to encouraging insight into root causes on an individual basis and seeking small incremental changes as important precursors of overall benefit.

Identifying root causes

The commitment to identifying and addressing the root causes of depression within the treatment process was a commonly expressed factor among both acupuncturists and counsellors. Acupuncturists commonly used the theoretical concept of "root" (ben) and "branch" (biao).

> *Within Chinese Medicine we talk about treating the root and the branch. And there is merit in treating both.*(acupuncturist2)
> *Looking for underlying causes. Obviously there's some symptomatic stuff, but always looking at the root causes and using that as where I would start to work out my treatment principles.*(acupuncturist3)

The counsellors were more interested in "going deeper" and "further back (in time)" with their clients as a way of getting to the root causes.

> *From my experience generally, you've got to get to the root causes of depression, so it's much deeper than a CBT approach, so I think if people don't do that when clients present depression, then perhaps they are failing the clients at some level.*(counsellor2)
> *I suppose for me the long term change generally stems from a clear understanding of just what's been at the root of it all.*(counsellor3)

The implications of this approach, as reported by several practitioners, are that unless the underlying causes are addressed, then it is likely that there will not be the sustained long-term change that is desired.

Individualisation

When practised within the theoretical framework of traditional Chinese medicine, acupuncture treatment has been customised to the individual, such that treatment varies not only between patients but also, for the same patient, it varies over time. Likewise for the counsellors in the trial, all of whom were committed to working within the humanistic tradition, a person-centred approach was provided.

Everybody's different, so whenever a patient comes in, obviously, you take their full medical history. And quite often there will be other key characteristics, so not everybody gets the same points diagnosis, because of the different underlying features of their condition.(acupuncturist4)
That the reason for depression for individuals and how it's processed is unique and therefore the process focuses on how the client experiences it. I also think it's useful to bear in mind the possible causes and theories to be shared with the client.(counsellor4)

Valuing incremental change

Practitioners reported a certain amount of caution about expecting sudden or cathartic changes in their patients. More common was a sense that positive benefit required a series of small incremental changes that when combined with self-help approaches would hopefully build a more sustained improvement.

Well long term change can even come about from even small changes, really. If somebody can just sleep all night, it's surprising.(acupuncturist5)
I think to try almost to help people take responsibility and realise that there maybe is something that they can do. I think sometimes people get trapped in feeling depressed and feeling unable to do anything. So almost helping empower them to find changes that they can start to make, to make those improvements for themselves, which over time build up and help them move forward.(counsellor5)

Addressing concurrent physical symptoms

Acupuncturists generally stressed the importance of addressing concurrent physical symptoms, for example helping patients relax or sleep better in order to be more receptive to change.

What I find really interesting about working on the trial is that a lot of time people came with depression but in reality there was a host of other signs and symptoms that they were not happy in their life. Just kind of bowel, musculoskeletal, anything. So when they got a sense that I was treating them as a whole person, rather than just treating the depression........ When I'd sorted out their back, their stomach, ulcers, bad knees, you know, suddenly their depression got better. To me, that's how Traditional Chinese Medicine should be – it works with everything. Rather than, you know, like depression as a standalone thing.(acupuncturist2)

By contrast, the counsellors were less focused on the physical symptoms, and worked more on the assumption that by treating the underlying causes of depression there should be a knock-on effect in terms of reducing physical symptoms.

I'm not particularly interested in just treating symptoms, but what I'm usually interested in and what people are usually asking for is that they want to understand why they're feeling the way that they are. If you can deal with that issue, then it should help them to rid themselves of the symptoms really.(counsellor6)

Lifestyle changes

Almost all of the acupuncturists highlighted the importance of giving advice about lifestyle change that was relevant to the Chinese medicine perspective.

Yeah, it's overall sort of aimed at the long-term and I think people, you know, if they get further along with the acupuncture, they realise that it's all to do with lifestyle change as well and that those things are going to be the ones that bring them lasting benefit. Because often people start to feel better after a few treatments and then when they build in the lifestyle thing, when they actually start to think, oh, this acupuncture seems to be working for me, maybe I'll follow some of the advice as well. (acupuncturist6)

Those acupuncturists who reported on the role of lifestyle change tended to stress the importance of tailoring the advice to the patient, both in terms of content related to acupuncture theory (e.g. diet, relaxation, exercise, etc) as well as likely acceptability.

The counsellors worked within a trial protocol that had a strong emphasis on working within the humanistic tradition, which included being non-directive. [11] The protocol therefore limited the extent that they could offer lifestyle advice within the trial. Some counsellors, who typically worked more eclectically elsewhere, said they might normally include lifestyle advice, especially when working with people with addictions.

Therapeutic relationship

Counsellors consistently stressed the importance of the therapeutic relationship.

I tend to think that lasting change requires a greater degree of insight [than CBT]. But I think the change often comes – I suppose this is what puts me very squarely in the humanistic camp, the existential camp, I think it's often the relationship itself – it's actually having a new experience of a relationship for some people can be transformative.(counsellor3)
But the essence of my approach is the relationship and building good levels of rapport and trust and helping the client to feel okay with you. So it's an okay space at the start and if that forms well, that's a springboard, hopefully, for sort of therapeutic practice and change for people.(counsellor2)

However for some acupuncturists, this was also reported as a component of the treatment process that helped engender longer-term gains.

And it's kind of like a trust relationship – if they believe in the acupuncture, they believe in what you're telling them. And that kind of gives them the impetus to carry on in the longer term.(acupuncturist6)

Careful "pacing" based on "readiness to change"

Many of the counsellors emphasised the need for careful "pacing" such that the process and tools employed were tailored and timed for each individual, depending on the "readiness" to change.

And what I'm very aware of in counselling is that people will come to therapy at different stages of readiness to change. And it's very difficult to measure how useful it's been. So for example, with one client I can think of in the trial, I think he would have – I think it was probably a first experience for him, from being listened to and from being taken seriously and I think that was huge. He was very stuck. In terms of how much that was going to affect outcomes, in terms of was he going to make the necessary changes, he might have been able to begin to identify, or briefly identify, what it was in his life that was making him depressed – in terms of outcomes he wasn't at the stage where he was going to make any massive changes. But I think just having that experience, that first experience. That kind of thing is so hard to measure, isn't it?(counsellor6)

I tend to go with the speed of the client. However, if I can – my personal approach would be to help them in as short a sessions as possible to get them to feel better. However, I'm very careful to work with their speed. So am I short or long term.(counsellor7)

A number of acupuncturists identified issues related to timing, expressing the point that as patients improve, ideally appointments should be spread out towards the end of the course of treatment and beyond, as a way of sustaining benefit over the longer term.

In summary, the themes capture both similarities and differences in approaches between acupuncture and counselling, with most practitioners of both interventions having a shared sense of the prerequisites for sustained long-term benefit. The impression formed from the interviews is that the various approaches do not operate in isolation. Although the emphasis may vary, the themes appear to be integrated into a coherent combination that uniquely informs the practice of each practitioner.

Generalisability issues

With regard to the extent that these findings are transferable to other settings, the majority of counsellors said that the severity of the depression amongst trial patients was not markedly dissimilar to the people they routinely saw. By contrast, the acupuncturists were generally less used to dealing with patients with moderate to severe depression, and many said that they less commonly saw patients who consulted primarily because of a diagnosis of depression. Several of the therapists reported that the trial patients had a different attitude towards treatment compared to their private patients, particularly a more limited knowledge of the therapeutic intervention and a lower level of motivation to help themselves. Therapists also noted that there were a greater proportion of patients in lower income brackets, with more long-standing depression, or with unmanaged drug/alcohol addictions.

Discussion

Principal findings

Both acupuncturists and counsellors generally delivered treatments with an eye to encouraging longer-term change with the intention that, ideally, any putative benefit would be sustained well beyond the 12 sessions that were provided within the trial. While both types of practitioners reported on the need to address the root causes, the approach differed. For the acupuncturists there was a focus drawn from Chinese medicine theory on treating the root cause (the *ben*) as well as the manifesting symptoms (the *biao*) with the precise details of the intervention customised to their patients at an individual level. Meanwhile the approach of the counsellors was to get below the surface of the clients' problems and to "go deeper" and "further back (in time)" as a way of getting a handle on the root cause and, as with the acupuncturists, this required an individualised approach.

There were further differences in approach to facilitating more sustained benefits. Acupuncturists were more focussed on physical symptoms, on whether these could be resolved by acupuncture in order to speed up the improvements in the symptoms of depression, and on providing lifestyle advice linked to the Chinese medicine diagnosis. Meanwhile counsellors were more explicit on the importance of a strong therapeutic relationship accompanied by a careful consideration of what might be a manageable pace of change.

Strengths and limitations

The sub-study is nested within the largest trial to date of acupuncture or counselling for depression, and provides unique access to clusters of practitioners who have reported here on the treatments that they provided. The patient group is clearly defined, all with "moderate" to "severe" depression as categorised by the Beck Depression Inventory (BDI-II). The methods used, involving interviews, verbatim transcripts, and thematic analysis, are consistent with many of the markers of quality in qualitative research. [12] We have helped establish the credibility and dependability of the results through involving an independent research team (LN and RC) to help conduct the study, by arranging meetings of stakeholders to review the research questions and the methods used, and by discussing the emerging themes and refining these through debate to agreement. A substantive report emerged from this process, from which a component is reported here. With regard to the transferability of the results, we have provided details of the practitioners as well as the patients who were the focus of our sub-study, such that readers can draw conclusions regarding relevance for other areas. In terms of limitations, our data is limited to patients receiving acupuncture as practised by those using the theories of traditional Chinese medicine and to clients receiving counselling as provided in the humanistic and non-directive and person-centred style.

Relationship to the wider literature

There is limited evidence in the literature for longer-term benefits associated with acupuncture for depression. [13] In a systematic review of RCTs, counselling for depression has been reported to be no better than GP care in the long term [14], though in a review of pre-post comparisons of client outcomes, benefits have been reported to last a year or more. [15] The trial, within which this sub-study was nested, provided some further evidence on longer-term effects beyond the period of treatment. [4] Within the wider literature there is a dearth of evidence on the acupuncture treatment factors that might be associated with longer-term change in the symptoms of depression. The findings from a small study involving interviews with six practitioners in a trial of acupuncture for back pain found that these acupuncturists had a goal of a positive long-term outcome, and developed a therapeutic partnership to support the active engagement of patients in their own recovery. [16] Consistent with many of the findings we report here, the authors reported that the key elements were: establishing rapport, using an interactive diagnostic process, matching treatment to the patient, and using explanatory models from Chinese medicine to aid a shared understanding and motivate lifestyle changes to reinforce the potential recovery.

In the counselling literature, a qualitative study reported on the long-term effects of counselling, with data drawn from 15 clients who had received counselling from between one and three years previously. [8] The authors' interpretation of the client interview data led them to describe a model of the change process and mechanisms that were perceived as essential to produce lasting benefit. They identified as key elements of the counselling process the active engagement of the client during and between sessions, and the acquisition of a "box of skills" to be built on further after the counselling was finished. Unlike in the current study, in which all clients of counsellors received humanistic counselling, the authors did not identify the counselling approach provided. Another difference between this study and ours, is that all patients in our study had been diagnosed with depression.

Implications for clinical practice and research

One implication for clinical practice is that, while both acupuncture and counselling for depression appear to be associated with longer-term benefits, the interventions seem to work in different ways. Further research is needed from the perspective of patients and clients on their experiences of treatment from these two modalities. To assist referral, a clearer understanding is needed of which type of person with depression would benefit from acupuncture and which from counselling. While taking into account patient preference, such a typology would provide referring clinicians with valuable guidance on suitability for referral.

Another question is in regard to the nature of depression, and the extent to which physical symptoms are also present. Evidence suggests that 69% of people experiencing depression in primary care initially present with physical symptoms [17] and 50% of people with depression are also in pain. [18] Our study has found that acupuncturists are interested in the physical symptoms that may accompany depression, and will routinely address these symptoms as part of the treatment.

One can speculate that this focus on physical symptoms may in part explain why the acupuncturists in this trial, who reported being less experienced in treating moderate to severe depression, nevertheless delivered just as good outcomes as the counsellors, who encountered this level of depression more commonly in routine practice. Further research is needed into the patient perspective on the treatment of depression with co-morbidities, and specifically the value they place on the comorbid symptoms being addressed concurrently.

Our research raises some important questions about the clinical practice of acupuncturists and counsellors when treating a population with depression when combined with unmanaged drug and alcohol addictions. Further research might be useful to explore appropriate strategies, which might be about ensuring the availability of options, including the involvement of other agencies, and practical support.

Conclusions

Long-term change appears to be an important focus within the practices of both acupuncturists and counsellors. Practitioners of both interventions generally stressed that, for longer-term benefit, there needs to be an individualised approach with a focus on root causes. Acupuncturists more often emphasised the importance of addressing concurrent physical symptoms and highlighted the importance of relevant lifestyle change. Counsellors commonly stressed the importance of the therapeutic relationship and emphasised the need for appropriate "pacing" such that the timing of the counselling process is geared to the "readiness" to change.

Supporting Information

Text S1 Consolidated criteria for reporting qualitative studies (COREQ): 32-item checklist.
(DOCX)

Acknowledgments

We acknowledge with appreciation the contributions of the practitioners who were interviewed or who attended the focus group, Janet Eldred for providing support for the management of both the trial and the sub-study, and Anne Burton for undertaking the transcriptions. This research is supported by the National Institute for Health Research (NIHR) under Programme Grants for Applied Research (Grant No. RP-PG-0707-10186). The views expressed in this presentation are those of the author(s) and not necessarily those of the NHS, the NIHR or the Department of Health. The funders had no role in study design, data collection and analysis, decision to publish, or preparation of the manuscript.

Author Contributions

Conceived and designed the experiments: HM LN RC SR HL SP AH KS. Performed the experiments: LN RC. Analyzed the data: HM LN RC. Contributed reagents/materials/analysis tools: HM LN RC KS. Contributed to the writing of the manuscript: HM LN RC. Revision of the manuscript: HM LN RC SR HL SP AH KS.

References

1. Parker G (2009) Antidepressants on trial: how valid is the evidence? Br J Psychiatry: 1–3.
2. Kirsch I, Deacon BJ, Huedo-Medina TB, Scoboria A, Moore TJ, et al. (2008) Initial severity and antidepressant benefits: a meta-analysis of data submitted to the Food and Drug Administration. PLoS Med 5: e45.
3. Mind (2002) My Choice: A Survey. Available: http://www.mind.org.uk/News+policy+and+campaigns/Press+archive/Mind+launches+campaign+for+more+choice+of+mental+health+services+at+GP+level.htm. Accessed 13 January 2008.
4. MacPherson H, Richmond S, Bland M, Brealey S, Gabe R, et al. (2013) Acupuncture and Counselling for Depression in Primary Care: A Randomised Controlled Trial. PLoS Medicine 10: e1001518. doi:10.1371/journal.pmed.1001518.
5. Centre for Outcomes Research & Effectiveness (CORE) (n.d.) Humanistic Psychological Therapies Competences Framework. Available: http://www.ucl.ac.uk/clinical-psychology/CORE/humanistic_framework.htm#. Accessed 30 September 2013.
6. MacPherson H, Elliot B, Hopton A, Lansdown H, Richmond S (2013) Acupuncture for Depression: Patterns of Diagnosis and Treatment within a Randomised Controlled Trial. Evid Based Complement Alternat Med 2013: 286048. doi:10.1155/2013/286048.
7. MacPherson H, Richmond S, Bland J, Lansdown H, Hopton A, et al. (2012) Acupuncture, Counselling, and Usual care for Depression (ACUDep): study protocol for a randomized controlled trial. Trials 13: 209.
8. Perren S, Godfrey M, Rowland N (2009) The long-term effects of counselling: The process and mechanisms that contribute to ongoing change from a user perspective. Counselling and Psychotherapy Research 9: 241–249. doi:10.1080/14733140903150745.
9. Braun V, Clarke V (2006) Using thematic analysis in psychology. Qualitative Research in Psychology 3: 77–101.

10. Ritchie J, Lewis J (2003) Qualitative Research Practice: A Guide for Social Science Students and Researchers. London:Sage.
11. Roth A, Hill A, Pilling S (2009) The competences required to deliver effective Humanistic Psychological Therapies. London, UK: University College London.
12. Hannes K (2011) Chapter 4: Critical appraisal of qualitative research. Supplementary Guidance for Inclusion of Qualitative Research in Cochrane Systematic Reviews of Interventions. Cochrane Collaboration Qualitative Methods Group. Available: http://cqrmg.cochrane.org/supplemental-handbook-guidance. Accessed 31 March 2014.
13. Smith CA, Hay PP, MacPherson H (2010) Acupuncture for depression. Cochrane Database Syst Rev: CD004046.
14. Bower P, Knowles S, Coventry PA, Rowland N (2011) Counselling for mental health and psychosocial problems in primary care. Cochrane Database Syst Rev: CD001025.
15. Research on humanistic-experiential psychotherapies (2013) Bergin and Garfield's handbook of psychotherapy and behavior change. Hoboken, N.J: John Wiley & Sons. pp. 495–538.
16. MacPherson H, Thorpe L, Thomas KJ (2006) Beyond needling - therapeutic processes in acupuncture care: a qualitative study nested within a low-back pain trial. J Altern Complement Med 12: 873–880.
17. Simon GE, VonKorff M, Piccinelli M, Fullerton C, Ormel J (1999) An international study of the relation between somatic symptoms and depression. N Engl J Med 341: 1329–1335. doi:10.1056/NEJM199910283411801.
18. Katona C, Peveler R, Dowrick C, Wessely S, Feinmann C, et al. (2005) Pain symptoms in depression: definition and clinical significance. ClinMed 5(4): 390–395.

PERMISSIONS

All chapters in this book were first published in PLOS ONE, by The Public Library of Science; hereby published with permission under the Creative Commons Attribution License or equivalent. Every chapter published in this book has been scrutinized by our experts. Their significance has been extensively debated. The topics covered herein carry significant findings which will fuel the growth of the discipline. They may even be implemented as practical applications or may be referred to as a beginning point for another development.

The contributors of this book come from diverse backgrounds, making this book a truly international effort. This book will bring forth new frontiers with its revolutionizing research information and detailed analysis of the nascent developments around the world.

We would like to thank all the contributing authors for lending their expertise to make the book truly unique. They have played a crucial role in the development of this book. Without their invaluable contributions this book wouldn't have been possible. They have made vital efforts to compile up to date information on the varied aspects of this subject to make this book a valuable addition to the collection of many professionals and students.

This book was conceptualized with the vision of imparting up-to-date information and advanced data in this field. To ensure the same, a matchless editorial board was set up. Every individual on the board went through rigorous rounds of assessment to prove their worth. After which they invested a large part of their time researching and compiling the most relevant data for our readers.

The editorial board has been involved in producing this book since its inception. They have spent rigorous hours researching and exploring the diverse topics which have resulted in the successful publishing of this book. They have passed on their knowledge of decades through this book. To expedite this challenging task, the publisher supported the team at every step. A small team of assistant editors was also appointed to further simplify the editing procedure and attain best results for the readers.

Apart from the editorial board, the designing team has also invested a significant amount of their time in understanding the subject and creating the most relevant covers. They scrutinized every image to scout for the most suitable representation of the subject and create an appropriate cover for the book.

The publishing team has been an ardent support to the editorial, designing and production team. Their endless efforts to recruit the best for this project, has resulted in the accomplishment of this book. They are a veteran in the field of academics and their pool of knowledge is as vast as their experience in printing. Their expertise and guidance has proved useful at every step. Their uncompromising quality standards have made this book an exceptional effort. Their encouragement from time to time has been an inspiration for everyone.

The publisher and the editorial board hope that this book will prove to be a valuable piece of knowledge for researchers, students, practitioners and scholars across the globe.

LIST OF CONTRIBUTORS

Calvin Yu-Chian Chen
School of Chinese Medicine, China Medical University, Taichung, Taiwan Department of Bioinformatics, Asia University, Taichung, Taiwan
Department of Computational and Systems Biology, Massachusetts Institute of Technology, Cambridge, Massachusetts, United States of America
Management Office for Health Data, China Medical University Hospital, Taichung, Taiwan

Ye Zhao, Xiaogang Wang, Jinhui Tian and Kehu Yang
Evidence-Based Medicine Center, Institute of Integrated Traditional Chinese and Western Medicine, School of Basic Medical Sciences, Lanzhou University, Lanzhou, Gansu, China

Jing Gu
Evidence-Based Medicine Center, Institute of Integrated Traditional Chinese and Western Medicine, School of Basic Medical Sciences, Lanzhou University, Lanzhou, Gansu, China
Institute of Integrated Traditional Chinese and Western Medicine, Gansu University of Traditional Chinese Medicine, Lanzhou, Gansu, China

Jianjun Jiang
Second School of Clinical Medicine of Lanzhou University, Lanzhou, Gansu, China

Chin-Chuan Tsai
The School of Chinese Medicine for Post-Baccalaureate, I-Shou University, Kaohsiung County, Taiwan

Chun-Chuan Shih
The School of Chinese Medicine for Post-Baccalaureate, I-Shou University, Kaohsiung County, Taiwan
Graduate Institute of Chinese Medicine, College of Chinese Medicine, China Medical University, Taichung, Taiwan
Taipei Chinese Medical Association, Taipei, Taiwan

Yi-Chang Su and Jaung-Geng Lin
Graduate Institute of Chinese Medicine, College of Chinese Medicine, China Medical University, Taichung, Taiwan

Chien-Chang Liao
Department of Anesthesiology, Taipei Medical University Hospital, Taipei, Taiwan School of Medicine, Taipei Medical University, Taipei, Taiwan
Center for Health Research, Taipei Medical University Hospital, Taipei, Taiwan

Herman A. van Wietmarschen
Division of Analytical Biosciences, LACDR, Leiden University, Leiden, The Netherlands
Sino-Dutch centre for Preventive and Personalized Medicine, Zeist, The Netherlands

Weidong Dai, Hongwei Kong and Guowang Xu
CAS Key Laboratory of Separation Science for Analytical Chemistry, Dalian Institute of Chemical Physics, Chinese Academy of Sciences, Dalian, China

Anita J. van der Kooij and Jacqueline J. Meulman
Mathematical Institute, Leiden University, Leiden, The Netherlands

Theo H. Reijmers and Thomas Hankemeier
Division of Analytical Biosciences, LACDR, Leiden University, Leiden, The Netherlands
Netherlands Metabolomics Centre, Leiden University, Leiden, The Netherlands

Yan Schroën
Sino-Dutch centre for Preventive and Personalized Medicine, Zeist, The
Netherlands
Oxrider, Education and Research, Nieuwegein, The Netherlands

Mei Wang
Sino-Dutch centre for Preventive and Personalized Medicine, Zeist, The Netherlands
SU BioMedicine, Utrechtseweg, Zeist, The Netherlands

Zhiliang Xu
College of Life Science Company Limited, Hangzhou, China

Xinchang Wang
Zhejiang Xinhua hospital Rheumatology and Immunology Department, HangZhou, China

Jan van der Greef
Division of Analytical Biosciences, LACDR, Leiden University, Leiden, The Netherlands
Sino-Dutch centre for Preventive and Personalized Medicine, Zeist, The Netherlands
SU BioMedicine, Utrechtseweg, Zeist, The Netherlands
TNO Netherlands Organization for Applied Scientific Research, TNO Pharma, Zeist, The Netherlands

Linong Ji and Yingli Chen
Peking University People's Hospital, Beijing, China

Xiaolin Tong
China Academy of Chinese Medicial Sciences Guang'anmen Hospital, Beijing, China

Hongyuan Wang
Peking University School of Public Health, Beijing China

Haoming Tian
Sichuan University West China Hospital, Chengdu, China

Huimin Zhou
The First Hospital of Hebei Medical University, Shijiazhuang, China

Lili Zhang
The Third Affiliated Hospital of Peking University of Traditional Chinese and Western Medicine, Beijing, China

Qifu Li
The First Affiliated Hospital of Chongqing Medical University, Chongqing, China

Yizhong Wang
The Central Hospital of China Aerospace Corporation, Beijing, China

Hongmei Li
China Meitan General Hospital, Beijing, China

Min Liu
The First Affiliated Hospital of Guangzhou University of Traditional Chinese Medicine, Guangzhou, China

Hongjie Yang
Shanghai University of Traditional Chinese Medicine Yueyang Hospital of Integrated
Traditional Chinese and Western Medicine, Shanghai, China

Yanbin Gao
Beijing University of Traditional Chinese Medicine Dongfang Hospital, Beijing, China

Yan Li
Zhongshan University Sun Yai-sen Memorial Hospital, Zhongshan, China

Quanmin Li
General Hospital of PLA Second Artillery, Beijing, China

Xiaohui Guo
Peking University First Hospital, Beijing, China
Gangyi Yang
The Second Affiliated Hospital of Chongqing Medical University, Chongqing, China

Zhongai Zhang
Nanjing Hospital of Traditional Chinese Medicine, Nanjing, China

Zhiguang Zhou
The Second Xiangya Hospital of Central South University, Changsha, China

Guang Ning
Shanghai Jiaotong University Ruijin Hospital, Shanghai, China

Sanjoy Paul
Queensland Clinical Trials and Biostatistics Centre, School of Population Health, University of Queensland, Queensland, Australia

Yao Tong, Hei Kiu Wong, Yi-Bin Feng and Di Wang
School of Chinese Medicine, Faculty of Medicine, the University of Hong Kong, Hong Kong, China

Zhang-Jin Zhang
School of Chinese Medicine, Faculty of Medicine, the University of Hong Kong, Hong Kong, China
Department of Psychiatry, Fourth Military Medical University, Xijing Hospital, Xi'an, Shaanxi, China

Qing-Rong Tan and Huai-Hai Wang
Department of Psychiatry, Fourth Military Medical University, Xijing Hospital, Xi'an, Shaanxi, China

Xue-Yi Wang
Mental Health Center, Hebei Medical University, Shijiazhuang, Hebei, China

Lai-Ming Ho
School of Public Health, the University of Hong Kong, Hong Kong, China

Roger Ng
Department of Psychiatry, Kowloon Hospital, Hong Kong, China

Grainne M. McAlonan
Department of Psychiatry, the University of Hong Kong, Hong Kong, China

Chuan-Yue Wang
Capital Medical University, Beijing Anding Hospital, Beijing, China

Vivian Taam Wong
Chinese Medicine Section, Hospital Authority, Hong Kong, China

Xun Li
Centre for Evidence-based Chinese Medicine, Beijing University of Chinese Medicine, Beijing, China
Centre for Complementary Medicine Research (CompleMED), University of Western Sydney, Sydney, New South Wales, Australia

Guoyan Yang, Xinxue Li and Jianping Liu
Centre for Evidence-based Chinese Medicine, Beijing University of Chinese Medicine, Beijing, China

Alan Bensoussan
Centre for Complementary Medicine Research (CompleMED), University of Western Sydney, Sydney, New South Wales, Australia

Yan Zhang, Jiu Chang and Xiaoxuan Sun
School of Preclinical Medicine, Beijing University of Chinese Medicine, Beijing, China

Jingli Yang
School of Management, Beijing University of Chinese Medicine, Beijing, China

Xiaoyun Zhou and Yu Guo
School of Acupuncture and Moxibustion, Beijing University of Chinese Medicine, Beijing, China

Yue Xu
School of Humanities, Beijing University of Chinese Medicine, Beijing, China

Jia-bo Wang, Xue-ru Zhang, Xiaohui Chu, Ping Zhang and Yan-ling Zhao
China Military Institute of Chinese Medicine, 302 Military Hospital, Beijing, China

Ling-na Zeng
China Military Institute of Chinese Medicine, 302 Military Hospital, Beijing, China,
Faculty of Life Science and Technology, Kunming University of Science and
Technology, Kunming, China

Qing-ce Zang
China Military Institute of Chinese Medicine, 302 Military Hospital, Beijing, China,
Pharmacy College, Jiangxi University of Traditional Chinese Medicine, Nanchang, China

Bao-cai Li
Faculty of Life Science and Technology, Kunming University of Science and Technology, Kunming, China

Qian-feng Gong
Pharmacy College, Jiangxi University of Traditional Chinese Medicine, Nanchang, China

Xiao-he Xiao
Integrative Medicine Center, 302 Military Hospital, Beijing, China

Youbo You, Lijun Bai, Ruwei Dai, Zhenyu Liu and Wenjuan Wei
Key Laboratory of Molecular Imaging and Functional Imaging, Institute of Automation, Chinese Academy of Sciences, Beijing, China

Hao Cheng
Department of Anesthesiology, Beijing Ditan Hospital affiliated to Capital Medical University, Beijing, China

Jie Tian
Key Laboratory of Molecular Imaging and Functional Imaging, Institute of Automation, Chinese Academy of Sciences, Beijing, China
Life Science Research Center, School of Electronic Engineering, Xidian University, Xi'an, Shaanxi, China

Weng Ieong Tou
School of Medicine, China Medical University, Taichung, Taiwan
Laboratory of Computational and Systems Biology, China Medical University, Taichung, Taiwan

Calvin Yu-Chian Chen
Laboratory of Computational and Systems Biology, China Medical University, Taichung, Taiwan
Department of Medical Research, China Medical University Hospital, Taichung, Taiwan
Department of Biotechnology, Asia University, Taichung, Taiwan
Department of Biomedical Informatics, Asia University, Taichung, Taiwan, 6 China Medical University Beigang Hospital, Yunlin, Taiwan

Xiao Lu and Shang Hongcai
Tianjin University of Traditional Chinese Medicine, Tianjin, China
MOE Virtual Research Center of Evidence-Based Medicine, Chengdu, China

Wang Jiaying
Evidence Based Medicine Center in Tianjin, Tianjin, China

Hu Jing
Peking University, Beijing, China

Xiong Jun
Department of Acupuncture, Jiang Xi Hospital of Traditional Chinese Medicine, Jiangxi Province, China

Hsienhsueh Elley Chiu
Department of TCM, Chang Gung University College of Medicine, Kaohsiung, Taiwan, Department of Neurology, Chang Gung University College of Medicine, Kaohsiung, Taiwan
Chang Gung Memorial Hospital, Chang Gung University College of Medicine, Kaohsiung, Taiwan

Chih-Cheng Huang
Department of TCM, Chang Gung University College of Medicine, Kaohsiung, Taiwan

Yu-Chiang Hong
Department of TCM, Chang Gung University College of Medicine, Kaohsiung, Taiwan,
Chang Gung Memorial Hospital, Chang Gung University College of Medicine, Kaohsiung, Taiwan

Ku-Chou Chang, Chia-Wei Liu and Teng-Yeow Tan
Department of Neurology, Chang Gung University College of Medicine, Kaohsiung, Taiwan
Chang Gung Memorial Hospital, Chang Gung University College of Medicine, Kaohsiung, Taiwan

Jen-Wen Hung
Department of Rehabilitation, Chang Gung University College of Medicine, Kaohsiung, Taiwan
Chang Gung Memorial Hospital, Chang Gung University College of Medicine, Kaohsiung, Taiwan

Chun-Chuan Shih
School of Chinese Medicine for Post-Baccalaureate, I-Shou University, Kaohsiung, Taiwan

Lee-Hsin Shaw
Institute of Traditional Medicine, National Yang-Ming University, Taipei, Taiwan,

Lie-Chwen Lin
Institute of Traditional Medicine, National Yang-Ming University, Taipei, Taiwan
National Research Institute of Chinese Medicine, Taipei, Taiwan

Tung-Hu Tsai
Institute of Traditional Medicine, National Yang-Ming University, Taipei, Taiwan,
Graduate Institute of Acupuncture Science, China Medical University, Taichung, Taiwan
Department of Education and Research, Taipei City Hospital, Taipei, Taiwan

Bin Ma, Guoqing Qi, Haimin Li, Yanqin Ding and Kehu Yang
Evidence-Based Medicine Center, Institute of Traditional Chinese and Western Medicine, School of Basic Medical Sciences, Lanzhou University, Lanzhou, Gansu, China

Jiwu Guo and Yulong Zhang
Evidence-Based Medicine Center, Institute of Traditional Chinese and Western Medicine, School of Basic Medical Sciences, Lanzhou University, Lanzhou, Gansu, China
Second School of Clinical Medicine of Lanzhou University, Lanzhou, Gansu, China

Jiye Peng
The Library of Lanzhou University, Lanzhou, Gansu, China

Yang Wang, Jinna Yu, Jiani Wu, Jing Wang and Zhishun Liu
Guang'anmen Hospital, China Academy of Chinese Medical Sciences, Beijing, China

Baoyan Liu
China Academy of Chinese Medical Sciences, Beijing, China

Herman A. van Wietmarschen
Division of Analytical Biosciences, LACDR, Leiden University, Leiden, The Netherlands
Sino-Dutch Centre for Preventive and Personalized Medicine, Zeist, The Netherlands

Theo H. Reijmers
Division of Analytical Biosciences, LACDR, Leiden University, Leiden, The Netherlands
Netherlands Metabolomics Centre, Leiden University, Leiden, The Netherlands

Anita J. van der Kooij and Jacqueline J. Meulman
Mathematical Institute, Leiden University, Leiden, The Netherlands,

Jan Schroën
Sino-Dutch Centre for Preventive and Personalized Medicine, Zeist, The Netherlands
Oxrider, Education and Research, Nieuwegein, The Netherlands

Heng Wei
Sino-Dutch Centre for Preventive and Personalized Medicine, Zeist, The Netherlands
TNO, Zeist, The Netherlands

Thomas Hankemeier
Division of Analytical Biosciences, LACDR, Leiden University, Leiden, The Netherlands
Sino-Dutch Centre for Preventive and Personalized Medicine, Zeist, The Netherlands
Netherlands Metabolomics Centre, Leiden University, Leiden, The Netherlands

Jan van der Greef
Division of Analytical Biosciences, LACDR, Leiden University, Leiden, The Netherlands
Sino-Dutch Centre for Preventive and Personalized Medicine, Zeist, The Netherlands
TNO, Zeist, The Netherlands

Fang-fang Fan, Sheng-jun Zhao and Ping Wang
Department of Pharmacy, The Affiliated Traditional Medical Hospital, Xinjiang Medical University, Urumqi, Xinjiang Uygur Autonomous Region, China

Qin Xu and Qi Sun
Medical Research Design and Data Analysis Center, The Affiliated Traditional Medical Hospital, Xinjiang Medical University, Urumqi, Xinjiang Uygur Autonomous Region, China

Xue-rui Guo
Department of Pediatrics, The Affiliated Traditional Medical Hospital, Xinjiang Medical University, Urumqi, Xinjiang Uygur Autonomous Region, China

Ailing Yin and Baochang Cai
College of Pharmacy, Nan'jing University of Chinese Medicine, Nan'jing, People's Republic of China

Wei Zhou and Liuqing D
College of Pharmacy, Nan'jing University of Chinese Medicine, Nan'jing, People's Republic of China
Jiang'su Engineering Research Center for Efficient Delivery System of TCM, Nan'jing, People's Republic of China
Nan'jing Engineering Research Center for Industrialization of Chinese Medicine Pellets, Nan'jing, People's Republic of China

Xiaobin Tan
Laboratory of New Drug Delivery System of Chinese Meteria Medica, Jiang'su Provinical Academy of Chinese Medicine, Nan'jing, People's Republic of China

Jinjun Shan and Shouchuan Wang
Jiangsu Key Laboratory of Pediatric Respiratory Disease, Institute of Paediatrics, Nan'jing University of Chinese Medicine, Nan'jing, People's Republic of China

Xiang Li, Leihong Wu, Wei Liu, Yecheng Jin, Qian Chen, Linli Wang, Xiaohui Fan and Yiyu Cheng
Pharmaceutical Informatics Institute, College of Pharmaceutical Sciences, Zhejiang University, Hangzhou, China

Zheng Li
State Key Laboratory of Modern Chinese Medicine, Tianjin University of Traditional Chinese Medicine, Tianjin, China

Na Lin, Shihuan Tang, Rixin Liang, Yan Ma, Defeng Li, Yi Zhang, Yanqiong Zhang and Hongjun Yang
Institute of Chinese Materia Medica, China Academy of Chinese Medical Sciences, Beijing, P.R. China

Haiyu Xu
Institute of Chinese Materia Medica, China Academy of Chinese Medical Sciences, Beijing, P.R. China
National resource center for Chinese Materia Medica, China Academy of Chinese Medical Sciences, Beijing, P.R. China

Luqi Huang
National resource center for Chinese Materia Medica, China Academy of Chinese Medical Sciences, Beijing, P.R. China

Yun Lei
Institute of Chinese Materia Medica, China Academy of Chinese Medical Sciences, Beijing, P.R. China
Beijing University of Chinese Medicine, Beijing, P.R. China

Huaqiang Zhai
Beijing University of Chinese Medicine, Beijing, P.R. China

Xiumei Gao
Institute of Chinese Materia Medica, China Academy of Chinese Medical Sciences, Beijing, P.R. China
Tianjin University of Traditional Chinese Medicine, Tianjin, P.R. China

Guangrong Zhu
Yunnan Datang Hanfang Pharmacy co.ltd, Yunnan, P.R. China

Zhijie Zhu, Xi Yu, Hailiang Liu, Huizhu Wang and Min Hong
National Standard Laboratory of Pharmacology for Chinese Materia Medica, Jiangsu Key Laboratory for Pharmacology and Safety Evaluation of Chinese Materia Medica,
Nanjing University of Chinese Medicine, Nanjing, China

Dandan Shen
National Standard Laboratory of Pharmacology for Chinese Materia Medica, Jiangsu Key Laboratory for Pharmacology and Safety Evaluation of Chinese Materia Medica,

Nanjing University of Chinese Medicine, Nanjing, China
Pharmacy Department, The First People's Hospital of Taicang, Taicang, China

Xuejian Xie
Nanjing General Hospital of Nanjing Military Command, Nanjing, China

Hongwei Fan
Department of Clinical Pharmacology Lab, Nanjing First Hospital, Nanjing Medical University, JiangSu Nanjing, China

Guorong Jiang
Suzhou Hospital of Tradional Chinese Medicine, Suzhou, China

Dawei Wang
Jiangsu Academy of Traditional Chinese Medicine, Nanjing, China

Qinli Ruan, Yanyan Chen, Meng Wang and Jinao Duan
Jiangsu Key Laboratory for High Technology Research of TCM Formulae, Nanjing University of Chinese Medicine, Nanjing, China

Yan Qiao
Jiangsu Key Laboratory for High Technology Research of TCM Formulae, Nanjing University of Chinese Medicine, Nanjing, China
Key Laboratory of Developmental Genes and Human Disease in Ministry of Education, Medical School of Southeast University, Nanjing, China

Yunli Zhao, Qiuli Wu, Lingmei Sun and Dayong Wang
Key Laboratory of Developmental Genes and Human Disease in Ministry of Education, Medical School of Southeast University, Nanjing, China

Chunhu Shi, Jinhui Tian and Kehu Yang
Evidence-Based Medicine Center, Lanzhou University, Lanzhou, China
Key Laboratory of Evidence Based Medicine and Knowledge Translation of Gansu Province, Lanzhou University, Lanzhou, China
School of Basic Medical Sciences, Lanzhou University, Lanzhou, China

Quan Wang
Evidence-Based Medicine Center, Lanzhou University, Lanzhou, China
Key Laboratory of Evidence Based Medicine and Knowledge Translation of Gansu Province, Lanzhou University, Lanzhou, China

Dan Ren
The First Clinical Medicine School, Lanzhou University, Lanzhou, China

Hongli Wei and Lihuan Zhang
The Second Clinical Medical School, Lanzhou University, Lanzhou, China

Hugh MacPherson, Stewart J. Richmond, Harriet Lansdown, Sara Perren, Ann Hopton and Karen Spilsbury
Department of Health Sciences, University of York, York, United Kingdom

Liz Newbronner
Department of Health Sciences, University of York, York, United Kingdom
Firefly Research & Evaluation, North Yorkshire, United Kingdom

Ruth Chamberlain
Firefly Research & Evaluation, North Yorkshire, United Kingdom

Index

A
Acupuncture Clinical Trials, 6, 8
Acupuncture Treatment, 21, 97-98, 101, 104, 133-135, 222-223
Alanine Aminotransferase (alt), 27
Allergic Inflammation, 191-192, 199-201
Allergic Sensitization, 191, 197
Antidepressants, 219, 224
Antipsychotics, 41, 43-44, 46-48
Assessment Of Multiple Systematic Reviews (amstar), 124
Atopic Contact Dermatitis (acd), 191
Aurantiamide, 82-87, 89-92, 94

B
Benign Prostate Hyperplasia (bph), 130
Binding Mechanisms, 82, 91
Breast Cancer, 22, 50, 52, 57, 59-60, 95, 178, 201
Bu-yang-huan-wu-tang (byhwt), 111

C
C-reactive Protein (crp), 23-24
Caenorhabditis Elegans, 202, 210-211
Cancer Care, 22, 50-51, 58-59
Categorical Principal Component Analysis (catpca), 136
Cerebrovascular Diseases, 103-104
Characterization, 23-24, 144-145, 189, 210
Chemical Analysis, 179, 181, 189
China National Knowledge Infrastructure (cnki), 51, 146-147
Chinese Journals, 58-59, 101, 124-125, 128-129, 218
Chinese Medicine, 1-2, 4, 6, 9, 12-14, 16-24, 26, 29-32, 40-42, 44-48, 50-51, 58-61, 69-70, 73, 82-83, 95, 97, 99, 101-104, 110-112, 115, 123-125, 129-132, 136-142, 144-147, 153-156, 167-168, 175-177, 179, 189-193, 197, 199-203, 208, 210, 217-219, 221-224
Circulatory System, 9, 21, 103, 110, 125-126
Clinical Chemistry, 23-27, 29
Colitis Treatment, 179, 181-182
Colorimetric Grading, 61-62, 66, 68-69
Complementary and Alternative Medicine (cam), 59
Computer-aided Drug Design (cadd), 1
Concomitant Use, 22, 41-43, 47
Controlled Clinical Studies, 50-53, 55-57, 59, 150
Coronary Heart Disease, 111, 122, 146-147, 153-154, 177, 190

D
Data Abstraction, 98
Data Screening, 4, 138
Default Mode Network, 70, 75, 78, 80-81
Disease-related Groups (drg), 103-104
Dissolution, 155-156, 166
Dragon's Blood Tablet, 179
Drug Screening, 1, 95, 189

E
Electroacupuncture, 130, 135
Electronic Database, 146-147
Epidemiological Study, 22, 41-42
Epidemiology, 60, 124, 126, 129, 132, 135, 153-154
Esophagus Cancer, 50, 59

F
Flos Lonicerae, 155, 167
Fructus Forsythiae, 155, 158, 167

G
Gender Differences, 16-17
Genkwa Flos, 202-207, 209-210
Glibenclamide, 31-35, 37-39
Glycemic Control, 31-33, 39-40

H
Herb-drug Interaction, 22, 41
Hub Configurations, 70-79
Hypoglycemia Rate, 31

I
In Silico Investigation, 82
Intention to Treat (itt), 130
International Clinical Trials Registry Platform (ictrp), 6, 14
Intestinal Absorption, 155, 163, 165-166, 179

L
Liquid Chromatography-tandem Mass Spectrometry, 111, 181
Liver Cancer, 50, 52, 57, 59

M
Main Components Interaction, 155
Metabolomics Measurements, 23, 25
Methodological Reporting, 212-213, 218
Mild Cognitive Impairment, 97-98, 101-102
Mild Hypoglycemic Episode, 31, 35
Molecular Mechanisms, 169, 176-179, 181, 189
Motor Neurons, 202-203, 205, 208-209

Multi-compound, 168-169, 172, 175-177
Multi-pathway Mode, 168, 172
Multi-target, 168-169, 175-177, 179
Multimodal Investigation, 70

N
Nasopharyngeal Cancer, 50, 52, 59
National Health Insurance (nhi), 16
National Health Insurance Research Database (nhird), 103
National Health Interview Survey (nhis), 16
Network Pharmacology, 168, 177, 179, 181, 188-189

O
Oral Administration, 69, 111-113, 121-123, 159, 161, 167, 177, 189

P
Pharmacokinetics, 111, 119, 122-123, 155-156, 159-160, 163-166, 177
Potential Src Kinase Ligands, 82
Prostatic Hyperplasia, 130, 135

Q
Quality Control, 25, 61-62, 68, 155, 213, 217
Quantitative-structural Activity Relationship (qsar), 82

R
Randomized Trials, 80, 101, 149, 151, 212-213, 218
Registration Quality Assessment, 6
Reporting Characteristics, 124, 127, 129
Reporting Quality, 14, 50, 54, 57, 59, 97, 100-101, 129, 146-147, 150-151, 153-154, 212-213, 217-218
Rheumatic Diseases, 27, 30, 136-138, 142, 144
Rheumatoid Arthritis, 23-25, 27-30, 136-138, 141-142, 144-145, 190
Rheumatoid Factor (rhf), 23

S
Schizophrenic Patients, 22, 41-42, 45-47
Screening Active Components, 191, 201
Sensory Evaluation, 61-62, 68-69
Somatosensory Stimulation, 70
Standardization, 33, 61-62, 68
Symptom Profiles, 23
Systems Biology, 1, 23-24, 82, 136, 144-145, 168, 177, 179, 181, 190
Systems Diagnosis Questionnaire, 136, 140, 144-145

T
Toxicity Assessment, 202-203, 207-208
Traditional Chinese Medicine, 1, 4, 6, 9, 12-14, 16-22, 29-32, 40, 48, 50, 59-61, 69-70, 73, 82-83, 95, 97, 99, 101-104, 110-112, 115, 124-125, 129-132, 145-147, 153-155, 167-168, 177, 179, 190-191, 201-202, 210, 218-219, 221-222

V
Virtual Screening, 1-2, 4, 95

W
Western Medicine, 6, 9, 11, 13, 17, 22, 29, 31-32, 53-55, 59, 99, 101, 105, 108, 110, 124-125, 135-137, 144-147, 149, 153-154, 189
World Health Organization (who), 6